Bronchoscopy and Central Airway Disorders

A Patient-Centered Approach

Bronchoscopy and Central Airway Disorders

A Patient-Centered Approach

Henri Colt, MD, FCCP

Professor Emeritus
University of California
Irvine, California

Septimiu Murgu, MD, FCCP

Assistant Professor of Medicine
University of Chicago
Chicago, Illinois

ELSEVIER
SAUNDERS

ELSEVIER
SAUNDERS

1600 John F. Kennedy Blvd.
Ste 1800
Philadelphia, PA 19103-2899

BRONCHOSCOPY AND CENTRAL AIRWAY DISORDERS: 978-1-4557-0320-3
A PATIENT-CENTERED APPROACH
Copyright © 2012 by Saunders, an imprint of Elsevier Inc.

Notices

Knowledge and best practice in this field are constantly changing. As new research and experience
broaden our understanding, changes in research methods, professional practices, or medical
treatment may become necessary.

Practitioners and researchers must always rely on their own experience and knowledge in
evaluating and using any information, methods, compounds, or experiments described herein. In
using such information or methods they should be mindful of their own safety and the safety of
others, including parties for whom they have a professional responsibility.

With respect to any drug or pharmaceutical products identified, readers are advised to check the
most current information provided (i) on procedures featured or (ii) by the manufacturer of each
product to be administered, to verify the recommended dose or formula, the method and duration
of administration, and contraindications. It is the responsibility of practitioners, relying on their
own experience and knowledge of their patients, to make diagnoses, to determine dosages and the
best treatment for each individual patient, and to take all appropriate safety precautions.

To the fullest extent of the law, neither the Publisher nor the authors, contributors, or editors,
assume any liability for any injury and/or damage to persons or property as a matter of products
liability, negligence or otherwise, or from any use or operation of any methods, products,
instructions, or ideas contained in the material herein.

Library of Congress Cataloging-in-Publication Data

Bronchoscopy and central airway disorders : a patient-centered approach / [edited by] Henri Colt,
Septimiu Murgu. — 1st ed.
   p. ; cm.
  Includes bibliographical references and index.
  ISBN 978-1-4557-0320-3 (hardback)
  I. Colt, Henri G. II. Murgu, Septimiu.
  [DNLM: 1. Bronchial Diseases–surgery. 2. Airway Obstruction–surgery.
3. Bronchoscopy–methods. WF 500]
  616.2'307545–dc23
                                             2012005768

Associate Acquisitions Editor: Julie Goolsby
Senior Content Development Specialist: Anne Snyder
Publishing Services Manager: Debbie L. Vogel
Project Manager: Jodi Willard/Kiruthiga Kasthuriswamy
Design Direction: Ellen Zanolle

Preface

This book is for all health care providers caring for patients with central airway disorders. It is particularly written for those practitioners known as interventional bronchoscopists, who perform procedures to restore and maintain airway patency in patients suffering from the effects of various forms of central airway obstruction. When one considers the number of patients with life-altering or life-threatening tracheobronchial disease either as a result of focal airway abnormalities or systemic illness, it is hard to believe there was once a time, just a few years ago, when these sub-subspecialists were few and far between. During those early years, interventional bronchoscopists were often perceived as proceduralists rather than as clinician-researchers, providing diagnosis via the bronchoscope, infrequently reflecting on how centrally obstructing airway disorders would fall into the realm of a multidisciplinary approach to patient care. As early adopters of technology, their move into therapeutics, primarily the relief of central airway obstruction using bronchoscopic resectional techniques, was accompanied by a need to convince their peers of the value of these activities. This required a focus on describing techniques and demonstrating results.

The past 10 years have seen an even greater flourish in what this specialty has to offer. Today interventional bronchoscopy has become the subject of increased recognition by international societies, medical journal editors, instrument manufacturers, basic scientists intrigued by airway pathology, physiologists, molecular biologists, biomedical engineers, and clinicians from numerous specialties. Tertiary care university training centers have recognized its value, and many whisper that in addition to sleep medicine and critical care, interventional pulmonology contributes to the triumvirate forming the future of pulmonary medicine. Technology remains at its forefront, such that the scope of practice has expanded to include early detection of lung cancer and other malignant disorders, mediastinal staging, incorporation of optical and acoustic imaging into multimodality platforms to enhance diagnosis and treatment, studies of airway dynamics, assistance with open surgical resection, minimally invasive image-guided access to peripheral nodules, bronchoscopic management of asthma, chronic obstructive lung disease, and fistulas and tracheomalacia. In addition, it has warranted collaborative efforts with surgical specialists, interventional radiologists, and cancer specialists to identify patients who might benefit from targeted therapy. Another major element of the bronchoscopist's practice is of course devoted to disease diagnosis, evaluation, and the relief of airway obstruction using a variety of minimally invasive instruments and techniques.

In addition to publishing original research and review papers and providing case demonstrations, didactic lectures, or hands-on workshops using low- and high-fidelity simulation, many experts in the field are devoting their surplus energies to education, enhancing overall competency, and augmenting opportunities for patients to have access to even more expert practitioners and novel technologies. The need for global dissemination of knowledge and techniques has now prompted a turn toward standardizing educational content and uniform teaching methodologies in addition to exploring ways in which social media and textbooks that include online access to learning materials (such as this one) might be used to assist in these tasks.

Several traditionally formatted books have been written, most of which describe quite well the technology and outcomes of many interventional procedures. However, none of these specifically addresses in a structured manner the multifaceted skills necessary to becoming a well-rounded, accomplished, and experienced practitioner of this highly technical and creative discipline. Some experts might argue that a book that addresses the consultative, reflective, procedural, and technical aspects of interventional bronchoscopy is not necessary or, if written, should consist of an abundance of chapters accompanied by a summary of the literature written by a multitude of specialists in the field, each providing his or her own point of view. To our knowledge, none of the existing books on interventional bronchoscopy has proposed to have the purpose we have set for *Bronchoscopy and Central Airway Disorders: A Patient-Centered Approach*.

The underlying premise of interventional bronchoscopy, in our opinion, is a product of two factors. The first is based on the acquisition of technical skills and might be referred to as its "artistic" component, cleverly addressed by Chevalier Jackson's famous "the bronchoscopist must have eyes on the tip of his fingers" and, more recently, by Shigeto Ikeda's mantra to "never give up." The second, we believe, is based on available published evidence. This could be viewed as the "scientific" component, in part alluded to by the 1997 Apple slogan "think different" and by the need to demonstrate that what might be technically achievable must also be in the best interest of the patient. Interventional bronchoscopists differ widely in regard to the proportions in which these two factors enter into their practice and teaching. We submit that the presence of both, to some degree, characterizes the mature and experienced interventional bronchoscopist. Therefore our goal in practice, in education, and in writing this book is to balance these components to the best of our ability and to convey this knowledge to others.

With very few exceptions, each and every topic we address in this book is probably better known to others than to us. Therefore we apologize to those specialists from various schools if this book escapes the severe censure that it surely deserves. We believe, however, that in this growing and increasingly exciting field, there is something lost when many authors cooperate independently. If there is any unity in the intellectual approach to interventional bronchoscopy, if there is any intimate relation between strategy and planning for a procedure, technical execution, and response to complications, it is necessary that these components be synthesized into a single school of thought.

We chose, therefore, to showcase our understanding of disease process and procedure-related consultation by using a "four box" approach to procedural decision-making through which readers may study the various elements of the initial evaluation, procedural strategies, procedural techniques and results, and long-term management issues that arise in daily practice. Using this template, learners may choose to reflect in greater or lesser detail on the major elements that are pertinent to a particular patient, as well as provide answers to specific questions that we ask at the end of each patient-centered scenario. To avoid redundancy, scenarios and their accompanying questions are structured to reinforce material that has been presented elsewhere in the book, while also introducing new information pertaining to medical management, techniques, literature reviews, and procedure-related concepts. Because we are distinctly aware that there may not be a single right way to approach an interventional case, we enlisted help from thirty-six internationally recognized experts representing eight different countries and thirteen different specialties. Their generosity has provided us with concise, second-opinion commentaries, similar to those one might obtain from second opinions in daily consultative practice. These expert opinions are not necessarily from interventional bronchoscopists and have the dual purpose of critiquing our approach and describing alternative strategies or techniques based on evidence and personal experiences.

Obviously, the problem of topic selection and choice of references in a book such as this is difficult. Needless to say, some scientific literature runs counter to many of our statements. We have done our best to select, without bias or harsh judgment, those references most pertinent to support or refute the approaches taken in our case resolutions and teaching points. Another obstacle is that a book without details becomes unsophisticated and uninteresting, whereas a book with too many details is in danger of becoming intolerably long. We have sought a compromise by addressing in some detail many topics that seem to us to have considerable importance for the interventional bronchoscopist, either because of disease prevalence or because of safety concerns related to certain procedures.

An interventional bronchoscopist's confidence grows gradually as he or she acquires technical skills, climbs the series of plateaus that make up the competency curve and, patient after patient, becomes better at identifying risks, benefits, and alternatives while rationally thinking through the decision-making process. We trust that learning from this collection of patient-centered scenarios will enhance the practitioner's self-assurance. We hope our efforts will also add to the reader's affective knowledge, which is defined as how one responds experientially and existentially to what often are life-threatening situations for patients. Over the years, we have expounded the virtues of decision, intention, control, and confidence. These four pillars form the basis of procedural expertise—there is no place for trial and error in the midst of palliating near-total central airway obstruction or resolving difficult patient management issues.

Although specific and lengthy training is necessary for many aspects of this procedure-related specialty, we do not believe that interventional bronchoscopy should be merely an affair of a few tertiary centers or a disputation among a handful of experts. Vast numbers of patients can benefit from the actions and experience of the thoughtful bronchoscopist, and many elements might and should come under the purview of a skilled practitioner. Interventional bronchoscopy can and undoubtedly will become an integral part of the practice of many specialists, and as such we have tried to consider it. Hence, we hope this book will help open the doors to expert management of patients with central airway disorders, expand the interested practitioner's scope of practice, and reinforce the rationales used by those already adept in interventional techniques.

Henri G. Colt
Septimiu D. Murgu

Acknowledgments

We are extremely grateful to the numerous experts from different specialties who shared their knowledge, experiences, and perspectives on the central airways disorders presented in this book.

Priscilla Alderson, BA, PhD
Professor Emerita
Social Science Research Unit
Institute of Education
University of London
London, England

Cristina Baldassari, MD
Assistant Professor
Department of Otolaryngology
Eastern Virginia Medical School
Children's Hospital of the King's Daughters
Norfolk, Virginia, USA

Heinrich D. Becker, MD, FCCP
Director
Department of Interdisciplinary Endoscopy
Thoraxklinik at Heidelberg University
Heidelberg, Germany

Chris T. Bolliger, MD, PhD
Professor of Medicine
Director of Respiratory Research
Co-Chairman Division of Pulmonology
Faculty of Health Sciences
University of Stellenbosch
Tygerberg/Cape Town, South Africa

Kenneth Chang, MD
Director
H.H. Chao Comprehensive Digestive Disease Center
Department of Medicine
University of California
Irvine, California, USA

Craig S. Derkay, MD, FACS, FAAP
Professor and Vice-Chairman
Department of Otolaryngology, Head and Neck Surgery
Eastern Virginia Medical School;
Director, Pediatric Otolaryngology
Children's Hospital of the King's Daughters
Norfolk, Virginia, USA

Gordon H. Downie, MD, PhD
Clinical Professor of Medicine
Louisiana State University—Shreveport
Shreveport, Louisiana, USA;
Department of Pulmonary Critical Medicine
NE Texas Interventional Medicine PA
Mt. Pleasant, Texas, USA

D. John Doyle, MD, PhD
Professor of Anesthesiology
Cleveland Clinic Lerner College of Medicine
Case Western Reserve University;
Staff Anesthesiologist, Department of General Anesthesiology
Cleveland Clinic Foundation
Cleveland, Ohio, USA

Eric Edell, MD
Professor of Medicine
Division of Pulmonary and Critical Care Medicine
Mayo Clinic
Rochester, Minnesota, USA

Armin Ernst, MD
Chief, Pulmonary, Critical Care and Sleep Medicine
St. Elizabeth Medical Center;
VP Thoracic Disease and Critical Care Service Line
Steward Health Care;
Professor of Medicine
Tufts School of Medicine
Boston, Massachusetts, USA

Laura Findeiss, MD, FSIR
Associate Professor of Radiology and Surgery
Chief of Vascular and Interventional Radiology
Department of Radiological Sciences
University of California, Irvine, School of Medicine
Orange, California, USA

Lutz Freitag, MD, FCCP
Professor of Pulmonary Medicine
Chief, Department of Interventional Pneumology
Ruhrlandklinik, University Hospital Essen
Essen, Germany

Kenji Hirooka
General Manager
Ultrasound Technology Department
R&D Division 2
Olympus Medical Systems Corporation
Hachioji-shi, Tokyo, Japan

Norihiko Ikeda, MD, PhD
Professor and Chairman
Department of Surgery
Tokyo Medical University
Shinjuku-ku, Tokyo, Japan

James R. Jett, MD
Professor of Medicine
National Jewish Health
Denver, Colorado, USA

Carlos A. Jimenez, MD
Associate Professor of Medicine
Department of Pulmonary Medicine
The University of Texas MD Anderson Cancer Center
Houston, Texas, USA

Kemp H. Kernstine, Sr., MD, PhD
Professor and Chairman, Division of Thoracic Surgery
Robert Tucker Hayes Foundation Distinguished Chair
  in Cardiothoracic Surgery
The Harold C. Simmons Comprehensive Cancer Center
University of Texas, Southwestern Medical Center and
  School of Medicine
Dallas, Texas, USA

Noriaki Kurimoto, MD, PhD, FCCP
Professor, Division of Chest Surgery
St. Marianna University
School of Medicine
Kawasaki, Kanagawa, Japan

Solomon Liao, MD, FAAHPM
Director of Palliative Care Services
Associate Clinical Professor
University of California, Irvine
Orange, California, USA

Ian Brent Masters, MB BS, FRACP, PhD
Associate Professor
Queensland Children's Respiratory Centre
Queensland Children's Medical Research Institute, The
  University of Queensland
Royal Children's Hospital
Brisbane, Queensland, Australia

Douglas J. Mathisen, MD
Chief, Thoracic Surgery
Massachusetts General Hospital;
Hermes Grillo Professor of Thoracic Surgery
Harvard Medical School
Boston, Massachusetts, USA

Atul C. Mehta, MBBS, FACP, FCCP
Professor of Medicine
Cleveland Clinic Lerner School of Medicine;
Staff, Respiratory Institute
Cleveland Clinic
Cleveland, Ohio, USA

Teruomi Miyazawa, MD, PhD, FCCP
Professor and Chairman
Division of Respiratory and Infectious Diseases
Department of Internal Medicine
St. Marianna University School of Medicine
Kawasaki, Japan

Ashok Muniappan, MD
Instructor in Surgery
Harvard Medical School;
Division of Thoracic Surgery
Massachusetts General Hospital
Boston, Massachusetts, USA

Kenichi Nishina
Master of Mechanical Engineering
Manager, Chief Product Engineer
Olympus Medical Systems Corporation
Ultrasound Technology Department
Hachioji-shi, Tokyo, Japan

Marc Noppen, MD, PhD
Chief Executive Officer
Former Head, Interventional Endoscopy Unit
Respiratory Division
University Hospital UZ Brussel
Brussels, Belgium

Reza Nouraei, MA (Cantab), MBBChir, MRCS
Specialist Registrar in Academic Otolaryngology
The National Centre for Airway Reconstruction
Imperial College Healthcare NHS Trust
Charing Cross Hospital
London, England

Hiroaki Osada, MD, PhD
Professor Emeritus
St. Marianna University School of Medicine
Kawasaki, Japan;
Consultant Chest Surgeon
Sho-nan Chu-oh Hosptial
Fujisawa, Japan

Martin J. Phillips, MBBS, MD, FRACP
Clinical Professor, University of Western Australia
Department of Respiratory Medicine
Sir Charles Gairdner Hospital
Nedlands, Perth, Australia

Udaya B. S. Prakash, MD
Scripps Professor of Medicine
Mayo Clinic College of Medicine
Rochester, Minnesota, USA

Ibrahim Ramzy, MD, FRCPC
Professor
Departments of Pathology-Laboratory Medicine and
  Obstetrics-Gynecology
University of California
Irvine, CA;
Adjunct Professor
Department of Pathology and Immunology
Baylor College of Medicine
Houston, Texas, USA

Federico Rea, MD
Professor of Thoracic Surgery
Department of Cardiologic, Thoracic and Vascular
  Sciences
Chief, Thoracic Surgery Division
University of Padua
Padua, Italy

Guri Sandhu, MD, FRCS, FRCS (ORL-HNS)
Consultant Otolaryngologist, Head & Neck Surgeon
Honorary Senior Lecturer
Imperial and University Colleges
London, England

Suresh Senan, MRCP, FRCR, PhD
Professor of Clinical Experimental Radiotherapy
VU University Medical Center
Amsterdam, The Netherlands

Sylvia Verbanck, PhD
Biomedical Research Unit
Respiratory Division
University Hospital UZ Brussel
Brussels, Belgium

Cameron D. Wright, MD
Professor of Surgery
Harvard Medical School;
Division of Thoracic Surgery
Massachusetts General Hospital
Boston, Massachusetts, USA

How to Use This Book: The "Four Box" Approach

This book was written to help physicians help patients. Central airway disorders, whether benign or malignant, can be chronic or acute, severely debilitating, life-threatening, and not easily curable or for that matter treatable. They adversely affect lifestyle, communication, quality of life, daily living activities, social interactions, co-morbidities, and survival. Patients with these disorders often require care from a variety of physician and non-physician specialists, ranging from primary health care provider teams to surgeons, medical internists and subspecialists, radiologists, pathologists, critical care specialists, experts in palliative care and oncology, social workers, speech therapists, respiratory therapists, advanced nurse practitioners and, of course, chest specialists and interventional pulmonologists.

Many of the diseases that comprise central airway disorders are seen infrequently during the course of one's medical career. Others are seen more often and may in some settings constitute the bulk of a physician's practice. Regardless of circumstance or practice environment, health care providers caring for patients with central airway disorders can benefit from the knowledge, experience (whether good or less good), and expertise of their colleagues. This is because, although it seems the symptoms of various central airway disorders have much in common, the specifics of each disease causing a central airway problem, including response to treatment, are different. Furthermore, universally accepted, reproducible, and generally available therapeutic strategies are not always accessible, and therefore patients are often subjected to the particular biases of their physicians or to the local availability of technology and expertise.

This leads to our second purpose for writing *Bronchoscopy and Central Airway Disorders: A Patient-Centered Approach*. We aspire to help interested and motivated learners acquire the cognitive, technical, affective, and experiential skills necessary to competently and efficiently perform minimally invasive bronchoscopic procedures in a patient-focused care environment. Readers may use all or part of this book in their studies of a disease process or procedure. Whether in practice or as part of a subspecialty training program, learners can use this book to refresh their memories or discover more about the specific techniques, treatments, behaviors, ethics, physics, and physiologic factors that might affect a management strategy. From a consultative perspective, readers may discern new issues that they wish to explore further with their patients, or they might increase their depth of knowledge pertaining to a specific disease process or disease-related problem.

In each chapter, competency, proficiency, and professionalism are sought in what we consider are the *three* major elements of a procedure: strategy and planning, technical execution, and response to procedure-related adverse events or complications. Cognitive skills

(knowledge of facts) are enhanced by reading, whereas technical skills (such as manual dexterity and instrument manipulation) are mastered using simulators as well as at the patient's bedside. These two forms of knowledge can be combined with the experiential learning gained from working through patient-centered exercises and accompanied by the review of pertinent photographs, figures, and a series of concise, illustrative videos. Similar to having an apprenticeship experience with a thoughtful and knowledgeable mentor, deconstructing a procedure-related consultation using a structured patient-centered approach helps learners contemplate on sets of patient, disease, and procedure-related issues in an orderly and more uniform fashion.

During the past several years, we have taught the four-box patient-centered practical approach methodology described in this book on five continents and in a variety of contexts. Although our methods are applied to airway procedures and central airway disorders and target mostly interventional pulmonologists and other specialists caring for patients with airway difficulties, we are pleased to note that the template is universal and easily generalizable to practitioners in other medical specialties and to other disease processes.

In truth, our four-box approach is inspired from Albert Jonsen's classic work in medical ethics. Our *Four Box Practical Approach exercises** help learners think about the "how" and "why" of their actions based on specifically designed patient-centered case scenarios that enhance one's ability to analyze background information, review the pertinent literature, and appraise one's own and others' experiences. Topics are addressed in ways that range from technical to ethical, from social commentary to evidence-based medicine, from descriptions of subjective assessments to the valued objective experience of expert opinion. Because the latter demands a mechanistic explanation based on available scientific knowledge, specific teaching points are made to answer certain questions provided at the end of each patient-centered scenario. This additional element of the four-box method further enriches this structural guide to an educational process. In addition, extensive footnotes are used throughout the text to expand on information provided without detracting from the flow of reading material. At the end of each chapter, a second opinion guest commentary is provided by an expert who may or may not be an interventional bronchoscopist but who has noted experience caring for patients with the central airway disorder in question.

We recognize that, although the interventional bronchoscopist's approach to patient care and procedure-related issues attempts to be genuinely scientific, it cannot

---

*Also available at www.Bronchoscopy.org.

always be. The approach must also be imaginative, vigorous, and filled with the delight of creativity and adventure. That has been our attitude in this book. To the best of our ability, we address everything that is more or less related to the bronchoscopic procedure that might impact a decision-making process: physical examination and complementary tests; procedure indications, risks and alternatives; anatomy, anesthesia, and perioperative care; results, complications, and outcomes assessments; patients' preferences, support systems, and expectations; ethics and palliative care; team experience; and quality improvement. Of course, sometimes the reader will not find everything in a single chapter and may wish to review other chapters in search of specific information. By encouraging the reader freedom to use the book in this fashion, rather than risking repetition, we were able to address many similar issues differently, and several different issues similarly. Thirty different patient-centered scenarios are presented, each describing a different disease process and procedural or therapeutic challenge.* This has provided us the opportunity to combine our own enthusiasm for learning with the penetrating intellect of the accomplished physician-scientist represented through published evidence and expert commentary.

An asterisk below the title of each chapter is meant to inform the reader of those elements within the four-box approach that receive particular attention in that particular chapter. Subheadings within the text allow the reader to peruse certain sections more easily while simultaneously reinforcing one's knowledge of the name for that particular element of "the box."

The last section of the book is comprised of a patient-centered scenario to provide the reader with an opportunity for self-evaluation while combining the information learned from studying previous chapters in response to questions asked. We hope the reader will find this exercise challenging as well as informative.

Henri G. Colt
Septimiu D. Murgu

---

*Although based on real patients, scenarios were modified to avoid any possibility for patient identification and to help us meet specific educational objectives.

THE "FOUR BOX" PRACTICAL APPROACH TO INTERVENTIONAL BRONCHOSCOPY

INITIAL EVALUATION

1. Physical examination, complementary tests, and functional status assessment
2. Patient's significant co-morbidities
3. Patient's support system (also includes family)
4. Patient preferences and expectations (also includes family)

PROCEDURAL STRATEGIES

1. Indications, contraindications, and expected results
2. Operator and team experience and expertise
3. Risk-benefits analysis and therapeutic alternatives
4. Respect for persons (Informed Consent)

PROCEDURAL TECHNIQUES AND RESULTS

1. Anesthesia and other perioperative care
2. Techniques and instrumentation
3. Anatomic dangers and other risks
4. Results and procedure-related complications

LONG-TERM MANAGEMENT PLAN

1. Outcome assessment
2. Follow-up tests, visits, and procedures
3. Referrals to medical, surgical, or palliative/end-of-life subspecialty care
4. Quality improvement and team evaluation of clinical encounter

The "Four Box" Practical Approach to Interventional Bronchoscopy© is an interactive learning program designed to complement a traditional apprenticeship subspecialty training model.[1] Its purpose is to help learners acquire the cognitive, technical, affective, and experiential skills necessary to perform minimally invasive bronchoscopic procedures in a patient- and family-centered care environment. Inspired from the four box approach to a medical ethics consultation by Al Jonsen,[2] the four boxes of a Practical Approach exercise pertain to the initial evaluation, procedural strategies and planning, procedural techniques and results, and long-term management components of a medical intervention. By working through a series of patient-centered case scenarios, learners are prompted to think about the how and why of their actions based on background information, medical history, results of physical examination, results of imaging studies, relevant literature, and experience.

Practical approach exercises can be completed alone or in a group, with or without the guidance of an instructor-mentor. Consistent with recommendations from the Accreditation Council for Graduate Medical Education (ACGME), practical approach patient-centered scenarios prompt learners to address major components of the procedure-related consultation and informed consent process, as well as outcomes and expectations consistent with professionalism and competency guidelines.[3-5] These include acquiring skills to:

- Gather essential and accurate information about patients.
- Make informed decisions about diagnostic and therapeutic interventions based on patient information and preferences, up-to-date scientific evidence, and clinical judgment.
- Use information technology to support patient care decisions and patient education.
- Develop patient management plans.
- Communicate effectively to counsel and educate patients and their families.
- Demonstrate caring and respect when interacting with patients and their families.
- Provide health care services aimed at preventing health problems or maintaining health.
- Work with other health care professionals, including those from other disciplines, to provide patient-focused care.

REFERENCES

1. Bronchoscopy International. The Practical Approach© Henri Colt, 2007-2011, Electronic On-Line Multimedia originally published 2007. May also be accessed at http://www.Bronchoscopy.org/Practical Approach /htm.
2. Jonsen AR, Siegler M, Winslade WJ. *Clinical ethics.* 6th Ed. New York: McGraw Hill; 2006.
3. ACGME website. http//www.acgme.org/outcome/comp/compfull.asp.
4. Apelgren K. ACGME e-Bulletin. August 2006.
5. ACGME Competencies at http://www.acgme.org.

Contents

SECTION 5
Practical Approach to Malignant Central Airway Obstruction

SECTION 6
Practical Approach to Other Central Airway Disease Processes

SECTION 7

Video Contents

SECTION 1

Practical Approach to Benign Exophytic Airway Obstruction

Chapter 1

Rigid Bronchoscopy with Laser Resection for Tracheal Obstruction from Recurrent Respiratory Papillomatosis

This chapter emphasizes the following elements of the Four Box Approach: techniques and instrumentation, and follow-up tests, visits, and procedures.

CASE DESCRIPTION

A 53-year-old male patient presented with progressive dyspnea on exertion for 6 months. He had a chronic cough with yellow phlegm but no hemoptysis. The patient was infected with human immunodeficiency virus (HIV) 25 years ago and had been on highly active antiretroviral therapy (HAART), which he was tolerating well. His most recent viral load before presentation was undetectable, and CD4 count was 1200/mm³. He had undergone several laryngeal procedures for laryngeal papillomas 13 years earlier, which resulted in residual hoarseness. His past medical history was significant for chronic obstructive pulmonary disease (COPD), for which he was on albuterol and tiotropium. Neck and chest computed tomography showed two masses in the upper trachea (Figure 1-1, A). He was not married, lived alone, and had a male partner. He worked as a real estate agent and enjoyed his work. He had a 90 pack-year history of smoking but no history of recreational drug or alcohol use. Examination revealed normal vital signs. No wheezing or stridor was observed, but decreased breath sounds were noted bilaterally. Hemoglobin was 15.8 g/dL and white blood cell count was 14,400/mm³. Other biochemical and coagulation markers were normal. Pulmonary function testing revealed a moderate obstructive ventilatory impairment (forced expiratory volume in 1 second [FEV₁] of 55% predicted without improvement after bronchodilators), a peak expiratory flow (PEF) of 45% predicted, scooping of the expiratory limb, and flattening of the inspiratory limb on the flow-volume loop (FVL; Figure 1-1, B). Maximal voluntary ventilation was 48% predicted. Residual volume was 130% predicted, and diffusing capacity of the lung for carbon monoxide (DLCO) was 53% predicted. Flexible bronchoscopy revealed two polypoid lesions in the upper trachea (Figure 1-1, C). Biopsy showed squamous papilloma, a central fibrovascular core covered by stratified squamous epithelium, and features of koilocytic atypia and squamous metaplasia but no evidence of malignant transformation. These findings were consistent with his previous diagnosis of recurrent respiratory papillomatosis (RRP) (Figure 1-2).

DISCUSSION POINTS

1. List four differential diagnoses of exophytic endoluminal tracheal lesions.
2. Describe three indications for adjuvant therapy in recurrent respiratory papillomatosis.
3. Describe the advantages and disadvantages of neodymium-doped yttrium aluminium garnet (Nd: YAG) laser therapy as compared with other laser therapies for treating this patient with RRP.

CASE RESOLUTION

Initial Evaluations

Physical Examination, Complementary Tests, and Functional Status Assessment

The diagnosis of tracheal obstruction was based on nonspecific symptoms and results from chest tomography. Pulmonary function tests showed moderate obstructive ventilatory impairment and mild hyperinflation with reduced DLCO—findings consistent with the patient's emphysema. The FVL did not reveal a classic pattern of flattening of both inspiratory and expiratory limbs as is seen in patients with fixed central and/or upper airway stenosis; instead, flattening of the inspiratory limb was evident, but the expiratory curve showed only a "scooped out" pattern as is usually seen in asthma and COPD (see Figure 1-1). Interpreting isolated flattening of the inspiratory limb as sign of a variable extrathoracic obstruction[1] would be erroneous and inconsistent with this patient's CT and bronchoscopic findings, which clearly showed intrathoracic obstruction (see Figure 1-1). Flattening of the expiratory limb, as was seen in our patient as well, may be masked by a significant reduction in PEF in patients with COPD.[2]

In general, the flow-volume loop is an insensitive test for tracheal obstruction because lesions must narrow the tracheal lumen to less than 8 mm before abnormalities can be detected.[2] Indeed, reports indicate that exertional dyspnea and reductions in PEF usually occur when the tracheal diameter falls to less than 8 mm.[3] In a study of more than 400 FVLs, the sensitivity of several quantitative and visual criteria for upper airway obstruction was 70%.[4] Another study showed that in cases of upper airway obstruction (i.e., vocal cord dysfunction), none of the spirometric data predicted disease. Authors concluded that normal FVLs should not influence the decision to

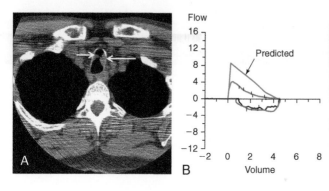

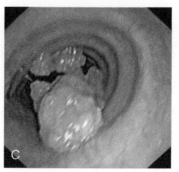

Figure 1-1 A, Neck and chest computed tomography shows two masses in the upper trachea, but no parenchymal lesions or mediastinal lymphadenopathy *(arrows)*. **B,** Flow-volume loop shows scooping of the expiratory limb and flattening of the inspiratory limb. **C,** Flexible bronchoscopy reveals two polypoid, "cauliflower"-like lesions in the upper trachea.

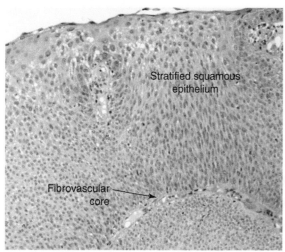

Figure 1-2 Biopsy shows squamous papilloma with features of koilocytic atypia and squamous metaplasia and a central fibrovascular core but no evidence of malignant transformation (magnification ×20, hematoxylin and eosin [H&E]).

perform laryngoscopy.[5] Even when the FVL pattern is characteristic, it offers only functional and inexact anatomic (location) information. Thus imaging studies are indicated.

One spirometry test that should not be ignored when patients with suspected tracheal obstruction are evaluated is maximal voluntary ventilation (MVV). The MVV is the largest volume of gas that can be moved into and out of the lungs in 1 minute by voluntary effort with vigorous coaching; normally it is measured as 125 to 170 L/min. The MVV depends on muscular force, compliance of the thoracic wall and lungs, and airway resistance. It is reduced in patients with emphysema or with central airway obstruction. A reduction in MVV, however, is nonspecific and is caused by upper or lower airways obstruction, restriction, or muscle weakness.[6] In a patient such as ours who showed good effort during the MVV maneuver and had no evidence of neuromuscular disease or restriction, the suspicion for airway obstruction is high. Although MVV is reduced in emphysema, a disproportionate reduction in measured MVV compared with the estimated value (MVV/FEV$_1$ of less than 25, such as that seen in our case), in fact, has a sensitivity of 66% for diagnosing upper airway obstruction.[7]

This patient had received a diagnosis of RRP and in the past required several procedures for laryngeal papillomas. In view of this, the likely diagnosis for the tracheal polypoid, "cauliflower-like" lesions was RRP. The differential diagnosis of this exophytic endoluminal lesion includes malignant and other benign processes. Tracheal malignant tumors are rare, constituting only 2% of all respiratory tract tumors.[8] These most commonly include squamous cell carcinoma and adenoid cystic carcinoma, which are responsible for 70% to 80% of tracheal tumors. Other tracheal tumors include carcinoid tumors, mucoepidermoid carcinomas, and a wide variety of carcinomas, sarcomas, lymphomas, and plasmacytomas.[9] Among lesions of sufficient severity to require intervention, malignant lesions have accounted for between 25% and 66% of cases; one third have been primary lesions and two thirds were secondary.[10] Cancers that can directly invade or metastasize to the airway and cause tracheal obstruction include renal cell, esophageal, lymphoma, melanoma, breast, colon, and thyroid carcinomas (Figure 1-3). For these reasons, biopsy is warranted to confirm diagnosis, even when "classic" polypoid, "cauliflower"-like lesions are seen during bronchoscopy.

Benign tumors account for less than 10% of tumors involving the trachea and mainstem bronchi.[11] Among histologically benign causes of tracheal exophytic endoluminal lesions, one should consider granulation tissue from endotracheal or tracheostomy tubes, airway stents, foreign bodies, hamartomas, solitary papillomas, lipomas, leiomyomas, chondromas, amyloidosis, exuberant tracheopathica osteochondroplastica, and inflammatory myofibroblastic tumor[12] (see Figure 1-3). Overall, most respiratory tract tumors are malignant, and benign tumors are rare (approximately 1.9% of all lung tumors); most of these are papillomas and hamartomas.[13]

Although RRP is considered by some investigators to be an uncommon tumor, secondary to infection with human papillomavirus (HPV) types 6 and 11, it is actually the most common benign tracheal neoplasm.[14] In our patient, the tracheal papillomas probably represented spread of disease from the original laryngeal site. The rate of tracheal involvement by laryngeal papilloma has been reported in the literature to be 2% to 17%.[15] Once in the tracheobronchial tree, RRP is difficult to control, causes significant morbidity, and in almost 2% of cases may undergo malignant transformation.[16] Malignant degeneration is aggressive and often is rapidly fatal, but it occurs infrequently in the absence of prior radiation therapy.[17]

Figure 1-3 Examples of malignant and benign exophytic endoluminal tracheal lesions. **A,** Squamous cell carcinoma in the lower trachea. **B,** Adenoid cystic carcinoma in the lower trachea completely occluding the left mainstem bronchus. **C,** Metastatic melanoma in the upper trachea. **D,** Invading esophageal cancer on the posterior membrane in the upper trachea. **E,** Exuberant cartilaginous nodules from tracheopathica osteochondroplastica. **F,** Post stent removal granulation tissue.

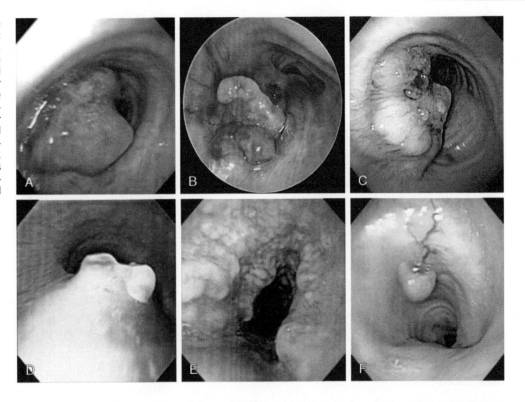

Comorbidities

The patient's comorbidities included moderate COPD and HIV infection. If interventions were provided with the patient under general anesthesia, these comorbidities could significantly increase the risk for COPD exacerbation or postoperative pneumonia. In a large retrospective study, however, HIV-infected patients were matched 1:1 with HIV-seronegative patients undergoing surgical procedures by type, location, age, and gender; findings showed that clinical outcomes, length of stay, and number of postoperative visits were similar among the matched patient pairs. Various complications were no more frequent among HIV-infected patients, except for pneumonia. Among the HIV-infected group of patients, a viral load of 30,000 copies/mL or greater was associated with a threefold increased risk of complications, but a CD4 cell count <200/mm^3 was not associated with increased risk.[18] Our patient's CD4 count was greater than 1000 and the viral load was undetectable, putting him in a low-risk group for developing postoperative pneumonia.

A patient's COPD should be treated so the best possible baseline level of function can be achieved before elective interventions are provided. A retrospective study of patients with COPD undergoing general anesthesia illustrated the importance of optimizing preoperative function.[19] In this report, 227 of 464 patients underwent some sort of preoperative preparation, including various combinations of bronchodilators, antibiotics, and systemic glucocorticoids. The incidence of pulmonary complications was lower in the prepared group than among those receiving no preoperative preparation (23% vs. 35%). Another study noted a reduction in the incidence of pulmonary complications from 60% to 22% in a group of high-risk patients prepared with bronchodilators, smoking cessation, antibiotics, and chest physical therapy.[20] Our patient had stable moderate COPD at the time of evaluation and was treated with short-acting β_2-agonists and long-acting anticholinergic agents according to international guidelines.[21]

Support System

This patient was living with HIV infection. Several of the attributes of HIV illness increase the likelihood that its victims will be stigmatized, for example, the illness is viewed in society as the result of individuals violating the moral order; the contagiousness of HIV is perceived to threaten society; HIV illness is viewed as a debilitating disease that results in death; and this disease has most frequently been associated with groups already marginalized in society. Of course, the HIV-acquired immunodeficiency syndrome (AIDS) stigma has the potential to influence health and health-seeking behaviors in a variety of ways and, therefore, should be an important consideration for health care professionals. Studies show disempowering health care practices occur within the health care encounter when persons living with HIV access health services.[22] The dominant and powerful role of health care professionals (in particular physicians) in the treatment decisions of persons living with HIV has been documented. Medical surveillance of an individual after an HIV-positive diagnosis was considered by some a "manifestation of paternalistic power in the guise of knowledge-seeking and in the name of beneficence."[23]

Our patient had a male partner who seemed very supportive. Study findings show heterogeneity in dyadic (i.e., relational level) support for illness management. In the context of HIV, a patient's social support may be particularly important in terms of adherence to medications.[24] Strict HAART adherence is required for treatment success and increased survival in patients living with HIV. Non-adherence can increase the risk of developing drug-resistant viral strains and transmitting drug-resistant strains to others. Regarding RRP, nonadherence could result in an inability to control the disease when adjuvant therapies are necessary. Although family and friends frequently provide support, relationship partners are a primary source of social support for gay male couples coping with HIV.[25]

Patient Preferences and Expectations

This patient had no evidence of cognitive dysfunction and was able to clearly express his desire for treatment. His partner was involved in these conversations per the patient's request, and they agreed to proceed with available therapeutic options for tracheal papillomatosis.* Thus rigid bronchoscopy under general anesthesia was offered to this patient.

Procedural Strategies

Indications

This symptomatic patient had tracheal obstruction due to RRP. A bronchoscopic procedure could be offered to restore airway patency and improve dyspnea. Hoarseness present for many years was likely caused by involvement of the vocal fold, usually the first and predominant site of papilloma lesions, causing hoarseness to be the principal presenting symptom. Hoarseness was unlikely to improve after rigid bronchoscopy.

Although no treatment has been consistently shown to eradicate RRP, removal of papilloma tissue as completely as possible without compromising normal airway wall structures may reduce recurrence and risk for malignant transformation. The pattern of obstruction was exophytic intraluminal, and no evidence of extrinsic compression was found. For endoluminal central airway obstruction, bronchoscopic therapies include electrosurgery, laser resection, microdebridement, rigid bronchoscopic de-bulking, cryotherapy, brachytherapy, and photodynamic

---

*The Centers for Disease Control and Prevention (CDC) estimates that tens of millions of people in the United States are infected with HPV, but the prevalence of RRP is low (10,000 to 25,000 people in the United States). The estimated incidence in adults is approximately 1.8 per 100,000, and it preferentially affects men by a ratio of 3:2. It is not known with certainty the manner in which adults acquire the virus, but it is speculated that sexual transmission is likely (http://www.rrpf.org). Patients with adult-onset RRP have lifetime sex partners and a higher frequency of oral sex than adult controls. *Genetic factors and impaired immune responses at the cellular level of the respiratory tract (e.g., tobacco use, exposure to radiation) appear to play a key role in determining who is susceptible to contracting this disease; the infectivity rate is not known but is considered very low;* otherwise, there would be many tens of millions of people in the United States with RRP. *This disease is not labeled contagious or a sexually transmitted disease;* some actively sexual adults, however, may risk infection by engaging in oral-genital sex with a person who has genital HPV. These individuals may wish to consider using a protective latex barrier when they have oral sex (http://www.rrpwebsite.org).

therapy. No stent insertion was planned unless airway lumen narrowing remained at 50% or greater.[26] Adjuvant treatments include potentially curative gene therapy (epidermal growth factor receptor [EGFR] tyrosine kinase inhibitors), retinoids (oral metabolites or analogs of vitamin A), and intralesional injection of antiviral agents in an attempt to induce growth arrest or apoptosis, or to inhibit the proliferation or promote the normal differentiation of HPV-infected cells.[27]

Contraindications

No absolute contraindications to rigid bronchoscopy were noted. However, the risk of perioperative cardiac complications should be considered in this patient with a history of HIV infection because diabetes mellitus, dyslipidemia, and coronary atherosclerosis are increasingly common among HIV-infected patients on long-term antiretroviral therapy.[28] One study found electrocardiographic (ECG) evidence of asymptomatic ischemic heart disease in 11% of HIV-infected patients.[29] Our patient had no clinical or electrocardiographic signs of coronary artery disease and had been cleared for general anesthesia by his internist.

Expected Results

Rigid intubation was planned using a 12-mm-diameter Efer-Dumon nonventilating rigid bronchoscope (Efer, La Ciotat, France) to allow passage of laser fiber, a rigid suction catheter, and forceps. Nd:YAG laser photocoagulation followed by rigid bronchoscopic debulking under general anesthesia was planned, along with spontaneous assisted ventilation. The goal was to reduce tumor burden, restore airway patency, and improve dyspnea, thus eventually decreasing regional dissemination of disease.[16]

Removal of HPV-involved tissues as completely as possible and without compromise of normal airway structures appears necessary to reduce recurrence. Most studies performed by otolaryngologists evaluated carbon dioxide (CO_2) or potassium-titanyl-phosphate (KTP) lasers because the disease is more commonly localized in the larynx. However, many reports have described successful use of Nd:YAG laser resection for RRP, especially when the trachea is involved.[30-34] One case series, for example, evaluated five patients with RRP; none had recurrence of disease after 1 year of follow-up post Nd:YAG laser treatment.[30] In urology, for instance, the Nd:YAG laser was used to effectively treat HPV-associated genital papillomas (caused by HPV 6 and HPV 11); its use led to a lower rate of recurrence compared with CO_2 laser treatment after 1 year of follow-up.[35] Moreover, tissue biopsies after Nd:YAG laser surgery demonstrated HPV recurrence mainly in nontreated areas, whereas after CO_2 laser treatment, viral recurrence was observed within and at the margins of treated tissue. This might be attributed to the fact that, in comparison with vaporizing (what you see is what you get) CO_2 laser energy, Nd:YAG laser energy provides deeper (what you don't see might hurt you) coagulation along with destruction of the HPV-infected basal cell layer of the mucosa. This region is usually responsible for the regeneration of papilloma tissue.[35] Nd:YAG laser coagulation of papilloma tissue in a noncontact mode may cause less smoke-containing toxic pyrolysis products and infectious HPV particles, and could potentially lower the risk of HPV transmission to adjoining healthy tissue compared with CO_2 laser surgery. In addition, effective suctioning during rigid bronchoscopy with the Nd:YAG laser offers fast and efficient removal of the unavoidable but small amount of potentially infectious laser plume. This might be another reason for the low rate of recurrence in a study of RRP lesions treated with the Nd:YAG laser.[30]

Team Experience

Nd:YAG laser treatment of RRP should be provided by physicians who are experienced in the application of non-contact Nd:YAG laser and able to estimate the thermal impact on treated tissue. The operator who is not aware of injury to deeper tissue layers caused by injudicious laser usage may encounter unacceptable scarring or even airway perforation and massive bleeding. Inappropriate and aggressive use of the laser may cause injury to nonaffected adjacent tissues and may create an environment suitable for implantation of viral particles. Procedures should not be performed in a facility that does not have the necessary complement of equipment for safe instrumentation of a patient's airway.[36]

Risk-Benefit Analysis

Although Nd:YAG laser may cause deep tissue damage, our patient had symptoms that required restoration of airway patency. No risk-benefit analysis has been performed to compare Nd:YAG laser versus other types of lasers or other treatment modalities, but several alternative techniques have been proposed for treating RRP. One survey showed that the microdebrider and the CO_2 laser were the preferred means for removal of laryngeal RRP; 52.7% of respondents preferred the microdebrider, and 41.9% the CO_2 laser.[37]

Therapeutic Alternatives for Restoring Airway Patency

- *CO_2 laser vaporization:* done under general anesthesia usually with muscle relaxants, with high-frequency supraglottic jet ventilation, and under suspension micro-laryngotracheoscopy. The CO_2 laser is believed to enhance precision and is preferred by some surgeons because of its short extinction coefficients and minimal thermal injury to adjacent tissues. The CO_2 laser has an emission wavelength of 10,600 nm and converts light to thermal energy that is absorbed by intracellular water; the result is controlled destruction of tissues by cell vaporization and cautery of tissue surfaces with minimal bleeding. Its use through a flexible broncho-scope has been described, but usually the CO_2 laser has to be coupled to an operating microscope, which allows treatment only with a rigid system; a high level of expertise and good coordination are needed to reach all affected areas while avoiding injury to healthy tissue adjacent to the papillomas. In one series of 244 patients with RRP treated over 2 months with the CO_2 laser, "remission" was achieved in 37%, "clearance" in 6%, and "cure" in 17% of cases.[38] However, CO_2 laser surgery may result in dissemination of infectious viral particles included in the laser plume with the potential for harmful effects on operating room personnel and patients.[39]

- *Microdebrider:* used by otolaryngologists as a laryngeal shaver for RRP. Advocates of this technique claim that the shaver is safer and more accurate and prevents thermal injury, and that postprocedure edema associated with use of the laser is minimized because tissue injury resulting from the shaver technique is confined to the superficial mucosa.[40] Some investigators used an endoscopic microdebrider to quickly debulk laryngeal disease. Pasquale et al. reported improved voice quality, less operating room time, less mucosal injury, and a cost benefit when the microdebrider was used compared with the CO_2 laser.[41] A Web-based survey of members of the American Society of Pediatric Otolaryngology found that most respondents favor the use of "shaver" technology.[37] Safety advantages include no risk of laser fire or burns and apparently no risk of aerosolized viral DNA particles. However, debilitating injury and scar with subsequent dysphonia have been reported.[42]

- *The KTP laser* with a 532 nm wavelength is very useful for cutting and coagulating tissues simultaneously; its incisional strength does not penetrate as deeply as the Nd:YAG laser, so less collateral tissue damage occurs. The KTP laser has been used successfully in treatment for tracheal papillomas.[32] Zeitels et al. reported that the use of a 532 nm pulsed KTP laser in the treatment of recurrent glottal papillomatosis and dysplasia led to 75% regression of disease in two thirds of patients; good results were also reported with a solid-state fiber-based thulium laser that functions similarly to a CO_2 laser, with the benefit that the laser beam is delivered through a small glass fiber.[43]

- *Pulsed-dye lasers* (wavelength 577 and 585 nm) are reportedly feasible and safe for treating patients with RRP[44]; McMillan et al. reported good preliminary results in three patients with use of the 585 nm pulsed-dye laser.[45] Rees et al. performed 328 pulsed-dye laser treatments in the office in 131 adult patients with upper airway RRP and reported that patients overwhelmingly preferred in-office surgery to a procedure received under general anesthesia.[46]

- *Argon plasma coagulation (APC):* allows controlled, limited penetration into tissues and good control of bleeding without carbonization or vaporization. APC has been used for RRP with good control of disease and no side effects or complications.[47]

- *Silicone stent insertion* may be useful in refractory endobronchial RRP when medical and other endobronchial therapies fail to restore airway patency. Case reports show that papilloma debulking and silicone stents can offer adequate control of symptoms.[48]

- *Tracheostomy* sometimes is performed to provide a secure airway for patients who require weekly or monthly surgical procedures (especially for laryngeal disease). It is noteworthy, however, that approximately 50% of tracheotomized patients develop peristomal and distal tracheal papillomas.[49]

- *Adjuvant therapy:* The decision to initiate adjuvant therapy should be individualized according to the frequency of surgical interventions, the morbidity of frequent surgeries, and the recurrence pattern of the papillomas. It has been suggested that adjuvant therapies are needed if surgery is required more frequently than 4 times a year for 2 years, or if papillomas begin to spread outside of the endolarynx. Adjuvant therapies include α-interferon, acyclovir, indole-3-carbinol, retinoic acid, photodynamic therapy, ribavirin, cidofovir, and cimetidine. Of note, few of these therapies have been evaluated in randomized prospective trials.

- α-*Interferon:* through its antiproliferative and immunomodulatory actions is the type of interferon most biologically active in treating RRP; results of studies show that it decreases the growth of papillomas and increases the time interval between surgical procedures. It may induce complete resolution of clinical disease in approximately 30% to 50% of patients and partial resolution in 20% to 42%.[50] It is administered initially at 5 million units/m^2 body surface area by subcutaneous injection daily for 30 days, and then 3 times weekly for a trial of at least 6 months. The dose can be reduced to 3 million units/m^2 given 3 times a week if side effects are severe. Patients on long-term interferon therapy should have their liver enzymes and leukocytes monitored at least on a quarterly basis. Weaning should be slow, to prevent a rebound effect.
- *Retinoic acid* is a vitamin A derivative that has been shown to modulate epithelial differentiation; however, a randomized study failed to demonstrate efficacy and found a high incidence of side effects such as dry skin, cheilitis, and arthralgia.[51] Results from a recent study suggest that concomitant administration of retinoic acid and α-interferon may have a synergistic effect on RRP control, and this combination may be useful for the treatment of patients with distal airway involvement.[52]
- *Indole-3-carbinol:* this derivative of cruciferous vegetables (cabbage, cauliflower, and broccoli) has been shown to alter the growth of papilloma in mice by altering estrogen metabolism, namely, by shifting production to antiproliferative estrogens. A third of patients who received indole-3-carbinol therapy showed remission, a third showed a slower rate of growth, and a third had no response. Indole-3-carbinol is best administered as a dietary supplement. The recommended daily dose is 200 to 400 mg for adults and 100 to 200 mg for children weighing less than 25 kg. Overall, indole-3-carbinol is very well tolerated and produces few side effects.
- *Photodynamic therapy (PDF):* may reduce surgical intervals, but photosensitivity limits its usefulness. The persistence of HPV DNA in normal-appearing mucosa after PDT indicates that the treatment is not curative, but it is reported to reduce the growth rate of papillomas by approximately 50% and may be particularly useful in endobronchial/endotracheal lesions. A randomized clinical trial in 23 patients ages 4 to 60 with severe RRP resulted in improvement in laryngeal disease; intravenous administration of meso-tetra (hydroxyphenyl) chlorine was performed 6 days before direct endoscopic PDT at 80 to 100 J of light for adults and 60 to 80 J for

children; however, papillomas recurred in 3 to 5 years, and the therapy was poorly tolerated by a quarter of the patients.[53]
- *Cidofovir:* this drug is designed to be injected into the papilloma bed after debulking surgery. Cidofovir is currently the most frequently used adjuvant drug in children with RRP. Snoeck et al. reported that in a series of 17 patients with severe RRP, injection of cidofovir 2.5 mg/mL directly into the papilloma bed after laser surgery was followed by a complete response in 14 days.[54] A more recent study found intralesional injections of cidofovir to be effective in a small cohort of adults with RRP.[55] Because animal studies demonstrated a high level of carcinogenicity for cidofovir, and because case reports have described progressive dysplasia in patients with RRP who received cidofovir, the RRP Task Force has published guidelines for clinicians interested in using cidofovir to treat RRP.[56] However, a randomized, double-blind, placebo-controlled trial evaluated intralesional cidofovir (0.3 mg/mL for children younger than 18 years and 0.75 mg/mL for patients older than 18 years; the dose was later increased to 5 mg/mL for both children and adults) after lesion resection (CO_2 laser or microresection) for severe recurrent RRP in 19 adults and children. Improvement in the Derkay severity score* was observed 12 months after therapy in both treated and placebo groups. The authors concluded that proof of efficacy of cidofovir in RRP is insufficient.[57] This study might change clinical practice; in a survey from 2004, more than 75% of respondents believed cidofovir had moderate to good efficacy. Only 4% reported that their patient's disease had worsened.[37]
- *Cimetidine:* in high doses (30 mg/kg for 4 months) has immunomodulatory effects and has been used successfully in a case of very advanced RRP with tracheo-bronchial-pulmonary involvement.[58] Only 15% of physicians, however, report routine use of reflux medications or precautions for RRP patients.[37] It is prudent to investigate and control reflux in RRP patients while this relationship is studied further.
- *Gefitinib:* an EGFR tyrosine kinase inhibitor, this drug was shown to elicit an immediate and dramatic response in patients with severe RRP refractory to other therapies.[59] The rationale for using this drug in RRP is based on the fact that respiratory papilloma cells have high levels of EGFR and respond to epidermal growth factor by a decrease in epithelial differentiation.
- *Intralesional bevacizumab:* appears to show some efficacy in prolonging the time between treatments, thereby reducing the number of treatments per year in children with severe RRP.[60] Bevacizumab, as a

---

*A staging system for assessing severity of disease and response to therapy in RRP based on the patient's clinical course (surgery-free interval, number of surgeries within a year, severity and location of papilloma lesions, and functional impairment as assessed by voice, stridor, respiratory distress, and the need for urgent intervention).

human monoclonal antibody, binds to and neutralizes the biologic activities of vascular endothelial growth factor (VEGF) isoforms, preventing them from interacting with their receptors. The rationale for using bevacizumab to treat aggressive RRP is based on the fact that VEGF receptors are present in papilloma specimens. Zeitels et al. successfully used bevacizumab to treat 10 adults with RRP. The authors concluded that this drug through its antiangiogenesis properties may enhance the photoangiolytic effect of laser therapy.[61]

Cost-Effectiveness

No formal cost-effectiveness evaluations of these bronchoscopic or adjuvant modalities have yet been published. Because currently no therapeutic regimen reliably eradicates HPV, it seems prudent to accept some residual papilloma rather than risking damage to normal tissue and producing excessive scarring. In children, the frequency of procedures and the severity of symptoms substantially impact quality of life and are associated with considerable economic cost, estimated at $150 million annually.[62]

Informed Consent

After he had been advised about all available alternatives, our patient elected to proceed with rigid bronchoscopy under general anesthesia. He was informed of potential risks for postoperative development of COPD exacerbation, as well as procedure-related complications such as airway edema and airway fire with use of the laser, hemorrhage, and long-term sequelae such as laser-induced tracheal stenosis or even distal spread of disease through laser plumes.

Techniques and Results

Anesthesia and Perioperative Care

The anesthesiologist should be properly informed about the patient's HAART regimen because protease inhibitors and non-nucleoside reverse transcriptase inhibitors are associated with significant drug–drug interactions. In general, HAART therapy should be continued through the perioperative period. If clinically necessary, however, stopping antiretroviral drugs for a few days should not have a harmful impact on their effectiveness. These drugs were continued in our patient. The stress of general anesthesia and surgery may unmask previously unsuspected adrenal suppression in patients with HIV infection, especially because symptoms of hypoadrenalism are nonspecific. This condition is seen mainly in patients with advanced HIV infection and in those with concurrent infection with *Mycobacterium avium* complex or cytomegalovirus. Hyponatremia, hyperkalemia, or hypotension should raise suspicion for this entity. These were not present in our patient, so we proceeded with rigid bronchoscopy under general anesthesia in the operating room (OR).

The OR should be set up in advance and equipment checked by the surgical team to ensure that bronchoscopes and telescopes of appropriate sizes are available, and that suction tubing and catheters are of proper length to fit through all available bronchoscopes, video equipment (desirable for education of patient and families, and to allow the treating team to follow the progress of the disease), light cables, and light sources. Laser equipment should be tested before the patient enters the room to ensure that it is functioning properly.[36]

Care must be taken to protect OR personnel because viral particles have been demonstrated in the laser plume. All rooms should be maintained at positive pressure. It is important to ensure that filters for the general ventilation system are maintained and changed as recommended by the manufacturer of the system. Dirty air filters will impede room air exchanges. Substantial evidence of viable virus (both HIV and HPV) has been identified in CO_2, erbium-doped yttrium aluminum garnet (Er : YAG), and Nd : YAG laser and electrocautery smoke generated at a range of power settings.[63,64] One study even showed a higher incidence of nasopharyngeal lesions among CO_2 laser surgeons in comparison with a control group.[65] Good suction of smoke and use of laser operating masks are usually sufficient,[50] but high-performance filtration masks, although very difficult to breathe through, may be more protective and are recommended by some investigators to reduce the risk of inhalation of particulate matter such as viral or bacterial contaminants.[66]

The most serious safety concern associated with use of the laser during rigid bronchoscopy is that the laser beam generates heat, which, in the oxygen-rich environment provided by anesthetic gases, could lead to an explosion or a fire in the airway. Acceptable techniques by which to avoid these complications for our patient included intermittent ventilation via rigid bronchoscopy with a fraction of inspired oxygen (FiO_2) less than 0.3 and jet ventilation. A survey of otolaryngologists in the United States showed the proportions of surgeons favoring the various techniques as follows: laser-safe tube 46%, jet ventilation 25%, apneic 16%, and spontaneous 12%.[67] Although jet ventilation generally is believed to be safe, concern has been raised that this method may lead to distal inoculation of the virus. The key is good communication between operator and anesthesiologist before and during the procedure so that approaches are coordinated. It is important to have an experienced anesthesiologist who is comfortable with managing the obstructed airway. If no such individual is available, then one should consider delaying the procedure or transferring the patient to a facility where one is available.[36]

Instrumentation

We chose a 12 mm Efer rigid nonventilating bronchoscope to allow passage of various instruments for laser-assisted papilloma debulking. A working suction tubing connected to an efficient smoke-evacuating device is essential to protect OR personnel from the hazards of surgical smoke. An efficient evacuation device must have a capture device that does not interfere with the surgeon's activities (e.g., the suction catheter), a vacuum source that has strong suction ability to remove the smoke properly, and a filtration system capable of filtering smoke and making the environment safer.[66] The surgeon and OR personnel should wear surgical masks and protective plastic eyeglasses.

Anatomic Dangers and Other Risks

When using laser resection for lesions in the upper-mid trachea, one should be aware of the vascular supply and adjacent vascular structures. The blood supply of the trachea is segmental, largely shared with the esophagus and derived principally from multiple branches of the inferior thyroid artery above and the subclavian and innominate arteries below. The innominate artery is adjacent to the trachea at the level of the right costoclavicular joint, and the right carotid artery is adjacent to the right tracheal wall of the cervical trachea. The vessels approach laterally, and only fine branches pass anterior to the trachea and posterior to the esophagus. Therefore it is probably safer to work anterior and posterior, when possible.

Laser-generated thermal energy can injure deeper tissues, leading to scarring with complications such as abnormal vocal cord function (when high subglottic or laryngeal lesions are treated), spread of viral particles to previously unaffected areas, and delayed local tissue damage.

Results and Procedure-Related Complications

The patient was atraumatically intubated with the rigid bronchoscope, and the stricture was reassessed in terms of precise location, extent, and associated mucosal changes. Exophytic endoluminal obstruction was seen for 4 cm, starting 4 cm below the vocal cords. Nd : YAG laser photocoagulation was performed; laser output power was set to 30 W, 1 second pulses for a total of 3379 Joules and 1 minute and 24 seconds. Laser light was applied in a noncontact mode at low power density (the tip of the fiber at 1 cm away from the lesion). After complete blanching of the papilloma, shrinkage of tissue was noted and resection was started using the beveled edge of the rigid bronchoscope (see video on ExpertConsult.com) (Video I.1.1). Suctioning capabilities through the rigid suction catheter at the distal part of the bronchoscope permitted a good view of the operating field and effective removal of laser plume. With regard to infection control in the setting of surgical smoke, during any endoscopic surgery, a chimney effect may cause a jet stream through the tube toward operating personnel. Moreover, smoke during endoscopic procedures is accumulated and then is released all at once in a relatively high-velocity jet in a particular direction. Consequently, the surgeon or OR personnel can be exposed to high concentrations of cells and infectious particles. To avoid this, the surgeon should ensure that the jet is not pointed in his or her direction.[68]

Development of carbonization zones and damage to healthy tissue was avoided during treatment. Specimens were sent to pathology for HPV typing, although its value in terms of predicting prognosis is currently limited. For subsequent surgeries, when needed, specimens should be sent for monitoring of progression to atypia and malignant transformation to squamous cell carcinoma. This practice, however, is controversial: in a survey, about one third of respondents performed re-biopsy of lesions at every surgery, presumably worried about the progression from squamous papilloma to papilloma with

atypia and possibly to squamous cell carcinoma About half of respondents perform a re-biopsy only when a change in the growth pattern is noted; the remainder do a re-biopsy yearly or use some other criteria.[37] Airway patency was completely restored. The procedure lasted 30 minutes. The patient tolerated the procedure well, and extubation was uneventful. The patient was transferred to the postanesthesia care unit for 2 hours, during which no complications were noted. He was discharged home the next day.

Long-Term Management

Outcome Assessment

The patient's airway obstruction was palliated. No immediate postoperative anesthesia or procedure-related complications were noted. No infectious complications were detected in the patient in the early postoperative period; in fact, in HIV-infected patients, bacterial sepsis occurs most often in advanced disease (with low CD4 count), poor nutrition, and neutropenia; this was not the case in our patient.

Referral

Because of his history of hoarseness and papillomas at the vocal cord level, we referred the patient to our otolaryngology colleagues. In adults, malignant degeneration usually involves the larynx, unlike in children, in whom cancer usually develops in the bronchopulmonary tree. Patients newly diagnosed with RRP warrant a substantial time commitment on the part of the otolaryngologist to engage the patient or the family (in case of children) in a frank and open discussion of the disease and its management. Support groups such as the Recurrent Respiratory Papilloma Foundation[36] and the International RRP ISA Center[69] can serve as a resource for information and support. Educational information, research updates, discussion groups, and announcements regarding new treatment modalities are discussed on these websites.

Follow-up Tests and Procedures

Once RRP has spread outside the larynx, computed tomography (CT) scans can be used to monitor development or worsening of pulmonary disease. However, less than 50% of surveyed otolaryngologists routinely use CT scans to monitor for progression. Of those who do use CT scans, 57% do so on a yearly basis, and 37% every 6 months. Information provided by spiral CT scanning with multiplanar reconstruction and virtual bronchoscopy may be used to monitor for recurrence of central airway obstruction.[70] The disease may undergo spontaneous remission, may persist in a stable state, requiring only periodic surgical treatment, or may be aggressive, requiring surgical treatment every few days to weeks and consideration of adjuvant medical therapy. Extralaryngeal spread of respiratory papillomas, as seen in our patient, has been identified in approximately 30% of children and in 16% of adults with RRP. The most frequent sites of extralaryngeal spread were, in decreasing order of frequency, the oral cavity, trachea and bronchi, and esophagus. Pulmonary parenchymal papilloma lesions begin as asymptomatic, noncalcified peripheral nodules, but they

Figure 1-4 **A** and **B,** Computed tomography from a different patient, who developed characteristic multiple, bilateral thin-walled cysts *(thin arrows)*. **C,** Post obstructive atelectasis potentially leading to infection and bronchiectasis is seen when the lobar bronchi are involved. **D,** The development of lymphadenopathy *(thick arrow)* should raise suspicion for potential malignant transformation.

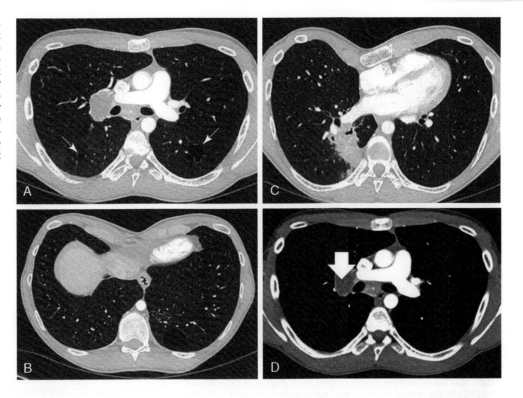

may enlarge and undergo central cavitation, liquefaction, and necrosis with evidence of multiple and bilateral thin-walled cysts (Figure 1-4). Patients later may develop atelectasis, recurrent bronchiectasis, pneumonia, and worsening pulmonary function. The clinical course of pulmonary parenchymal RRP is insidious and may progress over years. It eventually manifests as respiratory failure caused by severe destruction of lung parenchyma.[16] Our patient's CT scan showed no evidence of parenchymal abnormalities.

This patient's HPV typing showed HPV 6 and 11. Malignant transformation appears to be more likely with HPV 16, an unusual cause of RRP. Individualized follow-up was arranged between the patient and our team. Circumstances that would influence the timing and location of follow-up include travel distance to the medical center, the reliability of family (friends) accompanying the patient and the reliability of the patient's transportation, the rapidity with which papillomas recur, and the degree of airway compromise caused by the papilloma. A regimen proposed in children with RRP might include monthly follow-up in the office during the first year of disease diagnosis; airway evaluation is performed every other month and whenever the clinical situation warrants. Follow-up can be extended to every 2 to 4 months in subsequent years in a patient with stable disease and a reliable means of transportation. Surgical intervention would be planned according to clinical needs. In contrast, a patient who lives far from the hospital might be scheduled for interval examinations once a pattern of recurrence has been established. Email or phone contact between health care team and patients is helpful in monitoring the clinical situation between surgeries.[36]

In our patient, elective outpatient flexible bronchoscopy was scheduled for 30 days after the procedure to reassess airway patency and consider the need for additional therapies in case of papilloma recurrence. No obstruction was found, but residual "velvety"-like lesions suggested recurrence (Figure 1-5). No intervention was performed at that time. At 4 months after the initial procedure, however, recurrent obstruction caused symptoms that required intervention. We elected to repeat rigid bronchoscopy, but instead of laser, we used a rigid electrocautery suction catheter with output power of 20 W, in coagulation mode, accompanied by removal of tissues using grasping forceps (see video on ExpertConsult. com) (Video I.1.2). Airway patency was satisfactorily restored (see Figure 1-5), and although the patient showed progressive recurrence on follow-up surveillance flexible bronchoscopies, a repeat rigid bronchoscopic intervention was not needed until 1 year later.

Quality Improvement

Quality of care was considered satisfactory because airway patency had been safely restored and the patient had been discharged home within 24 hours. In our weekly team meeting, we discussed whether the patient should have received adjuvant therapy for his RRP. On the basis of current evidence and the fact that the patient required fewer than four interventions per year, we decided not to prescribe immunomodulatory or antiviral medications. We initiated an antireflux strategy because a history of gastroesophageal reflux is often reported in patients with RRP.

We discussed the fact that we had not applied a validated instrument to quantify this patient's disease severity before and after bronchoscopic interventions. Although

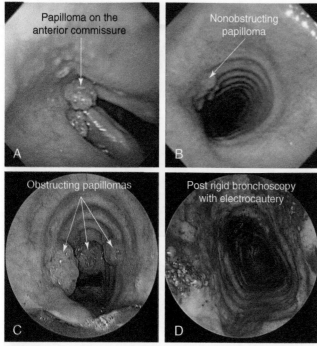

Figure 1-5 Follow-up bronchoscopy after 1 month showed **(A)** a small, nonobstructing papilloma present on the anterior commissure and **(B)** slightly raised "velvety" tracheal nodules consistent with RRP recurrence. Four months after the initial intervention, **(C)** obstructing papillomas were identified, causing worsening exertional dyspnea. **D,** Tracheal lumen after the rigid bronchoscopic intervention using an electrocautery suction catheter.

we objectively documented the extent and precise locations of the lesions, we did not officially document other parameters described in RRP staging systems (i.e., surgery-free interval, number of surgeries within a year, or functional impairment as assessed by voice, stridor, or respiratory distress and need for urgent intervention).[71] A consistent staging and severity scale is desirable for following the progression of RRP disease. Such a system would be ideally suited for tracking results of clinical trials of adjuvant therapies as well as physician-to-physician communications.

In addition, we discussed plans in case future interventions were required for this patient. Because significant recurrence of obstruction after use of the rigid electrocautery suction catheter was delayed for 1 year, we decided that this method would be repeated. Electrocautery produces high thermal energy, which creates fumes that very probably contain diffuse amounts of HPV, but we speculated that continuous and intimate contact of the suction catheter with the papilloma lesion (see video on ExpertConsult.com) (Video I.1.2) created less smoke and potentially reduced the spread of viral particles inside the airways. Although this is conjecture, we propose that studies are needed to compare laser therapy versus this electrocautery method in terms of time to disease recurrence and potential risk of transmission to the treating team. At the least, smoke evacuation policies should be the same for electrosurgery as for the use of lasers.[72]

DISCUSSION POINTS

1. List four differential diagnoses of exophytic endoluminal tracheal lesions.
   - Squamous cell carcinoma (see Figure 1-3, *A*)
   - Adenoid cystic carcinoma (see Figure 1-3, *B*)
     These two tumors are the most common primary tracheal cancers, accounting for 70% to 80% of all tracheal tumors.[9]
   - Hamartoma
   - Granulation tissue (see Figure 1-3, *F*)
     Most benign tracheal tumors are papillomas and hamartomas,[13] but in patients with a recent history of airway trauma (e.g., intubation, stent placement, rigid bronchoscopy), granulation tissue is a common cause of this type of central airway obstruction.[12]
2. Describe three indications for adjuvant therapy in recurrent respiratory papillomatosis.
   - Surgery required more frequently than 4 times a year for 2 years
   - Papillomas spreading outside of the larynx
   - Rapid recurrence of papillomas with airway compromise[67]
3. Describe the advantages and disadvantages of Nd:YAG laser therapy as compared with other laser therapies for treating this patient with RRP.
   - Advantages of Nd:YAG laser:
     - Better coagulating properties, thus minimizing the risk of excessive bleeding during resection
     - May reduce the risk for recurrence through deeper tissue effects and potential destruction of the HPV-infected basal cell layer of the mucosa[30,35]
     - May lower risk of HPV transmission to adjoining healthy tissue or operators because less smoke is generated by noncontact mode photocoagulation and effective suctioning during Nd:YAG laser surgery[30]
   - Disadvantages of Nd:YAG laser:
     - Deeper tissue effects, which may result in injury of the normal airway wall or even airway perforation and massive bleeding
     - Less precise than the CO_2 laser, thus potentially causing thermal injury to adjacent normal airway wall mucosa
     - May cause more carbonization or vaporization than the KTP laser, thus potentially altering histology in case biopsies are necessary for ruling out malignant transformation

Expert Commentary

provided by Craig S. Derkay, MD, FACS, FAAP, and Cristina Baldassari, MD

In our commentary on this review of the diagnosis and management of tracheal papillomatosis, we would like to highlight several additional points. The authors should take care in generalizing data from the urology literature on genital papillomas to recurrent respiratory papilloma (RRP). Furthermore, it is important to distinguish between juvenile-onset (JORRP) and adult-onset (AORRP) RRP. Most of the literature presented here focuses on JORRP, which typically is characterized by more aggressive disease. Children diagnosed at a young age and infected with HPV 11 typically experience more severe disease.[16]

In addition to progressive dyspnea, the patient in this case complained of hoarseness on presentation. He has obvious papilloma involving his larynx at the anterior commissure. Although the authors comment that bronchoscopy will not improve the patient's hoarseness, they fail to mention a treatment strategy for the laryngeal disease. Laryngeal papillomatosis requires excision. Caring for RRP patients often requires a multidisciplinary approach. In our opinion, it would have been prudent to attain an otolaryngology consult before taking the patient to the operating room for a bronchoscopy. The otolaryngologist might have chosen to excise the laryngeal lesions using a microdebrider through a microlaryngoscope with the patient under the same anesthesia.

RRP is a highly variable disease in terms of severity and progression. The patient and his partner, therefore, should be provided with further information regarding prognosis and disease course. Some patients, for example, will experience spontaneous remission, but others will suffer from aggressive papillomatosis and will require frequent surgical procedures. The variability inherent in RRP dictates the need for a standardized staging system that allows providers to effectively monitor a patient's course and response to therapy. The Derkay/Coltrera staging system (Figures 1-6 and 1-7) assigns a numeric grade based on the extent of papillomatosis at specific sites along the aerodigestive tract.[71] This staging system also grades the size of the lesions and the number of subsites involved, while taking into account functional parameters such as voice quality, stridor, and urgency of intervention. Elements of this system are effective in predicting the frequency of surgical intervention. For example, patients with anatomic scores greater than 20 will likely require their next surgical procedure sooner than those with scores lower than 10.[73]

We would like to emphasize the importance of obtaining a specimen for pathologic analysis each time the case patient has an operative intervention. This recommendation is specific to the case patient's human immunodeficiency virus (HIV) diagnosis and evidence of disease spread outside of the larynx. In children with stable RRP, we routinely send specimens to pathology yearly unless the established growth pattern has changed. However, the immunosuppression associated with HIV and acquired immunodeficiency syndrome (AIDS) has been linked to increased rates of respiratory malignancies.[74] Furthermore, malignant degeneration is more common in papillomas that have spread outside of the larynx.

The current standard of care for RRP is surgical therapy with a goal of complete removal of papilloma and preservation of normal structures. We prefer to treat patients with laryngeal RRP with the microdebrider. Advantages of this technique include decreased tissue edema, improved voice outcomes, less patient

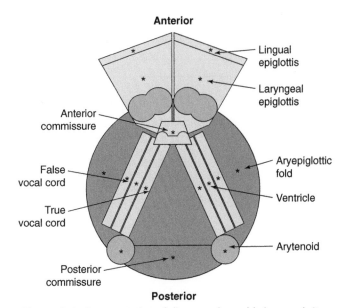

Figure 1-6 Representation of diagram of scorable laryngeal sites.

discomfort, faster operating time, and elimination of the risk of aerosolizing papilloma. Distal tracheal papillomatosis, however, can be challenging to access with the microdebrider in the absence of an indwelling tracheostomy tube.

The CO_2 laser is frequently used to treat patients with laryngeal papilloma using a microspot manipulator through the operating microscope. Until recently, this technique has had limited utility for distal tracheal disease, but new CO_2 laser probes are allowing it to be utilized through a flexible or rigid bronchoscope, thus providing access for its use in the distal airway. In patients with tracheal papillomatosis, therefore, our preferred management strategy is to use the Omni-Guide CO_2 laser (OmniGuide, Cambridge, Mass) delivered through a ventilating bronchoscope. In their review, the authors refer to a 15-year-old survey study conducted by the senior author regarding anesthesia techniques, wherein the preferred method at the time was use of a laser-safe endotracheal tube. Today, with the advent of the microdebrider, apneic and spontaneous ventilation techniques are preferred.

It is important to remember that RRP is a disease that is often characterized by relentless recurrence, no matter the treatment strategy. In this patient, the authors elected to utilize electrocautery during subsequent interventions, noting a slight decrease in surgical intervals once cautery was utilized. Any conclusions that electrocautery is superior to Nd:YAG in the treatment of tracheal papillomatosis, however, would be premature and are not yet justified by randomized studies.

Regardless of treatment methods used, care should be taken in applying treatment strategies that can result in thermal damage to surrounding tissues. Thermal damage can lead to significant complications such as granulation tissue overgrowth, scarring, and stenosis. Endobronchial electrocautery has been shown to result in mucosal ulceration and inflammation to

A Clinical Score

DATE OF SURGERY_____ SURGEON _____

INSTITUTION _____

1. Describe the patient's voice today:
   normal ___(0), abnormal ___(1), aphonic ___(2)
2. Describe the patient's stridor today:
   absent ___(0), present with activity ___(1), present at rest ___(2)
3. Describe the urgency of today's intervention:
   scheduled ___(0), elective ___(1), urgent ___(2), emergent ___(3)
4. Describe today's level of respiratory distress:
   none ___(0), mild ___(1), moderate ___(2), severe ___(3), extreme ___(4)
   Total score for Questions 1 through 4 = _____

B Anatomical Score

For each site, score as: 0 = none, 1 = surface lesion, 2 = raised lesion, 3 = bulky lesion

LARYNX:
    Epiglottis: Lingual surface ___   Laryngeal surface ___
    Aryepiglottic folds: Right ___ Left ___
    False vocal cords: Right ___ Left ___
    True vocal cords: Right ___ Left ___
    Arytenoids: Right ___ Left ___
    Anterior commissure _____
    Posterior commissure _____
    Subglottis _____
TRACHEA:
    Upper one-third _____
    Middle one-third _____
    Lower one-third _____
    Bronchi: Right ___ Left ___
Tracheotomy stoma _____
OTHER:
    Nose _____
    Palate _____
    Pharynx _____
    Esophagus _____
    Lungs _____
    Other _____   Total Score for Anatomical _____

C **Total Score**

Total Anatomical Score plus Total Clinical Score.

Figure 1-7 Laryngoscopic and clinical assessment scale for recurrent respiratory papillomatosis (RRP).

the depth of the perichondral spaces.[75] These changes can evolve into loss of chondrocyte viability and stenosis, especially if electrocautery is performed circumferentially. The authors took great care to remove papillomas without causing circumferential damage.

A surveillance bronchoscopy performed in the case patient 1 month after the initial intervention revealed recurrence. The authors chose to defer further intervention until the patient became symptomatic. Indeed, because of the variability of the RRP disease course, no standardized approach is available for follow-up in these patients. Our practice involves a 1 month follow-up procedure to assess for recurrence. We would plan to intervene at this time if evidence of disease was

noted. If disease was mild and nonobstructive at the 1 month bronchoscopy, as noted in the case patient, we would elect to lengthen the time to the next intervention. If no disease was noted at the next procedure, we would follow the patient clinically. CT scanning of the chest in a patient with disease in the trachea can be utilized at baseline and repeated at 6 to 12 month intervals to look for spread of disease into the lungs.

Systemic adjuvant therapy should be considered in patients with distal spread of papillomas. Although cidofovir is used most frequently for aggressive laryngeal disease, a recent Cochrane review did not support its routine use. Therefore pegylated interferon might be a reasonable choice for this patient.

REFERENCES

1. Stoller JK. Spirometry: a key diagnostic test in pulmonary medicine. *Cleveland Clin J Med.* 1992;59:75-78.
2. Miller RD, Hyatt RE. Obstructing lesions of the larynx and trachea: clinical and physiologic characteristics. *Mayo Clin Proc.* 1969;44:145-161.
3. Al-Bazzaz F, Grillo H, Kazemi H. Response to exercise in upper airway obstruction. *Am Rev Respir Dis.* 1975;111:631-640.
4. Modrykamien AM, Gudavalli R, McCarthy K, et al. Detection of upper airway obstruction with spirometry results and the flow-volume loop: a comparison of quantitative and visual inspection criteria. *Respir Care.* 2009;54:474-479.
5. Watson MA, King CS, Holley AB, et al. Clinical and lung-function variables associated with vocal cord dysfunction. *Respir Care.* 2009;54:467-473.
6. Enright PL, Hodgkin JE. Pulmonary function tests. In: George G, Burton JE, Hodgkin J, Ward J, eds. *Respiratory Care: A Guide to Clinical Practice.* 4th ed. Philadelphia: Lippincott; 1997:226-238.
7. Owens GR, Murphy DM. Spirometric diagnosis of upper airway obstruction. *Arch Intern Med.* 1983;143:1331-1334.
8. Faber LP, Warren WH. Benign and malignant tumors of the trachea. In: Shields TW, LoCicero J III, Ponn RB, eds. *General Thoracic Surgery.* 5th ed. Philadelphia: Lippincott Williams & Wilkins; 1999:899-917.
9. Regnard JF, Fourquier P, Levasseur P. Results and prognostic factors in resections of primary tracheal tumors: a multicenter retrospective study. The French Society of Cardiovascular Surgery. *J Thorac Cardiovasc Surg.* 1996;11:808-813.
10. Sharpe DA, Moghissi K. Tracheal resection and reconstruction: a review of 82 patients. *Eur J Cardiothorac Surg.* 1996;10:1040-1045.
11. Kwong JS, Muller NL, Miller RR. Diseases of the trachea and main-stem bronchi: correlation of CT with pathologic findings. *Radiographics.* 1992;12:645-657.
12. Ernst A, Feller-Kopman D, Becker HD, et al. Central airway obstruction. *Am J Respir Crit Care Med.* 2004;169:1278-1297.
13. Shah H, Garbe L, Nussbaum E, et al. Benign tumours of the tracheobronchial tree: endoscopic characteristics and role of laser resection. *Chest.* 1995;107:1744-1751.
14. Perelman MI, Koroleva NS. Primary tumors of the trachea. In: Grillo HC, Eschapasse H, eds. *International Trends in General Thoracic Surgery.* Vol 2. Philadelphia: Saunders; 1987:91-110.
15. Mounts P, Shah KV. Respiratory papillomatosis: etiological relation to genital tract papillomaviruses. *Prog Med Virol.* 1984;29:90-114.
16. Derkay CS, Wiatrak B. Recurrent respiratory papillomatosis: a review. *Laryngoscope.* 2008;118:1236-1247.
17. Shykhon M, Kuo M, Pearman K. Recurrent respiratory papillomatosis. *Clin Otolaryngol Allied Sci.* 2002;27:237-243.
18. Horberg MA, Hurley LB, Klein DB, et al. Surgical outcomes in human immunodeficiency virus-infected patients in the era of highly active antiretroviral therapy. *Arch Surg.* 2006;141:1238-1245.
19. Tarhan S, Moffitt EA, Sessler AD, et al. Risk of anesthesia and surgery in patients with chronic bronchitis and chronic obstructive pulmonary disease. *Surgery.* 1973;74:720-726.
20. Stein M, Cassara EL. Preoperative pulmonary evaluation and therapy for surgery patients. *JAMA.* 1970;211:787-790.
21. Global Initiative for Chronic Obstructive Pulmonary Disease. Executive summary: global strategy for the diagnosis, management, and prevention of COPD, 2006. www.goldcopd.com. Accessed September 5, 2010.
22. Mill J, Edwards N, Jackson R, et al. Stigmatization as a social control mechanism for persons living with HIV and AIDS. *Qual Health Res.* 2010;20:1469-1483.
23. Taylor B. HIV, stigma and health: integration of theoretical concepts and the lived experiences of individuals. *J Adv Nurs.* 2001;35:792-798.
24. Wrubel J, Stumbo S, Johnson MO. Male same sex couple dynamics and received social support for HIV medication adherence. *J Soc Pers Relat.* 2010;27:553-572.
25. Haas SM. Social support as relationship maintenance in gay male couples coping with HIV or AIDS. *J Soc Pers Relat.* 2002;19:87-111.
26. Bolliger CT. Laser bronchoscopy, electrosurgery, APC and microdebrider. In: Beamis JF Jr, Mathur P, Mehta AC, eds. Interventional Pulmonary Medicine. *Lung Biology in Health and Disease Series.* 2nd ed. Vol 230. New York: Informa; 2010:9-24.
27. Bollag W, Peck R, Frey JR. Inhibition of proliferation by retinoids, cytokines and their combination in four human transformed epithelial cell lines. *Cancer Lett.* 1992;62:167-172.
28. Lo J, Abbara S, Shturman L, et al. Increased prevalence of subclinical coronary atherosclerosis detected by coronary computed tomography angiography in HIV-infected men. *AIDS.* 2010;24:243-253.
29. Carr A, Grund B, Neuhaus J, et al. Asymptomatic myocardial ischaemia in HIV-infected adults. *AIDS.* 2008;22:257-267.
30. Janda P, Leunig A, Sroka R, et al. Preliminary report of endolaryngeal and endotracheal laser surgery of juvenile-onset recurrent respiratory papillomatosis by Nd:YAG laser and a new fiber guidance instrument. *Otolaryngol Head Neck Surg.* 2004;131:44-49.
31. Hirano T, Konaka C, Okada S, et al. Endoscopic diagnosis and treatment of a case of respiratory papillomatosis. *Diagn Ther Endosc.* 1997;3:183-187.
32. Komatsu T, Takahashi Y. Tracheal papilloma with exceptionally longer interval of recurrence. *Asian J Surg.* 2007;30:88-90.
33. Long YT, Sani A. Recurrent respiratory papillomatosis. *Asian J Surg.* 2003;26:112-116.
34. Hunt JM, Pierce RJ. Tracheal papillomatosis treated with Nd-Yag laser resection. *Aust N Z J Med.* 1988;18:781-784.
35. Schneede P, Meyer T, Ziller F, et al. Clinical and viral clearance of human papillomavirus (HPV)-associated genital lesions by Nd:YAG laser treatment. *Med Laser Appl.* 2000;16:38-42.
36. RRP Task Force. Practice guidelines for management of children with RRP. http://www.rrpf.org/RRPTaskForceGuidelines.html. Accessed September 5, 2010.
37. Schraff S, Derkay CS, Burke B, et al. American Society of Pediatric Otolaryngology members' experience with recurrent respiratory papillomatosis and the use of adjuvant therapy. *Arch Otolaryngol Head Neck Surg.* 2004;130:1039-1042.
38. Dedo HH, Yu KC. CO_2 laser treatment in 244 patients with respiratory papillomatosis. *Laryngoscope.* 2001;111:1639-1644.
39. Kashima HK, Kessis T, Mounts P, et al. Polymerase chain reaction identification of human papillomavirus DNA in CO_2 laser plume from recurrent respiratory papillomatosis. *Otolaryngol Head Neck Surg.* 1991;104:191-195.
40. Patel RS, Mackenzie K. Powered laryngeal shavers and laryngeal papillomatosis: a preliminary report. *Clin Otolaryngol.* 2000;25:358-360.
41. Pasquale K, Wiatrak B, Woolley A, et al. Microdebrider versus CO_2 laser removal of recurrent respiratory papillomas: a prospective analysis. *Laryngoscope.* 2003;113:139-143.
42. Mortensen M, Woo P. An underreported complication of laryngeal microdebrider: vocal fold web and granuloma: a case report. *Laryngoscope.* 2009;119:1848-1850.
43. Zeitels SM, Akst LM, Burns JA, et al. Office-based 532-nanometer pulsed KTP laser treatment of glottal papillomatosis and dysplasia. *Ann Otol Rhinol Laryngol.* 2006;115:679-685.
44. Valdez TA, McMillan K, Shapshay SM. A new treatment of vocal cord papilloma-585nm pulsed dye. *Otolaryngol Head Neck Surg.* 2001;124:421-425.
45. McMillan K, Shapshay SM, McGilligan JA, et al. A 585-nanometer pulsed dye laser treatment of laryngeal papillomas: preliminary report. *Laryngoscope.* 1998;108:968-972.
46. Rees CJ, Halum SL, Wijewickrama RC, et al. Patient tolerance of in-office pulsed dye laser treatments to the upper aerodigestive tract. *Otolaryngol Head Neck Surg.* 2006;134:1023-1027.
47. Bergler W, Honig M, Gotte K, et al. Treatment of recurrent respiratory papillomatosis with argon plasma coagulation. *J Laryngol Otol.* 1997;111:381-384.
48. Bondaryev A, Makris D, Breen DP, et al. Airway stenting for severe endobronchial papillomatosis. *Respiration.* 2009;77:455-458.
49. Cole RR, Myer CM, Cotton RT. Tracheostomy in children with recurrent respiratory papillomatosis. *Head Neck.* 1989;11:226-230.
50. Shykhon M, Kuo M, Pearman K. Recurrent respiratory papillomatosis. *Clin Otolaryngol Allied Sci.* 2002;27:237-243.
51. Bell R, Hong WK, Itril M, et al. The use of cis-retinoic acid in recurrent respiratory papillomatosis of the larynx: a randomized pilot study. *Am J Otolaryngol.* 1988;9:161-164.
52. Lippman SM, Donovan DT, Frankenthaler RA, et al. 13-Cis-retionic acid plus interferon-alpha 2a in recurrent respiratory papillomatosis. *J Natl Cancer Inst.* 1994;86:859-861.

53. Shikowitz MJ, Abramson AL, Steinberg BM, et al. Clinical trial of photodynamic therapy with meso-tetra (hydroxyphenyl) chlorine for respiratory papillomatosis. *Arch Otolaryngol Head Neck Surg.* 2005;131:99-105.

54. Snoeck R, Wellens W, Desloovere C, et al. Treatment of severe laryngeal papillomatosis with intralesional injections of cidofovir [(S)-1-(3-hydroxy-2-phosphonylmethoxypropyl)cytosine]. *J Med Virol.* 1998;54:219-225.

55. Co J, Woo P. Serial office-based intralesional injection of cidofovir in adult-onset recurrent respiratory papillomatosis. *Ann Otol Rhinol Laryngol.* 2004;113:859-862.

56. Derkay C. Cidofovir for recurrent respiratory papillomatosis (RRP): a re-assessment of risks. RRP Task Force Consensus Statement on Cidofovir. *Int J Pediatr Otolaryngol.* 2005;69:1465-1467.

57. McMurray JS, Connor N, Ford CN. Cidofovir efficacy in recurrent respiratory papillomatosis: a randomized, double-blind, placebo-controlled study. *Ann Otol Rhinol Laryngol.* 2008;117:477-483.

58. Harcourt JP, Worley G, Leighton SE. Cimetidine treatment for recurrent respiratory papillomatosis. *Int J Pediatr Otorhinolaryngol.* 1999;51:109-113.

59. Bostrom B, Sidman J, Marker S, et al. Gefitinib therapy for life-threatening laryngeal papillomatosis. *Arch Otolaryngol Head Neck Surg.* 2005;131:64-67.

60. Maturo S, Hartnick CJ. Use of 532-nm pulsed potassium titanyl phosphate laser and adjuvant intralesional bevacizumab for aggressive respiratory papillomatosis in children: initial experience. *Arch Otolaryngol Head Neck Surg.* 2010;136:561-565.

61. Zeitels SM, Lopez-Guerra G, Burns JA, et al. Microlaryngoscopic and office-based injection of bevacizumab (Avastin) to enhance 532-nm pulsed KTP laser treatment of glottal papillomatosis. *Ann Otol Rhinol Laryngol Suppl.* 2009;201:1-13.

62. Lindman JP, Lewis LS, Accortt N, et al. Use of the Pediatric Quality of Life Inventory to assess the health-related quality of life in children with recurrent respiratory papillomatosis. *Ann Otol Rhinol Laryngol.* 2005;114:499-503.

63. Baggish MS, Polesz BJ, Joret D, et al. Presence of human immuno-deficiency virus DNA in laser smoke. *Lasers Surg Med.* 1991;11:197-203.

64. Sawchuk WS, Weber PJ, Lowy DR, et al. Infectious papillomavirus in the vapor of warts treated with carbon dioxide laser or electrocoagulation: detection and protection. *J Am Acad Dermatol.* 1989;21:41-49.

65. Gloster H, Roenigk R. Risk of acquiring human papillomavirus from the plume produced by the carbon dioxide laser in the treatment of warts. *J Am Acad Dermatol.* 1995;32:436-441.

66. Biggins J, Renfree S. The hazards of surgical smoke: not to be sniffed at! *Br J Perioper Nurs.* 2002;12:136-138.

67. Derkay CS. Task force on recurrent respiratory papillomatosis. *Arch Otolaryngol Head Neck Surg.* 1995;121:1386-1391.

68. Alp E, Bijl D, Bleichrodt RP, et al. Surgical smoke and infection control. *J Hosp Infect.* 2006;62:1-5.

69. International RRP ISA Center. http://www.rrpwebsite.org. Accessed September 5, 2010.

70. Bauer TL, Steiner KV. Virtual bronchoscopy: clinical applications and limitations. *Surg Oncol Clin North Am.* 2007;16:323-328.

71. Derkay CS, Malis DF, Zalzal G, et al. A staging system for assessing severity of disease and response to therapy in recurrent respiratory papillomatosis. *Laryngoscope.* 1998;108:935-937.

72. Ulmer BC. The hazards of surgical smoke. *AORN J.* 2008;87:721-734.

73. Derkay CS, Hester RP, Burke B, et al. Analysis of a staging assessment system for prediction of surgical interval in recurrent respiratory papillomatosis. *Int J Pediatr Otorhinolaryngol.* 2004;68:1493-1498.

74. Frisch M, Biggar RJ, Engels EA, et al. Association of cancer with AIDS-related immunosuppression in adults. *JAMA.* 2001;285:1736-1745.

75. Tremblay A, Marquette CH. Endobronchial electrocautery and argon plasma coagulation: a practical approach. *Can Respir J.* 2004;11:305-310.

Chapter 2

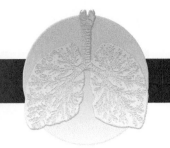

Endoscopic Therapy of Endobronchial Typical Carcinoid

This chapter emphasizes the following elements of the Four Box Approach: risk-benefit analysis and therapeutic alternatives, and follow-up tests, visits, and procedures.

CASE DESCRIPTION

A 47-year-old woman was hospitalized at an outside institution for hemoptysis and left lower lobe pneumonia. She had a history of wheezing for several months, which was unresponsive to bronchodilators and inhaled corticosteroids. Spirometry was normal. Three weeks before admission, she developed cough and fever. When she developed hemoptysis (half a cup of bright red blood within several hours), she presented to the emergency department. Vital signs showed a temperature of 38.5° C, heart rate of 120 bpm, respiratory rate of 28/min, and blood pressure of 150/75. She had no pain. Wheezing was noted on auscultation of the left hemithorax, and the patient had diminished air entry at the left base. The rest of the examination was unremarkable. Laboratory tests were normal except for a white blood cell count of 24,000/mm³. Chest radiography showed left lower lobe opacification (Figure 2-1, *A*). Computed tomography (CT) scan revealed left lower lobe atelectasis and a distal left main bronchial mass completely obstructing the left lower lobe bronchus and partially obstructing the entrance to the left upper lobe (see Figure 2-1, *B*). The patient was started on broad-spectrum antibiotics for pneumonia. Flexible bronchoscopy showed an exophytic endoluminal hypervascular distal left main bronchial lesion. Endobronchial biopsies revealed typical carcinoid.*

After bronchoscopy, hemoptysis increased, prompting transfer to our institution for palliation and bronchoscopic resection of the endobronchial tumor. Rigid bronchoscopy under general anesthesia confirmed the flexible bronchoscopic findings (see Figure 2-1). Neodymium-doped yttrium aluminium garnet (Nd:YAG) laser–assisted resection was performed to restore airway patency (Figure 2-2).

---

*World Health Organization (WHO) diagnostic criteria for typical carcinoid include a tumor with carcinoid morphology and <2 mitoses/2 mm² (10 high-power fields [HPFs]), lacking necrosis, and tumor 0.5 cm or larger. An atypical carcinoid is defined as a tumor with carcinoid morphology with 2 to 10 mitoses/2 mm² and/or necrosis (often punctate).

†Carcinoid syndrome is caused by systemic release of vasoactive substances. Acute symptoms include cutaneous flushing, diarrhea, and bronchospasm (10% to 20 % of patients with carcinoid syndrome); long-term sequelae of prolonged elevated hormone levels include venous telangiectasias, right-side predominant valvular heart disease, and fibrosis in the retroperitoneum and other sites.

DISCUSSION POINTS

1. Describe two strategies to decrease the risk of bleeding from bronchoscopic biopsy of this tumor.
2. Discuss the role of imaging studies in diagnosis and staging of carcinoid tumors.
3. List three open surgical treatment alternatives for endobronchial carcinoid.
4. Describe how tumor histology and morphology affect treatment decisions for carcinoid tumors.

CASE RESOLUTION

Initial Evaluations

Physical Examination, Complementary Tests, and Functional Status Assessment

Symptoms in patients with bronchial carcinoid depend on the tumor size, site, and growth pattern. For instance, a small peripheral carcinoid may be an incidental finding, and a large central tumor may result in symptoms similar to those found in our patient: cough, hemoptysis (due to its hypervascularity), and obstructive pneumonia. Some patients may also have shortness of breath.[1] The diagnosis is often delayed, and patients may receive several courses of antibiotics, bronchodilators, or inhaled corticosteroids to treat recurrent pneumonia or suspected asthma. In one study, 14% of patients had been treated for asthma for up to 3 years before the tumor was discovered.[2] The wheezing noted in our patient was localized to the left hemithorax, reflecting focal airway obstruction, not bronchoconstriction. In fact, diffuse wheezing is rare in patients with carcinoids, regardless of tumor location, because only 1% to 5% of patients exhibit hormone-related symptoms such as carcinoid syndrome.† In part, this reflects the low incidence of hepatic metastases—2% and 5%, respectively—for typical and atypical carcinoids.[2,3] In the setting of liver metastasis, however, more than 80% of patients have symptoms of carcinoid syndrome.[1] Bronchial and other extraintestinal carcinoids, whose bioactive products are not immediately cleared by the liver, may cause the syndrome in the absence of liver metastasis because of their direct access to the systemic circulation. However, bronchial carcinoids have low serotonin content because they often lack aromatic amino acid decarboxylase and cannot produce serotonin and its metabolites; they only occasionally secrete bioactive amines. Elevated plasma or urinary secretory product levels such as 5'-hydroxyindoleacetic acid (5'-HIAA) thus are rarely detected. Elevation of

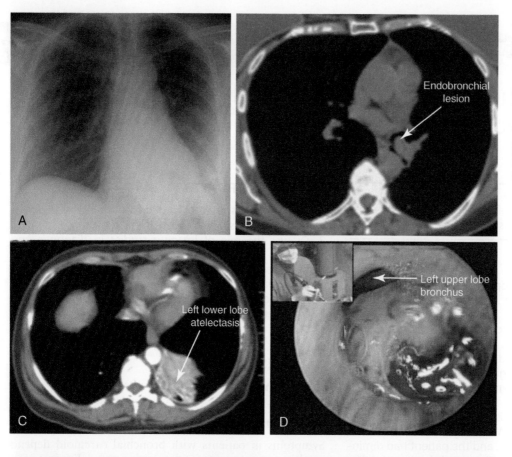

Figure 2-1 A, Preoperative chest radiograph shows left lower lobe opacification. **B,** Computed tomography (CT) scan reveals a distal left main bronchial mass completely obstructing the left lower lobe bronchus and partially obstructing the entrance to the left upper lobe. **C,** Left lower lobe atelectasis resulting from complete endobronchial obstruction. **D,** Hypervascular endobronchial lesion in the distal left main bronchus.

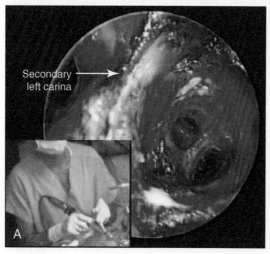

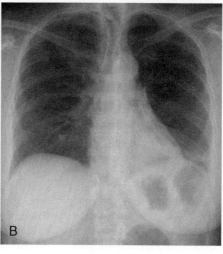

Figure 2-2 A, Rigid bronchoscopic view immediately after laser resection: the segments in the left lower lobe are patent. **B,** Chest radiograph after resection shows improved aeration in the left lower lobe.

plasma chromogranin A* is a relatively sensitive (≈75%) marker of bronchopulmonary carcinoids, but elevated levels are also seen in approximately 60% of patients with small cell carcinoma, and false-positive elevations can occur in renal impairment, in atrophic gastritis, and during proton pump inhibitor therapy.[4] Measurement of its levels is considered useful only in following disease activity in the setting of advanced or metastatic carcinoid.[5] No such serologic or urinary testing was performed in our patient before bronchoscopic intervention was provided.

With regard to radiographic studies, when the tumor is centrally located, as in our patient, bronchial obstruction may occur and atelectasis is noted (see Figure 2-1, C). Compared with chest x-ray, CT provides better resolution of tumor extent and location, as well as the presence or absence of mediastinal lymphadenopathy. High-resolution CT allows characterization of centrally located carcinoids, which may be purely intraluminal,

---

*Chromogranins (designated as A, B, and C) are proteins that are stored and released with peptides and amines in a variety of neuroendocrine tissues.

exclusively extraluminal, or, more frequently, a mixture of intraluminal and extraluminal components (the "iceberg" lesion). In the setting of post obstructive pneumonia, a clear distinction between intraluminal and extraluminal extension can be properly made only after post obstructive debris and atelectasis have been removed.[6] Tumor morphology impacts management because bronchoscopic treatments alone are considered by some investigators to be acceptable therapeutic alternatives for purely intraluminal typical carcinoids.[6] Chest CT scan should be performed as part of nodal staging for carcinoid tumors. Atypical carcinoids have a higher recurrence rate and present more often with hilar or mediastinal nodal metastases (20% to 60% vs. 4% to 27%), when compared with typical carcinoids.[1] This patient had no evidence of mediastinal or hilar lymphadenopathy on CT scan; because atelectasis and pneumonia were present, it was unclear whether the tumor had an extraluminal component (e.g., mixed obstruction, iceberg lesion).

The bronchoscopic appearance of this patient's carcinoid is classic: a pink to red vascular mass attached to the bronchus by a broad base. In one study, 41% of patients presented with evidence of bronchial obstruction.[3] These lesions occasionally can create a ball-valve effect (see video on ExpertConsult.com) (Video I.2.1). The hypervascular pattern has raised concern for bleeding following bronchoscopic biopsy. Some authors report bleeding in a quarter to two thirds of their patients, and some advise against biopsy when carcinoid is suspected.[7-9] In a review of 587 biopsies by flexible and rigid bronchoscopy, significant hemorrhage was seen in 15 (2.6%) patients, but 11 (1.9%) of these patients did not require transfusion or emergency surgery. In four patients (0.7%), emergency thoracotomy was necessary to address the problem of massive uncontrollable hemorrhage.[10] Other authors showed that biopsy is safe, significantly increases the diagnostic yield, and is not associated with significant hemorrhage.[3,11] It is wise to have electrocautery, argon plasma coagulation, or a laser readily available to control spontaneous or post biopsy hemorrhage if necessary (see video on ExpertConsult. com) (Video I.2.2).

Comorbidities

This patient had no signs or symptoms suggesting hormone-related disorders caused by carcinoid, such as Cushing's syndrome, acromegaly, or typical or atypical carcinoid syndrome.*

Support System

The patient lived with her husband, who was very supportive. Both were willing to proceed with treatment for curative intent.

Patient Preferences and Expectations

The patient had expressed fears of having lung cancer. She wanted clarification in terms of her diagnosis, prognosis, and follow-up after treatment. It was explained to her that bronchial carcinoid tumors are rare lung malignancies that rarely spread outside the chest.*[12,13] We were aware of data showing that the incidence of distant metastases at diagnosis for bronchopulmonary carcinoids is 5.5%[14]; that overall, 27.5% of bronchopulmonary carcinoids exhibit invasive growth or metastatic spread; and that the overall 5-year survival rate is 73.5%. Therefore we did not use the term *benign tumor* in our conversation with the patient.[12] Typical and atypical carcinoids, however, have different biologic behaviors and prognoses, causing them to be considered and reported as different tumors.[2] Typical carcinoids, as seen in this patient, usually have a good prognosis, with 5 year survival of 87% to 89%. Distant metastases from typical carcinoids may occur in approximately 10% of patients, even many years after radical resection of the primary tumor. Prolonged 10 year follow-up is therefore recommended. Atypical carcinoids are associated with 5 year survival of 44% to 78%.[1]

Procedural Strategies

Indications

In addition to being the procedure of choice to obtain a preoperative histologic diagnosis, bronchoscopy can be therapeutic in some cases when a polypoid exophytic tumor is entirely intraluminal. However, endobronchial resection with Nd:YAG laser is not considered curative for the vast majority of patients with central lesions, because most tumors extend into or through the wall of the bronchus. Bronchoscopic resection may be considered in the following clinical scenarios:

1. To palliate central airway obstruction in patients who are poor surgical candidates (Figure 2-3).[15] Our patient, although considered operable (normal spirometry and no comorbidities), was not a good candidate for open surgery at the time of admission, given her ongoing sepsis from post obstructive pneumonia.
2. To guide open surgical procedures after laser bronchoscopic removal of an obstructing lesion.[16] Investigators report that lung-preserving resections are facilitated by preoperative laser treatment in 10% to 12% of patients with central obstructing carcinoids. Treatment of airway obstruction before surgery allows the operator to estimate the extent of bronchoplastic surgery.[16,17]
3. As a reasonable alternative to immediate surgical resection in patients who present with an exophytic intraluminal tumor, good visualization of the distal tumor margin, and no evidence of bronchial wall involvement or suspicious lymphadenopathy by high-resolution CT. Close post-treatment follow-up is an integral component of such treatment.[6]

Contraindications

No contraindications to rigid bronchoscopy are known.

---

*Disorientation, anxiety, tremor, periorbital edema, lacrimation, salivation, hypotension, tachycardia, diarrhea, dyspnea, asthma, and edema.

*Bronchial carcinoids account for approximately 1% to 2% of all pulmonary malignancies in adults and in approximately 20% to 30% of all carcinoid tumors.

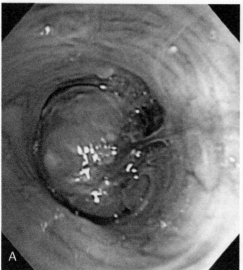
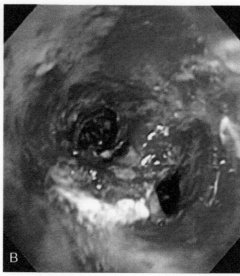

Figure 2-3 A, Right middle lobe typical carcinoid in a nonoperable elderly patient with significant cardiac comorbidities. **B,** Lateral and medial segments of the middle lobe bronchus are patent immediately after neodymium-doped yttrium aluminum garnet (Nd:YAG) laser–assisted bronchoscopic resection, with subsequent recurrence on follow-up bronchoscopy.

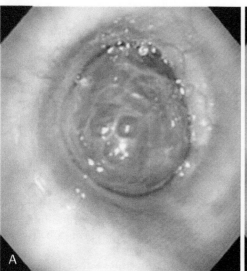
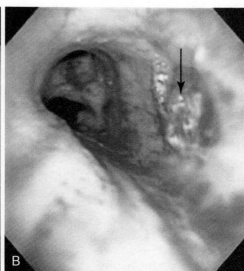

Figure 2-4 A, Typical bronchial carcinoid completely obstructing the mid-left mainstem bronchus. **B,** After laser resection, the base of implantation is seen extending for 1 cm along the medial wall of the left main bronchus *(arrow)*. Because this patient's high-resolution computed tomography (HRCT) scan showed no extraluminal disease and distal airways were patent, this patient was referred for a bronchoplastic intervention.

Expected Results

Bronchoscopic resection alone may provide prolonged recurrence-free survival for highly selected patients with a purely exophytic endoluminal bronchial carcinoid.[6,18-21] These patients present with a polypoid (exophytic) intraluminal tumor, good visualization of the distal tumor margin (usually less than 2 cm in extent), and no evidence of bronchial wall involvement or suspicious lymphadenopathy by high-resolution CT. In the largest series of 72 patients treated with this approach (57 typical and 15 atypical carcinoids), initial bronchoscopic management resulted in complete tumor eradication in 33 patients (46%). Surgery was required in 37 patients (including 11 of the 15 with atypical carcinoids)—2 for delayed recurrence at 9 and 10 years. At a median follow-up of 65 months, 66 patients (92%) remained alive, and only 1 of the deaths was tumor related.[6]

Team Experience

Rigid bronchoscopy with Nd:YAG laser resection is frequently performed in our referral center by a team of doctors and nurses experienced in managing critical central airway obstruction and hemoptysis. The goal of the operating team when this type of laser is used should be to remove unwanted tissue (tumor) with adequate hemostasis and minimum destruction of adjacent healthy tissue. Accurate removal of diseased tissue depends on the surgeon's ability to visualize tissues and feel and control the shape and size of target tissues in three dimensions. Thus experience is important because complete and clear visualization of the treated area, ensuring hemostasis and minimization of adjacent laser-induced thermal injury, requires skillful operation of the rigid bronchoscope and knowledge of laser physics and laser-tissue interaction. For example, in a patient with mid-left mainstem bronchial carcinoid (Figure 2-4), the goal is precise

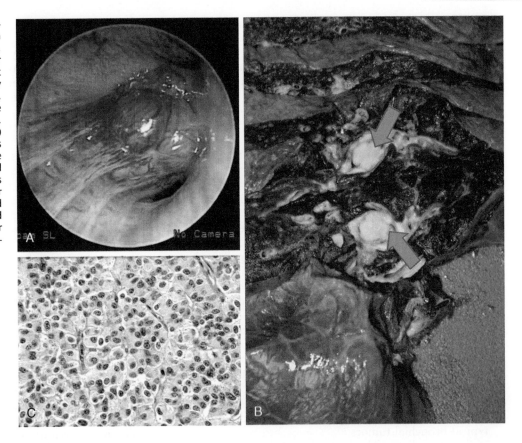

Figure 2-5 A, A polypoid wide-based hypervascular lesion in the distal bronchus intermedius, causing obstruction of the lower lobe bronchus from a different patient. **B,** After bilobectomy (right middle and lower lobes), the gross appearance of the resected tumor is a pale-tan, solid mass (1.1 × 0.9 × 0.8 cm) filling the bronchus intermedius *(arrows).* **C,** Histologically, the tumor was designated a typical carcinoid: uniform tumor cells forming solid nests with round or oval nuclei and evenly dispersed granular chromatin; mitoses and necrosis are absent. The tumor cells are traversed by fine fibrovascular septa.

removal of the lesion with minimal thermal trauma to the normal adjacent mucosa. Resection may be achieved in ways other than vaporization or widespread coagulation of blood vessels. Power density should be employed in ways that avoid damaging surrounding tissues to minimize interference, with consideration for future bronchoplastic procedures. If the tumor is completely removed, some investigators have suggested applying low-power density laser energy to residual bronchial surfaces to ablate and presumably kill residual tumor cells. Deep mucosal biopsies are warranted after a complete resection to ascertain the absence of disease.

Risk-Benefit Analysis

Open surgical resection is the preferred treatment approach for patients whose overall medical condition and pulmonary reserve will tolerate it. For patients whose condition does not permit complete resection, and for exceptional cases in which the lesion is entirely intraluminal, bronchoscopic resection may be an alternative.[6] Our patient had post obstructive pneumonia, so we opted for initial bronchoscopic treatment to restore airway patency to the left lower lobe.

Therapeutic Alternatives

1. Surgical resection with complete mediastinal lymph node dissection is, in general, considered the treatment of choice for carcinoid tumor because it offers a real chance of cure. The goal is en bloc resection of the entire neoplasm (Figure 2-5) with preservation of functional pulmonary parenchyma if possible.

Attempts to preserve lung parenchyma through the use of bronchoplastic techniques (e.g., sleeve, wedge, flap resection) to avoid lobectomy, bilobectomy, or pneumonectomy are justified and safe.[22-24] Parenchyma-sparing operations based on bronchoplastic or sleeve resection do not alter the oncologic result and lead to a better quality of life.[25] These procedures are possible only in the absence of "iceberg" lesions (in which the tumor appears entirely intraluminal bronchoscopically but has a significant extraluminal component that is evident with high-resolution computed tomography [HRCT]). The following surgical principles are recommended for bronchial carcinoids:

- For an exophytic polypoid tumor of the mainstem bronchus or bronchus intermedius, a bronchotomy with wedge or sleeve resection of the bronchial wall and complete preservation of distal lung parenchyma could be performed.[26]
- Tumors with more extensive central involvement are associated with severe distal parenchymal disease (i.e., nonfunctioning lung parenchyma), and atypical carcinoids require more extensive surgery (e.g., lobectomy, pneumonectomy).
- Complete mediastinal lymph node dissection is indicated at the time of initial treatment, along with surgical resection of nodal metastasis whenever feasible. Although between 5% and 20% of typical carcinoids, and 30% to 70% of atypical carcinoids, metastasize to lymph nodes, this does not preclude a full surgical resection or cure. Mediastinoscopy is rarely performed preoperatively; this practice is

justified by some by the fact that survival and recurrence may depend more on histology than on nodal status.[27] Larger studies show however, that N0 patients have much better survival than N1-N2 patients (10-year survival rates, 87% and 50%; $P = .00005$).[17]

2. Bronchoscopic treatment with argon plasma coagulation has been reported for recurrent typical bronchial carcinoids.[28]

3. Bronchoscopic treatment with electrocautery in one prospective study completely eradicated tumor in 14 of 19 patients with intraluminal typical bronchial carcinoid (complete response rate, 73%) after a median follow-up of 29 months. Most of these patients were treated with electrocautery, but it seems that there is no difference between this and Nd:YAG laser with regard to tumor control.[18] In a small study including 28 patients with intraluminal carcinoid, followed for a median duration of 8.8 years, five bronchoscopic resections on average were required to achieve complete removal. One and 10 year survival rates were 89% (range, 84% to 93%) and 84% (range, 77% to 91%), respectively. In this study, endoluminal tumor was removed piecemeal with biopsy forceps. Electrocautery was rarely required to control hemorrhage.[29]

4. Bronchoscopic cryotherapy was found to be successful and safe in a small series of 18 isolated endoluminal typical bronchial tumors.[30]

5. Definitive radiation therapy can provide palliation of a locally unresectable primary carcinoid.[31,32]

Cost-Effectiveness

No studies have evaluated the cost-effectiveness of bronchoscopic resection versus open surgical intervention for carcinoid tumor. Bronchoscopic interventions are cheaper and probably safer than open surgical resections. This may not be the case if, during the follow-up period, surgery was eventually needed in approximately 50% of patients who underwent bronchoscopic resection, as shown in one large series.[6] Even though most surgeries were needed for atypical carcinoids, primary surgical resection is recommended by most authorities for operable patients, regardless of histology.

Informed Consent

The patient and her husband showed understanding of the indication for the procedure, expected results, alternative treatments, potential associated complications, and additional management strategies once airway patency is restored. They were in agreement to proceed with rigid bronchoscopy under general anesthesia.

Techniques and Results

Anesthesia and Perioperative Care

Biopsy or manipulation of an actively secreting bronchial carcinoid can rarely induce acute carcinoid syndrome and cardiac arrest because of massive systemic release of bioactive mediators.[33,34] When this happens, patients acutely develop flushing, diarrhea, and bronchoconstriction, which can include acidosis, severe hypertension or hypotension, tachycardia, or myocardial infarction. Although not routinely used or recommended, somatostatin analog (octreotide) can be used perioperatively to prevent carcinoid crisis at the time of resection. Octreotide should be readily available during any surgical procedure in patients with carcinoids. Preoperative administration of octreotide (300 micrograms subcutaneously) can reduce the incidence of carcinoid crisis and is done routinely for carcinoid surgery, except with bronchial carcinoids, which only rarely secrete bioactive amines.[35] During a carcinoid crisis, blood pressure should be supported by infusion of plasma, and octreotide (300 micrograms IV) given immediately. A continuous IV drip of octreotide (50 to 150 micrograms per hour) may be needed.

Instrumentation

We chose an 11 mm Efer-Dumon rigid ventilating bronchoscope (Efer, La Ciotat, France) with an Nd:YAG laser on standby for management of bleeding and for tumor coagulation and debulking.

Anatomic Dangers and Other Risks

At the level of the distal left main bronchus, the left pulmonary artery is anterior, the descending aorta is posterior, and the inferior pulmonary vein and the left atrium are medial. Laser treatment should be performed carefully in this area to avoid direct application onto the posterior and medial walls. With hypervascular tumors such as this, absorption of laser energy is high for Nd:YAG laser, deep coagulation may be poor, and airway obstruction from blood and tumor debris may cause hypoxemia. Massive hemorrhage from laser-induced perforation of the airway and vascular rupture can be virtually impossible to stop, even if a thoracic surgeon is standing by, because intrathoracic exsanguination is accompanied by very rapid cardiopulmonary decline.

Results and Procedure-Related Complications

After induction of general anesthesia with propofol and ramifentanil, the patient was intubated with an 11 mm Efer-Dumon rigid ventilating bronchoscope. Complete obstruction of the left lower lobe bronchus and partial obstruction of the left upper lobe bronchus were noted (see Figure 2-1, B). There was no visibility of the distal airways in the left lower lobe, and it appeared that the tumor was involving the secondary left carina. The tumor was at least 2 cm long and was extending into the superior segment of the left lower lobe bronchus. Nd:YAG laser resection was initiated using 30 watt power, 1 second pulses for a total of 9519 joules. Parts of the tumor were coagulated, after which forceps and the bevel edge of the rigid bronchoscope were used to remove large pieces of tumor. Saline lavage was performed to remove large amounts of pus. Eventually, all bronchial segments of the lower lobe could be visualized (see video on ExpertConsult.com) (Video I.2.3). The patient was then extubated and transferred to the postanesthesia care unit, where no complications occurred.

Long-Term Management

Outcome Assessment

The patient was discharged home 2 days later and followed up with her referring pulmonologist. With regard to her long-term outcome, it is known that slow-growing typical carcinoids have a fairly good prognosis with an approximate 5-year survival rate of 88% (range, 80% to 96%), whereas atypical carcinoid has a 5-year survival of approximately 50%. Pulmonary carcinoids generally are staged using the tumor-node-metastasis (TNM) classification system for bronchogenic lung carcinoma. Typical carcinoid tumors most commonly present as stage I tumors, although more than half of atypical carcinoids are stage II (bronchopulmonary nodal involvement) or III (mediastinal nodal involvement) at presentation. Our patient was considered to have stage I tumor because no preoperative evidence of nodal involvement was noted.

Referral

Bronchoscopic resection is not considered standard curative treatment by many clinicians because of concerns about residual tumor within or beyond the endobronchial lumen. Because of the slow-growing nature of carcinoid tumors, recurrence may take years. Until more data become available, bronchoscopic treatment is best reserved for carefully selected elderly or debilitated patients, patients who refuse open surgery, and those whose symptoms (hemoptysis, pneumonia, or severe shortness of breath) require prompt bronchoscopic control. Our patient had a tumor with a long (>2 cm) base of implantation that extended into the segmental airways. In addition, the airway wall and the secondary left carina were involved. These findings made her a poor candidate for bronchoscopic treatment alone,[18] or for subsequent bronchoplastic interventions. Because it was believed that she was a candidate for conventional lung resection, thoracic surgery consultation was requested.

Follow-up Tests and Procedures

The patient was hospitalized overnight, and intravenous antibiotics were continued. Her hemoptysis and fever resolved, and she was discharged home 2 days later. Restored airway patency and treatment of her pneumonia improved her functional status. Octreoscan and hepatic imaging were negative. Residual tumor was known to be present at the secondary left carina. Several weeks later, therefore, the patient underwent left pneumonectomy without complications.

Some experts do not perform preoperative staging studies such as somatostatin receptor scintigraphy (octreoscan) or hepatic imaging unless there is clinical suspicion for metastatic disease. Others, however, include chest and upper abdomen CT, bronchoscopy, and the octreoscan in their routine preoperative evaluation.[17] The optimal posttreatment surveillance strategy has not been defined, and no consensus has been reached on what tests should be ordered. Some authorities perform history and physical examination and chest CT annually for patients with resected typical carcinoid, and every 6 months for resected atypical carcinoids for the first 2 years, then annually. Others perform chest CT every 6 months, regardless of histology. Somatostatin receptor scintigraphy could be performed in the follow-up of patients with bronchial carcinoid if there is suspicion for metastatic disease. Similarly, measurement of serum levels of chromogranin A (CGA) can be useful in following disease activity in the setting of advanced or metastatic disease.

Despite their low malignant potential, long-term follow-up of patients with typical bronchial carcinoids is warranted because local or distant disease recurrence may occur many years after initial treatment. In one large study, follow-up evaluation ranged from 6 months to 36 years (median, 121 months), during which 8% of patients had recurrences diagnosed, most commonly in the liver (55%), followed by lung (25%), bone (20%), adrenal gland (10%), pericardium (10%), and mediastinal lymph nodes (10%). No bronchial recurrences were seen. Recurrent cancer developed preferentially in atypical carcinoids (17.9%, vs. 3.4% in typical carcinoids; $P = .0001$) and in patients with positive nodes.[17]

In cases of sole bronchoscopic resection, one strategy is to perform HRCT and flexible bronchoscopy with endobronchial ultrasonography and tissue biopsy within 6 weeks after endobronchial resection. If the patient is operable, a referral for surgery is warranted if residual disease is evident. If no residual disease is present, repeat evaluation is performed every 6 months for 2 years, and annually thereafter.[6]

Quality Improvement

We referred this patient to surgery, but we were not sure if there was a role for adjuvant therapy after complete resection of a bronchial carcinoid. No prospective trials have directly addressed the benefit of adjuvant therapy for patients with typical or atypical bronchial carcinoids. Because of their favorable long-term outcomes, even in the presence of mediastinal nodal metastases, most experts agree that adjuvant therapy is not indicated for completely resected, typical bronchial carcinoids.[17,36] Despite lack of data and uncertainty as to benefit, guidelines from the National Comprehensive Cancer Network (NCCN) recommend chemotherapy and radiation therapy for resected stage II or III atypical carcinoids, but not for typical carcinoids.[37]

DISCUSSION POINTS

1. Describe two strategies to decrease the risk of bleeding from bronchoscopic biopsy of this tumor.
   - Administration of a diluted epinephrine solution before and after biopsy of a suspected endobronchial carcinoid may reduce the risk of severe bleeding.
   - Biopsy samples can be taken in the operating room with a rigid bronchoscope while the patient is under general anesthesia; with use of the rigid bronchoscope, large biopsy samples are obtained, and in cases of difficult to control bleeding, the Nd:YAG laser can be used for hemostasis.
2. Discuss the role of imaging studies in diagnosis and staging of carcinoid tumors.

No consensus has been reached on the need for preoperative staging imaging studies in patients who are thought to have an isolated bronchial carcinoid; typical carcinoids infrequently metastasize, and the diagnosis of nodal metastasis from atypical carcinoids is rarely made preoperatively. Whether increased availability of endobronchial ultrasound-guided mediastinal staging will alter this finding is an area for future research.

- Somatostatin receptor scintigraphy (SRS)* uses radiolabeled somatostatin analogs (octreotide, pentetreotide) to detect tumors expressing somatostatin receptors. Although approximately 80% of typical and 60% of atypical bronchial carcinoids express these receptors by immunohistochemistry, in patients with bronchial carcinoids the overall sensitivity of this test was found to be 81% for detecting the primary tumor, and 77.7% for revealing intrathoracic metastases/recurrences—results that were not superior to those of CT scanning.[38] A recent study with indium-111–octreotide showed all cases of primary tumors and all cases of recurrent or metastatic disease, sometimes even before symptoms appeared.[39] Specificity is limited because scintigraphy is also positive in gastroenteropancreatic tumors, granulomas, and autoimmune diseases. In a small study (n = 8) evaluating the role of SRS in the management of pulmonary carcinoid tumor, scans were strongly positive in the tumors and involved lymph nodes, correctly localized an occult secreting pulmonary carcinoid, and were accurate in ruling out distant metastases, with the caveat that granulomatous and reactive lymph nodes showed increased uptake.[40] Octreotide scans image the whole body and, although not universally accepted, are recommended by several authorities[38] and by the National Comprehensive Cancer Network (NCCN) to identify extrathoracic metastatic disease in patients with bronchial carcinoid.[14]
- Positron emission tomography (PET) scanning with fluorodeoxyglucose (FDG) for carcinoids has yielded conflicting results, probably because of the small size of these tumors and the fact that they often are hypometabolic. In a retrospective review of 16 patients with surgically resected bronchial carcinoids, PET detected 12 cases (75% of patients).[41] The use of other tracers, such as 11C-L-dopa and 11C-5-hydroxytryptophan (11C-5-HT), might improve sensitivity for imaging neuroendocrine tumors, but because of their extremely short half-life (≈20 minutes), they are not currently used in clinical practice.[42]
- Abdominal CT scanning before and after contrast is complementary to octreotide scanning in ruling out liver metastases and localizing tumor and can be used for staging according to some experts, because the most common metastatic site for all carcinoid tumors is the liver. In fact, a small study showed that CT detected liver metastasis in 14 patients, among whom only 9 (64%) had positive results on Octreoscan.[38]
- Magnetic resonance imaging (MRI) has greater sensitivity for liver metastases as compared with both Octreoscan and CT. This was shown in a prospective trial involving 66 consecutive patients with well-differentiated gastroenteropancreatic tumors, 40 of whom had histologically confirmed liver metastases.[43] MRI detected significantly more metastases than were detected by planar SRS or CT (sensitivity rates for MRI, planar SRS, and CT were 95%, 79%, and 49%, respectively). Although MRI may be the imaging study of choice for the detection of metastatic neuroendocrine tumors,[43] it has not been systematically used to detect extrathoracic metastasis from bronchial carcinoids.

3. List three open surgical treatment alternatives for endobronchial carcinoid.
   - Lung resection (lobectomy or pneumonectomy), parenchymal-sparing lung resection, and bronchoplasty. For typical carcinoid, several studies show that only surgery is curative, and that parenchymal-sparing surgery is favored. The relative frequency of various procedures for carcinoid is as follows: lobectomy (51% to 58%), bilobectomy (9% to 15%), segmentectomy or wedge resection (2% to 15%), bronchoplastic procedures (5% to 15%), and pneumonectomy (6% to 16%).[44]
   - For atypical carcinoid, parenchymal-sparing surgery is considered insufficient; the same surgical treatment as is used for non–small cell lung carcinoma is advocated.[7]

4. Describe how tumor histology and morphology affect treatment decisions for carcinoid tumors.
   - Bronchoscopic treatment improves presurgical conditions, allows tissue sampling for histologic classification, and provides information that might lead to less extensive parenchymal resection. It is also proposed for curative intent in selected patients with strictly intraluminal typical carcinoids.
   - Complete tumor removal with mediastinal lymph node dissection is the accepted practice for atypical carcinoids, extraluminal disease, and "iceberg" lesions, and in cases of residual disease or recurrence after intraluminal resection.

Expert Commentary

provided by Federico Rea, MD

Bronchial carcinoids are rare, well-differentiated neuroendocrine malignant tumors that account for 1% to 2% of all lung neoplasms.[44] As was discussed in the case, typical carcinoids have an excellent long-term prognosis, with 5 year survival ranging from 87% to 97%. Patients with atypical carcinoid, on the other hand, are at greater risk of developing metastases, and 5 year survival ranges from 56% to 77%.

---

*Administration of a radiolabeled form of the somatostatin analog octreotide results in normal uptake of the isotope in the spleen and bladder, and to a lesser extent in the liver.

The diagnostic and therapeutic management of carcinoids is still a matter of debate. In particular, three points are controversial:

1. Role and reliability of imaging techniques for diagnosis, staging, and follow-up
2. Role, safety, and efficacy of bronchoscopic procedures in diagnosis and treatment
3. Role of parenchymal-sparing surgery and lymphadenectomy

With regard to imaging techniques, high-resolution CT scanning is important for diagnosis of bronchial carcinoids and provides good information regarding tumor extent and location and lymph node involvement. However, particularly for centrally located tumors, the accuracy of this imaging technique may be low. For example, the presence of atelectasis makes it difficult to accurately differentiate tumor growth and the nature of any associated reactive or secondary lymphadenopathy. A second radiographic examination is usually required after resolution of any associated central airway obstruction or infection.

Carcinoid tumors express in high percentage one or more somatostatin receptors; therefore the use of somatostatin receptor scintigraphy, with radiolabeled somatostatin analog (^{111}In-octreotide), has become routine in most centers reporting this disease. The sensitivity of Octreoscan is greater than 90%. Its use has been suggested in the diagnosis of primary carcinoids and in the detection of early recurrences, even in asymptomatic patients.[45] Octreoscans suffer from low spatial resolution and are able to detect only subtype 2 somatostatin receptor. ^{18}F-FDG PET/CT has limited sensitivity for carcinoids because of low uptake of the marker. Recent progress is represented by ^{68}Ga-DOTATOC PET/CT, which seems to have high sensitivity for primary tumors and for secondary localizations, with better imaging resolution.[46] An additional indication for using these imaging techniques is to enhance the selection of ideal candidates for radiometabolic or somatostatin receptor–targeted anticancer therapy.[47]

Bronchoscopic procedures occupy a central role in the diagnosis and initial management of carcinoids. A significant proportion (at least 50% and up to 90% in typical histotypes) are centrally located in the bronchial tree, in which case tumors arise from the walls of medium to large airways. Central carcinoids are often symptomatic, so recurrent obstructive pneumonia or persistent cough or wheezing (frequently mistreated as asthma) should alert the physician. Although many authors have stressed the importance of such symptoms (including hemoptysis), many patients still undergo invasive diagnostic procedures too late, often after a symptomatic course of several months. In my opinion, early diagnosis is of fundamental importance because it allows treatment of obstructive symptoms, avoiding recurrent pneumonia, which can irreversibly damage the lung parenchyma such that parenchymal-sparing resection is no longer possible. Complications related to bronchoscopic biopsy of carcinoid tumors are rare, but in some cases, significant hemorrhage can occur. Its management can be difficult, so the availability of and ready access to instrumentation for rigid bronchoscopy should be verified before flexible bronchoscopic biopsy is performed in cases in which carcinoid tumor is suspected.

Bronchoscopy is also important as part of a management strategy. Careful preoperative bronchoscopic assessment is important in planning best surgical treatment and in determining the feasibility of a bronchoplastic procedure.[48] When major bronchi are obstructed, endoscopic debulking allows the physician to examine the airways beyond the tumor to evaluate its base of implantation and eventually to treat the airway obstruction. Endobronchial laser treatment (necessary in 34.3% of cases in my experience) has significantly increased the frequency with which parenchymal-sparing surgeries can be performed. Similar to the opinion expressed regarding the patient presented, I do not consider laser therapy curative. Usually, endobronchial carcinoids tend to spread extraluminally, and a correct approach should, in my opinion, consist of surgical removal. Moreover, the potential for lymph node involvement (5% to 20% in typical carcinoids), especially micrometastases not revealed by conventional imaging techniques, should require a complete systematic lymphadenectomy.

Some authors have proposed endobronchial laser therapy as definitive treatment for central typical carcinoids.[6,21,29] At the moment, very few studies are available, and conflicting results (recurrence rate, 2% to 5%) have been reported. No randomized studies have compared open and endobronchial approaches. Unfortunately, laser treatment rarely allows a radical resection because locally, the base of implantation is often large and deep, and the visible part in the bronchial tree can be only the tip of an iceberg. Radical local endoscopic treatment may be attempted in a highly select population with typical carcinoid tumors that are entirely endobronchial, forming a polypoid lesion with a small (less than 1 cm) base of implantation, a small dimension (probably less than 3 to 4 cm^2), no extraluminal growth, and no lymph node involvement noted by diagnostic imaging techniques. The procedure should be carried out by very experienced operators who are able to correctly use a laser, and who have access to high-resolution CT scanning and endobronchial ultrasound, which may prove helpful in monitoring biopsies to ensure complete bronchoscopic resection or in evaluating local recurrence. Surveillance should be prolonged because recurrence can occur even many years after the initial procedure, or spread to lymph nodes may be noted.

Surgery represents the treatment of choice for bronchial carcinoid, and parenchymal-sparing resections such as sleeve or bronchoplastic procedures have been suggested for central carcinoid tumors.[48] Despite this, a number of surgical aspects are still controversial. In my experience, a significantly increased number of sleeve resections or bronchoplastic procedures for centrally located carcinoids led to a significant reduction in the number of pneumonectomies in previous years.

These results were obtained as a result of improvements in surgical techniques, but also because of the popularization of parenchymal-sparing operations based on bronchoplastic or sleeve resections, which do not alter the oncologic result and obviously guarantee a better quality of life. Therefore I think that modern management of central carcinoids should privilege, when possible, sleeve resections, given that oncologic results are good and the rate of local recurrence is low in most experiences.[22-26,48-50] The need to avoid pneumonectomy gains greater weight when we consider that central typical carcinoid preferentially affects young people.[51]

Surgical resection of carcinoid tumors should always be combined with systematic lymph node dissection. The necessity for lymph node dissection is justified by the possibility of lymph node metastases, the incidence of which may range from 6% to 25%.[19,52] The prognostic relevance of lymph node involvement has been underlined by several authors[17,19,52,53]; therefore investigation into lymph node metastases seems an unavoidable prerequisite for establishing prognosis, and eventually for evaluating opportunities for adjuvant therapies. The accuracy of pathologic diagnosis can be enhanced, as demonstrated by Mineo et al., who described the relevance of lymph node micrometastases detected by immunohistochemical techniques.[54]

REFERENCES

1. Gustafsson BI, Kidd M, Chan A, et al. Bronchopulmonary neuroendocrine tumors. *Cancer.* 2008;113:5-21.
2. Filosso PL, Rena O, Donati G, et al. Bronchial carcinoid tumors: surgical management and long-term outcome. *J Thorac Cardiovasc Surg.* 2002;123:303-309.
3. Fink G, Krelbaum T, Yellin A, et al. Pulmonary carcinoid: presentation, diagnosis, and outcome in 142 cases in Israel and review of 640 cases from the literature. *Chest.* 2001;119:1647-1651.
4. Seregni E, Ferrari L, Bajetta E, et al. Clinical significance of blood chromogranin A measurement in neuroendocrine tumours. *Ann Oncol.* 2001;12(suppl 2):S69-S72.
5. Campana D, Nori F, Piscitelli L, et al. Chromogranin A: is it a useful marker of neuroendocrine tumors? *J Clin Oncol.* 2007;25:1967-1973.
6. Brokx HA, Risse EK, Paul MA, et al. Initial bronchoscopic treatment for patients with intraluminal bronchial carcinoids. *J Thorac Cardiovasc Surg.* 2007;133:973-978.
7. Marty-Ané C, Costes V, Pujol J, et al. Carcinoid tumors of the lung: do atypical features require aggressive management? *Ann Thorac Surg.* 1995;59:78-83.
8. Todd T, Cooper J, Weisberg D, et al. Bronchial carcinoid tumors: twenty years' experience. *J Thorac Cardiovasc Surg.* 1980;79: 32-36.
9. McCoughan BC, Martini N, Bains M. Bronchial carcinoids: review of 124 cases. *J Thorac Cardiovasc Surg.* 1985;89:8-17.
10. Dusmet ME, McKneally MF. Pulmonary and thymic carcinoid tumors. *World J Surg.* 1996;20:189-195.
11. Rea F, Binda R, Spreafico G, et al. Bronchial carcinoids: a review of 60 patients. *Ann Thorac Surg.* 1989;47:412-414.
12. Modlin IM, Lye KD, Kidd M. A 5-decade analysis of 13,715 carcinoid tumors. *Cancer.* 2003;97:934-959.
13. Hauso O, Gustafsson BI, Kidd M, et al. Neuroendocrine tumor epidemiology: contrasting Norway and North America. *Cancer.* 2008;113:2655-2664.
14. Quaedvlieg PF, Visser O, Lamers CB, et al. Epidemiology and survival in patients with carcinoid disease in The Netherlands: an epidemiological study with 2391 patients. *Ann Oncol.* 2001;12: 1295-1300.
15. Diaz-Jimenez JP, Canela-Cardona M, Maestre-Alcacer J. Nd:YAG laser photoresection of low-grade malignant tumors of the tracheobronchial tree. *Chest.* 1990;97:920-922.
16. Schreurs AJ, Westermann CJ, van den Bosch JM, et al. A twenty-five-year follow-up of ninety-three resected typical carcinoid tumors of the lung. *J Thorac Cardiovasc Surg.* 1992;104:1470-1475.
17. Rea F, Rizzardi G, Zuin A, et al. Outcome and surgical strategy in bronchial carcinoid tumors: single institution experience with 252 patients. *Eur J Cardiothorac Surg.* 2007;31:186-191.
18. van Boxem TJ, Venmans BJ, van Mourik JC, et al. Bronchoscopic treatment of intraluminal typical carcinoid: a pilot study. *J Thorac Cardiovasc Surg.* 1998;116:402-406.
19. Cardillo G, Sera F, Di Martino M, et al. Bronchial carcinoid tumors: nodal status and long-term survival after resection. *Ann Thorac Surg.* 2004;77:1781-1785.
20. Harpole DH Jr, Feldman JM, Buchanan S, et al. Bronchial carcinoid tumors: a retrospective analysis of 126 patients. *Ann Thorac Surg.* 1992;54:50-54.
21. Van Boxem TJ, Golding RP, Venmans BJ, et al. High-resolution CT in patients with intraluminal typical bronchial carcinoid tumors treated with bronchoscopic therapy. *Chest.* 2000;117: 125-128.
22. Terzi A, Lonardoni A, Feil B, et al. Bronchoplastic procedures for central carcinoid tumors: clinical experience. *Eur J Cardiothorac Surg.* 2004;26:1196-1199.
23. El Jamal M, Nicholson AG, Goldstraw P. The feasibility of conservative resection for carcinoid tumors: is pneumonectomy ever necessary for uncomplicated cases? *Eur J Cardiothorac Surg.* 2000; 18:301-306.
24. Lucchi M, Melfi F, Ribechini A, et al. Sleeve and wedge parenchyma-sparing bronchial resections in low-grade neoplasms of the bronchial airway. *J Thorac Cardiovasc Surg.* 2007;134:373-377.
25. Wilkins EW Jr, Grillo HC, Moncure AC, et al. Changing times in surgical management of bronchopulmonary carcinoid tumor. *Ann Thorac Surg.* 1984;38:339-344.
26. Cerfolio RJ, Deschamps C, Allen MS, et al. Mainstem bronchial sleeve resection with pulmonary preservation. *Ann Thorac Surg.* 1996;61:1458-1462.
27. Martini N, Zaman MB, Bains MS, et al. Treatment and prognosis in bronchial carcinoids involving regional lymph nodes. *J Thorac Cardiovasc Surg.* 1994;107:1-6.
28. Orino K, Kawai H, Ogawa J. Bronchoscopic treatment with argon plasma coagulation for recurrent typical carcinoids: report of a case. *Anticancer Res.* 2004;24:4073-4077.
29. Luckraz H, Amer K, Thomas L, et al. Long-term outcome of bronchoscopically resected endobronchial typical carcinoid tumors. *J Thorac Cardiovasc Surg.* 2006;132:113-115.
30. Bertoletti L, Elleuch R, Kaczmarek D, et al. Bronchoscopic cryotherapy treatment of isolated endoluminal typical carcinoid tumor. *Chest.* 2006;130:1405-1411.
31. Mackley HB, Videtic GM. Primary carcinoid tumors of the lung: a role for radiotherapy. *Oncology.* 2006;20:1537-1543.
32. Chakravarthy A, Abrams RA. Radiation therapy in the management of patients with malignant carcinoid tumors. *Cancer.* 1995; 75:1386-1390.
33. Karmy-Jones R, Vallieres E. Carcinoid crisis after biopsy of a bronchial carcinoid. *Ann Thorac Surg.* 1993;56:1403-1405.
34. Mehta AC, Rafanan AL, Bulkley R, et al. Coronary spasm and cardiac arrest from carcinoid crisis during laser bronchoscopy. *Chest.* 1999;115:598-600.
35. Kinney MA, Warner ME, Nagorney DM, et al. Perianaesthetic risks and outcomes of abdominal surgery for metastatic carcinoid tumours. *Br J Anaesth.* 2001;87:447-452.
36. Morandi U, Casali C, Rossi G. Bronchial typical carcinoid tumors. *Semin Thorac Cardiovasc Surg.* 2006;18:191-198.
37. NCCN Clinical Practice Guidelines in Oncology (NCCN Guidelines™). Neuroendocrine tumors. Version 2.2010. www.nccn.org. Accessed March 23, 2011.
38. Granberg D, Sundin A, Janson ET, et al. Octreoscan in patients with bronchial carcinoid tumours. *Clin Endocrinol* 2003;59: 793-799.

39. Musi M, Carbone RG, Bertocchi C, et al. Bronchial carcinoid tumors: a study on clinicopathological features and role of octreotide scintigraphy. *Lung Cancer.* 1998;22:97-102.

40. Yellin A, Zwas ST, Rozenman J, et al. Experience with somatostatin receptor scintigraphy in the management of pulmonary carcinoid tumors. *Isr Med Assoc J.* 2005;7:712-716.

41. Daniels CE, Lowe VJ, Aubry MC, et al. The utility of fluorodeoxyglucose positron emission tomography in the evaluation of carcinoid tumors presenting as pulmonary nodules. *Chest.* 2007;131:255-260.

42. Orlefors H, Sundin A, Garske U, et al. Whole-body (11)C-5-hydroxytryptophan positron emission tomography as a universal imaging technique for neuroendocrine tumors: comparison with somatostatin receptor scintigraphy and computed tomography. *J Clin Endocrinol Metab.* 2005;90:3392-3400.

43. Dromain C, de Baere T, Lumbroso J, et al. Detection of liver metastases from endocrine tumors: a prospective comparison of somatostatin receptor scintigraphy, computed tomography, and magnetic resonance imaging. *J Clin Oncol.* 2005;23:70-78.

44. Hage R, Brutel de la Riviere A, Seldenrijk CA, et al. Update in pulmonary carcinoid tumors: a review article. *Ann Surg Oncol.* 2003;10:697-704.

45. Gustafsson B, Kidd M, Modlin I. Neuroendorine tumors of the diffuse neuroendocrine system. *Curr Opin Oncol.* 2008;20:1-12.

46. Frilling A, Sotiropoulos GC, Radtke A, et al. The impact of 68Ga-DOTATOC positron emission tomography/computed tomography on the multimodal management of patients with neuroendocrine tumors. *Ann Surg.* 2010;252:850-856.

47. Sun LC, Coy DH. Somatostatin receptor-targeted anti-cancer therapy. *Curr Drug Deliv.* 2011;8:2-10.

48. Rizzardi G, Marulli G, Bortolotti L, et al. Sleeve resections and bronchoplastic procedures in typical central carcinoid tumours. *Thorac Cardiovasc Surg.* 2008;56:42-45.

49. Massard G, Ducrocq X, Thomas P, et al. Typical carcinoid tumors of the bronchi: an update. *J Cardiovasc Surg.* 2002;43:16-21.

50. Tastepe AI, Kurul IC, Demircan S, et al. Long-term survival following bronchotomy for polypoid bronchial carcinoid tumours. *Eur J Cardiothorac Surg.* 1998;14:575-577.

51. Rizzardi G, Marulli G, Calabrese F, et al. Bronchial carcinoid tumours in children: surgical treatment and outcome in a single institution. *Eur J Pediatr Surg.* 2009;19:228-231.

52. Thomas CF Jr, Tazelaar HD, Jett JR. Typical and atypical pulmonary carcinoids: outcome in patients presenting with regional lymph node involvement. *Chest.* 2001;119:1143-1150.

53. Garcia-Yuste M, Matilla JM, Alvarez-Gago T, et al. Prognostic factors in neuroendocrine lung tumors: a Spanish Multicenter Study. Spanish Multicenter Study of Neuroendocrine Tumors of the Lung of the Spanish Society of Pneumonology and Thoracic Surgery (EMETNE-SEPAR). *Ann Thorac Surg.* 2000;70:258-263.

54. Mineo TC, Guggino G, Mineo D, et al. Relevance of lymph node micrometastases in radically resected endobronchial carcinoid tumors. *Ann Thorac Surg.* 2005;80:428-432.

Chapter 3

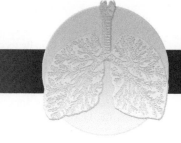

Bronchoscopic Treatment of Silicone Stent–Related Granulation Tissue

This chapter emphasizes the following elements of the Four Box Approach: risk-benefit analysis and therapeutic alternatives; anesthesia and other perioperative care; and techniques and instrumentation.

CASE DESCRIPTION

The patient was a 75-year-old man with post intubation tracheal stenosis. He had chronic obstructive pulmonary disease (COPD) (forced expiratory volume in 1 second [FEV$_1$] 40% of predicted) requiring home oxygen supplementation at 3 L/nasal cannula. He also suffered from coronary artery disease requiring coronary artery bypass graft (CABG) surgery 5 years previously, at which time he was intubated for 3 days. He had congestive heart failure (left ventricular ejection fraction [LVEF] 40%) and required placement of a pacemaker. Three months before our encounter, he began to complain of progressive dyspnea leading to stridor. Bronchoscopy revealed a severe (4 mm), complex (three cartilaginous rings), and multilevel "hourglass" tracheal stenosis (2.5 cm in extent), suggesting a post intubation origin (Figure 3-1). His stricture rapidly recurred after rigid bronchoscopy with dilation, prompting insertion of a 12 × 40 mm straight silicone stent in the patient's trachea 3 weeks later. The proximal aspect of the stent was located 4 cm below the vocal cords. Two months after stent placement, the patient developed progressive cough and dyspnea. On auscultation, he had rhonchi over the trachea, and stridor was heard with forced inspiration and expiration but not with tidal breathing. Bronchoscopy revealed a large amount of granulation tissue nearly completely obstructing the proximal aspect of the stent. Removal of the tissue was initiated using a flexible electrocautery probe during flexible bronchoscopy under moderate sedation (Figure 3-2).

DISCUSSION POINTS

1. Describe three indications for granulation tissue removal.
2. Describe the principles of cutting and coagulation when endobronchial electrocautery and argon plasma coagulation are used.
3. Describe two potential complications resulting from electrosurgery in this patient.

---

*An electrical current in which electron flow moves in only one direction; galvanic currents cause fibroblast proliferation and a resultant increase in collagen synthesis—a property used for wound healing and implicated in keloid formation.

†Benign hyperplastic granulation tissue can cause airway obstruction in up to 20% of patients after lung transplantation, typically occurring at the site of bronchial anastomosis a few months after surgery.

4. List and explain three mechanisms of pathogenesis for granulation tissue formation.

CASE RESOLUTION

Initial Evaluations

Physical Examination, Complementary Tests, and Functional Status Assessment

This patient presented with new exophytic endoluminal tracheal obstruction after stent placement, most likely consistent with hyperplastic granulation tissue formation, a benign form of central airway obstruction.[1] The main differential diagnosis of granulation tissue in patients with indwelling airway stents is tumor overgrowth, although mucus plugging and bacterial colonization can also cause firm, necrotic-appearing obstructive lesions. The exact prevalence of stent obstruction by granulation tissue versus tumor overgrowth is somewhat confounded by the fact that studies tend to report these events together rather than separately. With this caveat, the estimated frequency of recurrent obstruction from granulation tissue or tumor is 9% to 67% in patients with metal stents, and 6% to 15% in patients with silicone stents.[2] Tumor overgrowth tends to occur when only the tumor area is covered and no cancer therapy is offered; it is most often seen in patients with partially covered indwelling metal stents because malignant tissue grows through exposed wire mesh, causing obstruction (Figure 3-3). Our patient, however, had no history of cancer; his stent was placed for a benign post intubation stricture, and the rapid onset of exophytic tissue growth was not consistent with a malignant tumor growth rate.

Granulation tissue formation is less predictable. It seems that patients with known keloids or chronic airway infection are at higher risk.[3] Oversizing the stent has been suspected as a risk factor, especially when stents are placed in the upper trachea or subglottis (see video on ExpertConsult.com) (Video I.3.1). For silicone, as well as metal, friction between the sharp edges of the stent and the airway mucosa may cause granulation tissue formation. In addition, when electrocautery is used, the direct (aka galvanic) currents generated* around the metal wires may be cofactors in granulation tissue formation.[4] Shearing forces at the stent-mucosa interface created by differential motion of the stent relative to the airway contribute to constant stimulation of airway mucosa, further leading to reactive granulation tissue formation. Hyperplastic granulation tissue formation can be seen at the site of a lung transplant surgical anastomosis[†5,6] or at the anastomosis site after tracheal sleeve resection for

Figure 3-1 **A,** Post intubation stricture at initial bronchoscopy. Note the "hourglass" morphology and severely reduced airway diameter (4 mm). **B,** Potassium-titanyl-phosphate (KTP) laser–assisted rigid bronchoscopy restored airway patency to 10 mm (picture taken immediately post dilation). **C,** Stricture recurred 3 weeks later to its predilation severity. **D,** A 12 × 40 mm silicone stent was placed to restore airway patency.

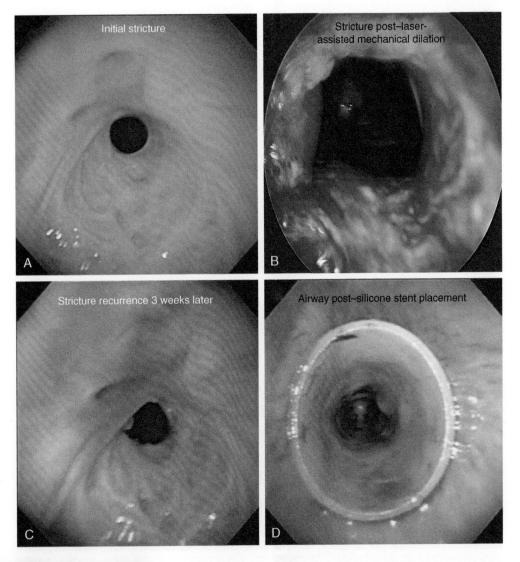

Initial stricture

Stricture post–laser-assisted mechanical dilation

Stricture recurrence 3 weeks later

Airway post–silicone stent placement

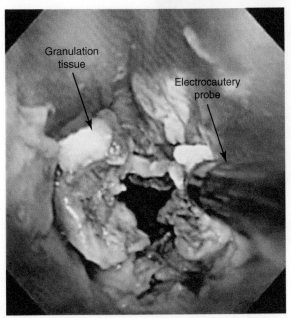

Granulation tissue

Electrocautery probe

Figure 3-2 Large amount of granulation tissue formed circumferentially around the proximal aspect of the stent. Note whitening of the tissues as an effect of electrocautery-induced coagulation.

tracheal stenosis (Figure 3-4). One study showed that 31% of patients with a lung transplant or benign disease developed granulation tissue after placement of a self-expandable metallic stent.[5]

Silicone stent insertion performed using rigid bronchoscopy under general anesthesia was considered an acceptable alternative to surgery for our inoperable patient with complex stenosis.* In fact, silicone stents provide long-term airway patency in nonsurgical candidates with a variety of central airway obstructive lesions.[†7-9] Stent-related complications, however, are not uncommon and in one series included migration (17.5%), obstruction from secretions (6.3%), and significant granulation tissue formation at the proximal or distal extremities of the stent (6.3%).[10] This latter complication may promote the development of secondary stenosis.[5] It is likely that other complications of stent insertion, such as kinking, fracture, or

---

*Most studies define complex stenoses as extensive scar ≥1 cm in vertical length, circumferential hourglass-like contraction scarring, or the presence of associated malacia.

†Coexistent diseases such as coronary heart disease, severe cardiac or respiratory insufficiency, or a poor general condition.

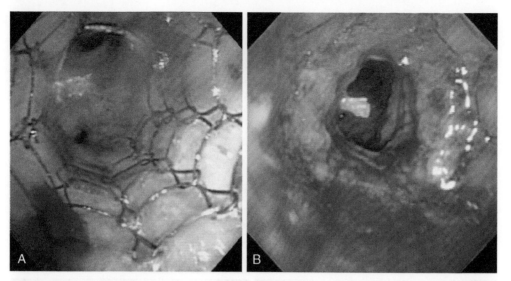

Figure 3-3 A, Partially covered 14 × 40 mm Ultraflex stent placed in the left main bronchus in a patient with extrinsic compression and mucosal infiltration from primary lung adenocarcinoma. **B,** Circumferential tumor growth through the uncovered portion of the stent was seen on follow-up bronchoscopy performed 3 weeks later.

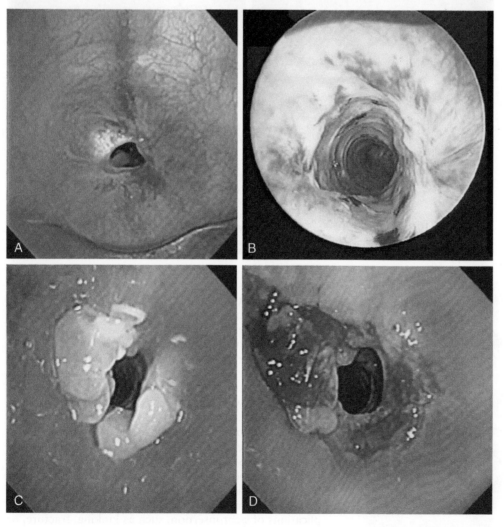

Figure 3-4 A, Patient with severe web-like tracheal stenosis underwent tracheal sleeve resection, **(B)** resulting in improved airway patency. **C,** Several weeks later, however, severe dyspnea triggered a flexible bronchoscopy, which revealed a large amount of obstruction granulation tissue at the anastomotic site. **D,** This tissue was very friable and bled easily just by gentle touch with the flexible bronchoscope.

compression of mucosal vasculature due to excessive centrifugal force exerted by expanding or self-expanding stents, also contribute to granulation tissue formation. As in our patient, diagnostic flexible bronchoscopy should always be performed when a stent-related adverse event is expected. This will confirm or rule out problems such as mucus plugging or stent migration and will allow an accurate reassessment of the stenosis, the degree of mucosal inflammation, associated cartilaginous collapse, and the relative amount and location of hypertrophic fibrotic tissue.[11] Bronchoscopy is the current standard for the detection and treatment of stent-related complications; in nonurgent situations, it usually involves a two-step procedure. Initially, diagnostic flexible bronchoscopy is performed to detect and characterize a stent complication; if a treatable complication is detected, rigid bronchoscopy may be required for therapeutic intervention. In our case, a large amount of obstructing granulation tissue was found proximal to the stent during flexible bronchoscopy* (see Figure 3-1).

This patient had developed significant granulation 2 months after stent placement, probably as a result of abnormal wound healing—a process that eventually led to hypertrophic fibrotic tissue formation and circumferential stenosis. The exact duration of indwelling stent placement necessary to cause airway injury and granulation is not known, and the exact molecular mechanisms responsible for this are only partially understood.[†] Some of the better studied mechanisms include overexpression of profibrotic transforming growth factor (TGF)-β_1 in the extracellular matrix[12] and the presence of high levels of vascular endothelial growth factor (VEGF) expression in the submucosal layers.[13] Wound healing also depends on local and systemic factors, such as infection, pressure, tissue necrosis, age, and comorbidities.[14] In this regard, patients with malignant disease develop less stent-related granulation tissue formation ($\approx 4\%$)—a phenomenon that can be explained in part by the use of radiotherapy and chemotherapy, leading to a less pronounced inflammatory response to the presence of the stent.[5]

Comorbidities

This patient suffered from several cardiovascular comorbidities. An assessment of risk for myocardial infarction or death and methods to reduce or eliminate these risks should be addressed before surgery is performed on such patients under general anesthesia.[15] Perioperative myocardial infarction causes substantial morbidity and prolonged hospitalization; mortality rates as high as 25% to 40% are associated. Noninvasive stress testing is widely used to help predict risk of perioperative complications, but the poor predictive power of these tests limits their usefulness. No data suggest benefits of percutaneous coronary intervention or CABG in reducing noncardiac surgical risk. In addition, angioplasty with stenting and its need for anticoagulation can expose patients to increased risk of perioperative bleeding. In general, stable patients who have previously undergone

coronary revascularization may safely undergo surgery, especially low cardiac risk procedures such as bronchoscopic interventions. In one study of patients who had undergone high-risk noncardiac surgeries, the revascularized patients experienced significantly fewer cardiac complications perioperatively when compared with patients without previous CABG.[16] It is currently recommended that asymptomatic patients who have undergone CABG in the previous 5 years should proceed directly to noncardiac surgery without further preoperative evaluation.[17] From a purely cardiac standpoint, our patient had no contraindication to rigid bronchoscopy under general anesthesia, making it a possible alternative for granulation tissue removal.

Postoperative pulmonary complications are at least equally prevalent and contribute similarly or more to morbidity, mortality, and length of stay in patients undergoing noncardiac surgery.[18] With regard to perioperative pulmonary risk stratification, patient-related risk factors for postoperative pulmonary complications* include advanced age,[†] American Society of Anesthesiologists class 2 or higher, functional dependence, COPD, and congestive heart failure (all were seen in our patient). Abnormal findings on chest examination (defined as decreased breath sounds, prolonged expiration, rales, wheezes, or rhonchi) were the strongest predictors of postoperative pulmonary complication rates (odds ratio, 5.8).[18] Evidence supports procedure-related risk factors for postoperative pulmonary complications, including general anesthesia and prolonged surgery (2.5 to 4 hours). The major procedure-related risk factors (vascular, abdominal, or thoracic surgery) confer higher risk for pulmonary complications than is associated with patient-related risk factors.[18] From a pulmonary standpoint, our patient was not an optimal candidate for general anesthesia, and granulation tissue was therefore removed using the flexible bronchoscope and moderate sedation.

Support System

This patient with advanced lung disease and his partner had to cope with a life limited by constant dyspnea. Although dyspnea may vary in severity from day to day, it invariably affects how patients and their partners see themselves and their place in society; people develop a feeling of isolation, helplessness, and fear.[19] Indeed, results of studies show that family caregivers voiced their feelings of helplessness and their sense of relief and security once they had decided to seek help (e.g., when the patient was admitted for acute care).[19] Interventions that target the family setting in which chronic disease management takes place have thus emerged as an alternative to traditional strategies that focus only on individual patients, or that consider family only as a peripheral source of positive or negative social support. When this approach is used, the educational, relational, and personal needs of all family members are emphasized with the aim of

---

*Of course, granulation tissue and other stent-related complications such as obstruction by tenuous secretions can be treated at the time of the initial diagnostic flexible bronchoscopy. One should be ready for procedure-related complications such as increasing hypoxemia or bleeding. These may be caused by the stent-related complication itself or during the course of treatment. For example, while tissues or secretions are removed with forceps, the loop sutures of a metal stent might be accidentally grasped, thereby mobilizing the stent and causing complete airway obstruction. On other occasions, tissue causing complete stent obstruction might not be removable. The bronchoscopist should be able to punch a hole through the tissue or secretions during the entire length of the stent, to create a passageway for ventilation, while other means of removing tissues, such as electrocautery or cryotherapy, are prepared.

[†]Normally, wound healing lasts up to 2 years, but malnutrition, hemodynamic status, tissue hypoxia, and metabolic factors (e.g., acidosis, diabetes mellitus) can cause a delay in the healing process.

---

*Atelectasis, pneumonia, respiratory failure, and exacerbation of underlying chronic lung disease.

[†]Advanced age (>65 years) is an important independent predictor of postoperative pulmonary complications even after adjustment for comorbidities.

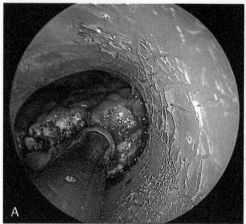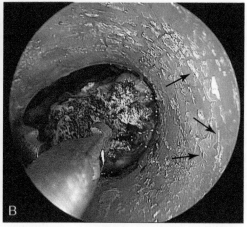

Figure 3-5 A, The rigid electrocautery probe is placed directly onto the granulation tissue formed distal to the stent, **(B)** once coagulated tissue is removed using the rigid forceps; despite minimal use of electrocautery (25 W, 3 second pulses) and lack of direct contact with the stent, collateral thermal stent damage characterized as a spontaneous break in the continuity of the silicone layer inside the stent was evident *(black arrows)*.

improving the quality of relationships among family members with respect to the disease.[20]

Patient Preferences and Expectations

During our preprocedure interview, our patient expressed his wish to avoid general anesthesia if possible. He was informed of available therapeutic options for his current airway problem, such as flexible bronchoscopy removal using laser, electrocautery, argon plasma coagulation, cryotherapy, or rigid bronchoscopy with stent revision, and removal of tissues by rigid bronchoscopic resection, laser, or electrosurgery. After he had been informed of the risks and benefits of available therapeutic alternatives for his situation, he elected to undergo flexible bronchoscopy with electrosurgery to improve symptoms acutely so that he could avoid rigid bronchoscopy.

Procedural Strategies

Indications

The obstructing granulation tissue resulted in stridor and respiratory distress at rest. The bronchoscopic procedure was indicated in an attempt to restore airway lumen patency and to improve airflow and symptoms.

Contraindications

This patient had no absolute contraindications to flexible bronchoscopy. In fact, the only contraindication to elective bronchoscopy is refractory hypoxemia.* Although hypoxemia is associated with cardiac arrhythmias in 11% to 40% of patients who undergo fiberoptic bronchoscopy, cardiac rhythm disturbances are rarely clinically important. The American Thoracic Society recommends avoiding bronchoscopy and bronchoalveolar lavage in patients with hypoxemia that cannot be corrected to at least a partial pressure of arterial oxygen (PaO_2) of 75 mm Hg or to a saturated oxygen level in hemoglobin (SaO_2) greater than 90% with supplemental oxygen. In case of use of electrosurgery, any high amount

of supplemental fraction of inspired oxygen (FiO_2) would pose a risk for airway fire and stent ignition. Our patient was on 3 L of oxygen at baseline, which is the equivalent of an FiO_2 of 0.32.*

Expected Results

Electrocautery uses high-frequency current, which leads to thermal tissue destruction. This bronchoscopic modality has been used successfully to remove granulation tissue [21] and can be performed using flexible or rigid bronchoscopy; when the rigid scope is used, the electrode tip must not be in contact with the rigid tube or other instruments or devices (e.g., forceps, stent) to avoid formation of an electrical circuit with the equipment or the operator (Figure 3-5). The main advantage of electrocautery over other techniques (photodynamic therapy, brachytherapy, or cryotherapy) is its rapid results. Care should be taken to avoid damaging normal airway wall structures or the indwelling airway stent. Necrosis caused by electrocautery depends on the voltage difference between the probe and the tissue, the surface area of contact, the duration energy is applied,† and the presence of blood or mucus.[22] For instance, in one study, superficial tissue damage was caused despite short duration of bronchoscopic electrocautery using 30 W power, use of a flexible electrocautery probe (2 mm² surface area) for less than 2 seconds. A longer duration of coagulation (3 or 5 seconds) caused damage to the underlying cartilage.[22]

Team Experience

The operating physician is responsible for settings, dosing of energy, and any decision regarding use of the electrosurgical unit. Although all staff members present should understand and confirm the settings used, the physician determines what modes, settings, and duration of delivery are used.

---

*By refractory, we mean persistent hypoxemia (<90%) despite administration of supplemental oxygen or noninvasive positive-pressure ventilation.

*The first liter is 0.03 FiO_2; thereafter it is 0.04 to each liter flow of oxygen. Therefore 3 L is the equivalent of approximately 0.32 FiO_2. Room air is 0.21 FiO_2.

†1 second coagulation resulted in a depth of necrosis of 0.2 ± 0.1 mm, and 0.2 ± 0.3 mm of tissue damage underneath; after 5 seconds, the depth of the crater with necrosis was 1.9 ± 0.8 mm, with clear damage to the underlying cartilage.

Therapeutic Alternatives to Granulation Tissue Removal

The choice of treatment modality is based on knowledge of its tissue effects, availability, operator experience, safety (e.g., electrocautery may not be possible in a patient who requires substantial supplemental oxygen to maintain oxygen saturation), and costs. Alternatives to granulation tissue removal include systemic and bronchoscopic therapies such as laser, electrocautery, argon plasma coagulation (APC), cryotherapy or rigid bronchoscopy with stent revision, and removal of tissues using rigid bronchoscopic forceps.

1. *Medical therapy:* Because wound healing is the source of the problem, researchers have tried to modulate and suppress this process.[13] Several agents have been tested for controlling the wound-healing process in airway stenosis: (1) inflammation phase: antibiotics, steroids, and hyperbaric oxygen (HBO)*; (2) proliferative phase: antibiotics, steroids, mitomycin,[†] 5-fluorouracil (5-FU)[‡]/triamcinolone, HBO; (3) maturation phase: halofuginone,[§] beta-aminopropionitrile , colchicine, penicillamine,[||] and N-acetyl-L-cysteine (NAC).[¶] Most of these agents were investigated in animal models. Three modalities were more thoroughly investigated: steroids and antibiotics, mitomycin, and antireflux medications.[13] Treatment with steroids and antibiotics did not have consistent results in different animal and human studies. Most studies demonstrated the superiority of mitomycin when compared with placebo if used immediately after tissue injury (i.e., on fresh, inflamed scar, containing mostly granulation tissue). Most of these studies show a tendency toward a favorable effect of mitomycin, yet results from the only prospective double-blind, randomized human study performed as of this writing did not demonstrate improvement when topical mitomycin was applied.[13] Reflux prevention includes education and behavioral changes, along with drugs such as proton pump inhibitors, H_2-receptor antagonists, and prokinetic agents.[13] Because of limited data supporting its efficacy and the severe nature of symptoms and the degree of obstruction, simple medical therapy was not offered to our patient.

2. *Neodymium-doped yttrium aluminum garnet (Nd:YAG) laser:* Effect is based on thermal tissue destruction resulting from light-tissue interaction. The distribution of energy depends on the optical properties of the material and the wavelength characteristic of the laser light. As absorbed energy is converted into heat, a rise in the temperature of the target tissue or material occurs; the temperature will rise above threshold levels only if the absorbed power density exceeds the capacity of the material to conduct heat away from the impact site. For example, at low power densities, the poor absorption of the Nd:YAG laser and its pronounced scattering result in slow homogeneous heating of a large volume of tissue without serious mechanical damage to the tissue surface.[23] At high power densities, however, the temperature 2 to 3 mm below the tissue surface rises rapidly, prompting vaporization of water content and a pocket of steam with pressure high enough to rupture overlying tissues.[24] Certain quantities of laser energy, defined by power density, would cause local heating without the extreme temperature elevation required to disrupt stent integrity or prompt stent ignition.[2] In these circumstances, laser-induced stent damage* may cause substantial morbidity from airway burn injury in case of stent ignition, or airway wall and vascular perforation in case of metal stent rupture. To identify margins of safety within which bronchoscopic Nd:YAG laser resection can be performed without damaging indwelling airway stents, an experimental in vitro study simulating a patient-care environment was conducted[†] using Nd:YAG laser performed at FiO_2 of 0.4 using fiber-to-target distances of 10 mm and 20 mm, and noncontact, continuous-mode, 1 second pulses at power settings of 10 W, 30 W, and 40 W. Results of this study showed that uncovered Wallstent and silicone stents were not damaged when Nd:YAG laser energy was delivered using power densities less than 172 W/cm^2 (10 W, 10 mm), but were damaged at power densities greater than 225 W/cm^2 (30 W, 20 mm); uncovered Wallstents, covered Wallstents, and silicone stents all were damaged at power densities greater than 225 W/cm^2 and at power settings greater than 30 W; covered Wallstents, however, had a high likelihood of ignition at all power densities studied (75 W/cm^2, 172 W/cm^2, 225 W/cm^2, 300 W/cm^2, 518 W/cm^2, and 690 W/cm^2).[‡,2,25] In fact, in another experimental study, investigators found that metal stents were destroyed after just

---

*HBO increases the oxygen flow and the arterial partial oxygen pressure in tissues, thus improving healing and re-epithelialization.

[†]Acts as an alkylating agent that inhibits DNA synthesis by cross-linking DNA; mitomycin also suppresses RNA and protein synthesis.

[‡]5-FU is a well-known antimetabolic drug that has an antiproliferative effect on human fibroblasts.

[§]Halofuginone is also an antifibrotic agent owing to a number of properties; it inhibits reversibly collagen1α synthesis.

[||]It completely blocks cross-linkage of newly formed collagen.

[¶]NAC interferes with disulfide bond formation.

---

*Stent damage was defined as visualization of blackish discoloration, blister formation, perforation, actual ignition, or rupture of the integrity of the stent. Rupture of the integrity of the metal stent was defined as a spontaneous break in the continuity of the metal mesh during laser application.

[†]In this study, however, the laser beam was focused on each stent, rather than on surrounding tissues, as is the case in clinical practice during removal of granulation tissue. Because laser energy is easily scattered and reflected, however, collateral absorption is frequent.

[‡]The average power density delivered for each setting was computed based on the formula: $Paw = 0.8635 \times power (watts)/\pi r^2$, where πr^2 is the spot size, and Paw is average power density. Because the laser beam diverges 11 degrees around the fiber core, the spot size at a distance was calculated using the following equation: Spot size = π ([fiber radius in centimeters] + [distance in centimeters] $\times$ tan 5.5 degrees).[2] When fiber-to-target distances of 10 mm and 20 mm were used, therefore, spot sizes were 0.05 cm^2 and 0.155 cm^2 (0.6 mm diameter coaxial fiber).

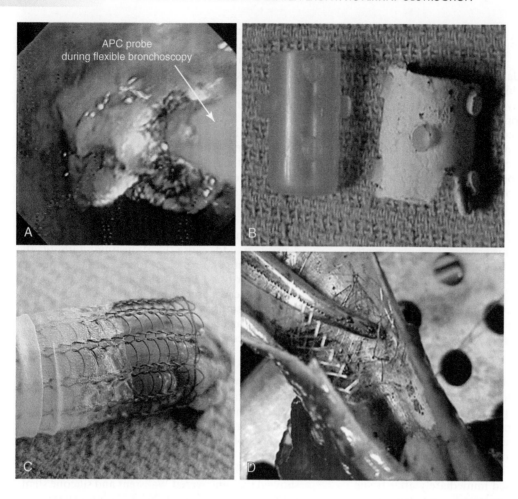

Figure 3-6 A, Argon plasma coagulation (APC) probe is seen in near contact mode with granulation tissue during flexible bronchoscopy in vivo. **B,** Damaged silicone stent after APC application at fraction of inspired oxygen (FiO₂) of 1.00. **C,** Melted Ultraflex stent membrane is noted after APC application. **D,** Broken stainless steel uncovered Wallstent wires can cause adjacent tissue damage through their conducting capabilities (note the charred tissue).

one 25 W pulse delivered 4 mm from the target, prompting authors to conclude that the Nd:YAG laser should not be used in patients with indwelling Wallstent, Strecker, and Palmaz metal stents[26] for fear of stent fracture. The importance of coexisting mucus or blood in the setting of indwelling airway stents was also well demonstrated in an in vitro study, in which investigators were able to ignite blood- or soot-covered silicone stents using multiple laser power settings. Clean silicone stents could not be ignited regardless of power density or oxygen concentration.[27]

3. *Argon plasma coagulation (APC):* This procedure is based on argon gas ionization by current, which will lead to thermal tissue destruction. Typically indicated for hemoptysis and malignant exophytic endoluminal obstruction,[28] APC has been used successfully for treating granulation tissue.[29] Because argon plasma is electrically conductive, an electrical spark jumps from the tip of the electrode to the target tissue, creating a thermal effect. The probe should not touch the tissue surface at any time (Figure 3-6); the distance between the probe's distal tip and conductive biologic tissue must be approximately 5 mm or less, and the target tissue must be conductive. Tissue that is dehydrated, carbonized, or denatured will resist the flow of electrical current. In a large prospective study of 364 patients treated

over a 4-year period, authors showed that APC is effective and safe in treating a variety of central airway disorders, including stent obstruction by tumor or granulation tissue (overall 67% success rate) with a complication rate of 3.7%.[30] In a small case series of three patients who developed strictures and stent-related granulation tissue after solid organ transplantation, the success rate of APC was 100% with no complications.[31] When this technique is used, however, a concern is that gas forced into the airway wall may collect within a blood vessel, causing gas embolism. Argon gas is heavy, inert, and 17 times less soluble in the body than carbon dioxide, and it may pass into the systemic circulation. Both cerebral gas embolism and cardiac arrest have been reported after airway applications of APC.[32,33]

Use of APC in the setting of indwelling airway stents was addressed in an experimental in vitro study simulating a patient-care environment where uncovered and covered nitinol (Ultraflex) stents, uncovered and covered Wallstents, and studded silicone stents were deployed in the tracheobronchial tree of a ventilated and oxygenated heart-lung block from an expired pig. APC was performed at power settings of 40 and 80 W using FiO₂ of 0.21, 0.40, and 1.00, and an argon gas flow rate of 0.8 L/min through the flexible bronchoscope. The primary outcome was the time taken for the APC to cause stent damage, defined as discoloration, ignition, or rupture. Airway fires involving all five types of stents consistently occurred in the presence of 100% oxygen at powers of 40 W and 80 W. At lower FiO_2 (0.21 and 0.40), silicone stents were not damaged at 40 W and 80 W. Uncovered Ultraflex stents were undamaged using 40 W at either FiO_2 (0.21 or 0.40), but could be damaged using both FiO_2 levels when the power was increased to 80 W. Covered Ultraflex and both uncovered and covered Wallstents were damaged at both power settings (40 W and 80 W) and FiO_2 (0.21 and 0.40) levels, with a trend toward earlier damage when higher FiO_2 and power were used (see Figure 3-6). When used within the parameters identified in this study (power 40 W, FiO_2 0.21, APC flow rate 0.8 L/min), APC could be a safe method for tissue destruction and could avoid the risk of airway stent ignition, especially if short bursts of APC are employed. The safety limits identified using FiO_2 of 0.4, however, are also important, because some patients undergoing APC may require supplemental oxygen therapy. Nitinol and stainless steel are metals that have high electrical conductivity in comparison with polyurethane and silicone, which are nonconductive plastic materials. These differences in stent properties also explain the easy combustibility of covered metal stents compared with uncovered metal and silicone stents.[34]

4. *Photodynamic therapy (PDT):* With this modality, tissues with the retained photosensitive agent are exposed to laser light. This results in nonthermal tissue destruction. PDT for nonmalignant airway obstruction is not well described, but in animal models of trauma-induced granulation tissue, rabbits that received PDT showed patchy granulation tissue that was only 20% to 30% of the volume of that seen in untreated animals. Although PDT may be a therapeutic alternative for airway stenosis originating from granulation tissue,[35] therapeutic effect is delayed, and multiple procedures may be necessary to remove necrotic debris. Furthermore, in a study comparing PDT versus electrocautery in the treatment of patients with early lung cancer, greater airway stenosis and increased subepithelial fibrosis were seen after treatment with PDT (and Nd:YAG laser).[36]

5. *Cryotherapy:* This treatment can be used for granulation tissue removal provided in a contact mode with cryoprobes. These are placed on target tissues in a succession of adjacent areas in such a way that the freeze zone margins overlap; repeated (usually three) freeze-thaw cycles, each lasting 30 seconds, will lead to tissue destruction. Tissues are subsequently removed with the use of forceps. In the search for an alternative to contact mode cryotherapy, a study of the human airway was performed using surgically resected specimens and noncontact spray cryotherapy to assess safety and histologic effects. Considerable cellular injury to the treated tissue was noted, but the supporting connective matrix was left intact. Long-term pathology findings (>100 days post-treatment) revealed a complete lack of scarring or stricture.[37] The technique consists of applying medical-grade liquid nitrogen (−196° C) directly to the tissue via a low-pressure, disposable 7-French cryocatheter introduced through the working channel of a therapeutic flexible bronchoscope.[38]

6. *Brachytherapy:* The rationale for the use of ionizing radiation in the setting of granulation tissue is based on its successful use in other benign diseases such as keloids, coronary artery restenosis, peripheral vascular restenosis, and heterotopic ossification.[6] Brachytherapy has been shown to successfully reduce the degree of nonmalignant airway obstruction.[39,40] In one study, 80% (15/19) of patients[41] with metal stent–induced granulation tissue responded favorably (a dose of 1000 cGy was applied in each treatment). In another study, investigators used one to two fractions of Ir-192 prescribed to 7.1 Gy at a radius of 1 cm in eight patients. However, the effect of brachytherapy is delayed, and repeat interventions may be necessary.[6]

7. *Stent removal and replacement with self-expanding metallic stents (SEMS):* In their uncovered form, these stents maintain epithelialization and mucociliary clearance but provide a major disadvantage in that they cause significant granulation tissue formation. Clinical reports have estimated that granulation tissue formation occurs in at least 25% to 30% of expanding metallic airway stents.[5,42] This tissue ingrowth can make removal difficult and can result in substantial airway wall trauma (see video on ExpertConsult.com) (Video I.3.2).[43] For our patient, we did not offer this therapy.

Cost-Effectiveness

The most cost-effective management of granulation tissue has not been identified. No direct comparative studies have investigated electrocautery versus any of the other techniques mentioned previously for this patient population, or for patients with malignant obstruction,[44] even though for malignancy, the effects of electrocautery seem to be equivalent to those of the Nd:YAG laser.[45]

Informed Consent

Informed consent was obtained before the procedure was performed, after the patient had been advised of the therapeutic alternatives described earlier; he agreed to proceed with flexible bronchoscopy under moderate sedation. He was informed of the potential need for emergent endotracheal intubation in case of worsening obstruction from edema, debris, or laryngospasm.

Techniques and Results

Anesthesia and Perioperative Care

Electromagnetic interference generated during electrosurgery has several effects on pacemakers and automatic implantable cardioverter-defibrillators (AICDs). Electrocautery can inhibit pacing of stimuli or trigger ventricular pacing. The presence of these devices warrants precautions because their deprogramming has been reported following electrocautery. If the patient's rhythm is not paced, the pacemaker can be inhibited* for the time of the procedure by applying a magnet over the pacemaker on the patient's chest. The magnet inhibits sensing of cardiac or noncardiac electrical events by the pacemaker, which reverts back to the programmed routine upon removal of the magnet. If, however, the patient has a paced rhythm, a technician with instruments required to reprogram the unit should be contacted before electrocautery is used. It is advisable to have the pacemaker's clinical support line number available, to maintain 15 cm between the active electrode and any electrocardiograph (ECG) electrode, and to have resuscitation equipment ready. Although most of these devices have a magnet response, some devices can be programmed to not respond to magnet application, and thus will need a device programmer to change the parameters. It is advisable to contact the manufacturing company to clarify these issues before beginning the procedure. For AICDs, the magnet can temporarily turn off defibrillation therapy without inhibiting pacing.† In addition to procedures requiring electrosurgery, indications for AICD deactivation include ongoing cardiac resuscitation, end-of-life care, inappropriate shocks, and transcutaneous pacing.[46] This patient's rythm was not paced, so a magnet was placed on his chest over the pacemaker site.

We performed the procedure with moderate sedation using 5 mg of midazolam intravenously. Careful management of supplemental oxygen is essential to avoid inadvertent airway injury due to ignition of gases by an electrical spark from a high-frequency generator during bronchoscopy. FiO_2 is maintained below 0.4 (translating to approximately 3 liters/minute or less with use of a nasal cannula) to avoid airway fire.‡

Techniques and Instrumentation

The power setting for electrosurgery is determined by the operator. The usual power is 15 to 30 W, but power may vary according to the physician's technique and the desired effect. For example, for deep coagulation, a 20 W power setting is selected with longer activation times. Increasing power to 40 W leads to higher energy levels at the tip of the probe, resulting in rapid but shallower effects (superficial coagulation). In our patient, we used coagulation mode at a 20 W power setting. The tissue effects of electrocautery depend not only on the settings, but also on patient-related factors. Patients have different tissue impedance according to their age and body mass, and depending on the specific disease process. To provide safe thermal effects without damage to tissue, most electrosurgical generators have an autostop function (it generates an audible tone when active),* which automatically ends current flow when tissue resistance is increased to a preset level, thus avoiding tissue charring and burning. Charred tissues have a tendency to adhere to the probe and interfere with further treatment.

Before the bronchoscope is inserted into the patient's airway, a grounding pad is placed on the patient (on the arm or hip closest to the treatment site). This ensures that a large area of the skin† is covered by the pad to avoid burns as the current exits the body. The grounding pad serves as a conductive plate to complete the electrical circuit between the electrosurgical unit and the active electrode. The surface area must be adequate to disperse the current, so that current density cannot collect in a single spot, causing a burn. Most units have alarms for when a current leak occurs or when the grounding pad is improperly positioned.

Anatomic Dangers and Other Risks

When working with electrosurgery in the upper trachea, one risks thermal injury to the normal mucosa, including the vocal cords, in case the patient coughs excessively or moves his or her head during the procedure. Local anesthesia may be a poor choice when risk of patient movement or coughing may jeopardize the procedure. A relatively immobile field or excellent coordination and scope control are needed for accurate direction of the electrocautery probe. In addition, the patient should be clear of electrically conductive objects, such as an intravenous stand. Padding (i.e., towels) should be placed between any metal and the patient's arms. Because electricity follows the path of least resistance, one should avoid direct skin-to-skin contact points (e.g., fingers to thighs). Jewelry probably should be removed during electrosurgery. Jewelry that must be left on (e.g., a ring that cannot be removed) should be isolated from skin using gauze with nonconductive tape. Attention should be paid to having a well-sedated patient who suddenly may twitch or move during the electrocautery application, because this may occur with neuromuscular stimulation; this can be caused by loose wires or connections on the front or back of the unit, broken wire bundles under insulation, or defective adapters that allow demodulation of current to below the 100 kHz threshold.

Results and Procedure-Related Complications

After induction of moderate sedation, with the patient receiving oxygen via face mask, the flexible bronchoscope (2.8 mm working channel) was introduced through the

---

*Placing a magnet over a permanent pacemaker does not turn the pacemaker off but temporarily "reprograms" the pacer into asynchronous mode.

†With some devices, application of a magnet produces a soft beep for each QRS complex. If the magnet is left on for approximately 30 seconds, the implantable cardioverter-defibrillator (ICD) is disabled and a continuous tone is generated. To reactivate the device, the magnet must be lifted off the area of the generator. After 30 seconds, the beep returns for each QRS complex.

‡Higher FiO_2 (up to 1.0) may be safely used in soft coagulation mode because no electrical arc formation occurs in this mode; therefore no risk of ignition is present.

---

*Without this function, coagulation is stopped by the operator as soon as vapors are seen, and the probe is cleaned of debris and charred tissue.

†Position the patient pad as close as possible to the operative site on a well-vascularized muscular area; one area is on the flank, over the kidney on the latissimus dorsi muscle, with the pad lateral and wrapping around the side; the pad should not be placed over bony prominences, tattoos, or scars or on hairy surfaces.

patient's right nostril. After local laryngeal analgesia was achieved with 300 mg of lidocaine, the scope was advanced through the cords in the patient's subglottis and upper trachea just proximal to the granulation tissue. The electrocautery probe was then inserted, oxygen flow was reduced to 3 L/min and coagulation of granulation tissue was initiated **(see video on ExpertConsult.com)** (Video I.3.3). The optimal activation time for electrocautery (including APC), if possible, is during the patient's exhalation phase or during apnea, when oxygen concentration is lowest. Electrocautery of short duration is applied because the probe is constantly moved along the tumor during the procedure and is mostly tangential to the mucosal surface. Repeat cleaning of the probe may be necessary during the procedure. Also, repeat cycles of coagulation and tissue removal with forceps are necessary when this technique is used. Withholding supplemental oxygen during actual activation avoids any increase in exposure of the electrical energy to high levels of oxygen. A patient with unstable oxygen saturation therefore may require significant time to treat. In our case, the procedure lasted 40 minutes. No procedure-related complications occurred, nor was evidence of airway wall perforation, pneumothorax, or airway fire noted.

Long-Term Management

Outcome Assessment

Granulation tissue removal resulted in immediate improvement in symptoms. The quality of care was satisfactory because restoring airway patency via flexible bronchoscopy allowed us to avoid the risk of general anesthesia and its potential complications.

Follow-up Tests and Procedures

Some operators perform surveillance flexible bronchoscopy every 3 to 6 months as part of routine evaluation of stent patency.[41] The value of this practice is questionable, and evidence indicates that routine follow-up bronchoscopy with lack of symptoms is not warranted in all patients with indwelling airway stents.[47] Clinical judgment has to be applied, however, on a case-by-case basis. In this patient, who had developed significant obstructing granulation tissue with stridor, we proceeded with surveillance flexible bronchoscopy after 8 weeks. At that time, the stent was still patent.

Quality Improvement

We did not objectively quantify the amount of granulation tissue. Some investigators grade the amount of granulation tissue on a 4-point scale: 0, no granulation tissue; 1, mild (less than 25%) obstruction; 2, moderate (25% to 50%) obstruction; and 3, severe (above 50%) obstruction.[41] Nor did we perform a multidetector computed tomography (MDCT) scan. MDCT might be a noninvasive imaging alternative to diagnostic bronchoscopy for the detection of stent complications. One study showed that MDCT accurately detected 29 of 30 (97%) complications diagnosed by bronchoscopy in 21 patients who underwent stent placement (11 of the 21 stents were metallic). In one false-negative case, MDCT failed to detect a stent fracture. No false-positive

diagnoses of stent complications were reported. However, this study examined granulation tissue and secretions, which together were responsible for 13 of 30 (43%) detected complications.[48] We propose that distinguishing between the two before bronchoscopy is important because procedural preparation may be different. For instance, if granulation tissue is the cause of obstruction, rigid bronchoscopy may be planned, or, alternatively, a therapeutic scope should be available to perform APC, cryotherapy, or electrocautery. On the other hand, if mucus plugging is the culprit for obstruction seen on MDCT, flexible bronchoscopy with therapeutic aspiration of secretions may suffice. MDCT may be useful if the stent needs to be replaced because a custom stent can be designed on the basis of measurements obtained by MDCT.[48]

DISCUSSION POINTS

1. Describe three indications for granulation tissue removal.
   - *Dyspnea:* results from airflow obstruction and increased work of breathing
   - *Hemoptysis:* a consequence of mechanical trauma caused by the stent (see Figures 3-3 and 3-4)
   - *Secretion retention:* results from inability to raise mucus caused by mucociliary impairment (stent-related) due to obstructing granulation tissue
2. Describe the principles of cutting and coagulation when endobronchial electrocautery and argon plasma coagulation are used.

   Endobronchial electrocautery is a monopolar technique because current passes from the electrode and completes the circuit through an electrical plate on the patient's skin. High-frequency generators are capable of producing temperatures that change cells. As current moves through tissue, electrons collide with molecules of the tissue, causing dissipation of energy in the form of heat, which is proportionate to the duration of application and the amount of energy and tissue resistance. Ideally, tissue is desiccated without carbonization, because carbonization can slow the cellular process of healing.
   - *Cutting:* This is done at high voltages (>200 V) to create an electrical arc between electrode and tissue, leading to immediate vaporization
   - *Coagulation:* This is achieved by heating tissues ($\approx 70°$ C) while avoiding vaporization (>100° C) and carbonization (>200° C)
     - *Soft coagulation:* Voltage currents are less than 200 V and unmodulated; the electrode is in direct contact with the tissue, avoiding electrical arc formation and carbonization.
     - *Forced coagulation (desiccation):* This procedure uses higher-voltage modulated currents (>500 V) but creates electrical arcs and may cause carbonization
     - *Spray coagulation (fulguration):* High-voltage (>2000 V), strongly modulated currents are used, leading to surface coagulation when used in a noncontact mode (in a contact mode, the effect is cutting).

- *APC:* This noncontact mode electrocautery is similar to spray coagulation, but the electrical arc between electrode and tissue is conducted via ionized argon gas continuously flowing from the tip of the probe. The usual settings for pulmonary applications include coagulation mode at 45 to 60 W and gas flow at 0.3 to 1 L/min.*
  - *Coagulation* is superficial (3 mm) and is more controlled than with spray coagulation in terms of smoke production and carbonization.[†]
  - *Cutting* is not an effect of APC; in fact, no risk of cutting is present because the actual tip of the electrode is inside the distal aspect of the probe and cannot be in direct contact with the tissues.[‡]

3. Describe two potential complications resulting from electrosurgery in this patient.
- Airway wall injury[22,49]
  - *Early:* This occurs as mucosal ulceration and inflammation potentially leading to cartilaginous destruction.
  - *Delayed:* This is seen as fibrosis and stenosis if the coagulation was performed circumferentially; it results from retractile scar formation and loss of cartilaginous support.
- Airway fire
  - Can be seen in all modes that generate an electrical arc (cutting, forced coagulation, APC[§]) but not in the soft coagulation mode
  - Tends to occur when the FiO_2 is above 0.4, or when electrosurgery is performed too close to a flammable material (stent, endotracheal tube, suction catheter)

4. List and explain three mechanisms of pathogenesis for granulation tissue formation.

   In granulation tissue formation, the balance between synthesis and breakdown of the matrix is lost in a sequence of events divided into three overlapping phases[14]:
- *Inflammation:* With edema and erythema in the thin mucosal layer, inflammation occurs within a few hours after subendothelial tissue exposure. The tracheal stretching and expansion that occur during respiration, head movement, and irritation may contribute to mechanical irritation of the mucosa and may produce cytokines that induce formation of granulation tissue. When the causative process persists, such as chronic irritation from the stent, ulceration develops. This phase includes release of inflammatory mediators (prostaglandins, interleukins 1 and 6, tumor necrosis factor [TNF]-α, and TGF-β) that increase blood vessel permeability and enhance inflammatory cell migration and accumulation.* The immunosuppression state, such as that seen in lung transplant recipients, may have an inhibitory effect on granulation tissue formation.[6] In fact, results of studies show that granulation tissue formation was significantly less in transplant recipients than in nontransplant patients at 3 months', 15 months', and 18 months' follow-up. During 2 years of follow-up, transplant recipients underwent significantly fewer laser resections and brachytherapy treatments for stent-related granulation.
- *Proliferation:* This phase is associated with epithelialization and angiogenesis. Cytokines involved are platelet-derived growth factor, VEGF, interleukin (IL)-1, IL-6, TGF-β, and fibroblast growth factor. During this phase, fibroblasts, macrophages, keratinocytes, and endothelial cells proliferate. Elastin and collagen proliferation leads to the formation of new connective tissue in which new vessels are present (granulation tissue). Indeed, microscopic examination of granulation tissue reveals an increase in angiogenesis and deposition of extracellular matrix. Studies show that $TGF-\beta_1$ released from epithelial cells stimulates fibroblasts to produce VEGF, which, in turn, induces angiogenesis and contributes to the formation of granulation tissue.[13] Production of VEGF indicates neovascularization, which characterizes tissue repair following injury. The highest levels of VEGF expression are noted in the submucosal layers.
- *Maturation:* This phase is controlled by epidermal growth factor and TGF-β. A mature scar is formed as remodeling occurs and tensile strength is gained. Microscopic examination of these tissues reveals deposition of extracellular matrix.[12] In biopsy specimens from stent stenoses, immunoreactive $TGF-\beta_1$[†] was principally localized extracellularly in association with subepithelial connective tissue. $TGF-\beta_1$ showed moderate to strong expression in the subepithelium but was rarely expressed in the epithelial cells. In contrast to $TGF-\beta_1$, Ki-67, which is a crucial marker for proliferation, could be detected, mainly in the epithelium but not in the subepithelium.

---

*APC should be avoided in an oxygen-rich environment; APC in the presence of foreign materials such as stents should be performed using short 1 to 2 second bursts and a lower 40 W power setting.

[†]Good technique with APC includes brief tissue rest time between activations. This cooling and shrinkage of tissue gives the physician a more accurate assessment of the depth of penetration from previous activations. Constant movement helps to assure that energy is not overly concentrated in one area.

[‡]Users may try manipulating the probe rather than the scope/probe continuum. The scope optical chip will set the correct viewing distance, allowing the physician consistent depth perception if the probe remains stationary. The physician may want to touch the tissue then pull back 1 to 3 mm before firing to set his visual cues for proximity to the tissue.

[§]Argon gas itself is not combustible, nor does it promote the combustion of combustible materials. Ignition is possible only if a combustion-promoting gas such as oxygen is also present or is mixed with the argon and applied to the combustible materials.

---

*These mediators are produced mainly by macrophages, which also accelerate nitric oxide synthesis by producing IL-1 and TNF-α.

[†]Enhanced $TGF-\beta_1$–mediated proliferation of human lung fibroblasts occurs in a dose-dependent manner in the presence of mitomycin-C. The local milieu with high-level, matrix-associated expression of $TGF-\beta_1$ in stenoses could therefore be one reason for the limited treatment effect of mitomycin-C.

Expert Commentary

provided by Martin J. Phillips, MBBS, MD, FRACP

This case illustrates the problem of stent obstruction with granulation tissue, a phenomenon that can occur with any stent but is more common with expandable metallic than with silicone stents. The patient was a 75-year-old man who had developed a severe complex post intubation tracheal stenosis, which was treated initially with laser-assisted mechanical dilation at rigid bronchoscopy. Within 3 weeks, the stricture had recurred and required further rigid bronchoscopy and insertion of a straight 12 × 40 mm silicone stent. After another 2 months, the proximal portion of the stent was almost completely obstructed with granulation tissue, which was removed with electrocautery via flexible bronchoscopy under moderate sedation.

I completely agree with the authors' decision to avoid using Nd:YAG laser in this patient. The authors rightly emphasize the precautions that need to be taken when granulation tissue adjacent to a stent is treated. Stent material is highly flammable at high temperatures in the presence of oxygen, and ignition may be further enhanced with increased absorption of laser energy by pigmented tissues, including by silicone when the stent itself is spotted with char tissue. Use of electrocautery to clear the granulation tissue is justified because it is a safe and effective modality if necessary precautions are taken.

An alternative approach worth considering is the use of argon plasma diathermy, also known as argon plasma coagulation (APC), at a power setting of 30 to 40 W delivered in short bursts. The electrical current, which is conducted in the argon plasma, arcs from the electrode to the nearest grounded conductive material, which in this case would be tissue. The silicone stent material is not a good conductor, and the current therefore preferentially goes to tissue, which becomes denatured. Nevertheless, it is possible for the stent to catch fire if tissue adjacent to it is flammable or reaches a high temperature.[34] The potential advantage of APC diathermy is that it may not penetrate so deeply as electrocautery* and therefore may be less likely to induce additional local fibrosis and inflammatory reactions. The risk of argon emboli is lessened if short bursts are used in a space that is not too confined so that excessive pressures are avoided. This should be possible in treating granulation tissue at the proximal end of the stent.

Another alternative is cryotherapy-assisted tissue removal. Rather than using the freeze-thaw technique generally employed for debulking endobronchial tumor—a technique with delayed action—a short freeze time of 3 to 5 seconds or so might allow granulation tissue to be pulled away from the stent orifice. Clearly no risk of thermal damage to the stent is present, and underlying cartilaginous structures within the trachea are protected. A little local bleeding may occur, although usually this is easily controlled.*

The authors used a flexible bronchoscope with moderate sedation, partly in accord with the patient's preference to avoid general anesthesia (GA), which clearly needs to be respected. The patient had a background history of COPD, as well as coronary artery disease and coronary artery bypass graft surgery. Bronchoscopy should be avoided if possible within 6 weeks of a myocardial infarction,[50] but this was not an issue for this patient. The patient had no history of ischemic symptoms following his cardiac surgery; it was therefore reasonable to proceed to bronchoscopy without further cardiac evaluation.[17] The patient's medication use would be checked to determine whether he was receiving anticoagulation, aspirin, or clopidogrel. Oral anticoagulation should be stopped 3 to 5 days before the procedure or reversed by vitamin K if the situation is more urgent and tissue removal is anticipated. Heparin can be given in the interim if necessary and stopped just before the procedure is performed. Procedures usually can be undertaken in the presence of aspirin therapy, but clopidogrel confers significant risks of bleeding[51] and should be ceased 5 to 7 days beforehand. Other common causes of prolonged bleeding include thrombocytopenia, which requires platelet transfusion if the platelet count is less than 50,000, and uremia. Apart from the use of electrocautery or APC diathermy, bleeding usually can be controlled with tamponade and topical application of 1:10,000 adrenaline (epinephrine) solution or cold saline.

It is difficult to estimate the severity of this patient's underlying COPD. If the reported FEV_1 of 40% predicted was taken in the context of his tracheal stenosis, the stenosis itself is likely to be the dominant factor, and treatment of the stenosis clearly would improve the patient's condition. In COPD with an FEV_1 of less than 40% predicted and hypoxemia, arterial blood gas tensions should be measured to determine whether the partial pressure of carbon dioxide (PCO_2) is elevated; this would necessitate caution with oxygen supplementation. A clue to the nature of this patient's problem could come from physiologic tests such as an inspiratory/expiratory flow-volume loop, which may show characteristic blunting, or computed tomography (CT) scans, which might demonstrate the structural abnormality. The severity of the obstruction with a stenosis of 4 mm diameter clearly necessitated intervention, regardless of COPD.

Had the patient been amenable to rigid bronchoscopy under GA, I would have been inclined to use this approach in view of the almost complete obstruction of the proximal end of the stent with granulation tissue. The patient had no cardiac contraindication to rigid bronchoscopy and had successfully undergone

---

*The depth of coagulation necrosis with electrocautery is 0.2 mm for 1 second bursts, but 1.9 mm with 5 second bursts. Tissue damage underneath the necrosis measures about 0.7 mm at 5 seconds. This results in overall histologic changes of ≈2.6 mm,[22] which is similar to APC (up to 3 mm). The pressure by which the electrocautery probe is pushed against the airway wall may affect the extent of tissue damage and, in practice, bronchoscopists use "soft palpation," a subjective parameter that is not an issue with APC, a noncontact modality.

---

*By local application of cold saline, epinephrine, and tamponade with the bronchoscope.

such procedures on two previous occasions. In my opinion, rigid bronchoscopy provides advantages in the presence of significant central airway obstruction because it allows the following:

1. Better ventilation (down a hollow tube rather than around a solid one).
2. Better control of bleeding (by tamponading of the bleeding area with the rigid scope; by aspiration of blood and clots with large suction catheters; and by maintenance of better vision with the ability to quickly clean the telescope or flexible scope).
3. Better removal of obstructing tissue with large forceps and suckers.

Granulation tissue developed rapidly after stent insertion in this patient's case. Such a reaction can occur as a result of movement of the stent relative to the airway during inspiration and expiration. Oversizing of the stent is a recognized contributing factor in the development of granulation tissue. In this instance, I wonder whether the stent may have been a little too short for the area of inflammation evident after the initial dilation. It might have been worth considering resizing the stent and replacing the current one with an hourglass silicone stent 50 mm in length. The hourglass configuration has a narrower central section, which would accommodate the area of maximal stenosis, and has wider diameter flanges, which might better approximate to the more normal dimensions of the trachea adjacent to the stenosed region. In my experience, this configuration also assists in preventing migration of the stent.

The authors mention the use of medical therapies in the treatment of granulation tissue. Such interventions are given with the intent of modulating the development of granulation tissue and fibrosis, rather than as a means of removal. As stated in the text, no conclusive evidence indicates that these therapies are of benefit, although mitomycin-C and intralesional steroids are frequently advocated, and of these, mitomycin-C has the most supportive evidence. Rojas-Solano and Becker[52] provide a good description of mitomycin-C applied by soaking a cotton swab in a solution of 0.4 mg/mL and using forceps to hold the swab for 5 minutes against the region to be treated. I have used this technique on occasion, as well as an alternative technique of local injections of 40 mg of Solu-Medrol, dissolved in 2 mL of saline, into the inflamed and treated area. This may be accomplished using a transbronchial aspiration needle without a side-hole and preferably short in length (i.e., 13 mm or less). The solution of methylprednisolone can be injected into the submucosa of the airway in small aliquots of 0.1 to 0.2 mL. The direction of the needle is coaxial with the airway, and a small mucosal bleb can often be seen, giving further reassurance that the needle is not perforating the wall of the airway (see video on Expert-Consult.com) (Video I.3.4). It is difficult to judge the potential benefits of such treatments on the basis of anecdotal experience, but I sometimes employ them when inflammation post dilation is significant, or when recurrence of stenosis occurs frequently.

REFERENCES

1. Ernst A, Feller-Kopman D, Becker HD, et al. Central airway obstruction. *Am J Respir Crit Care Med.* 2004;169:1278-1297.
2. Dalupang JJ, Shanks TG, Colt HG. Nd-YAG laser damage to metal and silicone endobronchial stents: delineation of margins of safety using an in vitro experimental model. *Chest.* 2001;120:934-940.
3. Matt BH, Myer CM 3rd, Harrison CJ, et al. Tracheal granulation tissue: a study of bacteriology. *Arch Otolaryngol Head Neck Surg.* 1991;117:538-541.
4. Freitag L. Airway stents. In: Strausz J, Bolliger CT, eds. *Interventional Pulmonology.* Lausanne, Switzerland: European Respiratory Society; 2010:190-217.
5. Saad CP, Murthy S, Krizmanich K, et al. Self-expandable metallic airway stents and flexible bronchoscopy: long-term outcomes analysis. *Chest.* 2003;124:1993-1999.
6. Tendulkar RD, Fleming PA, Reddy CA, et al. High-dose-rate endobronchial brachytherapy for recurrent airway obstruction from hyperplastic granulation tissue. *Int J Radiat Oncol Biol Phys.* 2008;70:701-706.
7. Brichet A, Verkindre C, Dupont J, et al. Multidisciplinary approach to management of postintubation tracheal stenoses. *Eur Respir J.* 1999;13:888-893.
8. Patelli M, Gasparini S. Post-intubation tracheal stenoses: what is the curative yield of the interventional pulmonology procedures? *Monaldi Arch Chest Dis.* 2007;67:71-72.
9. Zias N, Chroneou A, Tabba MK, et al. Post tracheostomy and post intubation tracheal stenosis: report of 31 cases and review of the literature. *BMC Pulm Med.* 2008;8:18.
10. Martinez-Ballarin JI, Diaz-Jimenez JP, Castro MJ, et al. Silicone stents in the management of benign tracheobronchial stenoses: tolerance and early results in 63 patients. *Chest.* 1996;109:626-629.
11. Colt HG. Functional evaluation before and after interventional bronchoscopy. In: Bolliger CT, Mathur PN, eds. *Interventional Bronchoscopy.* Basel, Switzerland: S. Karger; 2000:55-64.
12. Karagiannidis C, Velehorschi V, Obertrifter B, et al. High-level expression of matrix-associated transforming growth factor-beta1 in benign airway stenosis. *Chest.* 2006;129:1298-1304.
13. Lee YC, Hung MH, Liu LY, et al. The roles of transforming growth factor-β1 and vascular endothelial growth factor in the tracheal granulation formation. *Pulm Pharmacol Ther.* 2011;24:23-31.
14. Hirshoren N, Eliashar R. Wound-healing modulation in upper airway stenosis—myths and facts. *Head Neck.* 2009;31:111-126.
15. Maddox TM. Preoperative cardiovascular evaluation for noncardiac surgery. *Mt Sinai J Med.* 2005;72:185-192.
16. Eagle KA, Rihal CS, Mickel MC, et al. Cardiac risk of noncardiac surgery: influence of coronary disease and type of surgery in 3368 operations. CASS Investigators and University of Michigan Heart Care Program. Coronary Artery Surgery Study. *Circulation.* 1997;96:1882-1887.
17. Eagle KA, Berger PB, Calkins H, et al, American College of Cardiology, American Heart Association. ACC/AHA guideline update for perioperative cardiovascular evaluation for noncardiac surgery—executive summary: a report of the American College of Cardiology/American Heart Association Task Force on Practice Guidelines (Committee to Update the 1996 Guidelines on Perioperative Cardiovascular Evaluation for Noncardiac Surgery). *J Am Coll Cardiol.* 2002;39:542-553.
18. Smetana GW, Lawrence VA, Cornell JE, American College of Physicians. Preoperative pulmonary risk stratification for noncardiothoracic surgery: systematic review for the American College of Physicians. *Ann Intern Med.* 2006;144:581-595.
19. Harris S. COPD and coping with breathlessness at home: a review of the literature. *Br J Community Nurs.* 2007;12:411-415.
20. Fisher L, Weihs KL. Can addressing family relationships improve outcomes in chronic disease? Report of the National Working Group on Family-Based Interventions in Chronic Disease. *J Fam Pract.* 2000;49:561-566.
21. Coulter TD, Mehta AC. The heat is on: impact of endobronchial electrosurgery on the need for Nd-YAG laser photoresection. *Chest.* 2000;118:516-521.
22. van Boxem TJ, Westerga J, Venmans BJ, et al. Tissue effects of bronchoscopic electrocautery: bronchoscopic appearance and histologic changes of bronchial wall after electrocautery. *Chest.* 2000;117:887-891.

23. Staehler G, Halldorsson T, Langerholc J, et al. Dosimetry for neodymium:YAG laser applications in urology. *Lasers Surg Med.* 1980;1:191-197.
24. Halldorsson T, Langerholc J, Senatori L. Thermodynamic analysis of laser irradiation of biological tissue. *Appl Optics.* 1978;17: 3984-3985.
25. Fisher JC. The power density of a surgical laser beam: its meaning and measurement. *Lasers Surg Med.* 1983;2:301-315.
26. Witt C, Schmidt B, Liebetruth J, et al. Nd: YAG laser and tracheobronchial metallic stents: an experimental in vitro study. *Lasers Surg Med.* 1997;20:51-55.
27. Scherer TA. Nd:YAG laser ignition of silicone endobronchial stents. *Chest.* 2000;117:1449-1454.
28. Morice RC, Ece T, Ece F, et al. Endobronchial argon plasma coagulation for treatment of hemoptysis and neoplastic airway obstruction. *Chest.* 2001;119:781-787.
29. Colt HG. Bronchoscopic resection of Wallstent-associated granulation tissue using argon plasma coagulation. *J Bronchol.* 1998;5: 209-212.
30. Reichle G, Freitag L, Kullmann HJ, et al. Argon plasma coagulation in bronchology: a new method—alternative or complementary? *Pneumologie.* 2000;54:508-516.
31. Keller CA, Hinerman R, Singh A, et al. The use of endoscopic argon plasma coagulation in airway complications after solid organ transplantation. *Chest.* 2001;119:1968-1975.
32. Kono M, Yahagi N, Kitahara M, et al. Cardiac arrest associated with use of an argon beam coagulator during laparoscopic cholecystectomy. *Br J Anaesth.* 2001;87:644-646.
33. Reddy C, Majid A, Michaud G, et al. Gas embolism following bronchoscopic argon plasma coagulation: a case series. *Chest.* 2008;134:1066-1069.
34. Colt HG, Crawford SW. In vitro study of the safety limits of bronchoscopic argon plasma coagulation in the presence of airway stents. *Respirology.* 2006;11:643-647.
35. Nakagishi Y, Morimoto Y, Fujita M, et al. Photodynamic therapy for airway stenosis in rabbit models. *Chest.* 2008;133:123-130.
36. van Boxem AJ, Westerga J, Venmans BJ, et al. Photodynamic therapy, Nd-YAG laser and electrocautery for treating early-stage intraluminal cancer: which to choose? *Lung Cancer.* 2001;31:31-36.
37. Krimsky WS, Broussard JN, Sarkar SA, Harley DP. Bronchoscopic spray cryotherapy: assessment of safety and depth of airway injury. *J Thorac Cardiovasc Surg.* 2010;139:781-782.
38. Krimsky WS, Rodrigues MP, Malayaman N, et al. Spray cryotherapy for the treatment of glottic and subglottic stenosis. *Laryngoscope.* 2010;120:473-477.
39. Kramer MR, Katz A, Yarmolovsky A, et al. Successful use of high dose rate brachytherapy for nonmalignant bronchial obstruction. *Thorax.* 2001;56:415-416.
40. Kennedy AS, Sonett JR, Orens JB, et al. High dose rate brachytherapy to prevent recurrent benign hyperplasia in lung transplant bronchi: theoretical and clinical considerations. *J Heart Lung Transplant.* 2000;19:155-159.
41. Shlomi D, Peled N, Shitrit D, et al. Protective effect of immunosuppression on granulation tissue formation in metallic airway stents. *Laryngoscope.* 2008;118:1383-1388.
42. Burningham AR, Wax MK, Andersen PE, et al. Metallic tracheal stents: complications associated with long-term use in the upper airway. *Ann Otol Rhinol Laryngol.* 2002;111:285-290.
43. Alazemi S, Lunn W, Majid A, et al. Outcomes, health-care resources use, and costs of endoscopic removal of metallic airway stents. *Chest.* 2010;138:350-356.
44. Tremblay A, Marquette CH. Endobronchial electrocautery and argon plasma coagulation: a practical approach. *Can Respir J.* 2004;11:305-310.
45. Boxem T, Muller M, Venmans B, et al. Nd-YAG laser vs bronchoscopic electrocautery for palliation of symptomatic airway obstruction: a cost-effectiveness study. *Chest.* 1999;116:1108-1112.
46. Saraon TS. Pacemakers and implantable cardioverter defibrillators. http://emedicine.medscape.com/article/780825-overview# MagnetInhibition. Accessed March 6, 2011.
47. Matsuo T, Colt HG. Evidence against routine scheduling of surveillance bronchoscopy after stent insertion. *Chest.* 2000;118: 1455-1459.
48. Dialani V, Ernst A, Sun M, et al. MDCT detection of airway stent complications: comparison with bronchoscopy. *AJR Am J Roentgenol.* 2008;191:1576-1580.
49. Verkindre C, Brichet A, Maurage CA, et al. Morphological changes induced by extensive endobronchial electrocautery. *Eur Respir J.* 1999;14:796-799.
50. British Thoracic Society. Guidelines on diagnostic flexible bronchoscopy. *Thorax.* 2001;56(Suppl 1):i1-i21.
51. Ernst A, Eberhardt R, Wahidi M, et al. Effect of routine clopidogrel use on bleeding complications after transbronchial biopsy in humans. *Chest.* 2006;129:734-737.
52. Rojas-Solano J, Becker HD. Bronchoscopic application of mitomycin-C as adjuvant treatment for benign airway stenosis. *J Bronchol Intervent Pulmonol.* 2011;18:53-56.

Chapter 4

Bronchoscopic Removal of a Broncholith from the Lateral Wall of the Proximal Bronchus Intermedius

---

> This chapter emphasizes the following elements of the Four Box Approach: anatomic dangers and other risks, and results and procedure-related complications.

CASE DESCRIPTION

An 82-year-old woman presented with a 2 year history of chronic dry cough. She was treated empirically with antihistamines/decongestants, bronchodilators, inhaled corticosteroids, and proton pump inhibitors for post nasal drip syndrome, asthma, and gastroesophageal reflux disease (GERD), but her cough did not subside. No clinical evidence of aspiration or dysphagia was noted. The cough significantly affected her quality of life because she had developed urinary incontinence and recurrent syncope with severe coughing. She had no other complaints. She lived alone, and at the time of our encounter, she was accompanied by a friend. Physical examination and vital signs were normal. She had diabetes mellitus well controlled with once-daily long-acting insulin and was on no other medications. She had been exposed to tuberculosis when she was young, but she was never diagnosed or treated for active disease. Cardiac workup included dobutamine stress echocardiography, which was normal. Chest radiography and pulmonary function tests were normal. Videofluoroscopic swallow evaluation, 24 hour pH monitoring, and sinus computed tomography (CT) were normal. Noncontrast chest CT performed by her physician showed a calcified lymph node in the right hilum (Figure 4-1). Bronchoscopy revealed a hard, white-yellowish exophytic endobronchial lesion protruding from the lateral wall of the proximal bronchus intermedius (see Figure 4-1).

DISCUSSION POINTS

1. List and justify the instructions given to the patient before bronchoscopy regarding her nil per os (NPO) status.
2. List three disorders that could have been responsible for this patient's broncholith.
3. List three bronchoscopic methods of removing the broncholith.

---

*Chronic cough is defined as cough lasting longer than 8 weeks.

CASE RESOLUTION

Initial Evaluations

Physical Examination, Complementary Tests, and Functional Status Assessment

The diagnosis of broncholithiasis was made after 2 years of unsuccessful treatment for the most common causes of chronic cough. High intrathoracic pressures (up to 300 mm Hg) and velocities (up to 500 miles/hr) make cough an effective means of clearing the airways of excessive secretions and foreign material; however, these physiologic changes can cause a variety of profound physically and psychosocially adverse occurrences that may lead to a significant decrease in health-related quality of life (HRQL).[1] The spectrum of complications secondary to chronic cough is broad and includes cardiovascular, gastrointestinal, genitourinary, musculoskeletal, neurologic, ophthalmologic, psychosocial, and respiratory conditions, as well as reduced HRQL; our patient had already experienced loss of consciousness and urinary incontinence. Results of studies show that women with chronic cough are more inclined to seek medical attention than men because their HRQL is significantly more adversely affected, and because they are more likely to experience physical problems such as stress urinary incontinence.[2] It is important to exhaust all diagnostic and therapeutic modalities to eliminate cough, if possible, and to not minimize a patient's complaints.

Our patient underwent a thorough diagnostic evaluation for chronic cough* in accordance with American College of Chest Physicians (ACCP) guidelines.[3] She had no evidence of upper airway cough syndrome (aka post nasal drip syndrome), and she did not respond to empirical treatment with antihistamines and decongestants. No clinical or physiologic testing evidence or response to empirical therapy for asthma or GERD was noted. Many clinicians reserve bronchoscopy for patients with chronic cough and suspected lung cancer (based on age and smoking history) even when the chest x-ray is normal. Although bronchoscopy as a primary diagnostic modality is infrequently diagnostic in patients with chronic cough, it may detect laryngeal and tracheobronchial pathology, including broncholithiasis. In our patient, bronchoscopy was performed because the cough persisted after consideration of the most common causes, and because the CT scan suggested possible broncholithiasis, presenting as a

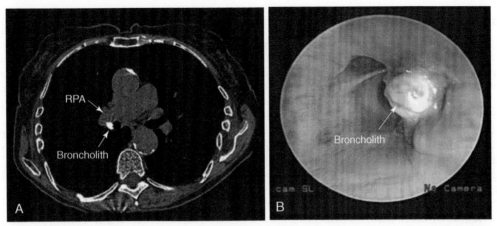

Figure 4-1 A, Axial non–contrast enhanced computed tomography (CT) scan view at the level of the proximal bronchus intermedius. The right pulmonary artery (RPA) is seen adjacent to the high attenuation material, suggesting broncholithiasis; airway involvement could not be confirmed in this study. **B,** Bronchoscopy reveals the penetrating broncholith on the lateral wall of the proximal bronchus intermedius; mild airway compression was noted posterior to the broncholith, but no evidence of granulation tissue or bleeding was observed.

high attenuation lesion; the differential diagnosis of such lesions seen on CT can be narrowed by carefully obtaining a patient history and evaluating other CT findings. In cases of broncholithiasis due to erosion by calcified peribronchial lymph nodes, CT usually shows lymph nodes with or without calcification at other locations and parenchymal changes due to previous infection. Our patient, however, had no such findings. Sometimes calcified peribronchial lymph nodes that do not erode into the bronchial lumen may mimic broncholithiasis. In these situations, diagnosis can be confirmed bronchoscopically. In fact, one study showed that bronchoscopy was diagnostic in 7 of 20 (35%) chronic cough patients with unremarkable chest x-ray and without pulmonary or extrapulmonary cancer.[4] Two of these seven patients (28%) had broncholithiasis. Although chest CT may be diagnostic, it rarely obviates the need for confirmatory bronchoscopy, especially if therapy is planned.

Although it is not a common cause of cough, studies show that patients with broncholithiasis most frequently present with chronic cough (67% of patients) followed by hemoptysis (38% to 66%), lithoptysis (13% to 19%), fever with sputum production (6% to 15%), dyspnea (15%), wheezing (11% to 15%), and chest pain (4%).[5] It is thought that repeated physical impingement of calcified peribronchial lymph nodes on the bronchial wall during respiratory motion is responsible for broncholith formation. When calcified lymph nodes compress or invade the bronchial lumen, changing the bronchial lumen shape, irritating the mucous membrane, and eroding the luminal wall, the previously mentioned clinical manifestations occur, which may lead to recurrent pneumonia or fistulas to the esophagus or the bronchial or even pulmonary artery.[6]

Our patient likely developed broncholithiasis after a pulmonary fungal infection or tuberculosis, even though the lung parenchyma showed no sequelae of prior lung disease. Some cases may be caused by histoplasmosis or by inflammatory stimuli such as silicosis and foreign bodies.[7] Although the most common sequelae of

histoplasmosis are asymptomatic pulmonary calcifications and calcified lymph nodes, for which no intervention is warranted, progressive complications such as pulmonary and mediastinal granulomatous disease, fibrosing mediastinitis, and broncholithiasis can occur. One study reported broncholithiasis in 27% (13/49) of patients with histoplasmosis-related complications.[8] Our patient had no other radiographic findings suggesting histoplasmosis such as calcified lung nodules or splenic granulomas. Consistent with results from published studies, our patient's broncholith was on the right side. Sites of predilection for broncholithiasis are on the right side owing to the greater number of pulmonary lymph nodes.[9] Some studies report that the bifurcation of the right middle lobe and right lower lobe and the bifurcation of the anterior segment of the left upper lobe and the lingular bronchus were also sites of predilection for broncholithiasis, because the bronchi form an acute angle and the bifurcation has no cartilage rings, making it easy for calcified lymph nodes to penetrate into the bronchial lumen.

When combined, CT scanning and bronchoscopy can clearly determine the type of broncholithiasis: intraluminal (free broncholiths) or penetrating (partially eroding broncholiths). This classification is not just of academic interest in that the type of broncholith identified guides management. Intraluminal broncholiths can lead to distal obstructive inflammation, and bronchial lumina might be obstructed by granulation tissues caused by broncholith-induced long-term airway irritation; these may be extracted by flexible or rigid bronchoscopy.[9] Penetrating broncholiths can cause damage to blood vessels and hemoptysis, sometimes even in death. For these patients, although bronchoscopy can be considered in cases of persistent hemoptysis combined with fistulas of trachea, bronchus, or esophagus, or severe secondary pulmonary infection, thoracotomy may be warranted.[5,10] On the basis of CT scan and bronchoscopy, our patient was diagnosed as having a penetrating broncholith with none of the already mentioned complications.

Comorbidities

This patient had diabetes mellitus. Interventions provided under general anesthesia can significantly increase risks for perioperative complications. Careful assessment of diabetic patients before surgery is required because of their high risk of coronary heart disease, which may be relatively asymptomatic compared with the nondiabetic population. Diabetes mellitus is also associated with increased risk of perioperative infection and postoperative cardiovascular morbidity and mortality.[11,12] Although the risk of surgical wound infection is real should thoracotomy be required, cardiac ischemia becomes unlikely in the presence of a negative dobutamine stress echocardiography. No evidence of other diabetes-associated conditions, such as hypertension, chronic kidney disease, cerebrovascular disease, and autonomic neuropathy, was noted; these conditions can complicate anesthesia and postoperative care.

Support System

The patient's age and diabetes mellitus status put her at risk for what is known as *geriatric syndrome,* which comprises functional disabilities, depression, falls, urinary incontinence, malnutrition, and cognitive impairment. Geriatric syndrome leads to frailty, loss of independence, and low quality of life.[13] This patient had no immediate family, but she was close to her friend, who was very supportive. In fact, although she was independent in activities of daily living and did not lack decision-making capacity, she did have an advance directive in the form of durable power of attorney for health care, identifying her friend as the surrogate decision maker for health care in case she lost decision-making capacity.

Patient Preferences and Expectations

Clinicians are not always obligated to grant requests for interventions that are clearly ineffective or that violate their conscience.[14] This patient was able to clearly express her desire for treatment and wanted her cough to improve so she could live a decent life. Her expectations were considered reasonable, and we decided to honor her request because it was within the standard of care. Her friend was involved in these conversations, and both agreed to proceed with available therapeutic options for broncholithiasis.

Procedural Strategies

Indications

A bronchoscopic procedure could be offered to remove the broncholith (broncholithectomy) and improve her disabling cough. Several treatment modalities have been shown to improve symptoms or manage complications related to broncholithiasis. Treatment ranges from nonoperative management (simple observation) to bronchoscopic broncholithectomy and even thoracotomy for patients in whom severe complications develop. Removal of the broncholith in this patient could prevent the development of hemoptysis, atelectasis, post obstructive pneumonia, bronchiectasis, and even bronchoarterial or bronchoesophageal fistulas.[15] Furthermore, removal of

the broncholith and its histologic evaluation would exclude alternative diagnoses that could be associated with or mimic broncholithiasis. For instance, primary endobronchial infection with dystrophic calcification (i.e., calcifications of fungus balls within ectatic bronchi), hypertrophied bronchial arteries with intramural protrusion, calcified endobronchial tumors, and tracheobronchial disease with mural calcification (i.e., tracheopathica osteochondroplastica) all can mimic broncholithiasis.[16]

1. Primary endobronchial actinomycosis could have similar images.[17]
2. Carcinoid tumors may show calcification. This is more common in central carcinoid tumors (39%) than in the peripheral type (8%).[18,19]
3. Hamartoma, when endobronchial, may show a central cartilaginous core and can mimic a broncholith.[20]
4. Tracheobronchial amyloidosis may be localized in the form of a polypoid nodule with calcification, thus mimicking a broncholith.[21]
5. Aspiration of radiopaque fragments or in situ calcification of foreign bodies may present with radiologic findings of tracheobronchial calcified nodules.[16]
6. Other less common calcified endobronchial tumors include osteomas, osteosarcomas, chondromas, and chondrosarcomas.
7. The bronchial arteries may become enlarged in various diseases, including acute or chronic pulmonary infection, pulmonary thromboembolism, and chronic obstructive pulmonary disease.[22] A hypertrophied bronchial artery may protrude into the bronchial lumen, thus mimicking a broncholith at contrast-enhanced CT.[22] Careful analysis of images obtained above and below the abnormality on unenhanced CT sometimes is needed to confirm the vascular nature of the lesion. At bronchoscopy, pulsations of the calcified endobronchial lesion should be carefully sought, before biopsy or removal is considered.

Contraindications

No absolute contraindications to rigid bronchoscopy are known. However, the risk of perioperative cardiac complications should be considered in this elderly patient with a history of diabetes mellitus. Our patient had no clinical signs or symptoms of coronary artery disease and had a normal dobutamine stress echocardiography. Endoscopic procedures (e.g., bronchoscopy) are considered to present low cardiac risk (reported risk of cardiac death or nonfatal myocardial infarction [MI] generally less than 1%), and intrathoracic surgery introduces intermediate risk (reported risk of cardiac death or nonfatal MI generally 1% to 5%).[23]

Expected Results

The objective of the procedure was to remove the endobronchial component of the calcified lymph node without perforating the airway wall and causing hemorrhage. We intended to leave one piece of broncholith embedded in the bronchial wall intact, if necessary, thus avoiding potential bleeding from the immediately adjacent pulmonary artery. Rigid bronchoscopic intubation was planned using a 12 mm diameter Efer-Dumon ventilating rigid bronchoscope (Efer Broncho, Marseilles, France); this scope allows passage of laser fiber, rigid suction catheter, and forceps, and because of the side-holes at its distal aspect, ventilation to the contralateral left lung would be possible while working in the right bronchial tree. Nd:YAG laser would be available should photocoagulation be needed at the area of insertion in the bronchial wall, coagulation of associated granulation tissue, or bleeding. Lasers (Nd:YAG, pulsed-dye, and holmium-yttrium aluminum garnet [Ho:YAG]) were reported to be useful for fragmenting an eroding broncholith that could not be dislodged with a rigid or a flexible bronchoscope, or for fragmenting a mobile broncholith that was too hard to be broken with the biopsy forceps and too large to be pulled through the upper airway.[24-26] Several reports describing use of the laser were limited to removing associated granulation tissue, not the broncholith per se.[27] Others used laser to shatter the broncholith when a significant part of the broncholith protruded into the lumen.[27] The shattering effect described in the literature can be achieved by applying high laser power (80 to 100 W) to the smallest surface area (high-power density) and very short pulses (0.2 to 0.3 second) interspaced by rest periods (2 to 5 seconds) to avoid overheating of the broncholith and the possible resulting popcorn* effect in adjacent tissues.

Success rates as high as 87% for bronchoscopic removal of broncholiths, without life-threatening complications, have been reported.[28,29] The outcome of bronchoscopy depends, however, on the type of broncholithiasis. Several surgical series have reported different outcomes of bronchoscopic broncholithectomy. Among 63 patients studied by Arrigoni et al., broncholiths were removed bronchoscopically from 40 patients (63%) whose bronchoscopies revealed visible broncholiths. The authors concluded that bronchoscopic extraction of a visualized broncholith was "reasonable" as long as irreversible distal bronchial and parenchymal damage had not occurred.[30] Based on their successful bronchoscopic removal of intraluminal broncholiths from eight patients without severe bleeding, Cole et al. likewise concluded that bronchoscopic broncholithectomy was a "useful adjunct" and should be thoughtfully attempted before complications of broncholithiasis occur.[29] Trastek et al. achieved complete bronchoscopic broncholith removal in 8 of 12 patients (66.7%) who underwent bronchoscopic extraction. Broncholithiasis recurred in three of these eight patients, for which one underwent repeat bronchoscopic broncholithectomy, one required right middle lobectomy, and one refused further intervention and died of massive hemoptysis. Three of four patients who underwent unsuccessful bronchoscopic removal attempts went on to surgery.[31] The authors concluded that bronchoscopic broncholithectomy "should probably be reserved for patients who are in poor medical condition." In an older case series, Faber et al. reported bronchoscopic removal in only 2 of 33 patients studied.[32] The authors concluded that bronchoscopic broncholith removal was indicated only if the broncholith was "loose and mobile" and extraction did "not require extensive manipulation."

In one of the largest published studies, bronchoscopic removal of 71 broncholiths (56% of total identified) was attempted in 48 patients (50.5%) during 61 bronchoscopy sessions. Forty-eight of the broncholiths selected for removal were partially eroding into the tracheobronchial lumen, and 23 were free. Forty-eight percent (23 of 48) of the partially eroding broncholiths were successfully removed bronchoscopically; a greater percentage of broncholiths were removed with the rigid bronchoscope (67%) than with the flexible bronchoscope (30%). All free broncholiths were completely extracted regardless of the type of bronchoscope used. Complications occurred in only two patients (4% of the bronchoscopic removal group), both with partially eroding broncholiths, and consisted of hemorrhage in one patient requiring thoracotomy and acute dyspnea in another patient, caused by a loose broncholith lodged in the trachea.[5]

Team Experience

Flexible and rigid bronchoscopic extractions of broncholiths are considered safe and effective.[5] However, when rigid bronchoscopy is performed, the operator needs to be skilled in gently manipulating the scope inside the airway during the broncholithectomy process to avoid airway wall perforation. Furthermore, because concern for hemorrhage is real in this type of broncholithiasis, the team needs to be ready to respond in case of massive intraoperative hemoptysis. This procedure should not be performed in a facility that does not have the necessary equipment to safely manage a patient's hemoptysis.

Risk-Benefit Analysis

Our patient had symptoms that significantly interfered with her quality of life and warranted intervention. No risk-benefit analysis has been performed to compare rigid bronchoscopy with other types of bronchoscopic treatment modalities. Also, no direct comparison studies have been conducted to evaluate bronchoscopy (rigid or flexible) versus thoracotomy. Results of retrospective studies show that a higher frequency of hemoptysis (66% vs. 38%) was seen in the group that did not undergo an attempt at bronchoscopic broncholith removal. Indeed, bleeding at initial bronchoscopic inspection and a firmly embedded broncholith seem to be the most common reasons for not attempting bronchoscopic removal and proceeding with thoracotomy. From the published literature, it is difficult to retrospectively interpret how bronchoscopists decided whether to attempt bronchoscopic removal, how vigorous the extraction efforts were, and why attempts were aborted.[5]

Selection of treatment depends on broncholith size, location, and proximity to the pulmonary artery on the chest CT scan, as well as the patient's symptoms. Similar characteristics of most patients who undergo successful endoscopic removal include a broncholith that is not fixed in the airway (or at least is partially mobile on

---

*Strong exposure of individual spots of tissue to the laser beam leading to strong absorption of laser light by the hemoglobin and vaporization of blood components and vascular walls in the irradiated area; this may cause vascular rupture and hemorrhage.

bronchoscopic probing), is small enough to be removed endoscopically, is proximal enough in the airway to facilitate removal, and is not contiguous with the pulmonary artery on the CT scan. If a broncholith is contiguous with the pulmonary artery, aggressive manipulation is dangerous, and thoracotomy should be considered instead.

Therapeutic Alternatives for Broncholith Removal

- *Observation:* Spontaneous broncholith expectoration (lithoptysis) may occasionally lead to resolution of symptoms, but overall, several studies show that this is rare. The 3 year natural history of asymptomatic patients with broncholithiasis appears to be benign (no progression of disease, either radiologically or by development of symptoms). The nodes do not necessarily rub their way into the airway, cause a fistula between mediastinal structures, or lead to superior vena cava syndrome. This suggests that patients can be followed yearly or perhaps even less stringently with CT scans. Intervention (bronchoscopy or thoracotomy) might not be warranted unless patients become symptomatic. These recommendations pertain to patients without active inflammatory disease and are reserved for those with asymptomatic burnt-out calcified nodal disease.[9] Our patient was symptomatic for 2 years, and simple observation was declined.
- *Flexible bronchoscopic extraction:* This approach seems just as efficacious as rigid bronchoscopy for free broncholiths (100% success rate). For penetrating broncholiths, however, it appears to be less effective than rigid bronchoscopy; a greater percentage of broncholiths are removed with the rigid bronchoscope (67%) than with the flexible bronchoscope (30%).[5] Flexible techniques are similar to foreign body extraction and utilize balloon catheters, forceps, and baskets. Complications include central airway obstruction due to loss of the broncholith during extraction, hemoptysis, and, rarely, death.[33-35]
- *Holmium:YAG laser:* This technique is often used in urology for stone removal, resection or vaporization of prostatic tissue, and treatment of urethral strictures; it has also been used to fragment broncholiths obstructing segmental and central airways. With a wavelength of 2010 nm, well into the infrared spectra, laser energy in part is absorbed by water contained within the stones, causing expansion and fragmentation in a process termed *microexplosion*.[36] The temperature rise in proximity to the laser tip appears to cause a chemical breakdown of the stone, resulting in weakening of the stone and allowing fragmentation without appreciable collateral mechanical or thermal damage. Application of the Ho:YAG laser directly to tissue will cause injury with a penetration depth of approximately 0.4 mm; this might provide some safety margin over the more familiar Nd:YAG laser with a depth of penetration up to 6 mm. The relatively low-energy photothermal effect of the Ho:YAG laser is well suited to destruction of stones in the bronchial tree. Small fragments resulting from laser-induced shattering can be irrigated and suctioned from the airway; larger fragments can be removed with baskets or forceps. The photothermal effect of the Ho:YAG slowly causes disintegration of the stone from within, resulting in smaller fragments and more controlled breakage.
- *Pulsed-dye laser:* This type of laser fragments calculi through a photoacoustic effect. Theoretically, the photoacoustic wave energy of pulsed-dye lasers could propel the stone farther into the airway, potentially causing mechanical collateral damage.
- *Cryotherapy:* This treatment is reported to be successful for partially attached broncholiths for which simple forceps extraction has failed.[37] Cryotherapy has been used for the removal of foreign objects, blood clots, granulation tissue, and mucous plugs, as well as for the management of endobronchial obstruction.[38] Advantages of cryotherapy include ease of use, lower cost compared with laser therapies, and reusability of the cryoprobe after disinfection. Complications include bleeding and airway perforation, especially when intervention includes manipulation of the broncholith stalk.
- *Thoracotomy:* This approach was proposed by clinicians who were concerned about the potential for significant hemorrhage, bronchial tears, or fistula formation when bronchoscopic extraction of broncholiths is attempted. To avoid such complications, on the basis of limited experience, some groups recommend that bronchoscopic removal be completely avoided[39] or limited to patients whose comorbidities preclude surgical intervention.[31] Thoracotomy is also offered when bronchoscopy (rigid and/or flexible) is unsuccessful. Types of surgeries depend on the location of the broncholith and the functionality of the distal lung parenchyma and include broncholithectomy, segmentectomy, lobectomy, bilobectomy, and even pneumonectomy.[5] Complications such as bleeding, fistula, and infection have been reported in 9% to 47% of cases, and death in 0% to 3% of cases. Long-term results usually are excellent with no reported recurrence in 68% to 100% of cases.[40] Most surgeries for broncholithiasis involve pulmonary resection; 80% to 95% of patients require segmentectomy or more extensive resection. Results of several surgical studies for broncholithiasis are summarized in Table 4-1. A review of these reports reveals several common themes. First, usual indications for surgery for broncholithiasis include chronic pulmonary suppurative disease (bronchiectasis), massive hemoptysis, bronchoesophageal fistula, and uncertainty about the diagnosis. Second, the mediastinal and hilar fibrocalcific reactions accompanying broncholithiasis can alter tissue planes, obscure anatomic landmarks, and increase blood vessel fragility in the operative field, making surgical dissection difficult and increasing the risk of complications. Third, long-term results of surgery are usually excellent (see Table 4-1).

Cost-Effectiveness

To our knowledge, no formal cost-effectiveness evaluations of bronchoscopic or surgical modalities have yet been published. In one series, 23 of 48 (48%) partly eroding broncholiths were completely removed

Table 4-1 Complications and Long-Term Outcomes of Surgical Interventions for Broncholithiasis

Reference	Number of Patients Who Underwent Surgery	Complications	Long-Term Outcome
30	n = 68 (of the total 253 patients with BL)	Two patients (3%) died in the immediate postoperative period. Twelve (18%) developed postoperative complications.	Follow-up was available for 59 surgical patients; 50 patients remained completely asymptomatic.
31	n = 40 (of the total 52 patients with BL)	Intraoperative complications occurred in five patients (13%), with one (2.5%) patient dying 3 days later. Postoperative complications occurred in another five (13%) patients.	No surgical patient had recurrent problems with BL, and 15 year survival for the surgical cohort was equivalent to that of a matched control group.
54	n = 20 (of the total 27 patients with BL)	Two (7%) postoperative deaths and two empyemas occurred.	N/A
32	n = 33	Only two patients (6%) developed postoperative morbidities, and no deaths occurred.	N/A
29	n = 25	No perioperative mortality	13 patients had follow-up; all were reported as being well from 3 to 30 years postoperatively.

BL, Broncholithiasis; *N/A*, not available.

bronchoscopically, and only two patients (4% of the bronchoscopic broncholithectomy group) experienced clinically significant complications. As compared with the morbidity and mortality of surgical intervention, bronchoscopic management is favorable in patients with loose or partly eroded broncholiths. Attempts at bronchoscopic extraction of a broncholith ideally should be conducted in a setting with capabilities for rigid and flexible bronchoscopy and immediate thoracic surgical support, and after the relationship of the broncholith to adjacent vascular structures has been studied tomographically. In uncomplicated and loose broncholithiasis, therapeutic bronchoscopy should be chosen first. Surgical resection should be considered when complications occur, and when bronchoscopic removal is unsuccessful.

Informed Consent

After she had been advised of all of the alternatives, our patient elected to proceed with rigid bronchoscopy under general anesthesia. She was informed of the potential risks for massive hemorrhage and the potential need for emergent thoracotomy.

Techniques and Results

Anesthesia and Perioperative Care

Surgery and general anesthesia cause a neuroendocrine stress response resulting in metabolic abnormalities that include insulin resistance, decreased peripheral glucose utilization, impaired insulin secretion, and increased lipolysis and protein catabolism; these may lead to hyperglycemia and even to ketosis in the perioperative period.[41] The hyperglycemic response to these factors may be attenuated by lack of caloric intake during and immediately after surgery (i.e., including NPO orders), making the final glycemic balance difficult to predict. Goals of perioperative diabetic management include maintenance of fluid and electrolyte balance, prevention of

ketoacidosis, avoidance of marked hyperglycemia, and avoidance of hypoglycemia. Patients with type 2 diabetes, as is seen in our patient, are susceptible to developing a nonketotic hyperosmolar state (NKH), which may lead to severe volume depletion and neurologic complications; they may also develop ketoacidosis in the setting of extreme stress. Hypoglycemia is another potentially life-threatening complication of poor perioperative metabolic control.

Even a few minutes of severe hypoglycemia (i.e., serum glucose concentration <40 mg/dL) can be harmful, possibly inducing arrhythmias and cognitive deficits. Hypoglycemia and subsequent neuroglucopenia can be difficult to detect in anesthetized or sedated patients. Ideally, all patients with diabetes mellitus should undergo surgery as early as possible in the morning to minimize disruption of their management routine while they are NPO. Generally, patients who use insulin (type 1 and insulin-dependent type 2) can continue with subcutaneous insulin (rather than an insulin infusion) perioperatively for procedures that are not long and complex. Some clinicians switch patients who are taking long-acting insulin (e.g., glargine) to intermediate-acting insulin 1 to 2 days before surgery because of potentially increased risk for hypoglycemia with the former. However, if the basal insulin is correctly calibrated, it is reasonable to continue long-acting insulin while the patient is NPO and is on intravenous dextrose. No data are available to support one approach over the other. For our patient, who underwent a morning procedure for which breakfast and lunch were likely to be missed, we did not administer any short-acting insulin on the morning of surgery; also, we gave two thirds of a dose of long-acting insulin to provide basal insulin during the procedure and to prevent ketosis. Dextrose-containing intravenous solution (dextrose with water or one half isotonic saline) at a rate of 75 to 125 mL/hr is used to provide 3.75 to 6.25 g glucose/hr to avoid the metabolic changes of starvation.[42] Postoperatively, in this elderly patient with

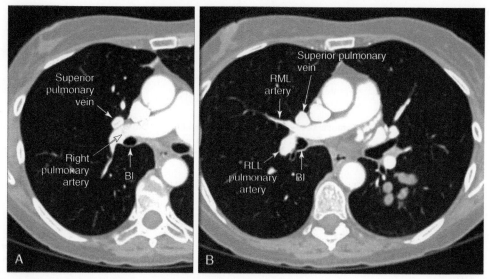

Figure 4-2 Anatomic relationships between bronchus intermedius (BI) and adjacent vessels on contrast-enhanced high-resolution computed tomography (CT). **A,** At the proximal BI level, CT shows the right pulmonary artery just above and to the right of the bronchus; the superior pulmonary vein is above the pulmonary artery. **B,** At the distal BI level, CT shows the right lower lobe artery lateral and the middle lobe artery anterior to the bronchus.

NPO status, frequent, small doses of short-acting insulin (sliding scales) could be used to correct elevated glucose levels, if present.

The operating room should be set up in advance and equipment checked by the surgical team. Because massive bleeding may be encountered, the airway surgeon should make sure that laser equipment is available and that the team has easy access to absorbable hemostats for local hemorrhage control, endobronchial blockers, and double-lumen endotracheal tubes for isolating the right lung and providing ventilation to the left lung. Also, some operators may prefer to consult a thoracic surgeon before intervention in case emergent thoracotomy becomes necessary.

Techniques and Instrumentation

The exact bronchoscopic technique used to remove a particular broncholith (i.e., chipping, crushing, probing, pulling, etc.) is operator dependent. We first use a 12-mm rigid bronchoscope. A flexible bronchoscope can then be easily placed down through the rigid scope, and the entire airway evaluated. The broncholith is identified and probed to determine whether it is fixed to the sides of the airway, or whether it is mobile (see Figure 4-1). If bleeding occurs from vascular granulation tissue or from areas adjacent to the broncholith, Nd:YAG or holmium laser can be used, as previously described. In addition, laser can be used to directly shatter the broncholith in selected patients. Suction catheter and a forceps should be ready to remove the broncholith if it becomes loose after manipulation.

Anatomic Dangers and Other Risks

The risk for complications may be lessened by judicious use of advanced imaging techniques, which enhance the bronchoscopist's knowledge of the relationships of target lesions to critical structures. These techniques may also improve the efficiency of the application of specific endobronchial therapies. Although uncommon, one of the most serious complications that can occur during rigid bronchoscopy with or without the use of lasers includes perforation of the bronchial wall into an adjacent vascular structure and resultant hemorrhage. For a penetrating broncholith, high-resolution CT scanning is needed before extraction to clarify the relationships of the broncholith to the blood vessels. With regard to our patient, at the level of the proximal bronchus intermedius (BI), the interlobar pulmonary artery lies anterior and lateral to the bronchus. The right superior pulmonary vein lies anterior to the right interlobar pulmonary artery (Figure 4-2). Frequently, two veins may be seen in this location and should not be mistaken for lymph node enlargement. Infrequently, a small vein branch draining a portion of the posterior segment of the upper lobe could pass posterior to the BI, then medially at lower levels to join the inferior pulmonary vein.

Results and Procedure-Related Complications

This patient underwent general anesthesia, the neck was extended, and the rigid bronchoscope was inserted through the vocal cords under direct vision. Once the rigid bronchoscope was in the upper trachea, ventilation was carried out through a side channel of the rigid bronchoscope, thus allowing sufficient room to work through the end of the scope concomitantly while still oxygenating and ventilating the patient. The broncholith was reassessed in terms of precise location, extent, and associated mucosal changes. The exophytic endoluminal component extended for 0.5 cm on the lateral wall of the proximal BI, right below the primary right carina. Nd:YAG laser output power was set to 30 W, with 1 second pulses, but the laser was not necessary because no bleeding occurred after resection of the broncholith with the beveled edge of the rigid bronchoscope (see video on

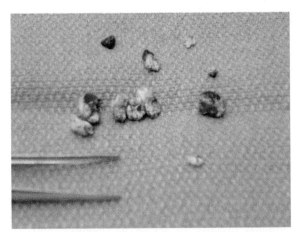

Figure 4-3 Fragments of broncholith composed of calcium phosphate and carbonate. Because fragmentation is common during removal, a complete examination with the flexible bronchoscope is warranted at the end of the procedure to exclude fragment migration in the distal segmental airways.

ExpertConsult.com) (Video I.4.1). No associated granulation tissue was noted; this finding precluded the need for laser treatment. The procedure lasted 30 minutes. The patient tolerated the procedure well and was transferred to the postanesthesia care unit for 2 hours, during which no complications were noted. She was discharged home the next day.

Long-Term Management

Outcome Assessment

The patient's endobronchial broncholith was completely removed (Figure 4-3). No immediate postoperative anesthesia- or procedure-related complications were noted. No bleeding was noticed intraoperatively or in the postoperative period. No perioperative hypoglycemic or hyperglycemic episodes occurred.

Referral

Because the broncholith was removed completely and no evidence of bronchoarterial fistula was observed, a postoperative thoracic surgery consultation was not needed.

Follow-up Tests and Procedures

This patient was scheduled for follow-up on an outpatient basis to monitor for recurrence of respiratory symptoms. At 2 weeks' follow-up, the patient's cough had nearly completely resolved. If her cough should return, a follow-up bronchoscopy would be performed to detect the recurrence of broncholithiasis. Because the exact cause of her broncholithiasis remained undetermined, chest CT scan could be repeated based on clinical grounds to assess the potential for histoplasmosis-associated complications such as progressive mediastinal fibrosis. Although *Histoplasma* is commonly cultured from calcified lymph nodes and broncholiths in asymptomatic patients, no antimicrobial treatment is recommended unless evidence of chronic histoplasmosis or other complications such as granulomatous mediastinitis is noted

in the patient.[43] Our patient's broncholith showed only calcium carbonate. Microbiology was negative for mycobacterial, bacterial, or fungal organisms.

Quality Improvement

Quality of care was considered satisfactory because airway patency had been safely restored, and the patient was discharged home within 24 hours. In our weekly team meeting, we discussed the fact that we did not apply a validated instrument to quantify this patient's HRQL owing to her chronic cough. HRQL may be defined as a patient's perception of the impact of health and disease on multiple domains of his or her life (e.g., physical function, psychosocial state). One cough-specific quality of life questionnaire (CQLQ) has been developed; it includes the subscales of physical complaints, psychosocial issues, functional abilities, emotional well-being, extreme physical complaints, and personal safety fears. This CQLQ was shown to be a valid and reliable method by which to assess the impact of cough on the quality of life of patients with cough, as well as the efficacy of therapies administered to patients with chronic cough.[44] This instrument was studied in 154 patients suffering from chronic cough, among whom 0.6% of patients had broncholithiasis; it is considered a valid method by which to assess the efficacy of cough therapies in patients with chronic cough. We should have used the CQLQ to quantify objectively this patient's HRQL before and after the intervention.

DISCUSSION POINTS

1. List and justify the instructions given to the patient before bronchoscopy regarding her nil per os (NPO) status.
   - Water and other clear liquids, including tea, coffee, soda water, apple, and pulp-free orange juice, are allowed up to 2 hours before anesthesia in otherwise healthy adults, children, and pregnant women not in labor scheduled for elective surgery.[45]
   - The fasting period after intake of solids should not be less than 6 hours.
     - Restrictions for solids include soups, yogurt, and sour milk– or milk-containing drinks.
     - The fasting period is 8 hours for a regular or heavy meal (may include fried or fatty foods, meat) based on American Society of Anesthesiologists (ASA) recommendations.[46]
   - Chewing gum or tobacco in the immediate preoperative period (last 2 hours before induction) is discouraged because these have been shown to increase gastric content.
   - Up to 150 mL of water together with oral medication up to 1 hour before induction of anesthesia is safe in adults.[47]
   - These guidelines are justified by controlled studies and meta-analyses done in different countries in both adult males and adult females[45]; these NPO recommendations were shown to be safe and do not increase gastric fluid volume or acidity.
   - Some patients are more likely to regurgitate under anesthesia, including those who are pregnant,

elderly, or obese, and those who have stomach disorders (obstruction, hiatal hernia, gastroparesis from diabetes mellitus). More research is needed to determine whether these people can safely drink up to a few hours before surgery[48]; patients probably should be fasted after intake of solids for longer than 6 hours.

2. List three disorders that could have been responsible for this patient's broncholith.
   - Previous mycobacterial or fungal infections could result in calcified hilar and mediastinal lymph nodes and potentially in broncholithiasis[7]; among these, the most common are:
     - Tuberculosis
     - Histoplasmosis
     - Coccidioidomycosis

3. List three bronchoscopic methods of removing the broncholith.
   - Flexible bronchoscopy extraction using balloons and forceps
     - For free broncholiths (100% success)
     - For penetrating broncholiths (30% success)[5]
   - Flexible bronchoscopy with cryotherapy: reported to be successful for partially attached broncholiths that failed forceps extraction[37]
   - Rigid or flexible bronchoscopy with laser: used to fragment a mobile broncholith that was too hard to be broken with the biopsy forceps and was too large to be pulled through the upper airway
     - Pulsed-dye[24]
     - Nd:YAG[25]
     - Ho:YAG[26]

Expert Commentary

provided by Udaya B. S. Prakash, MD

To summarize, the case described is that of an 82-year-old woman with a 2 year history of troublesome chronic dry cough leading to urinary incontinence and recurrent post-tussive syncope. Her cough was refractory to empirical treatment, which included antihistamines/decongestants, bronchodilators, inhaled corticosteroids, and proton pump inhibitors for post nasal drip syndrome, asthma, and GERD. Her only active comorbid condition, diabetes mellitus, was well controlled with once-daily insulin.

Apparently, the chest radiograph was reported to be normal. On the other hand, noncontrast chest CT showed a calcified lymph node in the right hilum (see Figure 4-1). This led to the possibility of broncholithiasis, which was confirmed by bronchoscopy (see Figure 4-1). Following appropriate preoperative preparation of the patient, she was subjected to general anesthesia, and the broncholith was successfully extracted using a rigid bronchoscope.

This case should alert clinicians to consider a number of issues. These include the difficulty and hence the delay in diagnosis, the causes of broncholithiasis, clinical and diagnostic aspects, and treatment options. All of these are covered in detail in the case discussion. The following require emphasis:

1. Was this patient's chronic cough caused by the broncholith?
   The answer is clear in that her cough resolved after the broncholith was successfully extracted.

2. Why did it take longer than 2 years to arrive at the proper diagnosis?
   Broncholithiasis is an uncommon cause of cough and is seldom considered in the differential diagnosis of chronic cough.[49] In the absence of roentgenologic abnormalities, etiologic considerations of chronic cough frequently follow the well-known clinical practice of trying to diagnose and treat common causes such as asthma, post nasal drainage, postinfectious cough, and gastroesophageal reflux. A commonly overlooked but nonetheless important fact is that radiologists and clinicians alike often ignore calcified granulomas on chest roentgenographs. The common occurrence of this abnormality causes it to not be considered in the causation of undiagnosed chronic cough. Even when chest CT reveals calcified lymph nodes or calcified granulomas adjacent to a bronchial lumen, broncholithiasis is rarely taken into account.

3. What caused broncholithiasis in this patient?
   Broncholiths are calcified peribronchial lymph nodes that partially erode the bronchial lumen or become loose foreign bodies in the airway. In the United States, the most common cause of broncholith formation is previous fungal granulomatous lymphadenitis due to infection by *Histoplasma capsulatum*. Other causes are discussed in detail in the case discussion. The patient discussed in the chapter most likely had histoplasmosis-induced broncholithiasis.

4. What are the mechanisms that cause symptoms?
   When a calcified lymph node or a pulmonary parenchymal granuloma is located away from the vicinity of the bronchus, it is sometimes referred to as a *pulmolith* or a *pneumolith*. These abnormalities, when anatomically located closer to a bronchial lumen, have the potential to become broncholiths. Gradual tracheobronchial impingement occurs as a result of the interaction of fibrocalcific changes with the repetitive visceral motions of respiration, circulation, and deglutition.[32,50] Asymptomatic broncholithiasis is extremely uncommon. Indeed, symptoms appear when the calcified lymph node impinges on or erodes into the airway lumen. Bronchial distortion, irritation, and erosion by broncholiths can cause chronic cough, hemoptysis, stone expectoration (lithoptysis), recurrent pneumonia, and fistulas between bronchi and adjacent mediastinal structures.[5] It is important to note that the history of lithoptysis is rarely forthcoming unless the patient is specifically asked about it.

5. How is broncholithiasis diagnosed?
   The singularly important step is to suspect the diagnosis when radiologic images show calcified

densities close to the central airways. Chest CT may be necessary for acquiring a better understanding of the relationship between the calcified lesion, airways, and vascular structures. Bronchoscopy often is the only test given to document a diagnosis of broncholithiasis; it should not be withheld when clinical suspicions are strong.

6. Is an invasive therapeutic approach required?

Most symptomatic patients require an invasive bronchoscopic or surgical technique to remove the broncholith. Occasionally, patients cough out fragments of a broken broncholith over a period of time until the entire calcified lesion is expectorated. In this case, most of the broncholith resides outside the bronchial lumen; with frequent coughing, the endoluminal portion breaks off and is expectorated. Until the next piece of the broncholith enters the airway lumen, symptoms may disappear, albeit briefly. Minimally symptomatic patients may not require immediate therapy, and periodic observation seems prudent. Massive hemoptysis caused by broncholithiasis is a rare complication; only three cases of death from broncholith-associated massive hemoptysis have been reported in the literature.[51-53]

7. Was rigid bronchoscopy necessary in this patient?

The decision to use the rigid bronchoscope is debatable. If the initial flexible bronchoscopic examination had revealed a loose endoluminal broncholith, I would have attempted flexible bronchoscopic extraction under deep sedation. Gentle nudging of the broncholith with the tip of the flexible bronchoscope may loosen a loosely adherent broncholith, which then can be extracted using a wire basket without resorting to rigid bronchoscopy. If the broncholith is more firmly attached, however, the latter instrument is required. Experience at the Mayo Clinic has shown that the success rate in extracting the loose broncholith is the same whether the bronchoscope used is flexible or rigid.[54]

8. What complications are associated with bronchoscopic extraction?

Earlier literature stressed that surgical extraction is preferable to a bronchoscopic approach. With the advent of improved equipment and technique, bronchoscopic extraction of loose and mobile endobronchial broncholiths is highly successful and should be attempted before resorting to surgical treatment. Initial consideration for surgery is required for broncholithiasis complicated by chronic pulmonary suppurative disease (bronchiectasis), massive hemoptysis, bronchoesophageal fistulas, and uncertainty about the diagnosis.[32]

In conclusion, the patient described exemplifies the typical features of broncholithiasis. From a clinician's perspective, it is worth remembering the effects of delay in diagnosis, the importance of radiologic imaging, and the crucial role of bronchoscopy in diagnosis and treatment of this disorder. The rarity of the condition frequently excludes it from consideration by physicians who are managing a most common respiratory symptom, chronic cough.

REFERENCES

1. Irwin RS. Complications of cough: ACCP evidence-based clinical practice guidelines. *Chest.* 2006;129:54S-58S.
2. French CT, Fletcher KE, Irwin RS. Gender differences in health-related quality of life in patients complaining of chronic cough. *Chest.* 2004;125:482-488.
3. Irwin RS, Baumann MH, Bolser DC, et al. American College of Chest Physicians (ACCP). Diagnosis and management of cough executive summary: ACCP evidence-based clinical practice guidelines. *Chest.* 2006;129:1S-23S.
4. Sen RP, Walsh TE. Fiberoptic bronchoscopy for refractory cough. *Chest.* 1991;99:33-35.
5. Olson EJ, Utz JP, Prakash UB. Therapeutic bronchoscopy in broncholithiasis. *Am J Respir Crit Care Med.* 1999;160:766-770.
6. Shang Y, Bai C, Huang HD, et al. Images for diagnosis: broncholithiasis-induced bronchial artery fistula and pulmonary artery fistula in an aged female: a case report. *Chin Med J.* 2010;123:507-509.
7. Tsubochi H, Endo S, Suhara K, et al. Endobronchial aspergillosis and actinomycosis associated with broncholithiasis. *Eur J Cardiothorac Surg.* 2007;31:1144-1146.
8. Hammoud ZT, Rose AS, Hage CA, et al. Surgical management of pulmonary and mediastinal sequelae of histoplasmosis: a challenging spectrum. *Ann Thorac Surg.* 2009;88:399-404.
9. Cerfolio RJ, Bryant AS, Maniscalco L. Rigid bronchoscopy and surgical resection for broncholithiasis and calcified mediastinal lymph nodes. *J Thorac Cardiovasc Surg.* 2008;136:186-190.
10. Chujo M, Yamashita S, Kawano Y, et al. Left sleeve basal segmentectomy for broncholithiasis. *Ann Thorac Cardiovasc Surg.* 2008;14:101-104.
11. Malone DL, Genuit T, Tracy JK, et al. Surgical site infections: reanalysis of risk factors. *J Surg Res.* 2002;103:89-95.
12. Lee TH, Marcantonio ER, Mangione CM, et al. Derivation and prospective validation of a simple index for prediction of cardiac risk of major noncardiac surgery. *Circulation.* 1999;100:1043-1049.
13. Araki A, Ito H. Diabetes mellitus and geriatric syndromes. *Geriatr Gerontol Int.* 2009;9:105-114.
14. Weijer C, Singer PA, Dickens BM, et al. Bioethics for clinicians: dealing with demands for inappropriate treatment. *CMAJ.* 1998;159:817-821.
15. Meyer M, Regan A. Broncholithiasis. *N Engl J Med.* 2003;348:318.
16. Seo JB, Song KS, Lee JS, et al. Broncholithiasis: review of the causes with radiologic-pathologic correlation. *Radiographics.* 2002;22:S199-S213.
17. Seo JB, Lee JW, Ha SY, et al. Primary endobronchial actinomycosis associated with broncholithiasis. *Respiration.* 2003;70:110-113.
18. Zwiebel BR, Austin JH, Grimes MM. Bronchial carcinoid tumors: assessment with CT of location and intratumoral calcification in 31 patients. *Radiology.* 1991;179:483-486.
19. Shin MS, Berland LL, Myers JL, et al. CT demonstration of an ossifying bronchial carcinoid simulating broncholithiasis. *AJR Am J Roentgenol.* 1989;153:51-52.
20. Ahn JM, Im JG, Seo JW, et al. Endobronchial hamartoma: CT findings in three patients. *AJR Am J Roentgenol.* 1994;163:49-50.
21. Kim HY, Im JG, Song KS, et al. Localized amyloidosis of the respiratory system: CT features. *J Comput Assist Tomogr.* 1999;23:627-631.
22. Song JW, Im JG, Shim YS, et al. Hypertrophied bronchial artery at thin-section CT in patients with bronchiectasis: correlation with CT angiographic findings. *Radiology.* 1998;208:187-191.
23. Fleisher LA, Beckman JA, Brown KA, et al. ACC/AHA 2007 guidelines on perioperative cardiovascular evaluation and care for noncardiac surgery: a report of the American College of Cardiology/American Heart Association Task Force on Practice Guidelines. *J Am Coll Cardiol.* 2007;50:e159-e241.
24. Aust MR, Prakash UB, McDougall JC, et al. Bronchoscopic bronchothotripsy. *J Bronchol.* 1994;1:37-41.
25. Miks VM, Kvale PA, Riddle JM, et al. Broncholith removal using the YAG laser. *Chest.* 1986;90:293-297.
26. Ferguson JS, Rippentrop JM, Fallon B, et al. Management of obstructing pulmonary broncholithiasis with three-dimensional imaging and holmium laser lithotripsy. *Chest.* 2006;130:909-912.

27. Snyder RW, Unger M, Sawicki RW. Bilateral partial bronchial obstruction due to broncholithiasis treated with laser therapy. *Chest.* 1998;113:240-242.

28. Moersch HJ, Schmidt HW. Broncholithiasis. *Ann Otol Rhinol Laryngol.* 1959;68:548-563.

29. Cole FH, Cole FH Jr, Khandekar A, et al. Management of broncholithiasis: is thoracotomy necessary? *Ann Thorac Surg.* 1986;42:255-257.

30. Arrigoni MG, Bernatz PE, Donoghue FE. Broncholithiasis. *J Thorac Cardiovasc Surg.* 1971;62:231-237.

31. Trastek VF, Pairolero PC, Ceithaml EL, et al. Surgical management of broncholithiasis. *J Thorac Cardiovasc Surg.* 1985;90:842-848.

32. Faber LP, Jensik RJ, Chawla SK, et al. The surgical implication of broncholithiasis. *J Thorac Cardiovasc Surg.* 1975;70:779-789.

33. Yi K, Lee H, Park S, et al. Two cases of broncholith removal under the guidance of flexible bronchoscopy. *Korean J Intern Med.* 2005;20:90-91.

34. Menivale F, Deslee G, Vallerand H, et al. Therapeutic management of broncholithiasis. *Ann Thorac Surg.* 2005;79:1774-1776.

35. Potaris K, Miller DL, Trastek VF, et al. Role of surgical resection in broncholithiasis. *Ann Thorac Surg.* 2000;70:248-252.

36. Larizgoitia I, Pons JM. A systematic review of the clinical efficacy and effectiveness of the holmium:YAG laser in urology. *BJU Int.* 1999;84:1-9.

37. Reddy AJ, Govert JA, Sporn TA, et al. Broncholith removal using cryotherapy during flexible bronchoscopy: a case report. *Chest.* 2007;132:1661-1663.

38. Mathur PN, Wolf KM, Busk MF, et al. Fiberoptic bronchoscopic cryotherapy in the management of tracheobronchial obstruction. *Chest.* 1996;110:718-723.

39. Brantigan CO. Endoscopy for broncholith. *JAMA.* 1978;240:1483.

40. Menivale F, Deslee G, Vallerand H, et al. Therapeutic management of broncholithiasis. *Ann Thorac Surg.* 2005;79:1774-1776.

41. Gavin LA. Perioperative management of the diabetic patient. *Endocrinol Metab Clin North Am.* 1992;21:457-475.

42. Hoogwerf BJ. Perioperative management of diabetes mellitus: how should we act on the limited evidence? *Cleve Clin J Med.* 2006;73(suppl 1):S95-S99.

43. Kauffman CA. Histoplasmosis: a clinical and laboratory update. *Clin Micr Rev.* 2007;20:115-132.

44. French CT, Irwin RS, Fletcher KE, et al. Evaluation of a cough-specific quality-of-life questionnaire. *Chest.* 2002;121:1123-1131.

45. Søreide E, Eriksson LI, Hirlekar G, et al. Pre-operative fasting guidelines: an update. *Acta Anaesthesiol Scand.* 2005;49:1041-1047.

46. Practice guidelines for preoperative fasting and the use of pharmacologic agents to reduce the risk of pulmonary aspiration: application to healthy patients undergoing elective procedures: a report by the American Society of Anesthesiologist Task Force on Preoperative Fasting. *Anesthesiology.* 1999;90:896-905.

47. Søreide E, Holst-Larsen H, Reite K, et al. Effects of giving water 20-450 ml with oral diazepam premedication 1-2 h before operation. *Br J Anaesth.* 1993;71:503-506.

48. Brady M, Kinn S, Stuart P. Preoperative fasting for adults to prevent perioperative complications. *Cochrane Database Syst Rev.* 2003;CD004423.

49. Prakash UBS. Uncommon causes of cough. ACCP Evidence-Based Clinical Practice Guidelines. *Chest.* 2006;129:206S-219S.

50. Baum GL, Bernstein L, Schwarz J. Broncholithiasis produced by histoplasmosis. *Am Rev Tuberc.* 1958;77:162-167.

51. Lin CS, Becker WH. Broncholith as a cause of fatal hemoptysis. *JAMA.* 1978;239:2153.

52. McLean TR, Beall AC, Jones JW. Massive hemoptysis due to broncholithiasis. *Ann Thorac Surg.* 1991;52:1173-1175.

53. Bollengier WE, Guernsey JM. Broncholithiasis with aorto-tracheal fistula. *J Thorac Cardiovasc Surg.* 1974;68:588-592.

54. Groves LK, Effler DB. Broncholithiasis: a review of twenty-seven cases. *Am Rev Tuberc.* 1956;73:19-30.

Chapter 5

Treatment of Tracheobronchial Aspergillosis Superimposed on Post Tuberculosis–Related Tracheal Stricture

This chapter emphasizes the following elements of the Four Box Approach: physical examination, complementary tests, functional status assessment, and follow-up tests, visits, and procedures.

CASE DESCRIPTION

The patient was a 59-year-old female with a remote history of pulmonary tuberculosis with tracheobronchial involvement (details unknown). She had been appropriately treated with antituberculosis drugs for 9 months. Several years before our encounter, but well after her bout with tuberculosis, she had been diagnosed with asthma, but her dyspnea had never truly improved back to her baseline. Within the 2 weeks just before admission to our institution, she had increasing productive cough of yellowish-green sputum, dyspnea, fever with chills, and gradual hoarseness. She did not respond to a 2 week course of levofloxacin and prednisone (40 mg/day with tapering regimen). She was also using inhaled fluticasone 100 µg twice daily. The patient was hospitalized with severe respiratory distress and stridor suggestive of severe airway obstruction and then was transferred to our institution for further management when she developed worsening cough, dyspnea at rest, and complete loss of her voice. She was not married, was not a smoker, and had no other medical problems. Her wish was clearly to relieve the dyspnea and cough and return to work as an office manager. Physical examination revealed blood pressure of 168/86 mm Hg, heart rate of 110 bpm, temperature of 36.9° C, and respiratory rate of 22, along with saturation of 95% (room air). On chest examination, she had coarse breath sounds, wheezing bilaterally, and stridor over tracheal auscultation. Otherwise, her examination was normal. Initial laboratory data were unremarkable. Computed tomography (CT) with external three-dimensional reformation showed a 2 cm long, "hourglass"-shaped tracheal stenosis with a diameter of 7 mm (Figure 5-1). Complete atelectasis of the right upper lobe was noted (see Figure 5-1). Flexible bronchoscopy performed in the intensive care unit showed thick yellow material on the vocal cords and subglottis and white-yellowish pseudomembranes extending down the posterior membrane of the left main bronchus and on the spur of the left upper and left lower lobe bronchi. The right upper lobe bronchus was completely closed; this was probably a sequel of her tuberculosis. Bronchoscopy confirmed the location and degree of stenosis (Figure 5-2).

DISCUSSION POINTS

1. List three differential diagnoses for the "pseudomembrane" pattern seen on bronchoscopy.
2. Describe the airway findings in acute tracheobronchial aspergillosis.
3. Describe some of the issues to be considered in cases of airway stent insertion in the setting of tracheal stenosis and concurrent active *Aspergillus* tracheobronchitis.
4. Describe the medical treatment of acute tracheobronchial aspergillosis.

CASE RESOLUTION

Initial Evaluations

Physical Examination, Complementary Tests, and Functional Status Assessment

This patient likely had infectious tracheobronchitis on a background of previous tracheal stenosis. In the setting of tracheal stenosis, mucosal inflammation associated with even mild respiratory tract infection can cause edema and mucus production, which may further occlude the lumen. In this patient, the presence of white-yellowish necrotic material was contributory to stenosis and likely was responsible for worsening symptoms. Without a confirmatory test such as CT or bronchoscopy, patients with previously undiagnosed tracheal stenosis and acute worsening due to respiratory tract infection may be misdiagnosed as having an exacerbation of chronic obstructive pulmonary disease or asthma. This is especially true when symptoms improve temporarily after therapy with antibiotics or corticosteroids because they reduce mucosal swelling and inflammation, thereby improving airway caliber. Recurrent or persistent symptoms minimally responsive or unresponsive to bronchodilators should raise suspicion for central airway obstruction before the development of critical stenosis requiring intensive care unit (ICU) admission.[1]

Regarding other diagnostic tests that could have been performed during the initial evaluation, the classic flattening of inspiratory and expiratory curves seen with severe tracheal obstruction on flow-volume loop would not have offered relevant treatment information; this pattern, although specific for fixed upper/central airway obstruction, in a patient with stridor and respiratory distress not only is not necessary but is

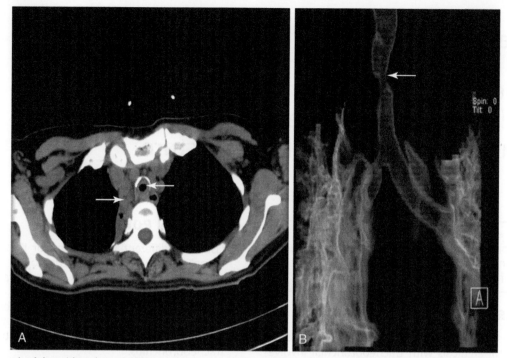

Figure 5-1   Stenosis of the mid-trachea on **(A)** axial chest computed tomography (CT) and **(B)** three-dimensional (3D) CT external rendering. Axial images reveal the 7 mm tracheal diameter and the atelectatic right upper lobe; 3D imaging shows the hourglass morphology and the 2 cm extent of the tracheal stenosis.

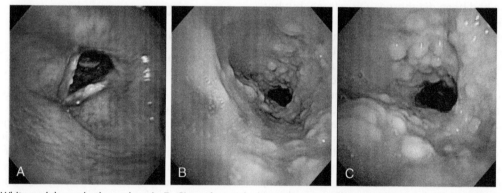

Figure 5-2   **A,** White nodules on both vocal cords. **B,** Circumferential white-yellowish pseudomembranes covering and narrowing the trachea, starting in the subglottis. **C,** The critical stenosis was located in mid-trachea at 5 cm below the vocal cords, narrowing the trachea to 7 mm.

potentially dangerous because it can precipitate respiratory failure.

CT scanning* might thus be preferred for the initial evaluation of patients with suspected severe central airway narrowing to assess the length of the stenosis and the distal airways, which may not be accessible by flexible bronchoscopy in cases of severe airway lumen narrowing. In our patient, CT images quantified the degree of obstruction (i.e., severe, >70% reduction in cross-sectional area) and the extent of the narrowed tracheal segment (i.e., 2 cm), revealed the morphology of the stricture (i.e., hourglass), ruled out extrinsic compression as being responsible for the tracheal narrowing, and revealed other associated parenchymal findings (e.g., right upper lobe [RUL] atelectasis). CT is preferably performed before

bronchoscopy because it might guide additional diagnostic procedures when parenchymal abnormalities or mediastinal lymphadenopathy is present. However, CT does not offer information about mucosal abnormalities that can be detected only on bronchoscopy (e.g., pseudomembranous tracheobronchitis).

Given the frail status of this patient, bronchoscopy was performed in the ICU. We were prepared to endotracheally intubate and stabilize her airway had she developed worsening respiratory failure during or after the procedure. To avoid a decrease in respiratory drive and potential hypercarbic respiratory failure, bronchoscopy was performed with only local laryngeal analgesia.* Bronchoscopy revealed large, "cheese-like," white-yellowish necrotic pseudomembranes on a background of hourglass

---

*Of note, conventional tracheal radiographs with a high kilovoltage technique accentuate the air–soft tissue interface, soften bone shadows, and are useful in evaluating the glottis and the subglottic larynx.

*A total of 200 mg of 1% lidocaine was used to prevent laryngospasm and laryngeal reflexes such as trismus, bradycardia, tachycardia, hypotension, and hypertension.

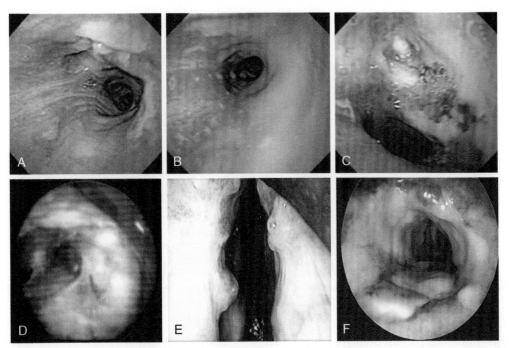

Figure 5-3   White "cheese-like" pseudomembranes are seen in the **(A)** lower trachea, **(B)** left main bronchus, and **(C)** left upper lobe in a patient with active caseating endobronchial tuberculosis. Circumferentially infiltrated upper tracheal wall by **(D)** thick white-yellowish pseudomembranes and **(E)** laryngeal nodules caused by rhinoscleroma. **F,** Acute necrotizing tracheitis is seen in a patient with *Staphylococcus aureus* infection.

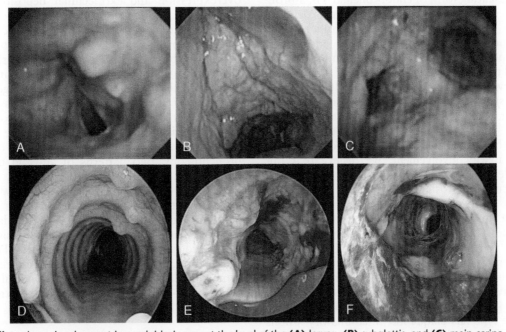

Figure 5-4   Diffuse airway involvement in amyloidosis seen at the level of the **(A)** larynx, **(B)** subglottis, and **(C)** main carina. **D,** Several focal, raised, firm nodules are noted overlying the cartilaginous rings and covered by normal mucosa in a patient with tracheopathica osteochondroplastica (TPO). **E,** TPO nodules may sometimes be irregular and covered by edematous airway mucosa. **F,** Acute tracheitis causes white necrotic pseudomembranes in a patient undergoing radiation therapy for non–small cell lung cancer.

(funnel-shaped) tracheal stenosis (see Figure 5-2). This type of mucosal abnormality can be seen in patients with mycobacterial or fungal infection, including tuberculosis, aspergillosis, candidiasis, mucormycosis, *Pseudallescheria boydii,* and *Scedosporium prolificans* (Figure 5-3)[2]; in addition, necrotizing bacterial tracheobronchitis, severe smoke inhalation injury with superimposed infection,

infiltrating adenocarcinoma, and sometimes aggressive active tracheobronchial Wegener's granulomatosis or radiation tracheatis present in a similar fashion (Figure 5-4).[3,4] Awareness of these diagnoses is important when approaching a patient with pseudomembranous tracheobronchitis because airway biopsies are necessary to confirm most of these disorders, and treatments are disease specific.

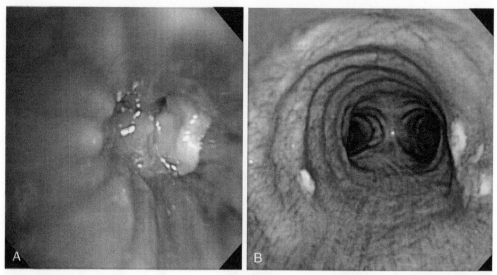

Figure 5-5   A, Obstructing type and **(B)** ulcerative type of tracheobronchial aspergillosis (images obtained from two different patients).

This pseudomembranous pattern of airway mucosa in fact is commonly seen in the actively caseating type of endobronchial tuberculosis (TB).* This form of TB appears to be highly contagious, with a reported rate of AFB sputum positivity that exceeds 50%.[5] In addition to this actively caseating form of endobronchial TB, a bronchitic type identified as airway erythema and edema, a granular type with associated submucosal tubercle formation, a mucosal ulcerative type, an edematous-hyperemic type with significant mucosal inflammation and bronchial narrowing, and a fibrostenotic type causing cicatricial airway strictures may occur.[5] It is unclear whether true stepwise progression occurs from one type to another, or whether each particular type may occur independently without required passage through the other histopathologic forms.[5] Given her history of tuberculosis with airway involvement, we believe that our patient had developed acute infection on a background of post tuberculosis fibrostenotic stricture.

Aspergillus tracheobronchitis is an uncommon but well-described manifestation of *Aspergillus* infection, occurring in less than 7% of patients with pulmonary aspergillosis.[6,7] Three types of tracheobronchial aspergillosis have been identified on the basis of bronchoscopic pattern: obstructive, ulcerative, and pseudomembranous. The obstructive type is characterized by thick mucus plugs without gross evidence of bronchial inflammation.[8] The ulcerative type has plaque-like inflammatory lesions (Figure 5-5). The pseudomembranous type is characterized by extensive inflammation with formation of a pseudomembrane overlying the mucosa and containing *Aspergillus* organisms.[9] This type is most prevalent in immunocompromised patients,[8] is diagnosed by evidence of *Aspergillus* on microscopic specimens of material obtained at bronchoscopy, and has been reported to be refractory to antifungal therapy.[9]

Other differential diagnoses of diffuse infiltrating white-yellowish central airway lesions may include amyloidosis, infiltrating adenocarcinoma, tracheobronchial amyloidosis, atypical forms of tracheopathica osteochondroplastica, and rhinoscleroma. Amyloidosis is caused by overexpression and extracellular deposition of specific proteins.*[10] Airway involvement in amyloidosis (AL) is seen with the AL type in which the specific protein deposition comprises κ and λ light chains of monoclonal immunoglobulins. Women are affected earlier (52 vs. 59 years of age), slightly more often (10:9 ratio), and more extensively than men, and cough, wheezing, dyspnea, and occasionally hemoptysis are the usual symptoms that precede histologic diagnosis by an average of 17 months.[11] In fact, patients are often treated before diagnosis for recurrent pneumonia, tracheobronchitis, or asthma. At bronchoscopy, two patterns of amyloid deposition are described: a nodular or unifocal disease, and a diffuse submucosal disease (see Figure 5-4).†[12] Low-dose external beam radiation is a reported treatment alternative‡[13]; however, excisional therapy is the standard treatment for upper and central airway amyloidosis, which may often progress to respiratory failure. Frequent laser excisions (≈5 treatments/yr) sometimes are necessary. In some nodular forms of tracheobronchial amyloidosis, neodymium-doped yttrium aluminum garnet (Nd:YAG)

---

*Amyloid deposits may be systemic or organ limited; in systemic amyloidosis, the composition of subunit proteins dictates the pattern of organ involvement, the rapidity of disease progression, and outcome.

†Diagnosis of amyloidosis rests on apple-green birefringence conferred by Congo red staining. Once amyloid has been identified, the extent of disease and the protein subunit must be defined. The extent of disease is most easily determined by performing a fat pad aspirate and by staining with Congo red dye. Median survival with untreated systemic AL disease is 13 months.

‡Because plasma cells are radiosensitive, low-dose external beam radiation was attempted in five published cases of tracheobronchial amyloidosis. Regression of endobronchial deposits was reported after delivery of 20 Gy in 10 fractions.

---

*This is the most common form of endobronchial tuberculosis and is reported in 5.8% of patients with pulmonary tuberculosis.

laser treatment removes tissue and eliminates further amyloid deposition in the field. However, the diffuse form usually recurs after laser treatment, and repeated rigid laser bronchoscopies denude airways and promote collagen scar formation. Repeated airway debridement may trade one obstructing disease (amyloidosis) for another (scar stenosis).

Tracheopathica osteochondroplastica (TPO) is another rare nonmalignant disorder of the central airways characterized by multiple dense nodules localized in the submucosa of the tracheobronchial wall.*[14,15] TPO is a slowly progressive disease of adulthood with a mean time from presentation to diagnosis of approximately 4 years; it is usually detected incidentally upon intubation, or when CT or bronchoscopy is performed for airway symptoms or for unrelated conditions.[16,17] Although TPO may involve the larynx, the disease is usually limited to the central airways (trachea and mainstem bronchi) and does not involve the lung parenchyma or other organs. Mucosal changes (edema, hyperemia), impaired clearance of secretions, and enlarged submucosal nodules may lead to recurrent inflammation, infection, and central airway obstruction. Cough, hoarseness, exertional dyspnea, wheezing, and recurrent lower airway infections are the usual symptoms, and stridor and rhonchi are present in advanced obstructive cases, which can even lead to respiratory failure.[14] The disease is usually distinguishable from other disorders, however, because it does not involve the posterior membranous portion of the trachea. In addition, bronchoscopy findings are often considered to be characteristic when focal or diffuse raised, firm nodules overlying the cartilaginous rings are noted (see Figure 5-4).[15] Occasionally, however, atypical irregular nodules[†] and mucosal inflammation may mimic carcinoma or airway infection.[15] Although no obvious relationship to malignancy has been noted, a large case series showed that 24 (19%) of 126 patients had associated cancers, especially bronchogenic adenocarcinoma.[18] For this reason, bronchoscopic biopsies may still be needed.

Infiltrated tracheobronchial wall by diffuse polypoid lesions covered with thick white secretions, bulging into and narrowing the lumen, can be seen with a chronic, slowly progressive, infectious disease of the respiratory tract caused by the bacterium *Klebsiella rhinoscleromatis*, a subspecies of *Klebsiella pneumoniae* that has special affinity for the nasal mucosa.[19] In many patients, the disease process (aka scleroma) remains confined to the nasal cavity (thus the name *rhinoscleroma*), but involvement of other parts of the respiratory tract has been reported (see Figure 5-3). The presentation, similar to that of our patient, is nonspecific and includes chronic productive cough, stridor, and dysphonia.*[20,21] The incidence of laryngeal involvement in rhinoscleroma varies between 15% and 80%, but tracheobronchial involvement is far less common. A report from the United States showed that 13 of 22 patients with rhinoscleroma had laryngotracheal disease; of these, 9 had subglottic stenosis and/or glottic stenosis, and only 2 had tracheal involvement limited to the first two tracheal rings.[22] In a different study of 56 patients, the nose was affected in 100% of patients; other affected regions were nasopharynx in 13 patients, palate in 7 patients, skin in 2 patients, larynx in 3 patients, trachea in 17 patients, nasolacrimal duct in 2 patients, and premaxilla in 1 patient.[21] Given its geographic prevalence in Central America, the Middle East, and central Europe, and its usual nasal involvement, rhinoscleroma was unlikely in our patient. Biopsies are warranted because Gram stains will identify tiny bacilli consistent with *K. rhinoscleromatis* in the cell cytoplasm.[21]

Comorbidities

This patient had no other conditions that would have precluded flexible or rigid bronchoscopic interventions under moderate sedation or general anesthesia.

Support System

This patient lived alone and had a limited circle of acquaintances. The news that she suffered from tracheal stenosis caused her anxiety, worry, and frustration that her disease was not diagnosed earlier. She did not show any signs of denial; in fact, she wanted to know everything about her illness and discuss it in detail. In an attempt to alleviate her confusion and state of anxiety, we explained to her the nature of her airway disease and the possible diagnostic and treatment alternatives.

Patient Preferences and Expectations

The patient shared with us her emotions and expressed her wish to breathe better so she could go back to work. She desired to stay active and independent. She had no close friends or family, and she did not feel comfortable sharing her illness with her few acquaintances from work. She shared with us her concern that she would lose her job because of her breathing problems and frequent absences. Furthermore, she was terrified by the thought that without a job she would surely lose her insurance and would not be able to undergo further treatment. We made a treatment plan together by deciding to initially

---

*Histopathologic studies suggest that bone morphogenetic protein-2 acts synergistically with transforming growth factor-β₁ in promotion of nodule formation within the tracheal submucosa.

†Nodules are actually calcifications, chondrifications, or ossifications of the upper layer of the airway. These abnormalities may have foci of bone marrow with active areas of hematopoiesis. Ossifications consist of lamellar-type bone covered by normal mucosa or squamous metaplasia that may connect by bone, cartilage, or connective tissue to the perichondrium of the tracheal rings. Biopsies are often difficult because of the bony nature of the nodules.

---

*Medical treatment using antibiotics and corticosteroids is the basic approach, although surgical treatment may be needed for fibrosclerosis unresponsive to medical treatment. Untreated rhinoscleroma tends to progress slowly over many years and might involve any part of the respiratory system. Tetracycline or quinolones (e.g., ciprofloxacin 500 mg twice daily) are recommended for a period of 6 months or until nasal biopsies are negative. Surgical debridement is limited to patients with acute life-threatening complications or, alternatively, to patients with chronic debilitating respiratory symptoms and upper airway obstruction due to airway scarring. A high incidence of recurrence is reported, reaching up to 25% within 10 years.

determine the exact cause of her problem and to alleviate dyspnea by performing rigid bronchoscopic dilation. We explained that the treating team works to provide care to all individuals, regardless of their socioeconomic status, and that from a medical ethics perspective, we believe that as human beings we are all valuable social entities who have the right, not the privilege, to health care access.[23] From a pragmatic standpoint, however, we referred her to a case manager to discuss additional medical insurance options.

Procedural Strategies

Indications

Rigid bronchoscopy was planned to perform biopsies for diagnosis and to restore airway patency because the patient had stridor and respiratory distress due to severe tracheal narrowing. We also intended to perform bronchoscopic debridement of the pseudomembranes to prevent acute life-threatening occlusion of the airway from sloughing of the necrotic airway mucosa.

Contraindications

No contraindications to rigid bronchoscopy were identified.

Expected Results

Debridement of the pseudomembranes and dilation of the underlying stenosis were expected to improve airflow and relieve dyspnea; once a firm diagnosis was obtained, medical treatment using antibiotics or antifungals (depending on the final results) would be initiated. We were aware that further surgical or bronchoscopic treatment might have been required for the fibrostenosis if it was unresponsive to the initial bronchoscopy.

Team Experience

Rigid and flexible bronchoscopies are performed routinely in this facility, but severe tracheobronchitis causing airway obstruction is only rarely seen in our center. Infectious obstructing airway processes are more commonly seen in endemic areas for tuberculosis or rhinoscleroma or in lung transplant centers managing patients who develop anastomotic complications. Although we were confident that airway patency could be restored during rigid bronchoscopy, we were not convinced about the need or benefit for airway stent insertion or about the natural course of her airway disease process.

Therapeutic Alternatives

Laser therapy, dilation, and stent insertion all have been employed with varying success to deal with airway stenoses, but these therapies usually are offered when a mature stenosis is seen, not in the setting of severe necrotizing airway infection.

Flexible bronchoscopy with laser or electrocautery and balloon dilation is an alternative to rigid bronchoscopy for patients with tracheal stenosis. In this patient with unstable respiratory status, however, we considered that control of the airway during rigid bronchoscopy was a safer method to restore airway lumen patency. A variety of silicone and expandable metallic airway stents are available to palliate airway stenosis and malacia, but in the setting of infection, simple dilation may be preferred as the initial therapy. Exuberant granulation tissue may form in the setting of stent insertion for an active inflammatory stricture.[24] Initial balloon or rigid bronchoscopic dilation in this situation allows time for the inflammatory lesion to mature into a fibrous stricture that is more suitable for stent placement.

Tracheostomy has to be considered in any patient with critical airway obstruction, but in our patient, we believed it was not justified for at least four reasons: first, the tracheostomy tube may not have been able to bypass the severe stenosis; second, the severe inflammation could have been worsened by chronic irritation from the tracheostomy tube; third, airway narrowing, thick secretions, and sloughing of the pseudomembranes could result in acute fatal airway obstruction and death; and fourth, less invasive alternatives are available.

Cost-Effectiveness

This patient had an unusual presentation of likely infectious tracheobronchitis complicating long-standing tracheal stenosis. Optimal management in this scenario, to our knowledge, has never been systematically studied. Furthermore, as of this writing, no guidelines are available on the cost-effectiveness of various treatments for tracheal stenosis with or without superimposed infection. The interventional bronchoscopy profession has not yet participated in systematic measurement of quality for this disease, whether patient satisfaction or other outcome measures, in a way that is truly demonstrative of mature professional commitment. In this regard, we recognize that physicians can work on behalf of quality only if they combine organizationally and work on systems systematically. An individual physician's commitment to excellence, although habitual and commendable, is not necessarily sufficient to ensure high-quality care[25] from a societal perspective. As professions mature—after all, the subspecialty organizational work of interventional pulmonology has been ongoing for less than two decades—collaborative work can be increasingly devoted to ensuring uniform education, establishing guidelines and recommended algorithms of care, and determining strategies that allow improved access and more rapid bedside availability of technology-driven discoveries. By applying our clinical judgment and respecting our patient's values, we considered that restoration of airway patency in the presence of severe life-threatening symptoms was a priority.

Informed Consent

The patient showed good understanding of her illness, indications for treatment, risks, and potential alternatives.

Techniques and Results

Anesthesia and Perioperative Care

The primary concern from an anesthesia standpoint was the extent and degree of airway narrowing. Pertinent information usually can and should be obtained by the anesthesiologist during the preoperative period by a careful history, physical examination, and review of diagnostic imaging studies. In this patient, dyspnea, subjective stridor, and the fixed stridor noted on auscultation during both respiratory phases were consistent with CT and bronchoscopy studies showing a fixed airway obstruction. The exact location, extent of stenosis, or degree of airway obstruction accurately established by chest CT and bronchoscopy should be shared with the anesthesiologist before the procedure is performed. This information will help determine what size endotracheal tube (ETT) should be used, if necessary, the safe depth for ETT placement, and, for very high lesions, whether an ETT can be used at all.[26]

We did not administer sedative premedication because of the potential for hypoventilation and further airway obstruction. For a very anxious patient, these drugs should be considered only in a closely monitored environment.

General anesthesia using spontaneous assisted ventilation was planned for this patient as for most of our patients with central airway obstruction undergoing rigid bronchoscopy. During emergence from anesthesia, airway patency may temporarily worsen because edema in the upper airway may manifest itself once the bronchoscope is removed. Furthermore, excessive coughing can increase bleeding. At the completion of the procedure, therefore, the patient should be fully awake. Because we decided to use a rigid bronchoscope, at the end of the procedure a decision had to be made as to whether to replace it with an ETT. We decided that if the patient were not breathing adequately (i.e., hypoventilation, paradoxical abdominal movement), or if the airway had been traumatized, the trachea should remain intubated. A tube exchanger could be placed in the trachea through a rigid bronchoscope to be used as a guide for placement of a new ETT if reintubation became necessary. Otherwise, the patient should receive mask oxygen after extubation, during transport, and while in the postanesthesia care unit. Post procedure stridor, if present, might require treatment with humidified oxygen, nebulized epinephrine, steroids, or heliox, or may even warrant reintubation.[26] Decisions regarding reintubation ideally are made during the day, in a controlled setting—not in the middle of the night at the time of an emergency.*

Instrumentation

A 12 mm Efer-Dumon rigid ventilating bronchoscope was chosen for the initial intubation. An Nd:YAG laser was ready in case of bleeding requiring photocoagulation. A variety of silicone stents and stent introducers and the stent loading system were available for possible stent placement. Large forceps† were also available for removal of the pseudomembranes.

---

*Indeed, we believe that careful assessment and planning substantially avoid problems. We therefore heed the idea that there "should be no surprises," and that one should never "trust the airway."

†An alternative, not available to us at the time of this procedure, is the optical forceps. This forceps has a centrally located 5.5 mm telescope that ensures optimal visualization and stability.

Anatomic Dangers and Other Risks

Imminent airway obstruction in this case could result from secretions or sloughing of the necrotic mucosa occluding the airway lumen already narrowed from the underlying stenosis. Removing the pseudomembranes by bronchoscopic procedures may be useful because of the poor penetration of antifungal or antibacterial agents into the abnormal pseudomembranous tissues; however, the friable and inflamed airway wall may bleed, and bronchoscopic debridement might inadvertently cause tracheal wall perforation.

Results and Procedure-Related Complications

The patient was intubated with the rigid bronchoscope without difficulty (see video on ExpertConsult.com) (Video I.5.1). The white-yellowish material was noted extending from subglottis to carina and mainstem bronchi (Figure 5-6). The tracheal lumen in mid-trachea was reduced to 7 mm. With the rigid bronchoscope, we subsequently performed dilation and removed the pseudomembranes at the level of critical narrowing, thus restoring airway patency. Bronchial washing and biopsies were performed for microbiology, cytology, and histopathology. Minimal bleeding was controlled by laser photocoagulation (Nd:YAG laser; 436 joules total energy, 1 second, 30 W pulse) (see video on ExpertConsult.com) (Video I.5.2). A stent was not placed because of concern for worsening infection potentially caused by covering the abnormal necrotic mucosa and because of possible poor penetration of nebulized antifungal or antibacterial agents through the stent. Once bleeding was controlled post dilation to 12 mm, the rigid bronchoscope was removed and the procedure was terminated. The patient was transferred back to the ICU for overnight monitoring.

Long-Term Management

Outcome Assessment

Restoration of airway patency improved dyspnea and relieved respiratory distress at rest. Washings and biopsy specimens showed negative acid-fast stains and bacteriologic cultures, thus making mycobacterial infection and rhinoscleroma unlikely.

Septate, branching fungal hyphae consistent with *Aspergillus* and mucosal necrosis were evident (see Figure 5-6).

Follow-up Tests and Procedures

Comprehensive testing showed no evidence of immunodeficiency or malignancy. The patient was started on oral voriconazole 200 mg twice a day and nebulized amphotericin B 10 mg every 8 hours. Flexible bronchoscopy 1 week later showed improvement of airway mucosa with residual pseudomembranes (Figure 5-7). Her symptoms gradually improved, and the patient was discharged home. Flexible bronchoscopy performed 3 weeks after the procedure showed no further evidence of disease on the vocal cords and substantial improvement of airway mucosa in the trachea and mainstem bronchi (see Figure 5-7). Dyspnea improved, and her voice

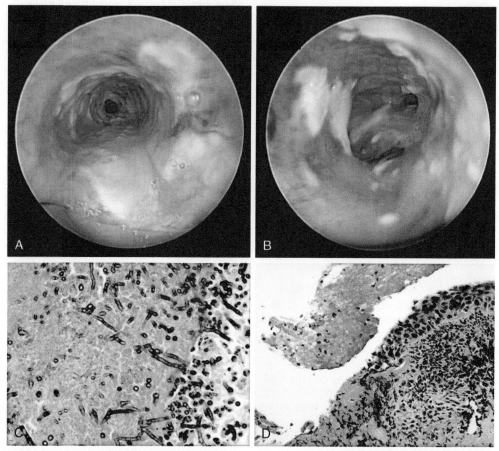

Figure 5-6 Tracheal lumen during rigid bronchoscopy shows diffuse pseudomembranes **(A)** above and **(B)** below the critical airway narrowing. Photomicrograph of tissue from tracheal biopsies showing **(C)** *Aspergillus* organisms with branching and septate hyphae (hematoxylin and eosin [H&E] stain, original magnification, ×100) and **(D)** necrotic mucosal tissue (H&E stain, original magnification, ×40).

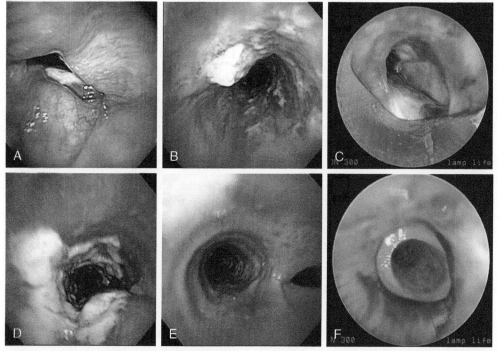

Figure 5-7 Flexible bronchoscopy 1 week after rigid bronchoscopy showed **(A)** resolution of vocal cord lesions and **(B)** persistent but improved airway mucosa with residual pseudomembranes in the trachea. Three weeks after the procedure, **(C)** bronchoscopy showed substantial improvement of airway mucosa in the trachea and right main and left main bronchus **(D)** without distal airway involvement. Nine weeks later, **(E)** no evidence of pseudomembranes was found, but a complex stricture was noted at mid-trachea extending for approximately 2.5 cm and narrowing the airway to 7 mm. **F,** A ringed Hood silicone stent (35 mm long × 16 mm wide) was inserted to restore airway patency.

returned to normal, but the patient continued to have cough and had not returned to work. Nine weeks later, she came to the emergency department with worsening dyspnea. Bronchoscopy revealed a recurrent stricture of the mid-trachea 7 mm in diameter and 2.5 cm in length with no evidence of pseudomembranes (see Figure 5-7). Rigid bronchoscopy was performed, and the tracheal stricture was dilated with the 13 mm rigid bronchoscope. This time we decided to proceed with silicone stent insertion. Optimal stent length was estimated by withdrawing the telescope from the distal to the proximal end of the stricture. The estimated stent diameter was extrapolated from the outer diameter of the largest rigid bronchoscope (13 mm in this case). A silicone ringed stent (Hood, Woburn, Mass), 35 mm long × 16 mm wide, was inserted within the mid-trachea such that the distal aspect of the stent was approximately 2.5 cm above the carina, and the proximal aspect of the stent was 5 cm below the vocal cords (see Figure 5-7). The patient's symptoms improved, and she was continued on voriconazole for an additional 6 months. Follow-up bronchoscopy at 5 months showed no evidence of recurrent *Aspergillus* infection. The patient went back to work 3 months after her initial presentation.

Referrals

Because she had expressed a need for support with emotional issues, we offered her a consultation with a psychologist, which she declined. Depression and anxiety are common in people with chronic illnesses, as are all sorts of other emotions and relationship issues. Patients might also be having problems coping with their illness, or with symptoms or treatments, and a psychologist can assist with this. Other individuals and organizations may offer counseling, but it is important that patients make sure they see someone who is properly qualified and accredited.

Quality Improvement

We wondered whether our patient should have undergone flexible bronchoscopy after her initial diagnosis of tuberculosis, especially when "asthma" symptoms developed.

It is known that 10% of patients with endobronchial tuberculosis are, in fact, eventually diagnosed with fibrostenosis[5]; in one study, 65% of patients with actively caseating tuberculosis had developed fibrostenosis within 3 months of treatment. On the other hand, most granular, bronchitic, and ulcerative types of endobronchial tuberculosis resolve completely without sequelae.[5] Most experts agree that routine bronchoscopic follow-up is warranted during and after treatment for endobronchial tuberculosis, because patients with airway strictures may be asymptomatic until critical airway narrowing is reached, and because strictures may develop despite efficacious antituberculosis chemotherapy.[27] Furthermore, when present, airway strictures can be effectively treated by surgery or interventional bronchoscopic procedures.[28] We therefore believed that because this patient was known to have a history of endobronchial TB, follow-up bronchoscopy was warranted following her TB diagnosis, to detect possible stricture in a timely fashion, and

before the advent of potentially life-threatening symptoms related to critical airway narrowing. However, we were aware that essential issues in assessment and improvement in quality of care have to do with the ways that physicians think, rather than with the ways that they are controlled or judged.[25] To address quality assurance concerns in health care, physicians, as professionals, should maintain medical knowledge and pursue lifelong learning through continuous professional development.[25]

We also questioned why this patient developed such an aggressive form of fungal disease with lack of obvious immunosuppression. The cause of *Aspergillus* tracheobronchitis in this patient remained unclear and could have been multifactorial. Probably altered local defense mechanisms resulting from inhaled corticosteroids, a mildly immunocompromised state caused by antibiotic and systemic corticosteroid usage, and susceptibility to an abnormal airway resulting from preexisting stenosis facilitated the local invasion of *Aspergillus*[29,30] and the formation of pseudomembranes. We did not think that *Aspergillus* infection by itself was responsible for the patient's fibrotic stenosis, even though data from lung transplantation show that *Aspergillus* infection and airway necrosis are associated with the development of airway complications* (24.4% per patient and 23.8% per anastomosis).[31] This strong association between isolation of *Aspergillus* and subsequent development of anastomotic bronchial complications has been noted, however, in a different population than our patient; the patient with lung transplant is sometimes profoundly immunosuppressed, and bronchial ischemia at the anastomotic site may predispose to necrosis and saprophytic fungal infection.[†32] Bronchial anastomosis is particularly susceptible to such infections owing to its relative devascularization after transplant, defense impairment (mucociliary clearance and cough reflex), disruption of lymphatic drainage, and altered alveolar phagocytic function.[2]

DISCUSSION POINTS

1. List three differential diagnoses for the "pseudomembrane" pattern seen on bronchoscopy (see Figure 5-3).
   - Active caseating endobronchial tuberculosis
   - Necrotizing bacterial tracheobronchitis
   - Active tracheobronchial rhinoscleroma
2. Describe the airway findings in acute tracheobronchial aspergillosis.
   - Obstructive (see Figure 5-5)
   - Ulcerative (see Figure 5-5)
   - Pseudomembranous (see Figure 5-2)

---

*Anastomotic airway complications can be classified as (1) partial- or full-thickness necrosis or (2) airway obstruction. Necrosis includes bronchial dehiscence (with or without pleural fistula), anastomotic ulceration, and sloughing of mucosal tissue. Obstruction includes mechanical airway stenosis from granulation tissue, cicatricial fibrosis, and dynamic collapse secondary to bronchomalacia.

†Saprophytic fungal organisms are airborne and obtain their nourishment from nonliving organic matter, making ischemic and necrotic debris at the anastomosis the ideal environment for their proliferation and potentially facilitating an invasive infection.

3. Describe some of the issues to be considered in cases of airway stent insertion in the setting of tracheal stenosis and concurrent active *Aspergillus* tracheobronchitis.
   - Extrapolating from the lung transplant population, for stenotic lesions with significant inflammation, stent placement probably should be undertaken after dilation and after the lesion has matured into a fibrous stricture.[33] In fact, the presence of indwelling airway stents may, in itself, increase the risk for endobronchial infections and complications.
4. Describe the medical treatment of acute tracheobronchial aspergillosis.

   In lung transplant patients (from whom most evidence comes), the estimated mortality rate of *Aspergillus*-related tracheobronchitis or anastomotic infection is between 14% and 24%.[2] Aggressive and early treatment of *Aspergillus* infection, or the use of prophylaxis to reduce the incidence of these infections in transplant patients, may lead to a reduction in the incidence of airway complications.
   - Antifungal prophylaxis, frequent bronchoscopic surveillance, and aggressive early empirical therapy are among the approaches commonly undertaken. The duration of antifungal prophylaxis is controversial but is not less than 3 months and can be as long as 18 months. Prophylactic agents used include itraconazole, inhaled amphotericin B, and voriconazole.
   - For an *Aspergillus* infection, systemic plus inhaled antifungals combined with bronchoscopic management are used. Endobronchial amphotericin B application has been also described.[2] On the basis of published reports, patients usually are treated with antifungal agents such as amphotericin B (conventional, nebulized), liposomal amphotericin, and voriconazole. The latter has been shown to have greater efficacy in immunocompromised patients and acceptable tolerability for prolonged oral administration.[34] Only conventional amphotericin B and voriconazole are licensed for the primary treatment of invasive aspergillosis.[35] Itraconazole appears to be used in nonimmunocompromised hosts and as adjunctive treatment. Debridement may be warranted in some patients with *Aspergillus* pseudomembranous tracheobronchitis and necrosis, as described in this case.

Expert Commentary

provided by Atul C. Mehta, MBBS, FACP, FCCP

This interesting case highlights several clinical vignettes pertaining to diagnosis and management of patients with central airway obstruction from a known or suspected infectious cause. The first is that endobronchial tuberculosis (EB-TB) is much more frequent than what is reported because the diagnosis of TB is usually established by sputum studies. Flexible bronchoscopy rightfully is not required to establish its diagnosis in most cases, but it should be considered in patients with airway symptoms such as wheezing or shortness of breath. Endobronchial tuberculosis may heal with scar formation (stenosis). Obviously, this patient's "asthma" symptoms were related to her stenosis because they failed to improve with conventional treatment. In my opinion, patients with a known history of EB-TB should undergo a follow-up bronchoscopy to assess progression or resolution of airway abnormalities. Had it been performed during the course of this patient's medical management, it is possible that therapeutic bronchoscopy might have been successful in preventing right upper lobe collapse.[5]

This case also highlights the value of three-dimensional (3D) reconstruction in the evaluation of central airway obstruction. This radiologic modality complements flexible bronchoscopy by providing details on the extent and nature of the ailment. When and where available, I believe that every elective bronchoscopy should be preceded by a CT scan of the chest,[36] especially if airway obstruction is suspected. This leads to a third point that I would like to make: "All that wheezes is not asthma." When asthma symptoms fail to respond to conventional treatment, very close attention should be paid to the quality and shape of the flow-volume loop obtained during pulmonary function testing. Spirometry is readily available worldwide and could have been performed while this patient was stable. It may have clearly shown fixed upper airway obstruction. On the basis of these findings, flexible bronchoscopy would have been considered at an earlier stage. I agree with the authors that this test should be avoided during acute exacerbations.

Another point I would like to make pertains to infectious origins. In their case resolution, the authors provide an exhaustive differential diagnosis, yet for the sake of completion, I would add a condition known as pseudomembranous stenosis, which is encountered following intubation.[37] Consideration should also be given to fungal infections such as *Cryptococcus neoformans* and *Aspergillus niger*.[38,39] The former organism is seen mainly in immunocompromised hosts. The latter organism is resistant to conventional antifungal treatment, including aerosolized amphotericin B and oral voriconazole. It is generally found among patients, usually lung transplant recipients, who are receiving these drugs as prophylaxis against *Aspergillus fumigatus*. The patient presented in this case was not reported to be immunocompromised, yet her use of inhaled corticosteroids might have contributed to colonization with this ubiquitous fungus, while short-term use of high-dose prednisone and broad-spectrum antibiotics led to an invasive infective stage. Nevertheless, a high degree of suspicion is required to detect any form of *Aspergillus* tracheobronchitis. Fortunately, this disease is being recognized with increased frequency as judged by the number of publications available in the peer-reviewed literature.

The management strategy for this patient certainly requires a two-step approach: temporizing measures followed by definitive treatment. The basis for selection of the instrument used—a rigid or a flexible bronchoscope—to perform debridement and to relieve symptoms remains institution and physician specific. In my experience, balloon bronchoplasty can be as effective as dilation with a rigid instrument. Once optimal patency of the trachea is established, an attempt should be made to probe the right upper lobe with a balloon catheter, and, if the stricture does not appear to be overly stiff and patent segmental airways are found beyond the stenosis, dilation might be attempted.

Medical measures, including inhaled bronchodilators and antifungal agents, as well as oral antifungals, should be continued. Corticosteroids should be avoided. Metal stents are clearly contraindicated in this case, even though there is a great likelihood of migration of silicone stents. This latter type of stent could be tried if the patient is deemed unsuitable for open surgical resection. In my opinion, 3D CT of the airway is very helpful because it clearly defines the extent (2 cm) and the nature (complex) of the stenosis. Following proper treatment of her tracheobronchial aspergillosis, this patient should be considered for tracheal reconstruction. A time-proven approach using Montgomery T-tube placement could also be a valid consideration if the complications of corrective surgery are deemed unacceptable. Prolonged surveillance is warranted, and topical as well as systemic antifungal treatment may need to be continued until total healing is established.

REFERENCES

1. Brichet A, Verkindre C, Dupont J, et al. Multidisciplinary approach to management of postintubation tracheal stenosis. *Eur Respir J.* 1999;13:888-893.
2. Santacruz JF, Mehta AC. Airway complications and management after lung transplantation: ischemia, dehiscence, and stenosis. *Proc Am Thorac Soc.* 2009;6:79-93.
3. Matthews JI, Matarese SL, Carpenter JL. Endobronchial tuberculosis simulating lung cancer. *Chest.* 1984;86:642-644.
4. Van den Brande P, Lambrechts M, Tack J, et al. Endobronchial tuberculosis mimicking lung cancer in elderly patients. *Respir Med.* 1991;85:107-109.
5. Chung HS, Lee JH. Bronchoscopic assessment of the evolution of endobronchial tuberculosis. *Chest.* 2000;117:385-392.
6. Kemper CA, Hosteler JS, Follansbee SE, et al. Ulcerative and plaque-like tracheobronchitis due to infection with *Aspergillus* in patients with AIDS. *Clin Infect Dis.* 1993;7:344-352.
7. Hines DW, Haber MH, Yaremko L, et al. Pseudomembranous tracheobronchitis caused by *Aspergillus. Am Rev Respir Dis.* 1991;143:1408-1411.
8. Denning DW. Commentary: unusual manifestation of aspergillosis. *Thorax.* 1995;50:812-813.
9. Tasci S, Glasmacher A, Lentini S, et al. Pseudomembranous and obstructive *Aspergillus* tracheobronchitis—optimal diagnostic strategy and outcome. *Mycoses.* 2006;49:37-42.
10. Berk JL, O'Regan A, Skinner M. Pulmonary and tracheobronchial amyloidosis. *Semin Respir Crit Care Med.* 2002;23:155-165.
11. Thompson PJ, Citron KM. Amyloid and the lower respiratory tract. *Thorax.* 1983;38:84-87.
12. Berg AM, Troxler RF, Grillone G, et al. Localized amyloidosis of the larynx: evidence for light chain composition. *Ann Otol Rhinol Laryngol.* 1993;102:884-889.
13. Kurrus JA, Hayes JK, Hoidal JR, et al. Radiation therapy for tracheobronchial amyloidosis. *Chest.* 1998;114:1489-1492.
14. Hussain K, Gilbert S. Tracheopathia osteochondroplastica. *Clin Med Res.* 2003;1:239-242.
15. Lazor R, Cordier JF. Tracheobronchopathia osteochondroplastica. *Orphanet Encyclopedia*, June 2004. http://www.orpha.net/data/patho/GB/uk-TO.pdf. Accessed May 25, 2011.
16. Birzgalis AR, Farrington WT, O'Keefe L, et al. Localized tracheopathia osteoplastica of the subglottis. *J Laryngol Otol.* 1993; 107:352-353.
17. Neumann A, Kasper D, Schultz-Coulon HJ. Clinical aspects of tracheopathia osteoplastica. *HNO.* 2001;49:41-47.
18. Yokoyama ST. Bronchial science. *Japan Research Institute Bronchial Magazine.* 1996;18:558-562.
19. Shum TK, Whitker CW, Meyer PR. Clinical update on rhinoscleroma. *Laryngoscope.* 1982;92:1149-1155.
20. Andreca R, Edson RS, Kern EB. Rhinoscleroma: a growing concern in the United States? Mayo Clinic experience. *Mayo Clin Proc.* 1993;68:1151-1157.
21. Gaafar HA, Gaafar AH, Nour YA. Rhinoscleroma: an updated experience through the last 10 years. *Acta Otolaryngol.* 2011; 131:440-446.
22. Amoils CP, Shindo ML. Laryngotracheal manifestations of rhinoscleroma. *Ann Otol Laryngol.* 1996;106:336-340.
23. Papadimos TJ. Healthcare access as a right, not a privilege: a construct of Western thought. *Philos Ethics Humanit Med.* 2007;2:2.
24. Murthy SC, Gildea TR, Mehta AC. Removal of self-expandable metallic stents: is it possible? *Semin Respir Crit Care Med.* 2004; 25:381-385.
25. Brennan TA. Physicians' professional responsibility to improve the quality of care. *Acad Med.* 2002;77:973-980.
26. Brodsky JB. Bronchoscopic procedures for central airway obstruction. *J Cardiothorac Vasc Anesth.* 2003;17:638-646.
27. Albert RK, Petty TL. Endobronchial tuberculosis progressing to bronchial stenosis. *Chest.* 1976;70:537-539.
28. Hoheisel G, Chan BK, Chan CH, et al. Endobronchial tuberculosis: diagnostic features and therapeutic outcome. *Respir Med.* 1994; 88:593-659.
29. Mehrad B, Paciocco G, Martinez FJ, et al. Spectrum of *Aspergillus* infection in lung transplant recipients: case series and review of the literature. *Chest.* 2001;119:169-175.
30. Saraceno JL, Phelps DT, Ferro TJ, et al. Chronic necrotizing pulmonary aspergillosis: approach to management. *Chest.* 1997; 112:541-548.
31. Herrera JM, McNeil KD, Higgins RS, et al. Airway complications after lung transplantation: treatment and long-term outcome. *Ann Thorac Surg.* 2001;71:989-994.
32. Nunley DR, Gal AA, Vega JD, et al. Saprophytic fungal infections and complications involving the bronchial anastomosis following human lung transplantation. *Chest.* 2002;122:1185-1191.
33. Chhajed PN, Malouf MA, Tamm M, et al. Interventional bronchoscopy for the management of airway complications following lung transplantation. *Chest.* 2001;120;1894-1899.
34. Herbrecht R, Denning DW, Patterson TF, et al. Randomized comparison of voriconazole and amphotericin B in primary therapy of invasive aspergillosis. *N Engl J Med.* 2002;347:408-415.
35. Denning DW, Kibbler CC, Barnes RA. British Society for Medical Mycology. British Society for Medical Mycology proposed standards of care for patients with invasive fungal infections. *Lancet Inf Dis.* 2003;3:230-240.
36. Lee KS, Boiselle PM. Update on multidetector computed tomography imaging of the airways. *J Thorac Imaging.* 2010;25: 112-124.
37. Deslée G, Brichet A, Lebuffe G, et al. Obstructive fibrinous tracheal pseudomembrane: a potentially fatal complication of tracheal intubation. *Am J Respir Crit Care Med.* 2000;162:1169-1171.
38. Peikert T, Tazelaar HD, Prakash U. Endobronchial cryptococcosis. *J Bronchol.* 2005;12:59-61.
39. Karnak D, Avery RK, Gildea TR, et al. Endobronchial fungal disease: an under-recognized entity. *Respiration.* 2007;74: 88-104.

SECTION 2

Practical Approach to Benign Tracheal Stenosis

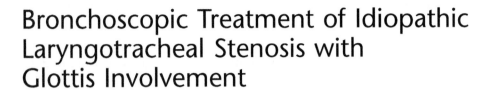

Chapter 6

Bronchoscopic Treatment of Idiopathic Laryngotracheal Stenosis with Glottis Involvement

This chapter emphasizes the following elements of the Four Box Approach: patient preferences and expectations (also includes family), anesthesia and other perioperative care, results and procedure-related complications, and referrals to medical, surgical, or palliative/end-of-life subspecialty care.

CASE DESCRIPTION

The patient is a 29-year-old woman who had developed mild hoarseness and progressive shortness of breath with exertion. These symptoms interfered with her life to the point that she had to stop working as a teacher because of impaired phonation. Intermittent sensations of nocturnal suffocation improved after coughing up thick mucus. She had no history, clinical signs, or symptoms of connective tissue disorders, and no history of endotracheal intubation. Other findings included asymptomatic mild mitral valve prolapse diagnosed after a routine cardiac examination revealed a 2/6 systolic ejection murmur. The patient had type 2 diabetes mellitus, which was well controlled with metformin. Her physical examination was unremarkable except for a mouth opening of 2 fingerbreadths. After 6 months of unsuccessful antiasthma treatment, a flexible bronchoscopy had revealed a circumferential subglottic stenosis extending for 1 cm with associated inflamed hyperemic mucosa (Figure 6-1). A fibrotic band extended to but did not involve the right vocal cord. The degree of airway narrowing was calculated at 60% on computed tomography and morphometric bronchoscopic analysis (Figure 6-2). No posterior glottis stenosis or cicatricial fusion of the vocal cords was noted.

DISCUSSION POINTS

1. Mention two demonstrably accurate methods for assessing functional impairment in this patient.

2. Describe how the extent of laryngotracheal stenosis (LTS) affects whether this patient should be referred for surgical intervention.
3. Describe existing evidence for using adjuvant therapies to potentially decrease the rate of recurrence of this type of stricture.

CASE RESOLUTION

Initial Evaluations

Physical Examination, Complementary Tests, and Functional Status Assessment

The clinical presentation of this patient is classic for idiopathic laryngotracheal stenosis (LTS). Most patients who suffer from this disease are females in their third, fourth, or fifth decade. Currently, it is not clear why idiopathic LTS is restricted to females, but estrogen and progesterone receptor studies in resected surgical specimens showed positive staining of fibroblasts, suggesting a hormonal role in pathogenesis.[1] Many patients will have been misdiagnosed with asthma for months to years before an LTS is discovered. The duration of symptoms in one study was less than 2 years in 28% of patients, 2 to 10 years in 61% of patients, and longer than 10 years in 11% of patients.[1] Symptoms at rest in LTS usually are not present until a 70% reduction in tracheal lumen diameter is attained, and stridor, at rest, can be noticed only when the tracheal lumen becomes smaller than 5 mm in diameter.[2] Effort intolerance caused by exertional dyspnea is the primary cause of morbidity and early disability in LTS. Its presence in this patient is consistent with moderate stenosis using a bronchoscopic classification, signaled by 50% to 70% airway lumen narrowing.[3-5] Under the Myer-Cotton System* for LTS, she would be classified as having a grade II lesion, because her stenotic index (SI)[†] was 60% (Figure 6-3).[6] The patient's functional status, which probably should be part of a multidimensional evaluation of LTS, can be objectively measured using, for example, the Medical Research Council (MRC) dyspnea scale, which has been shown to be sensitive to the presence of varying degrees of LTS.[7]

Bronchoscopy, in addition to contributing to an assessment of the severity of airway narrowing, allows precise determination of the extent (craniocaudal length) and location of the stenosis. According to the McCaffrey

---

*A widely used staging system for classifying tracheal stenosis based on the degree of airway narrowing.

†The SI represents the cross-sectional area (CSA) of the obstructed area relative to that of normal airway lumen proximal or distal to the stenosis. $SI = (CSA_{normal} - CSA_{abnormal})/(CSA_{normal} \times 100\%)$; the greater the SI, the greater the degree of airway narrowing and the more severe the obstruction.

67

system,* the patient's stricture, with extension to the glottis, was stage IV. This system is based on the site and extent of an airway stenosis. Four stages are thus defined: I: lesions confined to the subglottis or trachea that are less than 1 cm in length; II: subglottic stenoses longer

*McCaffrey system classifies LTS based on the subsites involved and on the length of the stenosis; sites of stenosis in this system are defined as follows: subglottic, when stenosis is in the region bounded superiorly by a plane 0.5 cm below the glottis and inferiorly by the lower edge of the cricoid cartilage; tracheal, when the stenosis is below the lower edge of the cricoid; and glottis stenosis, when stenosis of the interarytenoid space is present.

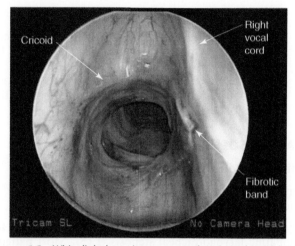

Figure 6-1 White light bronchoscopy reveals a circumferential stricture, extending 1 cm, with associated inflamed hyperemic mucosa but without malacia. A fibrotic band extends to but does not involve the right vocal cord.

than 1 cm within the cricoid and not extending to the glottis or trachea; III: subglottic stenoses that extend into the upper trachea but do not involve the glottis; and IV: lesions involving the glottis. Almost 20% of patients with LTS have combined subglottic and glottis stenosis.[8]

Comorbidities

Other than having diabetes and mitral valve prolapse without significant mitral regurgitation, confirmed by echocardiography, our patient was healthy. Diabetes is known to impair microcirculation with resultant deleterious effects on wound healing. Diabetes was found to be an important risk factor for anastomotic complications (odds ratio of 3) in patients who undergo laryngotracheoplasty or cricotracheal resection.[9] This may be a consequence of impairment of an already compromised collateral circulation at the end of the divided airway. Tension at the anastomosis further increases risk.

Support System

The patient was married to a very supportive husband; her knowledge of the diagnosis was minimal. In addition to receiving information from us during the initial encounter, she was advised to search for support groups, chat rooms, and reliable Internet websites for patients suffering from the same disorder.[10,11]

Patient Preferences and Expectations

Although the patient was asymptomatic at rest, her disease interfered with her ability to work, exercise, and enjoy outdoor activities. She wanted to have a child and was worried that pregnancy could worsen her symptoms and compromise both her and her baby's health. She was

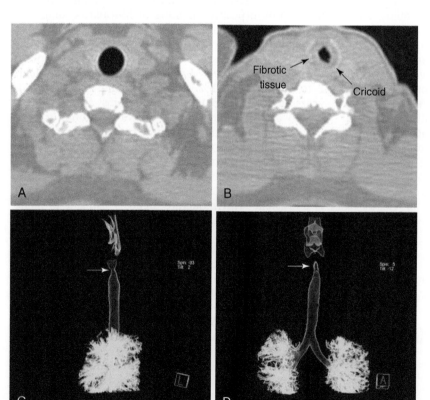

Figure 6-2 Axial computed tomography (CT) scan view shows **(A)** the normal tracheal lumen distal to the stricture and **(B)** circumferential fibrotic stenotic tissue at the level of the cricoid. External three-dimensional reconstructions **(C)** in the left lateral and anterior views show the 1 cm long stricture and **(D)** normal tracheal lumen beyond the stenosis.

Grade	
I: 0%-50% obstruction	
II: 51%-70% obstruction	
III: 71%-99% obstruction	
IV: 100% obstruction	

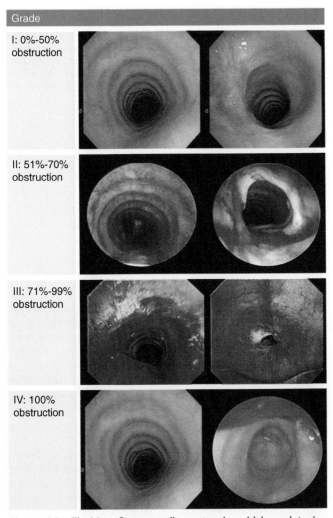

Figure 6-3 The Myer-Cotton grading system is a widely used staging system for classifying laryngotracheal stenosis based on the degree of airway narrowing. Grade IV strictures are rarely seen and only in patients with indwelling tracheostomies because 100% obstruction is not compatible with life in a nontracheostomized patient.

informed of available therapeutic options for LTS, including flexible or rigid bronchoscopic dilation, laser-assisted mechanical dilation (LAMD), surgery, and even tracheostomy. Because tracheostomy would further compromise her quality of life, this was considered only as a last resort in case of disease progression. She was terrified about the possibility of losing her voice, which would preclude her from working as a teacher. After her symptoms, personal values, and expectations were considered, the likelihood of complications resulting from open surgical resection was believed to outweigh the benefits, in part because of her very high stenosis extending to the glottis, diabetes, and the possibility of dysphonia postsurgical interventions.[9] Rigid bronchoscopy with dilation and laser resection under general anesthesia, therefore, appeared to be a reasonable initial therapeutic alternative.

Procedural Strategies

Indications

This patient's stricture was considered idiopathic because no history of intubation, autoimmune disease,

relapsing polychondritis, radiation, trauma, or prior surgery was elicited; therefore, systemic medical therapy with immunosuppressive drugs had no role. A bronchoscopic procedure or open surgery could restore satisfactory airway lumen patency and improve symptoms.[4,9]

Her active lifestyle caused routinely high flow velocity through her moderately stenotic airway. Improving airway patency to less than 50% narrowing could alleviate her exertional dyspnea.[12] In a large series of idiopathic strictures, the point of maximal stenosis was found to be almost always located in the region extending from the upper edge of the cricoid to the lower edge of the first tracheal ring.[13] Our patient's stricture was only 1 cm in length. From a flow dynamics standpoint, longer stenoses (>1 cm) show only a small difference in pressure profiles, with a slightly smaller magnitude of total pressure drop across the stricture and shorter (<1 cm) strictures of comparable diameter.[12] Strictures up to 1 cm long are considered of mild extent and, if uncomplicated by malacia, appear to respond well to bronchoscopic laser-assisted dilation. On the other hand, operable patients with longer strictures and patients with associated malacia may be better managed with open surgical interventions.[8]

The morphology of the stricture, however, was circumferential. Results from studies show that patients with circumferential stenosis require a second endoscopic intervention more often than those with purely eccentric localized hypertrophic tissue (75% vs. 43%) (Figure 6-4). This would support referral for primary surgical resection.[14,15] Risks of surgical resection and reanastomosis, however, must be carefully weighed because of the fibrotic band extending to the right vocal cord and the patient's fear of voice alteration. An incomplete surgical resection could leave behind residual fibrotic tissue, leading to restenosis.[16] In addition to the length of the resection, the fixed morphology of the stricture plays an important role in anastomotic tension: Fibrous retracting strictures (i.e., circumferential and hourglass strictures) are very different from dynamic, malacic stenoses (pseudoglottic, triangular stomal strictures); in the former, the healthy trachea is already tractioned, whereas in the latter, it is the normal elasticity of the trachea that tends to worsen the stenosis. Just because stenoses are of the same length, therefore, does not mean that traction across the suture line after surgical resections is the same.[9] Taking into account the circumferential and fixed morphology, its extension to the glottis, the patient's preferences, and her diabetes, we chose to proceed initially with a rigid bronchoscopic intervention.

Contraindications

No absolute contraindications to rigid bronchoscopy were identified. No history of lung disease that could potentially increase the risk for hemodynamic instability or oxygenation or ventilation difficulties during general anesthesia was reported. Her mitral valve prolapse was asymptomatic, and no history of renal or liver disease that would increase the risk for bleeding was elicited.

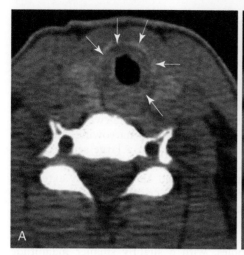 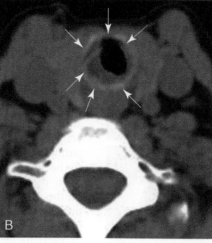

Figure 6-4 Morphologies of idiopathic laryngotracheal stenosis at the level of the cricoid cartilage from two different patients. **A,** Circumferential: Hypertrophic tissue overlies the cricoid cartilage *(arrows)* over its entire circumference. **B,** Eccentric: Hypertrophic tissue is localized and noncircumferential.

Expected Results

Our patient's 1 cm, fixed, circumferential stenosis with hypertrophic fibrotic tissue could initially respond to laser-assisted dilation with an increase in airway cross-sectional area. In patients with idiopathic LTS, however, the therapeutic success of rigid bronchoscopic interventions is variable. Factors impacting success include stenoses that (1) were not completely circumferential (eccentric) (see Figure 6-4), (2) measured less than 1.0 cm in the vertical extent, and (3) were not associated with significant loss of cartilage or remodeling.[14] In a retrospective analysis of 16 patients with mean follow-up time of 75.5 months, 14 patients required treatment: 9 patients were controlled effectively using endoscopic laser techniques; endoscopic management failed, however, in 5 patients (noted to have stenosis thicker than 1 cm).[17]

In a larger study of 30 patients, endoscopic treatment by CO_2 (in 4 patients) or neodymium-doped yttrium aluminum garnet (Nd : YAG) laser–assisted dilation (in 26 patients) without or with temporary airway stent insertion (in 4 patients) was considered to be the treatment of choice for initial management of idiopathic LTS. After repeated endoscopic failures (mean, 6.2), open neck surgery by laryngotracheoplasty or reconstruction and anastomosis was performed in 17% of patients, particularly for lesions longer than 1 cm.[18] In another series, all patients were treated bronchoscopically. Sixty percent required a second procedure, with a mean interval between procedures of 9 months, and no need for tracheotomy or open surgical intervention was reported.[15] Similar results have been reported in several nonrandomized studies of bronchoscopic management.[18-20]

Team Experience

Laser-tissue interactions are based on biologic, photochemical, or thermal reactions. The treating team's knowledge of tissue effects in specific settings is important because choosing the wrong laser (e.g., using the Nd : YAG laser to cut or the potassium-titanyl-phosphate [KTP] laser to coagulate) or inappropriate laser settings or resection techniques (e.g., inappropriate use of power

density*) in the subglottic area can enhance laser-related adverse effects. Laser-related adverse effects might alter local anatomy. We suggest, therefore, that patients with idiopathic LTS should be managed within the context of a multidisciplinary airway disease program, or, at the least, that their condition should be discussed with surgical colleagues whenever possible before bronchoscopic treatments are initiated.

Risk-Benefit Analysis

A stricture in the subglottic larynx[†] poses a challenge because of its proximity to the vocal cords, and because this region is the narrowest segment of the airway. Although no prospective randomized studies are available from which to draw conclusions with regard to the best therapeutic intervention, several investigators have retrospectively compared the outcomes of open airway surgery versus endoscopic treatments (laser, dilation) in idiopathic LTS. Initial endoscopic treatment is recommended for lesions less than 1 cm in length and without cartilage collapse because of the high rate of symptomatic relief and the minimal complications reported in this group.[17,18] Many proponents of surgical therapies advocate bronchoscopic treatment initially, provided that it is not repeated if the stenosis returns to its initial grade afterward.[21] Others propose that primary resection and reanastomosis should be offered to patients with disease refractory to three (not one) bronchoscopic procedures.[17]

Although treatment algorithms may be helpful in providing guidance, treatment decisions should be individualized according to causes, functional impairment,

---

*Power density or irradiance represents the quotient of the power incident on an element of surface and is expressed in watts per square centimeter. This is controlled by the surgeon: the power setting in watts and the spot size on the tissue (determined by the distance of the laser fiber from the target).

†The larynx, located at the level of the C3-C6 vertebrae, extends from the tip of the epiglottis to the inferior border of the cricoid cartilage; *subglottic larynx* refers to the space extending from the glottis (vocal cords and the space between them) to the inferior border of the cricoid cartilage.

Figure 6-5 **A,** Suspension apparatus in a patient with laryngotracheal stenosis (LTS) undergoing CO_2 laser–assisted dilation. **B,** Rigid bronchoscopy in a different patient with LTS undergoing dilation.

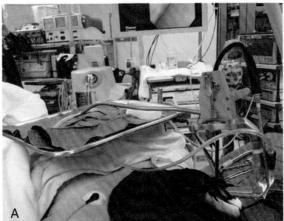
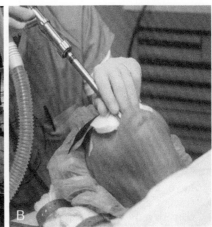

comorbidities, the site and severity of stenosis, and the function of the vocal cords.[21] Our patient, for example, has a very high lesion with glottic extension, associated inflammation, and diabetes. These increase her risk for postoperative complications.[13] At the same time, although bronchoscopic treatment is justifiable as an initial treatment, repeated procedures probably should be reserved for patients in whom definitive resection is deemed inappropriate because of unresectability, inoperability, patient choice, or surgeon preference in light of excessive risk for restenosis or procedure-related complications due to anatomy, surgical inexperience, severe inflammation, or proximity to the glottis.

Therapeutic Alternatives for Restoring Airway Patency

- *Dilation:* One study analyzed a total of 384 procedures performed in 127 patients with multifactorial LTS: 91 (72%) patients underwent primary dilation, of whom 12 (13%) were cured, 4 (4%) had evidence of persistent LTS but did not require further treatment, and 11 (12%) were lost to follow-up.[22] Dilation can be performed with tapered Savary-Gilliard dilators, Jackson dilators, bougies, or angioplasty balloons after radial laser or electrocautery incisions.[23]
- *KTP laser:* As compared with the CO_2 laser, its tissue penetration is significantly deeper, so that special attention must be paid to avoid perforation of the airway.
- *Nd:YAG laser:* This approach is used in conjunction with dilation to release the tension of the stricture by performing radial incisions in the stenotic tissues.[24] Use of Nd:YAG at a low power density in a noncontact mode, however, is considered by some experts to be unacceptable primary treatment that could cause more scarring and could preclude or complicate further open surgical interventions.[21]
- *CO_2 laser:* This technique is used in suspension laryngoscopy for laryngeal and subglottic stenoses (Figure 6-5), or with a rigid bronchoscope and a CO_2 laser coupler for tracheal and bronchial stenoses. In one study, 49 patients with laryngeal stenosis, 6 patients with tracheal stenosis, and 5 patients with combined laryngeal and tracheal stenosis underwent CO_2 laser resection (total, 60 patients); follow-up was provided for 1 month to 8 years. Multiple procedures were required in 35 of 49 (71%) patients with laryngeal stenosis. Thirty-nine (80%) of these patients with laryngeal stenosis were successfully managed (average number of procedures in successful cases, 2.18). Factors found to be associated with poor results or failure include circumferential stricture longer than 1 cm in vertical dimension, tracheomalacia, previous history of severe bacterial infection associated with tracheostomy, and posterior laryngeal inlet scarring with arytenoid fixation.[14,25] Based on laser-tissue interactions, the CO_2 laser (10,600 nm) is the preferred laser for treating benign stenosis, because no scatter and no deep penetration occur; therefore, the risk for collateral mucosal damage or airway perforation, respectively, is lower[26]; it is used in the ultrapulse mode with a fluence* of 150 mJ/cm^2 at a frequency of 10 Hz to avoid charring and heat diffusion into surrounding tissues.[21]
- *Spray cryotherapy:* Liquid nitrogen (−196° C) is applied directly to the tissue via a low-pressure, disposable 7-French catheter; the published experience is still very limited for airway applications. In a case series, three patients were successfully treated using balloon dilation and four cycles of 5 second spray cryotherapy with complete thaw of the treated area between applications; no further interventions were required at 9 months' follow-up.[27]
- *Metal stent insertion* is associated with significant complications, including granulation tissue, extension of stenoses, perforation, and hemoptysis.[28,29] The Food and Drug Administration (FDA) warns that metallic tracheal stents in patients with benign airway disorders should be used only after all other treatment options (such as surgical procedures or placement of silicone stents) have been thoroughly explored. Use of these stents as a bridging therapy to surgery is not recommended, because removal of these stents is associated with significant complications.[29] In one study, all patients with LTS who had undergone covered or uncovered metallic stent placement developed new strictures or granulation tissue, which precluded definitive surgical treatment or required more extensive resections.[30]

---

*Energy fluence represents total energy incident on the tissue per unit area.

- *Silicone stents* are placed under rigid bronchoscopy or suspension laryngoscopy for inoperable or unresectable patients with recurrent high LTS despite repeated dilations. When sitting in the subglottic regions, the proximal end of the stent may induce ulceration and granulation tissue formation with subsequent glotto-subglottic restenosis.
- *Airway reconstruction,* such as laryngotracheoplasty, cricotracheal resection, or tracheal resection, could be the primary treatment considered for patients who become operable candidates after bronchoscopic intervention, as well as for operable candidates who have failed bronchoscopic treatment. Cricotracheal resection with primary thyrotracheal anastomosis is considered by some to be the procedure of choice for the treatment of severe idiopathic LTS (>70% luminal obstruction).[31,32] Data suggest that fewer patients required subsequent intervention after primary airway reconstruction (27%) than after a dilation treatment (70%).[33] Resection is usually successful. Mortality among patients who had anastomotic complications was 7.4% (6/81), whereas it was 0.01% among those without anastomotic complications. Anastomotic complications are uncommon in idiopathic LTS. Important risk factors are reoperation, diabetes, lengthy resections, laryngotracheal resections, young patient age (pediatric patients), and the need for tracheostomy before operation.[9] A laryngotracheal resection with anastomosis to the larynx was also associated with a higher anastomotic failure rate (odds ratio, 1.8). Advantages of major airway reconstruction are that it consists of single-stage, definitive treatments. However, these treatments are associated with higher mortality and morbidity than dilation, including unilateral recurrent laryngeal nerve palsy, neck abscess, pneumothorax, and subcutaneous emphysema. This surgery can also significantly impact the adult female voice, lowering the pitch of the speaking voice into the male range and reducing pitch range. The change in voice that potentially accompanies this procedure should be discussed with patients during a preoperative counseling session.[33]
  - Grillo et al. treated 35 patients by both laryngotracheal reconstruction (LTR) and laryngotracheoplasty (LTP) or cricotracheal resection (CTR). Ten patients had excellent results and 22 had good outcomes with respect to airway and voice preservation and did not require further dilations; two cases had fair results and underwent dilation annually, and one patient required a permanent tracheostomy.[34]
  - Ashiku et al. evaluated 73 patients with idiopathic LTS; all patients were treated with LTR. Twenty-eight of 73 (38%) had undergone a previous procedure with laser, dilation, tracheostomy, T-tube, or laryngotracheal operations. No perioperative mortality was reported; temporary tracheostomies were needed in 7 patients. Sixty-seven of 73 (91%) patients had good to excellent long-term results with voice and breathing quality and did not require further intervention.[13]
- *Permanent tracheostomy* is warranted in the few patients with critical stenoses who are candidates for neither surgery nor stent insertion, who develop recurrence after such interventions, or who have failed multiple bronchoscopic treatments. Tracheostomy, particularly when performed emergently, can render subsequent laryngotracheal resection and anastomosis impossible because of lengthening of the damaged tract of airway to be resected. Intubation is preferable until a long-term treatment plan is chosen.

Cost-Effectiveness

To our knowledge, no prospective randomized studies have evaluated the outcomes or cost-effectiveness of endoscopic versus open surgical interventions for this disease.

Informed Consent

After they were advised of all therapeutic alternatives, the patient and her husband elected to proceed with rigid bronchoscopy under general anesthesia. She was informed of potential risks for postoperative development of laryngeal edema, stridor, and possible respiratory failure. She was informed that the stricture may recur, and that she may require subsequent interventions. Feedback communication techniques were used, and both she and her spouse were able to accurately describe the proposed procedure, expected results, alternatives, and potential associated complications.

Techniques and Results

Anesthesia and Perioperative Care

The need for antibiotics is routinely addressed during the preprocedural pause. For this patient, this issue is important given her mitral valve prolapse. Although two studies showed that bacteremia is seen in more than 30% of patients undergoing rigid bronchoscopy,[35,36] according to current recommendations from the American Heart Association, patients with mitral valve prolapse no longer require endocarditis prophylaxis.[37]

The anesthesiologist should be informed about the procedure plan: use of the rigid bronchoscope and spontaneous assisted ventilation; the potential for air leak while working through an open system as compared with a closed system with jet ventilation; difficulty in recording end-tidal CO_2; the rules of laser use; and the need to reduce the fraction of inspired oxygen (FiO_2) to less than 0.4 during resection to avoid airway fire. Although muscle relaxants usually are not necessary, a smooth induction is warranted in patients with high LTS to avoid "bucking" and trauma to the larynx during the intubation process. When general anesthesia with inhaled gases is employed, the nose and mouth must be sealed, usually with gauze packing, to avoid gas leakage. Packing, however, restricts manipulation of the rigid bronchoscope within the airway.

We routinely use spontaneous assisted ventilation after induction and intubation with the rigid scope in our patients with upper and central airway obstruction. Spontaneous ventilation, however, creates negative inspiratory intraluminal pressure that exacerbates an extrathoracic lesion. With inspiration, negative intra-luminal pressure causes inward movement of collapsible airway segments, further narrowing the lumen and limiting inspiratory airflow. During expiration, positive intraluminal pressure improves airway dimensions and airflow.

In patients with extrathoracic LTS, therefore, muscle paralysis and positive-pressure ventilation (PPV) may be preferred because this approach generates positive intra-luminal pressure that improves ventilation. This helps explain the apparent improvement in certain airway obstructive lesions after PPV. For example, the degree of upper airway obstruction is lessened when flow-volume loops are recorded under conditions of muscle relaxation and PPV in comparison with spontaneous ventilation.[38]

After removal of the rigid bronchoscope, transient but potentially severe laryngeal or subglottic edema can occur.[39] In these cases, laryngoscopy-guided endotracheal reintubation can be difficult, so a flexible bronchoscope should be readily available. In addition, it is advisable that the rigid bronchoscope not be dismantled until the operator and the anesthesiologist agree that laryngotra-cheal patency is ensured and reintubation is not needed.

We routinely administer dexamethasone 8 to 10 mg intravenously after rigid bronchoscopic interventions in patients with LTS. Given that procedure-related laryngeal edema can occur within 2 to 24 hours after extubation, patients are monitored and are often kept overnight in a short-stay unit. No clear evidence suggests that periop-erative administration of corticosteroids prevents laryn-geal edema in patients undergoing rigid bronchoscopy; however, experimental animal studies of induced laryn-geal injury have shown that dexamethasone given before extubation resulted in reduced submucosal edema.[40]

Instrumentation

We used a 12 mm EFER rigid open ventilating broncho-scope. The necessary accessory instruments for this case included suction tubing and a bare laser fiber. KTP laser was used for this stenosis because it has greater tissue absorption* than Nd:YAG (but less than CO_2), resulting in more shallow tissue penetration than is attained with Nd:YAG (but deeper than with CO_2). In addition, its low scattering characteristics minimize collateral airway wall injury.[41] Gauze pads, foam rubber, or plastic mouth guards can be used to protect the teeth. Depending on the position of the glottis and the laryngotracheal axis, one, two, or no pillows may be necessary beneath the patient's head resting on the operating table.

Anatomic Dangers and Other Risks

Structures neighboring the larynx (carotid arteries, jugular and thyroid veins) and superior and recurrent laryngeal nerves can be injured during a bronchoscopic procedure with laser resection if the laser beam is not directed

parallel to the airway. Excessive tension on the larynx from a large rigid bronchoscope may cause edema, vocal cord damage, or arytenoid cartilage dislocation, resulting in postoperative stridor, laryngospasm, and respiratory distress.

Results and Procedure-Related Complications

Direct intubation using a rigid telescope through the rigid tube is our method of choice for rigid broncho-scopic intubation. The bronchoscope was inserted with its beveled edge facing forward. Upon looking through the telescope, the bronchoscopist can see the uvula pos-teriorly; the bronchoscope is advanced along the base of the tongue, and the rigid bronchoscope is gently lifted anteriorly and upward, bringing the epiglottis into view (see video on ExpertConsult.com) (Video II.6.1). The anterior aspect of the beveled tip of the bronchoscope is then slid beneath the epiglottis. Gentle advancement of the rigid tube provides visualization of the arytenoids; the rigid tube is lifted more anteriorly so that the vocal cords are seen. As they are approached, the tip of the bronchoscope is rotated 90 degrees laterally so that the bevel lies between them. The bronchoscope is advanced without traumatizing the vocal cords or the arytenoids and is rotated to enter the subglottis so that the beveled tip lies along the posterior wall of the trachea (see video on ExpertConsult.com) (Video II.6.1). The extent of the stricture, its location, associated mucosal changes, and the presence or absence of malacia and infection were assessed. Its distance with respect to the vocal folds and the carina was measured in millimeters and in number of residual normal tracheal rings above and below the stenosis (see video on ExpertConsult.com) (Video II.6.2).

Extension was 1 cm, starting at 0.5 cm below the vocal cords, with most severe narrowing at 1.5 cm below the glottis at the level of the cricoid cartilage. A KTP laser was used at high power density in near contact mode with 1 second, 6 W pulses (total energy delivered, 100 Joules). A single 3 mm long and 0.5 to 1.0 mm deep radial inci-sion was made through the hypertrophic tissue to reach the plane of the normal lumen of the tracheal wall before dilation (see video on ExpertConsult.com) (Video II.6.3). When two or more incisions are performed, care is taken to preserve mucosa between the incisions.[15] Airway patency was restored. The procedure lasted 45 minutes, after which the patient was extubated and was transferred to the postanesthesia care unit for 24 hours; no complications were noted up to the time of discharge the next morning. The morphometric bronchoscopy-calculated post-treatment stenotic index was 20%.[5]

Long-Term Management

Outcome Assessment

Objective measurements revealed improved airway patency, and the history suggested improved exertional dyspnea. Symptomatic improvement was not assessed using the MRC dyspnea scale validated for LTS,[42] nor was a voice assessment tool used to identify procedure-related changes. Both are now used before and after treatment for idiopathic LTS.[43]

*Absorption is the key phenomenon in effective laser use and is defined as the transformation of radiant energy to a different form of energy through the interaction of matter. When photons enter the tissue, those that are not reflected, scattered, or transmitted are absorbed, and their energy is transferred to molecules within the tissues and is normally dissipated as heat, responsible for the clinical effects of lasers.

Referral

Multidisciplinary assessment involved thoracic surgeons; ear, nose, and throat surgeons; pulmonary physicians; and radiologists. Open surgical intervention remained a treatment option in cases of symptomatic recurrence. We therefore insisted on referral to an experienced tracheal surgeon for consultation.

Follow-up Tests and Procedures

Elective outpatient follow-up with flexible bronchoscopy was not recommended unless symptoms recurred,[44] which, in fact, happened 6 months later. This prompted out-of-state referral to a thoracic surgeon for resection, but the surgeon recommended repeat rigid bronchoscopic resection and dilation. We added a prescription for proton pump inhibitors because a history of gastroesophageal reflux is often present in patients with idiopathic LTS.[45] Reflux is considered a probable cause of idiopathic LTS because healing of subglottic injury is impaired by gastric juices in experimental animal research.

With regard to future interventions, in case our patient becomes pregnant as intended, the literature suggests that pregnant patients with subglottic stenosis usually present with symptoms during the third trimester.[46,47] Worsening symptoms may not be related to recurrence of the disease process itself, but rather may be caused by pregnancy-induced airway mucosal hyperemia and edema. Procedures often can be postponed until after delivery, given that labor-induced hyperventilation can potentially contribute to severe flow limitation. If strictures are present and airflow limitation is a concern, general anesthesia should be avoided, if possible, and the stenosis palliated using flexible bronchoscopy with moderate sedation, electrocautery, and dilation.[46] We believe that patients with advanced pregnancy requiring therapeutic bronchoscopic intervention should be assessed by an obstetrician, and obstetrics should be on standby during the procedure in case the woman goes into labor.

Quality Improvement

We judge outcomes of interventions for LTS on the basis of restored airway patency, resolution of symptoms, preservation of a satisfactory voice, and absence of symptomatic recurrence requiring reintervention. Objective voice assessment tools have been validated for use in females suffering from idiopathic LTS who are undergoing open tracheal resection.[48] Results are considered *excellent* if voice (including singing voice) and respiration are viewed as normal by the patient, and *good* if only a mild change in vocal characteristics is noted. This usually indicates some degree of weakness in the ability to project the voice and an inability to sing as well as before the surgery. Mild dyspnea on major exertion is accepted as a *good* result because the maximum airway attainable in such cases is the anatomically narrower diameter of the immediate subglottis. A result is considered *fair* in cases of hoarseness, an intermittently weak voice, or exercise tolerance limited by postoperative airway stenosis requiring dilations.[13] Repeat rigid bronchoscopic treatment satisfactorily restored airway patency without causing voice changes, but this remains a concern for both the patient and the treating team in case subsequent intervention is needed.

DISCUSSION POINTS

1. Mention two demonstrably accurate methods for assessing functional impairment in this patient.
   - *Single-domain assessment:* MRC dyspnea scale is more sensitive to the presence of varying degrees of tracheal stenosis than are peak expiratory flow and forced expiratory volume in 1 second.[7]
   - *Multiple-domain assessment:*
     - The Clinical COPD Questionnaire is a 10-item patient-administered scale that assesses symptom severity, functional limitation, and mental function. This is a valid and sensitive patient-centered disease-specific outcome measure instrument that is used to assess symptom severity, levels of function, and well-being in adult patients with LTS.[49]
     - The A-D-V-S System documents functional outcomes of interventions for adult LTS. It addresses airway status (A) with regard to the presence or absence of tracheostomy or airway stent, as well as dyspnea (D), voice quality (V), and swallowing ability (S).[50]
2. Describe how the extent of LTS affects whether this patient should be referred for surgical intervention.
   - A craniocaudal length greater than 1 cm is predictive for failure of bronchoscopic intervention[14,17,18] and therefore is indicative of a preference for surgical resection in many instances.
3. Describe existing evidence for using adjuvant therapies to potentially decrease the rate of recurrence of this type of stricture.
   - *Antireflux medication:* The impact of treating reflux on outcomes of LTS is not yet known, but personal and published anecdotal evidence supports this strategy.[51]
   - *Intralesional corticosteroid injection:* potentially beneficial in Wegener's granulomatosis (WG) or post intubation LTS, but studies show no benefit in idiopathic LTS.[52]
   - *Topical application of mitomycin-C:* This alkylating agent inhibits fibroblast proliferation and extracellular matrix protein synthesis. Performed during bronchoscopic treatment with the hope of reducing fibrosis and restenosis, its use is debated.
     - *Positive studies:* a retrospective study of 50 patients and no controls: 93 endoscopic procedures (dilations) with mitomycin application were performed; 75% to 93% success rate (airway stenosis relief) with one major complication (fungal infection)[53]; in another study of 16 patients who underwent laser-assisted dilation, mitomycin was superior to both placebo and intralesional steroids.[52]
     - *Negative studies:* 16 patients with idiopathic LTS underwent laser dilations with and without mitomycin; results were inconclusive after a mean follow-up of 76 months.[17] A randomized,

placebo-controlled trial of patients with LTS compared restenosis rates of two applications of mitomycin-C given 3 to 4 weeks apart, versus one application immediately after surgery[54]; relapse occurred at a slower rate in the two-application group during the first 3 years, and recurrence 5 years after surgery was similarly high (70%) in both groups.* The local milieu with high-level, matrix-associated expression of transforming growth factor (TGF)-β_1 in stenoses could be one reason for the limited treatment effect of mitomycin-C.[55]

- Other antiproliferative agents
  - *5-Fluorouracil:* This agent has antiproliferative effects on fibroblasts. Although no human studies have been reported to date, injection in soft tissue adjacent to induced subglottic stenosis in rabbits led to lower rates of stenosis formation.[56]
  - *Halofuginone:* This antibiotic agent has antifibrotic properties. No human studies have been conducted to date, but in vitro, its effects are comparable with those of mitomycin-C for fibroblast inhibition. No subglottic stenosis was seen in 10 dogs treated with oral halofuginone compared with a 72% rate of stenosis in controls.[57]

Expert Commentary

provided by Guri Sandhu, MD, FRCS, FRCS (ORL-HNS), and Reza Nouraei, MA, MBBChir, MRCS

The authors describe a case of idiopathic subglottic stenosis treated with rigid bronchoscopy and KTP laser. This progressive fibro-inflammatory condition exclusively affects females, in our experience, of European ancestry, most commonly during the third and fourth decades of life. It is, by definition, a diagnosis of exclusion, and we agree with the authors' diagnostic evaluation.

Our diagnostic criteria for idiopathic subglottic stenosis are given in Table 6-1. Because patients with vasculitis sequentially and additively present with different manifestations of their disease over several years, we keep this diagnosis under regular review with histology and periodic clinical and biochemical screenings.

We would add to the authors' initial assessment objective assessments of airway physiology and symptom severity. In particular, we would globally assess the degree of dyspnea, dysphonia, and dysphagia using the ADVS system[43] and individual symptom domains using the Clinical COPD Questionnaire[49] for airway, the Voice Handicap Index (VHI)-10 for voice,[58] and the Eating Assessment Tool (EAT)-10 scale for swallowing.[59]

We would perform flexible pharyngolaryngoscopy to assess the vocal folds for mobility impairment and

Table 6-1 Diagnostic Criteria for Idiopathic Subglottic Stenosis

Clinical Features
- Female patient
- No history of laryngotracheal injury
  - No endotracheal intubation or tracheotomy/no occurrence of exertional dyspnea within 3 years of intubation/tracheotomy
  - No thyroid/anterior neck surgery
  - No neck irradiation
  - No caustic or thermal injuries
  - No significant anterior neck trauma (blunt or penetrating)
- No history of autoimmunity
  - Negative history for vasculitis, formally ascertained through a vasculitis-specific systemic inquiry and semi-quantified using the Birmingham Vasculitis Activity Scale (BVAS)
  - No history to suggest sarcoidosis or amyloidosis

Serum Biochemistry
- Negative titers for:
  - Angiotensin-converting enzyme (ACE)
  - Antinuclear antibody (ANA), rheumatoid factor (RF)
  - Antineutrophil cytoplasmic antibody (ANCA)

Gross Lesion Morphology
- Stenosis must include the subglottis.

*Histopathology**
- Exclusion of other pathologic entities (e.g. tumors, vasculitides, amyloidosis)
- Fibrosis restricted to lamina propria with normal perichondrium/cartilage
- Mixture of granulation and fibrosis with prominence of keloidal pattern fibrosis

*This is established with a deep endoscopic biopsy at the time of first treatment.

the hypopharynx for pooling of secretions, but never flexible tracheoscopy/bronchoscopy in a symptomatic spontaneously breathing patient, because this can readily precipitate acute airway obstruction in the presence of a tight stenosis (Figure 6-6).

We have a low threshold for investigating laryngopharyngeal reflux, and most patients receive antireflux therapy. Where any concern is raised about laryngeal dysfunction and dysphagia, we would also perform video fluoroscopy. In this case a fibrous band was noted to extend to the undersurface of the right vocal fold, but both vocal folds were mobile. Therefore we would consider this case a type I and not a type IV McCaffrey stenosis.

Assessment of airflow physiology using flow-volume loop examination is a routine part of our initial and ongoing assessment of patients with airway stenosis. Flow-volume loops provide detailed information about

---

*This study may be confounded by various causes of LTS (idiopathic tracheal stenosis [ITS], post-intubation tracheal stenosis [PITS], and WG).

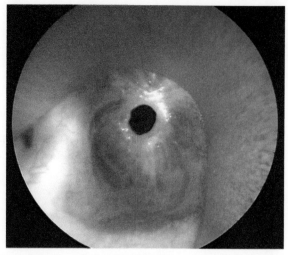

Figure 6-6 A patient with idiopathic subglottic stenosis and a maximum cross-sectional airway diameter of 4 mm.

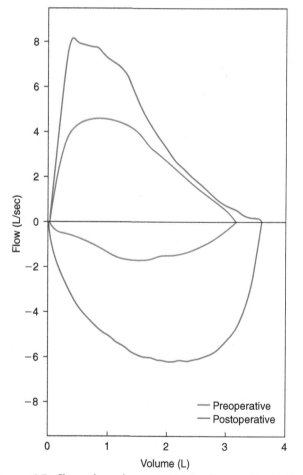

Figure 6-7 Flow-volume loop examination in a patient before *(blue line)* and after *(green line)* endoscopic laryngotracheoplasty.

Table 6-2 Outcome Assessment in Airway Stenosis

Level of Assessment	Outcome Measures
Anatomy	• Myer-Cotton Scale for cross-section narrowing
	• Craniocaudal extent (vertical height) of the lesion
	• Distance from glottis
Flow physiology	• Spirometry
	• Flow-volume loop
Exercise physiology	• Incremental shuttle walk test
	• Cardiopulmonary exercise
Airway status	• "A" domain of ADVS
Symptoms: dyspnea and effort intolerance	• "D" domain of ADVS
	• Clinical COPD Questionnaire (CCQ)
Symptoms: voice	• "V" domain of ADVS
	• VHI-10
Symptoms: swallowing	• "S" domain of ADVS
	• EAT-10 Instrument
Quality of life	• Short-Form 36 (SF-36)

COPD, Chronic obstructive pulmonary disease; *EAT,* Eating Assessment Tool; *VHI,* Voice Handicap Index.

We do not routinely perform imaging studies for idiopathic subglottic stenosis because once airway stenosis is diagnosed, our next step is to perform examination under anesthesia, at which time lesion anatomy is further assessed and, in most cases, endoscopic laryngotracheoplasty is performed. Anatomic assessment consists of determining the craniocaudal height of the lesion, the distance from the glottis, and minimum airway cross-section. These are determined by using a quantitative endoscopic technique,[60] although airway cross-section is now summarized using the Myer-Cotton System, given that precise knowledge of cross-sectional impairment does not affect treatment or prognosis. The panel of outcome measures used in our assessment of patients with airway stenosis is provided in Table 6-2.

In patients with idiopathic subglottic stenosis, the airway is highly reactive, and injudicious attempts at endoscopic laser photoresection of the stenosis, pushing a rigid bronchoscope through it, or stenting will almost invariably produce aggressive scar reformation, which can wholly close up the airway (Figure 6-8). Similarly, long-term tracheostomy is not a solution because the airway above the tracheostomy will scar and close down, causing aphonia.

We always perform airway surgery via suspension laryngoscopy. This gives unencumbered no-touch access to the laryngotracheal complex (Figure 6-9) and allows two-handed minimally traumatic rigid instrumentation, microscope visualization, and line-of-sight CO_2 laser surgery. All patients receive intravenous induction of anesthesia and supraglottic jet ventilation. Total intravenous technique is used for anesthesia maintenance. This method of anesthesia induction and maintenance is based on studies demonstrating

the presence, nature, severity, and postsurgical relief of upper airway stenosis (Figure 6-7).[42] Recently, we have begun to use cardiopulmonary exercise testing, in particular, measures of incremental inspiratory reserve depletion, as a way of quantifying stenosis-related effort intolerance.

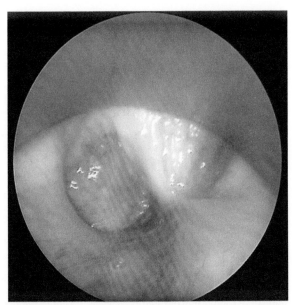

Figure 6-8 Total laryngotracheal stenosis following circumferential laser photoresection of idiopathic subglottic stenosis.

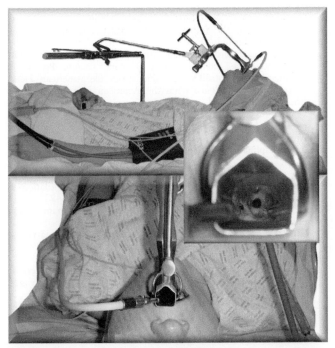

Figure 6-9 *Top,* Side view of suspension laryngoscopy. *Bottom,* Bird's-eye view of suspension laryngoscopy. *Inset,* Microscope (surgical) view of the laryngotracheal complex in a case of idiopathic subglottic stenosis.

favorable physiology and an improved safety profile compared with spontaneous ventilation.[38] At the first treatment, we obtain a deep wedge-shaped biopsy specimen, including the perichondrium, to look for characteristic histopathologic features of this condition (see Table 6-1). Patients then receive 80 to 120 mg

circumferential intralesional depot injections of methylprednisolone acetate, followed by three or four radial incisions using CO_2 laser at 8 to 10 W, deployed through a micromanipulator attached to the operating microscope. This is followed by controlled dilation using the CRE™ Pulmonary Balloon Dilation System to 15 to 16 mm (Boston Scientific, Natick, Mass). We have never used a KTP laser to treat idiopathic subglottic stenosis, given its deeper tissue penetration and more aggressive collateral tissue injury compared with the CO_2 laser.

Idiopathic subglottic stenosis is a progressive condition, and its natural history is recurrent. Therefore we do not equate recurrence following endoscopic treatment with treatment failure and, in our practice, the need to perform repeat endoscopic treatment is not an indication for open laryngotracheal surgery. Most patients require a repeat endoscopic procedure usually once or twice per year. Only 2 of 60 patients in our series did not require repeat endoscopic procedures. Our patients are informed of the relative merits and risks of endoscopic or open surgery and are offered the option of repeat endoscopic surgery or open laryngotracheal reconstruction. To date, around 50 patients have elected to have repeat endoscopic surgery, and 10 patients so far have chosen to undergo open surgery.

Our approach to open surgery for this condition differs from the orthodoxy of cricotracheal resection and anastomosis. We reason that idiopathic subglottic stenosis is a primary mucosal disease that overlies healthy perichondrium and cartilage.[1] Laryngotracheal framework resection therefore is unnecessary; notwithstanding the fact that the excellent cure rates reported in one study with cricotracheal resection[13] have not been replicated, this procedure necessarily destroys the cricothyroid pitch manipulation mechanism and will cause most female patients to have male voices after surgery.[33] Moreover, cricotracheal resection conceptually treats this condition as a benign neoplasm, and, in cases like the one presented, where the disease extends to the glottis, the rational "complete" treatment would be a laryngectomy.

We perform a laryngotracheal fissure with posterior cricoid split, excise mucosal disease off perichondrium, expand the posterior cricoid with costal cartilage, place a skin graft–covered closed Silastic stent with the dermis placed outward through the glottis, and augment the anterior airway using a sternohyoid muscle flap. The stent and the temporary tracheostomy are removed at 2 weeks. The areas where the stenosis was excised will be colonized with keratinocytes, as will a longitudinal strip anteriorly and posteriorly at the site of the rib graft and at the site of the anterior laryngotracheal split. This provides a biologic mechanism for inhibition of further fibrosis in the same way as has been demonstrated in Dupuytren's disease, which is also an idiopathic fibroinflammatory condition.[61] To date this surgery has been performed on 10 patients with complete resolution of airway symptoms in all cases and follow-up of up to 3 years, with one case of suboptimal voice outcome.

REFERENCES

1. Mark EJ, Meng F, Kradin RL, et al. Idiopathic tracheal stenosis: a clinicopathologic study of 63 cases and comparison of the pathology with chondromalacia. *Am J Surg Pathol.* 2008;32:1138-1143.
2. Heffner JE, Miller KS, Sahn SA. Tracheostomy in the intensive care unit. Part 2. Complications. *Chest.* 1986;90:430-436.
3. Hollingsworth HM. Wheezing and stridor. *Clin Chest Med.* 1987;8:231-240.
4. Brichet A, Verkindre C, Dupont J, et al. Multidisciplinary approach to management of postintubation tracheal stenoses. *Eur Respir J.* 1999;13:888-893.
5. Murgu S, Colt HG. Morphometric bronchoscopy in adults with central airway obstruction: case illustrations and review of the literature. *Laryngoscope.* 2009;119:1318-1324.
6. Myer CM, O'Connor DM, Cotton RT. Proposed grading system for subglottic stenosis based on endotracheal tube sizes. *Ann Otol Rhinol Laryngol.* 1994;103:319-323.
7. Nouraei SA, Nouraei SM, Randhawa PS, et al. Sensitivity and responsiveness of the Medical Research Council dyspnoea scale to the presence and treatment of adult laryngotracheal stenosis. *Clin Otolaryngol.* 2008;33:575-580.
8. McCaffrey TV. Classification of laryngotracheal stenosis. *Laryngoscope.* 1992;102:1335-1340.
9. Wright CD, Grillo HC, Wain JC, et al. Anastomotic complications after tracheal resection: prognostic factors and management. *J Thorac Cardiovasc Surg.* 2004;128:731-739.
10. Tracheal stenosis. http://health.groups.yahoo.com/group/tracheal_stenosis. Accessed February 22, 2011.
11. Laryngotracheal stenosis. The National Center for Airway Reconstruction. http://www.airwaystenosis.com. Accessed February 22, 2011.
12. Brouns M, Jayaraju ST, Lacor C, et al. Tracheal stenosis: a flow dynamics study. *J Appl Physiol.* 2007;102:1178-1184.
13. Ashiku SK, Kuzucu A, Grillo HC, et al. Idiopathic laryngotracheal stenosis: effective definitive treatment with laryngotracheal resection. *J Thorac Cardiovasc Surg.* 2004;127:99-107.
14. Simpson GT, Strong MS, Healy GB, et al. Predictive factors of success or failure in the endoscopic management of laryngeal and tracheal stenosis. *Ann Otol Rhinol Laryngol.* 1982;91:384-388.
15. Roediger FC, Orloff LA, Courey MS. Adult subglottic stenosis: management with laser incisions and mitomycin-C. *Laryngoscope.* 2008;118:1542-1546.
16. Couraud L, Moreau JM, Velly JF. The growth of circumferential scars of the major airways from infancy to adulthood. *Eur J Cardiothorac Surg.* 1990;4:521-525.
17. Valdez TA, Shapshay SM. Idiopathic subglottic stenosis revisited. *Ann Otol Rhinol Laryngol.* 2002;111:690-695.
18. Giudice M, Piazza C, Foccoli P, et al. Idiopathic subglottic stenosis: management by endoscopic and open-neck surgery in a series of 30 patients. *Eur Arch Otorhinolaryngol.* 2003;260:235-238.
19. Dedo HH, Catten MD. Idiopathic progressive subglottic stenosis: findings and treatment in 52 patients. *Ann Otol Rhinol Laryngol.* 2001;110:305-311.
20. Simpson CB, James JC. The efficacy of mitomycin-C in the treatment of laryngotracheal stenosis. *Laryngoscope.* 2006;116:1923-1925.
21. Monnier P, George M, Monod ML, et al. The role of the CO_2 laser in the management of laryngotracheal stenosis: a survey of 100 cases. *Eur Arch Otorhinolaryngol.* 2005;262:602-608.
22. Herrington HC, Weber SM, Andersen PE. Modern management of laryngotracheal stenosis. *Laryngoscope.* 2006;116:1553-1557.
23. Shapshay SM, Beamis JFG, Hybels RL, et al. Endoscopic treatment of subglottic and tracheal stenosis by radial laser incision and dilatation. *Ann Otol Rhinol Laryngol.* 1987;96:661-664.
24. Mehta AC, Lee FY, Cordasco EM, et al. Concentric tracheal and subglottic stenosis: management using the Nd-YAG laser for mucosal sparing followed by gentle dilatation. *Chest.* 1993;104:673-677.
25. Werkhaven JA, Weed DT, Ossoff RH. Carbon dioxide laser serial micro trap door flap excision of subglottic stenosis. *Arch Otolaryngol Head Neck Surg.* 1993;119:676-679.
26. Moseley H, Oswal V. Laser biophysics, Chapter 2. In: Oswal V, Remacle M, eds. *Principles and Practice of Lasers in Otorhinolaryngology and Head and Neck Surgery.* The Hague: Kugler; 2002:5-30.
27. Krimsky WS, Rodrigues MP, Malayaman N, et al. Spray cryotherapy for the treatment of glottic and subglottic stenosis. *Laryngoscope.* 2010;120:473-477.
28. Saad CP, Murthy S, Krizmanich G, et al. Self-expandable metallic airway stents and flexible bronchoscopy: long-term outcomes analysis. *Chest.* 2003;124:1993-1999.
29. U.S. Food and Drug Administration. Metallic tracheal stents in patients with benign airway disorders. http://www.fda.gov/Safety/MedWatch/SafetyInformation/SafetyAlertsforHumanMedicalProducts/ucm153009.htm. Accessed February 22, 2011.
30. Gaissert HA, Grillo HC, Wright CD, et al. Complication of benign tracheobronchial strictures by self-expanding metal stents. *J Thorac Cardiovasc Surg.* 2003;126:744-747.
31. Sandu K, Monnier P. Cricotracheal resection. *Otolaryngol Clin N Am.* 2008;41:981-998.
32. Marulli G, Rizzardi G, Bortolotti L, et al. Single-staged laryngotracheal resection and reconstruction for benign strictures in adults. *Interactive CardioVascular and Thoracic Surgery.* 2008;7:227-230.
33. Smith ME, Roy N, Stoddard K, Barton M. How does cricotracheal resection affect the female voice? *Ann Otol Rhinol Laryngol.* 2008;117:85-89.
34. Grillo HC, Mark EM, Mathisen DJ, et al. Idiopathic laryngotracheal stenosis and its management. *Ann Thorac Surg.* 1993;56:80-87.
35. Burman SO. Bronchoscopy and bacteremia. *J Thorac Cardiovasc Surg.* 1960;40:635-639.
36. Nayci A, Atis S, Talas DU, et al. Rigid bronchoscopy induces bacterial translocation: an experimental study in rats. *Eur Respir J.* 2003;21:749-752.
37. Wilson W, Taubert KA, Gewitz M, et al. American Heart Association Rheumatic Fever, Endocarditis, and Kawasaki Disease Committee; American Heart Association Council on Cardiovascular Disease in the Young; American Heart Association Council on Clinical Cardiology; American Heart Association Council on Cardiovascular Surgery and Anesthesia; Quality of Care and Outcomes Research Interdisciplinary Working Group. Prevention of infective endocarditis: guidelines from the American Heart Association: a guideline from the American Heart Association Rheumatic Fever, Endocarditis, and Kawasaki Disease Committee, Council on Cardiovascular Disease in the Young, and the Council on Clinical Cardiology, Council on Cardiovascular Surgery and Anesthesia, and the Quality of Care and Outcomes Research Interdisciplinary Working Group. *Circulation.* 2007;116:1736-1754.
38. Nouraei SAR, Giussani DA, Howard DJ, et al. Physiological comparison of spontaneous and positive-pressure ventilation in laryngotracheal stenosis. *Br J Anaesth.* 2008;101:419-423.
39. Mathisen DJ, Grillo HC. Endoscopic relief of malignant airway obstruction. *Ann Thorac Surg.* 1989;48:469-473.
40. Kil HK, Kim WO, Koh SO. Effects of dexamethasone on laryngeal edema following short-term intubation. *Yonsei Med J.* 1995;36:515-520.
41. Ishman SL, Kerschner JE, Rudolph CD. The KTP laser: an emerging tool in pediatric otolaryngology. *Int J Pediatr Otorhinolaryngol.* 2006;70:677-682.
42. Nouraei SAR, Winterborn C, Nouraei SM, et al. Quantifying the physiology of laryngotracheal stenosis: changes in pulmonary dynamics in response to graded extrathoracic resistive loading. *Laryngoscope.* 2007;117:581-588.
43. Nouraei SAR, Nouraei SM, Upile T, et al. A proposed system for documenting the functional outcome of adult laryngotracheal stenosis. *Clin Otolaryngol.* 2007;32:407-409.
44. Matsuo T, Colt HG. Evidence against routine scheduling of surveillance bronchoscopy after stent insertion. *Chest.* 2000;118:1455-1459.
45. Maronian NC, Azadeh H, Waugh P, Hillel A. Association of laryngopharyngeal reflux disease and subglottic stenosis. *Ann Otol Rhinol Laryngol.* 2001;110:606-612.
46. Rumbak M, Dryer J, Padhya T, et al. Successful management of subglottic stenosis during the third trimester of pregnancy. *J Bronchol Intervent Pulmonol.* 2010;17:342-344.
47. Scholz A, Srinivas K, Stacey MR, et al. Subglottic stenosis in pregnancy. *Br J Anaesth.* 2008;100:385-388.
48. Smith ME, Roy N, Stoddard K, Barton M. How does cricotracheal resection affect the female voice? *Ann Otol Rhinol Laryngol.* 2008;117:85-89.

49. Nouraei SAR, Randhawa PS, Koury EF, et al. Validation of the clinical COPD questionnaire as a psychophysical outcome measure in adult laryngotracheal stenosis. *Clin Otolaryngol.* 2008;34: 343-348.

50. Nouraei SAR, Nouraei SM, Howard DJ, et al. A proposed system for documenting the functional outcome of adult laryngotracheal stenosis. *Clin Otolaryngol.* 2007;32:407-409.

51. Terra RM, de Medeiros IL, Minamoto H, et al. Idiopathic tracheal stenosis: successful outcome with antigastroesophageal reflux therapy. *Ann Thorac Surg.* 2008;85:1438-1439.

52. Perepelitsyn I, Shapshay SM. Endoscopic treatment of laryngeal and tracheal stenosis—has mitomycin C improved the outcome? *Otolaryngol Head Neck Surg.* 2004;131:16-20.

53. Ubell ML, Ettema SL, Toohill RJ, et al. Mitomycin-C application in airway stenosis surgery: analysis of safety and costs. *Otolaryngol Head Neck Surg.* 2006;134:403-406.

54. Smith ME, Elstad M. Mitomycin C and the endoscopic treatment of laryngotracheal stenosis: are two applications better than one? *Laryngoscope.* 2009;119:272-283.

55. Karagiannidis C, Velehorschi V, Obertrifter B, et al. High-level expression of matrix-associated transforming growth factor-beta1 in benign airway stenosis. *Chest.* 2006;129:1298-1304.

56. Cincik H, Gungor A, Cakmak A, et al. The effects of mitomycin C and 5-fluorouracil/triamcinolone on fibrosis/scar tissue formation secondary to subglottic trauma (experimental study). *Am J Otolaryngol.* 2005;26:45-50.

57. Eliashar R, Ochana M, Maly B, et al. Halofuginone prevents subglottic stenosis in a canine model. *Ann Otol Rhinol Laryngol.* 2006;115:382-386.

58. Rosen CA, Lee AS, Osborne J, et al. Development and validation of the voice handicap index-10. *Laryngoscope.* 2004;114: 1549-1556.

59. Belafsky PC, Mouadeb DA, Rees CJ, et al. Validity and reliability of the Eating Assessment Tool (EAT-10). *Ann Otol Rhinol Laryngol.* 2008;117:919-924.

60. Nouraei SAR, McPartlin DW, Nouraei SM, et al. Objective sizing of upper airway stenosis: a quantitative endoscopic approach. *Laryngoscope.* 2006;116:12-17.

61. Tonkin MA, Burke FD, Varian JP. Dupuytren's contracture: a comparative study of fasciectomy and dermofasciectomy in one hundred patients. *J Hand Surg Br.* 1984;9:156-162.

Chapter 7

Idiopathic Subglottic Stenosis Without Glottis Involvement

This chapter emphasizes the following elements of the Four Box Approach: physical examination, complementary tests, and functional status assessment; patient preferences and expectations (also includes family); and techniques and instrumentation.

CASE DESCRIPTION

The patient was a 40-year-old female with a 2-year history of progressive shortness of breath and new complaints of exertional stridor and difficulty performing daily activities. These symptoms had prompted a working diagnosis of adult-onset asthma, but her response to bronchodilator and inhaled corticosteroids was unsatisfactory. No history of endotracheal intubation, connective tissue or autoimmune disorders, tuberculosis, or fungal infections was reported. On physical examination, stridor was heard on auscultation over the trachea. Computed tomography revealed a circumferential stricture in the subglottis, which narrowed the airway cross-sectional area by 60% and extending for 1.5 cm (Figure 7-1). Spirometry was normal except for flattening of the inspiratory and expiratory limbs of the flow-volume loop, suggestive of a fixed upper airway stenosis (see Figure 7-1). The workup for connective tissue disease was unremarkable. Flexible bronchoscopy showed a circumferential subglottic stenosis 1.5 cm below the cords at the level of the cricoid (see Figure 7-1). The stricture appeared simple because no evidence of malacia was noted, but its exact extent could not be measured bronchoscopically because the estimated diameter was only 5 mm, prohibiting the bronchoscope from being advanced beyond the stenosis (see video on ExpertConsult.com) (Video II.7.1). The patient was scheduled for rigid bronchoscopic laser-assisted dilation to temporarily restore airway patency, resolve symptoms, and avoid a potential airway emergency while more definitive treatment was planned.

DISCUSSION POINTS

1. Describe the features of this lesion based on the McCaffrey and Myer-Cotton classification systems.
2. Describe the impact of the stricture on airflow limitation and symptoms in this patient.

3. Describe the role of impulse oscillometry in patients with tracheal stenosis.

CASE RESOLUTION

Initial Evaluations

Physical Examination, Complementary Tests, and Functional Status Assessment

This patient had symptomatic idiopathic subglottis stenosis of moderate severity with a stenotic index* of 60% based on computed tomography (CT) measurements. The severity, extent, and possibly the morphology (shape) of the airway narrowing determine the magnitude of ventilatory impairment and the likelihood of response to a particular treatment strategy.[1] Cutoff values have been proposed to qualify the degree of narrowing as mild (<50%), moderate (51% to 70%), or severe (>71%).[1] Rather than relying on a subjective assessment of severity made at the time of white light flexible bronchoscopy, CT and morphometric bronchoscopy have been used to obtain objective measures that might assist in classifying stricture severity. With this latter technique, still images are captured with the bronchoscope in the center of the airway lumen proximal, distal, and directly at the level of the target abnormality while the tip of the scope is kept at a constant distance from the target area.[1] Images are then saved on CD-ROM or USB device. Cross-sectional area (CSA) of the airway is calculated by using image processing software such as the ImageJ analysis program (National Institutes of Health, Bethesda, Md; available free of charge at http://rsb.info.nih.gov/ij/) (Figure 7-2). As of this writing, however, it is unclear whether morphometric bronchoscopy measurements correlate with subjective estimations of airway narrowing, and whether objective measurement assessments of airway lumen impact decision making and outcomes. Relying on morphometric bronchoscopic measurements also has its disadvantages. For example, in our patient, the method could not be applied because normal tracheal lumen beyond the stricture could not be visualized. Passing the bronchoscope (outside diameter, 5.2 mm) through the stenotic lesion could have caused mucosal edema, worsened respiratory distress, and potentially precipitated respiratory failure. In our case, therefore, the degree of airway narrowing was calculated on the basis of CT images obtained at end inspiration.

White light bronchoscopy (WLB) is very useful in the evaluation of subglottic stenosis because it can detect inflammation and identify hypertrophic stenotic tissues.

---

*For fixed airway stenosis, a stenosis index (SI) represents the cross-sectional area (CSA) of the obstructed area relative to that of normal airway proximal or distal to the stenosis. $SI = (CSA_{normal} - CSA_{abnormal})/CSA_{normal} \times 100\%$; the greater the SI, the greater the degree of airway narrowing and the more severe the obstruction.

Figure 7-1 Axial computed tomography (CT) scan view reveals the circumferential stenosis **(A)** and the normal tracheal diameter distal to it **(C)**. The flow-volume loop shows flattening of the inspiratory and expiratory limbs consistent with upper airway obstruction **(B)**. Flexible bronchoscopy, performed from the front of the patient, reveals the subglottic stricture, which was seen before passing the vocal cords **(D)**. Once in the subglottis, the diameter of the stricture was noted to be smaller than that of the bronchoscope **(E)**. The extent of the stricture was therefore assessed only on the basis of the sagittal CT scan view **(F)** because the scope was not passed distal to the stricture.

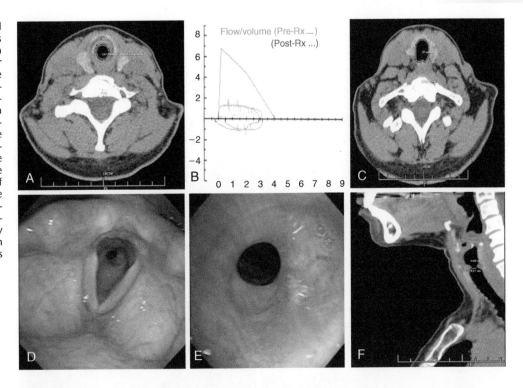

Figure 7-2 Manual method of morphometric bronchoscopy using the ImageJ analysis program. The region of interest (ROI) manager function can be used to measure the area that is selected using the "polygon selection" function (the operator selects the area to be measured). The airway lumen cross-sectional area is measured in pixels.

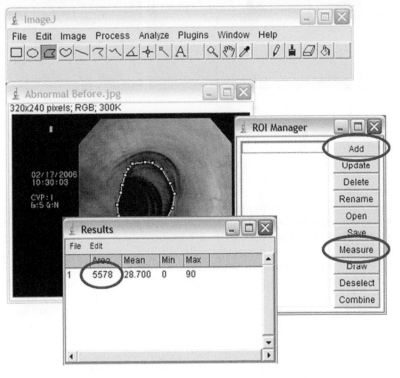

The airways, however, cannot be studied in cross-section; therefore WLB cannot be used to accurately assess the depth of hypertrophic tissues that make up the circumferential stricture, or to judge the integrity of cartilaginous airway structures. For this purpose, high-frequency endobronchial ultrasonography (EBUS) is useful because the radial EBUS (20 MHz) identifies hypoechoic and hyperechoic layers that correlate with laminar histologic structures of the central airways.[2] In fact, structural central airway wall abnormalities have been identified in patients with Wegener's granulomatosis, tuberculosis, relapsing polychondritis, lung cancer,* or compression by vascular rings, and in patients with excessive dynamic airway collapse.[2-4] Endobronchial ultrasound examination using a 20 MHz radial probe can be performed at the time of initial diagnosis or at the time of treatment during flexible or rigid

---

*The depth of tumor and cartilage invasion and destruction can be assessed by EBUS.

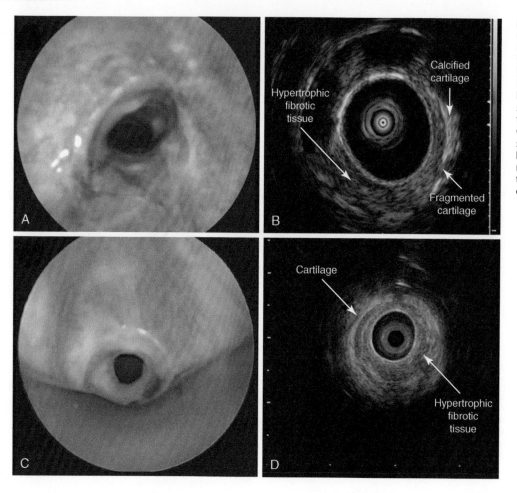

Figure 7-3 White light bronchoscopy and high-frequency endobronchial ultrasound (EBUS) images in tracheal stenosis. **A,** Post intubation tracheal stenosis showing a circumferential stricture. **B,** The corresponding EBUS image shows hypertrophic tissues and the disrupted calcified cartilage. **C,** Idiopathic subglottic stenosis seen on white light bronchoscopy. **D,** The corresponding EBUS image reveals prominent hypertrophic tissues and the integrity of the cartilage.

bronchoscopy to visualize airway wall structures at the level of stenosis and potentially to guide treatment decisions.[5] For instance, for patients who are not surgical candidates, or if tracheal surgical expertise is not available, a simple stricture characterized solely by hypertrophic fibrotic tissue can be successfully dilated (with or without laser assistance) and will not require a stent; on the other hand, for a complex stenosis, in which the cartilage is destroyed, dilation alone will not be long-lasting, making stent insertion almost obligatory to maintain airway rigidity and patency.[6]

In the absence of obvious cartilaginous collapse, however, it is impossible to assess the integrity of the cartilage by WLB alone if prominent hypertrophic stenotic tissue is present (Figure 7-3). High-frequency endobronchial ultrasound, with its high resolution, allows visualization of stenotic tissue and cartilaginous structures (see Figure 7-3). In idiopathic tracheal stenosis, histologic studies of resected specimens showed integrity of the cartilage; in complex stenoses such as those after tracheostomy or intubation, histologic evidence revealed partial or total destruction of cartilage.[7] Abnormal cartilaginous structures may be identified by EBUS (see Figure 7-3). Furthermore, results from EBUS can help determine the extent to which a lesion might be dilated or ablated by helping avoid damage to normal cartilage and damage to the peribronchial blood vessels[5,8] during dilation or bronchoscopic resection. EBUS can also be used to measure the diameters of both the normal airway and the stenosis, thereby potentially facilitating accurate assessment of the degree of narrowing and stent size selection.*[8] EBUS is a minimally invasive procedure performed under moderate sedation or general anesthesia that adds extra time to a diagnostic bronchoscopic procedure.

Experimental studies of nonpulmonary tissues have shown that a novel optical technology, optical coherence tomography (OCT), may detect laser-induced tissue changes.[9] Because laser-induced thermal injury disrupts the normal optical properties of tissues, OCT is capable of visualizing architectural features of the airway wall and may be a useful tool to define therapeutic target volumes in situ and to monitor tissue coagulation, cutting, and ablation intraoperatively. This may result in subsequent reduction of the iatrogenic collateral airway wall injury well described in experimental studies. The physical principles of OCT are analogous to ultrasound: When a beam of sound or light is directed onto a tissue, it is back-reflected (backscattered) differently from structures that have different acoustic or optical properties. The principal difference between ultrasound and OCT is that

---

*When the EBUS probe is retrieved from the distal end of the stenosis to the proximal side with the balloon inflated, the diameter of the balloon changes according to the degree of narrowing. In this way, normal and abnormal areas can be measured to accurately determine the degree of stenosis and to potentially impact stent size selection.

the speed of light (3×10^8 m/s) is many orders of magnitude faster than that of sound (1500 m/s). With OCT, light is emitted from the source, directed into tissues, and reflected off internal structures. The longer the distance traveled, the longer the delay in returning to a detector. The delay in returning light from deeper structures compared with shallow structures is used to reconstruct images. With time domain OCT systems (currently commercially available for clinical use), in-depth profiling is performed by measuring echo time delay and the intensity of backscattered or reflected light.* The system we intended to use in this patient measured OCT echo time delays by comparing the backscattered or back-reflected light signal versus a controlled reference signal. The resolution of OCT is much higher than that of ultrasonography, and in studying central airway wall microstructures, it is possible to visualize upper airway wall layers (mucosa and submucosa) but not the entire human cartilage, because the depth of penetration in tissues is approximately 1.7 mm.[10] OCT systems are also used during bronchoscopy (flexible or rigid) to prolong diagnostic and therapeutic procedures. In our patient, we considered that OCT could become part of our minimally invasive armamentarium for evaluating patients with tracheal stenosis. We therefore planned to use this technology as part of an internal review board–approved research protocol.

Another imaging technique, which is noninvasive, is vibration response imaging (VRI).† This technology requires minimal patient cooperation and can be repeated as often as necessary.[11] VRI has been used in the evaluation of patients with asthma, chronic obstructive pulmonary disease (COPD), foreign body aspiration, and central airway obstruction.[11] Results from experimental studies suggest that different sound frequencies are generated by airways of different sizes, such that differential analysis of VRI might allow precise localization of pathologic processes in different compartments of the lung.[11,12] This is important in patients with central and concurrent peripheral airway obstruction, such as those with asthma/COPD and tracheal or subglottic stenosis. For instance, when a patient with COPD and post intubation tracheal stenosis develops nonspecific respiratory symptoms (cough, dyspnea, inability to raise secretions), VRI might be able to noninvasively localize the pathogenic process to the peripheral airway (e.g., COPD) or the central airway (e.g., tracheal stenosis), thus potentially avoiding the need for diagnostic computed tomography or bronchoscopy. This technology, however, was not available to us at the time of this patient's evaluation.

With regard to physiologic studies, in this patient, the flow-volume loop was characteristic of fixed upper/central airway obstruction, revealing a "square" pattern caused by limitation of both inspiratory and expiratory flow. Published findings demonstrate absence of correlation between severity of obstruction as determined by the flow-volume loop and symptoms,[13] or between spirometry-derived indices and radiologic assessment of airway obstruction.[14] Furthermore, spirometry and flow-volume loops do not localize the anatomic level of the obstruction. Impulse oscillometry (IOS) can be used to localize the region of flow limitation in patients with concurrent central and peripheral airway obstruction. IOS is an effort-independent test during which brief pressure pulses of 5 to 35 Hz are applied during tidal breathing. Pressure-flow oscillations are superimposed on the subject's tidal breaths, and real-time recordings are used to provide an estimate of total respiratory system impedance, including measurements of resistance* (R) and reactance† (X) at different frequencies that might differentiate between central and peripheral components of airway obstruction.[15] Resistance of lung tissue, caused by its viscoelastic properties, decreases with increasing oscillation frequency and becomes essentially negligible at 5 Hz. This means that resistance at 5 Hz relates mainly to flow resistance in the tracheobronchial tree. Increased R at a low oscillation frequency (5 Hz) reflects an increase in total respiratory resistance suggestive of airway obstruction. This is noted, for example, in patients with COPD. In these patients, no flow dependence of resistance is observed in the absence of upper or central airway obstruction.[16]

By contrast, the occurrence of upper/central airway stenosis is expected to generate increases in flow dependence of resistance,‡ both in normal subjects and in COPD patients with peripheral airway obstruction.[17] With an airway of decreasing size, a gradual increase in resistance is noted, as well as a gradual increase in the flow dependence of resistance ($\Delta R/\Delta V$). Furthermore, an increase in resistance at a higher frequency (20 Hz) reflects specifically increased central airway resistance.[18] The IOS maneuver, which provides the advantages of requiring only passive cooperation during tidal breathing and does not cause respiratory fatigue,[15] may in fact be more sensitive than spirometry for detecting upper/central airway stenosis. In one study, for eight patients who could be assessed after bronchoscopic intervention, R values were lower than before the intervention, but only one patient showed a post intervention R value within normal limits. By contrast, in 6 of 8 patients, post intervention $\Delta R/\Delta V$ (flow dependence of resistance) values fell within normal limits, suggesting that the flow dependence of R ($\Delta R/\Delta V$), which is more specific of upper/central airway obstruction, should also be considered during examination of patients with tracheal stenosis and/or for whom R is expected to be increased owing to peripheral airway obstruction.[16] This is probably the case for patients with concurrent stenosis and smoking histories, COPD, or asthma when it is otherwise unclear which part of R is

---

*Distance or spatial information is determined from the time delay of reflected echoes according to the formula $z = \Delta T \bullet v$, where z is the distance the echo travels, ΔT is the echo delay, and v is the wave propagation velocity of wave.

†This novel imaging technique can be described as an electronic stethoscope that picks up sounds from the chest using 40 piezo-acoustic sensors. Analog signals are transformed into dynamic gray scale images, similar to the process involved in ultrasound imaging.

---

*Attributed to the airways and tissue resistance.

†Determined by inertial and compliant properties of the respiratory system.

‡The basic principle of fluid dynamics in the trachea is that upper/central airway resistance generated by excessive narrowing should increase with airflow.

due to tracheal obstruction and which part arises from more peripheral airway obstruction. At the time our patient was seen, IOS was not available at our facility. In view of the patient's stridor and dyspnea, we chose to forgo additional testing and proceeded instead with rigid bronchoscopic dilation.

Comorbidities

The patient had uncontrolled "asthma" on inhaled corticosteroids and rescue albuterol, which had offered only partial relief. No other comorbidities interfered with general anesthesia or bronchoscopy.

Support System

The patient was married, and her husband was very involved in her care. In fact, he had expressed his concerns that the research project into which we intended to enroll his wife was just meant to advance the careers of treating team members and had nothing to do with his wife's care. Indeed, it is not uncommon to encounter such opinions; surveys show that about one third of respondents among cancer trial participants, for example, and a quarter of nonparticipants fully or partially agreed with the statement that medical research is performed primarily to promote doctors' careers.[19]

Patient Preferences and Expectations

The patient herself believed that our main motive in conducting medical research was our wish to find new treatments or tests that would help other patients like her; in general, this is the opinion of most participants in both cancer and noncancer trials.[20] Data on patients' attitudes toward research in benign tracheal stenosis are not yet available. However, bioethicists believe that biomedical knowledge is a public good (i.e., it is available to any individual even if that individual does not contribute to it); therefore participation in biomedical research is an important way to support the public good, suggesting, at least from a utilitarian perspective, that we all have the duty to participate in it,*[21] assuming that the risks of participation are not excessive. Another reason why it might be morally wrong to refuse to participate is that from a principle-based ethic (i.e., beneficence), if a person can prevent something bad or can produce something good, then that person has a duty to perform that action. In fact, failure to participate in research could be considered a form of free-riding, in other words, similar to when a person receives a benefit that others pay for, thereby taking advantage of those who contributed but refusing to share the burden of obtaining it.[21] Of course, the obligation to participate in research is not absolute or legally mandated, and circumstances or reasons may prevail or diminish the force of duty.†

---

*The public good argument implies that people should participate unless they have a good reason NOT to. Such a shift in mentality would be of great benefit for the progress of biomedical research, but it requires strict adherence to informed consent and full disclosure policies and practices on the part of researchers.

†Reasons why people refrain from participating in medical research include sincere religious beliefs about bodily integrity, fear of adverse effects, a need to avoid the "unknown," and a feeling of lacking information.

The purpose of our research protocol was to explore whether novel acoustic and optical imaging technologies could complement traditional diagnostic studies such as WLB and CT, by identifying in vivo airway wall changes before and after laser-assisted dilation of circumferential tracheal strictures. This study was approved by the Institutional Review Board (IRB). Disclosure of IRB approval may be important in helping patients choose to participate in research, as demonstrated in a study from Denmark showing that most patients stated that research ethics committee oversight had had an impact on their decision to participate.[20] The fact that a clinical study has been reviewed and approved by an ethics committee apparently gives patients a sense of security and increases their willingness to participate. Sharing such information with patients is essential during the informed consent process. Well-functioning IRBs ensure that patient risks will not be excessive relative to the benefits of participating in the research endeavor. A patient's moral obligation to participate may be weaker if potential risks to the individual far outweigh potential expected benefits of the research project.

Procedural Strategies

Indications

Bronchoscopic procedures or open surgery is clinically indicated to restore satisfactory airway lumen patency and improve symptoms.[22,23] This patient had symptomatic stenosis. Improving airway patency to less than 50% narrowing could lead to alleviation of her exertional dyspnea.[17]

Contraindications

No absolute contraindications to rigid bronchoscopy were identified. No history of heart or lung disease was elicited that could have potentially increased the risk for hemodynamic instability during general anesthesia. No history of renal or liver disease was revealed that would have increased the risk for bleeding.

Expected Results

The morphology of the stricture was circumferential. In this setting, results from studies show that a second endoscopic intervention is required more often than for patients with strictures due to purely eccentric localized hypertrophic tissue.[24,25] In patients with idiopathic subglottic stenosis, however, the therapeutic success of rigid bronchoscopic interventions is variable. In addition to morphology, a major factor impacting success includes stenoses less than 1.0 cm in length and not associated with significant loss of cartilage. In one series, patients were treated bronchoscopically; 60% of them required a second procedure, with a mean interval between procedures of 9 months.[25] Similar results have been reported in several other nonrandomized studies of bronchoscopic treatments.[26-28]

Team Experience

In our institution, second to malignant central airway obstruction, benign tracheal strictures are the most common diagnoses prompting interventional bronchoscopic procedures. Our patients are managed within the context of a multidisciplinary airway disease program and are routinely discussed with surgical colleagues before bronchoscopic treatments are initiated.

Therapeutic Alternatives

Simple mechanical dilation (with balloons, bougies, or rigid bronchoscope), CO_2 or potassium-titanyl-phosphate (KTP) laser–assisted mechanical dilations, and surgical interventions such as laryngotracheoplasty were discussed with the patient and her husband. Surgical treatment consisting of cricotracheal resection and primary thyro-tracheal anastomosis is considered by some to be the procedure of choice for the treatment of severe idiopathic subglottic stenosis (>70% luminal obstruction).[29] Our patient had a lesser degree of obstruction and refused open surgery because the success rate of bronchoscopic interventions was acceptable to her. We did not offer her stent placement because of the known frequency of stent-related complications when stents are placed in the subglottic regions (the proximal end of the stent may induce ulceration and granulation tissue formation with subsequent glottis or subglottic restenosis), and because complications from stent insertion might increase the complexity of a stricture or increase the length of the stenotic segment. These two factors might adversely affect open surgical resection at a later date.

Cost-Effectiveness

To our knowledge, no randomized studies have evaluated outcomes or the cost-effectiveness of endoscopic versus open surgical interventions for this disease.

Informed Consent

After they had been advised of all therapeutic alternatives, the patient and her husband elected to proceed with rigid bronchoscopy under general anesthesia. A separate informed consent was obtained for the research protocol.

Techniques and Results

Anesthesia and Perioperative Care

In general, when the patient is taken to the operating room, the treating team verifies the patient's name using at least two identifiers (in addition to reading the patient's name bracelet) and the written history and physical and the informed consent form, thereby ensuring that the patient, the surgeon, and the procedure being performed are correctly identified. The patient or caretaker is asked to confirm the type of procedure being performed. The individual responsible for this communication correlates site marking (when necessary), consent, printed operating room schedule, and history and physical with the patient's name. If any part is not matching, the process is stopped until it is validated.* In our institution, the person performing the procedure must document in the medical record the appropriate procedure before the procedure takes place.

Many institutions also apply the so-called time-out or preprocedure pause process. This is performed immediately before the procedure for the purpose of preventing medical error by conducting a final verification of correct patient, procedure, and site (when applicable).* This is done by active (two-way) communication among all surgical/procedural team members and is consistently performed before all procedures, that is, before the incision, or if no incision is planned, as for rigid bronchoscopy, then before the procedure (e.g., rigid bronchoscopic intubation) is initiated. A practical way to do this is to utilize a visual checklist posted in the operating room (Figure 7-4).† At our institution, the circulating nurse documents in the medical record that the time-out was completed. In general, the health care facility defines who is responsible to initiate the time-out, but all those present are accountable for it and must participate in the time-out, including the surgeon, the anesthesia provider, the circulating nurse, and house staff when present. In certain institutions in the United States, if a surgical procedure begins without first completing the time-out, this must be reported for peer review and quality improvement analysis.[30]

We routinely use spontaneous assisted ventilation after induction and intubation with the rigid scope in patients with upper and central airway obstruction. Spontaneous ventilation, however, may create negative inspiratory intraluminal pressure that exacerbates an extrathoracic lesion; therefore, with inspiration, negative intraluminal pressure worsens the collapse of the airway, thus further limiting inspiratory airflow and potentially leading to hypoventilation.‡

At the end of the procedure, after removal of the rigid bronchoscope, transient but potentially severe laryngeal or subglottic edema can occur,[31] in addition to laryngospasm or aspiration of gastric contents. In patients at high risk for aspiration because of retention of gastric contents caused by inadequate preoperative starvation, gastroesophageal reflux, or reduced gastric emptying due to gastrointestinal pathology, an H_2-blocker (e.g., ranitidine 50 mg) or a proton pump inhibitor (e.g., omeprazole 40 mg) can be given 6 to 12 hours before surgery and repeated at least 30 minutes before anesthesia induction to reduce the acidity or the volume of gastric contents. Preoperative gastric emptying with an orogastric or nasogastric tube is not routinely recommended before surgery, even when done on an emergent basis. When aspiration occurs, however, the operating table should be immediately tilted to a 30 degree head-down position, thus positioning the larynx at a higher level than the pharynx,

---

*If a discrepancy occurs, the next step is to call the surgeon to provide adequate documentation to resolve discrepancy.

---

*Site marking should be done for any procedure that involves laterality or multiple structures or levels (even if the procedure takes place outside an operating room).

†During a time-out, the following elements are to be verified, as appropriate: patient's name using two identifiers, site (including marking, when indicated), procedure, correct position, equipment/implants present, allergies, American Society of Anesthesiologists (ASA) status, and type of anesthesia. Any differences/discrepancies must be reconciled immediately; the procedure cannot start until discrepancies are corrected.

‡This is a real possibility in patients with subglottic or upper tracheal stenosis when in supine position and under general anesthesia, because the patient's hyperextended neck position causes a significant length (≈50%) of the trachea to be extrathoracic.

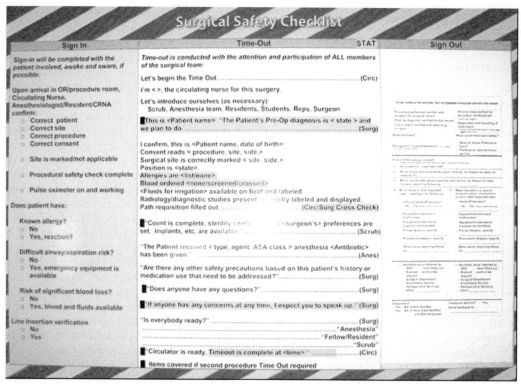

Figure 7-4 Example of surgical safety checklist posted in the operating room.

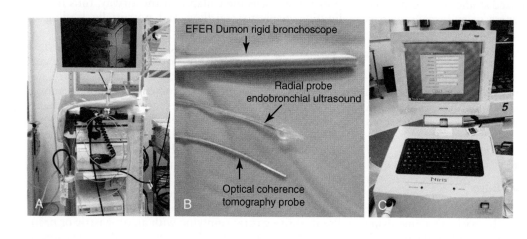

Figure 7-5 Equipment used in this patient. **A,** The white light bronchoscopy tower and the radial endobronchial ultrasound probe. **B,** Close view of the 9.5 mm EFER-Dumon rigid bronchoscope, the radial ultrasound probe with its water-inflated balloon, and the optical coherence tomography (OCT) probe. **C,** The OCT console.

allowing gastric contents to drain externally. Once the mouth and the pharynx are suctioned, the airway is secured by endotracheal intubation if necessary. A nasogastric tube to empty the stomach should be inserted once the airway is secured. Endotracheal suctioning before positive-pressure ventilation is essential to avoid forcing the aspirated material deeper inside the lungs. In view of these rare but potentially life-threatening complications, careful observation of the patient's vital signs and respiratory status is warranted until the patient is fully awake and communicative.

Instrumentation

We chose to perform rigid bronchoscopy using the EFER-Dumon rigid bronchoscope (Bryan Corp, Woburn, Mass) and the KTP laser (Laserscope, San Jose, Calif) for ablation and dilation of the stricture. Commercial two-dimensional, time domain OCT (Niris Imaging System, Imalux Corp, Cleveland, Ohio) and radial EBUS systems (Olympus Optical Co. Ltd., Tokyo, Japan) (Figure 7-5) were used to evaluate airway wall microstructures in the region of hypertrophic tissue constituting the stenosis. This OCT system has a depth resolution of 10 to 20 μm (in air), a lateral resolution of 25 μm, an imaging depth of approximately 1.7 mm (in tissue), a lateral scanning range of 2 mm, and a probe diameter of 2.7 mm. EBUS was performed using a 20 MHz radial mechanical-type probe with resolutions that typically are below 100 μm (Model UM-3R, Olympus, Tokyo, Japan) and an ultrasound unit (EU-M 20 Endoscopic Ultrasound System, Olympus) (see Figure 7-5).

Figure 7-6 A, Optical coherence tomography (OCT) probe onto hypertrophic stenotic tissues at the left incision site before laser and dilation. **B,** The corresponding OCT tomogram reveals a homogeneous light backscattering layer, and resultant loss of layer structures is visible. **C,** Endobrachial ultrasound (EBUS) probe with the water-filled balloon occludes the lumen inside the stricture. **D,** EBUS image of the stricture before treatment shows the thick layer of the hypertrophic tissue visualized overlying the cartilage. OCT image size is 2 mm horizontal and 2.2 mm (in air) vertical.

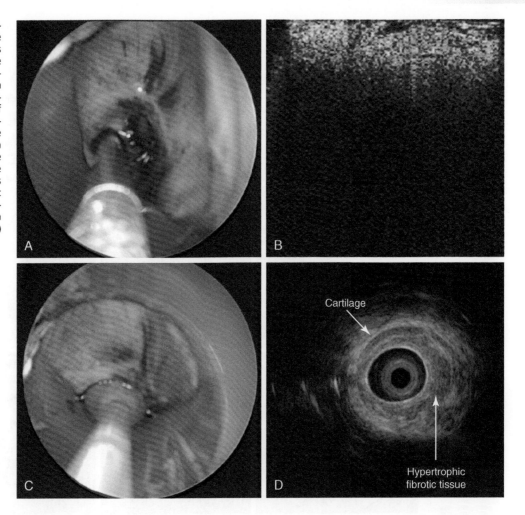

Anatomic Dangers and Other Risks

During work in the subglottis, risks for vocal cord trauma, laryngeal edema, and arytenoid dislocation all potentially contribute to stridor and respiratory distress in the postoperative period. Therefore, a careful, atraumatic intubation is warranted, for which the patient must be properly anesthetized.* Bucking, coughing, or laryngospasm during rigid bronchoscopic intubation could traumatize the stenotic lesion, causing edema and hyperemia, thus interfering with laser application.† It is therefore important for the operator to carefully manipulate the rigid scope in the larynx to avoid inadvertent trauma to the normal mucosa or the stenotic lesion. The scope therefore should be kept aligned with the airway and "off the wall." When making a radial incision on hypertrophic stenotic tissues, the operator should use the laser at the highest power density that is compatible with his or her level of eye-mind-hand coordination and minimize total laser beam exposure time.‡

_____

*Patients ideally should be in stage 3 of anesthesia, also known as *surgical anesthesia*; during this stage, the skeletal muscles are relaxed, the patient's breathing is regular, and loss of laryngeal reflexes occurs.

†High energy absorption by the hyperemic mucosa will reduce penetration and increase collateral thermal damage.

‡Longer exposure times result in higher total energy density and greater risk for laser-induced thermal damage.

Results and Procedure-Related Complications

After induction, the patient was atraumatically intubated with a 9.5 mm EFER-Dumon rigid nonventilating bronchoscope (aka tracheoscope). The circumferential stricture was seen 1.5 cm below the cords with the most prominent hypertrophic tissue on the right lateral and posterior tracheal wall. The stricture was estimated at 5 mm, being of the same size as the rigid telescope. OCT images of the stricture were obtained on the right and left sides of the stricture (Figure 7-6). The high-frequency endobronchial ultrasound probe was introduced, revealing hypertrophic tissues in a circumferential manner with the most prominent component on the right and posteriorly **(see video on ExpertConsult.com)** (Video II.7.2) (see Figure 7-6). KTP laser incisions were performed using a power setting of 6 W and 1 second pulses for a total of 1 minute and 10 seconds and a total energy of 424 joules. Two incisions were performed: one at 5 o'clock (right posterolateral) and one at 1 o'clock (right anterolateral). The OCT probe was reinserted to capture images of laser effects on tissues (Figure 7-7). Then the stricture was dilated, and once bypassed, measurements were performed. The stricture was 1.5 cm long, consistent with CT measurements. Examination of the patient's lower airways showed no other abnormalities. The scope was removed, and the patient was reintubated with a

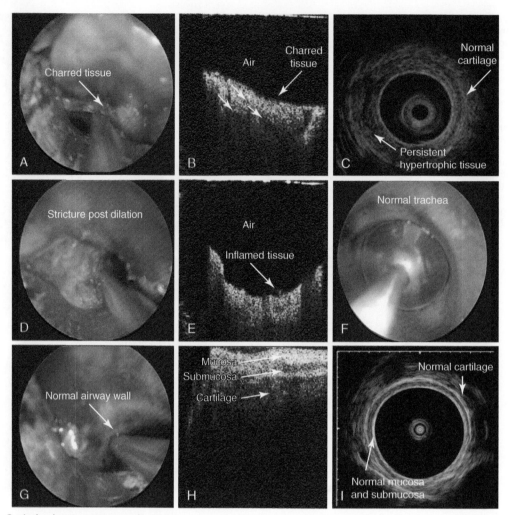

Figure 7-7 **A,** Optical coherence tomography (OCT) probe overlying an area with laser-induced charred tissue. **B,** The corresponding OCT tomogram shows a high backscattering layer; the carbonized layer at the surface absorbs, and the incident OCT beam results in reduced penetration and causes shadowing artifacts, identified by vertical low backscattering streaks *(arrows)*. **C,** OCT probe overlying fibrotic tissue without charring post dilation. **D,** The corresponding OCT tomogram reveals a bright homogeneous light backscattering layer, probably explained by inflammation, which disrupts tissue boundaries and shows a bland image. **E,** OCT probe overlying the normal tracheal wall. **F,** The OCT tomogram reveals normal airway wall layers: Mucosa has enhanced reflectivity compared with underlying submucosa; the extracellular matrix of cartilage decreases scattering of incident light and reflects as a dark region on the OCT image. **G,** Post treatment, radial probe endobrachial ultrasound (EBUS) shows thinner but persistent hypertrophic tissues. **H,** EBUS probe with the water-filled balloon in the normal trachea distal to the stricture. **I,** EBUS image of the normal tracheal wall: Submucosa and cartilaginous layers are clearly identified overlying the water-filled balloon. OCT image size is 2 mm horizontal and 2.2 mm (in air) vertical. Note that in images **A** and **C**, the OCT probe is not in intimate contact with the airway wall, so that OCT tomograms also show a layer of low light backscattering consistent with air.

10.5 mm EFER-Dumon nonventilating scope to further dilate the stricture. The EBUS probe was reinserted and the balloon was inflated at the level of the stricture for 10 seconds (see video on ExpertConsult.com) (Video II.7.3). EBUS images obtained post dilation revealed continued evidence of residual but less prominent hypertrophic tissue (see Figure 7-7). OCT images were obtained at the level of the stricture post dilation and of the normal airway wall, after which the procedure was terminated (see Figure 7-7).

EBUS of hypertrophic tissues revealed a homogeneous layer overlying normal tracheal cartilage. The right posterior hypertrophic tissue was thick and indistinguishable from the posterior trachealis muscle (see Figure 7-6), which usually is characterized by three layers.[32] In vivo

OCT of hypertrophic tissues showed a bland image consisting of a homogeneous light backscattering layer and absence of normal airway wall–layered microstructures (see Figure 7-6). After the radial laser incision, OCT of charred tissue showed high backscattering, reduced imaging penetration, and shadowing artifacts identified as vertical low backscattering streaks (see Figure 7-7). After dilation, OCT in noncharred areas showed a bland pattern confirming continued absence of normal airway wall proximity. A bright light backscattering layer suggested the presence of acute inflammation (see Figure 7-7). EBUS showed thinner but persistent hypertrophic tissue overlying the cartilage and unchanged thick posterior hypertrophic tissue (see Figure 7-7) after resection and dilatation. Because airway

Figure 7-8 **A,** Follow-up flexible bronchoscopy at 10 weeks detects recurrent circumferential stricture of 6 mm diameter. **B,** During rigid bronchoscopy, the stricture was dilated to 12 mm; note the mucosal hyperemia induced by mechanical dilation.

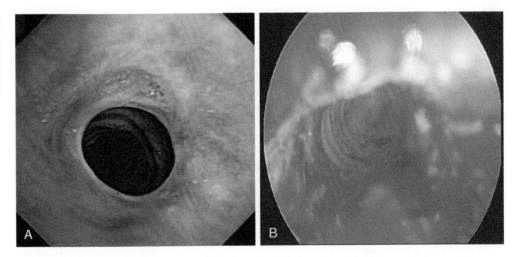

patency was considered satisfactory at 10 mm,* the patient was extubated.

After extubation, the bronchoscopist was talking with the circulating nurse, documenting the procedure performed while the bronchoscopy team was removing the instruments for sterilization. The anesthesiologist was preoccupied with documentation of the procedure in the electronic medical record. The pulmonary trainee was teaching some medical students and residents present in the operating room, explaining to them some basic physiology of tracheal stenosis. Suddenly, while on the gurney and ready to be transported from the operating room, the patient's oxygen saturation suddenly dropped to 80% as noticed by a medical student who was keeping an eye on the patient. The pulse oximetry wave was optimal, and examination revealed inspiratory stridor. The patient was still obtunded. It is well known that airway patency can be temporarily worsened as patients recover from general anesthesia. Edema in the upper airway may manifest itself after the bronchoscope is removed. Laryngospasm was suspected in our patient, so a chin lift and jaw thrust maneuver was immediately performed, and positive-pressure ventilation assistance using the resuscitation mask was promptly applied. The patient's oxygen saturation improved within seconds, laryngospasm immediately resolved, and 10 minutes later, after she was fully awake, the patient was safely transported to the recovery area. It is noteworthy that when these events occurred, the bronchoscopist verbally scolded the anesthesiologist for not paying attention to "my patient," reprimanding a bureaucratic system that obliges us to be "busy with paperwork, rather than taking care of our patients." The anesthesiologist, similarly frustrated, accused the treating team of prematurely removing the bronchoscopy equipment, stating, "it is your procedure, since when do your nurses remove equipment from the room before we remove the patient?" Subsequently, the patient was accompanied to the recovery area uneventfully. No post

procedure stridor was noted, but had it occurred, treatment with humidified oxygen, nebulized epinephrine, steroids, or even reintubation may have been required.

Long-Term Management

Outcome Assessment

Airway patency was restored to 10 mm. The presence of residual hypertrophic tissues and inflammation, although predictable after bronchoscopic interventions, could not be easily appreciated using white light bronchoscopy in terms of extent in cross-section. The presence of residual hypertrophic tissue after treatment is considered a predictive factor for recurrence, as suggested by published histopathologic and surgical data.[33-35] We continue to hypothesize that in vivo application of an EBUS radial probe during bronchoscopic resection may be useful for identification of such residual hypertrophic tissue and could predict recurrence.[5] OCT may allow identification of normal airway wall microstructures and may identify their absence at the level of the stricture; once charring occurs, however, OCT images are compromised owing to high absorption and reduced penetration,[5] allowing us to learn that once charring occurs, this optical technology probably plays no role. Future studies may clarify the exact role of these technologies in guiding treatment decisions. It is noteworthy to mention that EBUS findings are not specific for idiopathic tracheal stenosis, however, and similar circumferential thickening of the submucosa with intact bronchial cartilage has been described in cases of Wegener's granulomatosis.[8]*

Referrals

The patient was scheduled to see a thoracic surgeon on an outpatient basis because she had required two rigid bronchoscopic dilations and remained at risk for recurrence.

---

*This patient's sagittal tracheal diameter was estimated at 12 mm; in fact, in women, 10 mm is considered the lower limit of normal for both sagittal and coronal diameters. Her post procedure stenotic index was 20%—a degree of airway narrowing that does not cause airflow limitation.

---

*We noted these findings in some cases of post intubation tracheal stenosis without cartilage disruption.

Follow-up Tests and Procedures

Four months later, the patient developed progressive dyspnea (World Health Organization [WHO] class III) and stridor with minimal exertion. Flexible bronchoscopy showed recurrent moderate stenosis (Figure 7-8). Rigid bronchoscopic dilation was performed again with restoration of airway patency to 12 mm and improvement in symptoms (see Figure 7-8). Because the patient lived far from the hospital, and to potentially detect early recurrence before severe symptoms developed, we had chosen to prescribe a peak flow meter* and had asked the patient to keep a log of daily peak flows and to call us when more than 20% reduction from baseline occurred.

It is known that after an airway intervention, some residual obstruction persists or some mucosal edema develops as a result of the procedure itself (e.g., granulation tissue, sputum impaction), impairing complete return of airway resistance to normal values. In fact, possible edema post intervention implies that the lumen area at the time of post intervention functional testing could be slightly smaller than that estimated in vivo at the time of termination of the intervention. In addition, the narrowest passage in the upper airway, including the trachea, is in fact the glottis, with a typical lumen area of 100 mm^2 during normal breathing.[36] This explains why, in the case of lumen area exceeding 100 mm^2, $\Delta R/\Delta V$ values generally fall to within limits of normal. Therefore, follow-up protocols in patients such as ours, at risk for stenosis recurrence, could include IOS monitoring to determine clinically relevant threshold values for R and $\Delta R/\Delta V$. We continued the patient's inhaled corticosteroids (which may help with reducing inflammation at the level of the stricture) and prescribed proton pump inhibitors in an attempt to potentially reduce the risk for recurrence by diminishing potential adverse effects from reflux, as suggested by anecdotal published evidence.[37]

Quality Improvement

The episode of stridor that occurred during emergence from anesthesia made us reflect on patient safety and quality of care. Because the potential need for emergency reintubation is always present during this phase of anesthesia (especially in a patient with recent dilation of the subglottic stricture), we concluded that all necessary airway equipment and a bronchoscopist with the proper equipment should remain immediately available in the operating theater until the patient is fully awake. We chose to make this an official entry in our department's policy and procedure manual and to incorporate this into our procedural checklist.

Events in the operating room also prompted us to reflect on the issue of professionalism. We believed that at the time of laryngospasm and transient hypoxemia, the operating room noise level was unacceptably high, and that distraction was contributory to the adverse event that might have been prevented had mask ventilation been prolonged after extubation, or had everyone not been busy teaching, talking, and doing other things. Although induction of anesthesia and, before that, the period of attention required when performing a time-out tend to be calm, quiet, and focused moments, with operating rooms providing an excellent barrier to noise, interruption, and distraction, emergence from anesthesia in the operating room often seems to be a noisier moment. The procedure is over, and people are anxious to move on to whatever needs to be done next; prepare the room for the next patient, finish charting, teach, or ask about a colleague's weekend activities. Indeed, data demonstrate increased distraction during emergence from anesthesia compared with the induction or maintenance phase of anesthesia. One study for instance found that the mean noise level* during emergence (58.3 dB) was significantly higher than during induction (46.4 dB) and maintenance (52 dB), and that sudden loud noises,† greater than 70 dB,‡ occurred more frequently at emergence (34 times) than at induction (9 times) or maintenance (13 times). The median (range) of staff entrances into the operating room or exits from the room were 0 (0 to 7), 6 (1 to 18), and 10 (1 to 20) for induction, maintenance, and emergence, respectively ($P < .001$). Furthermore, conversations unrelated to the procedure occurred in 28 of 30 (93%) emergences from anesthesia.

These findings are especially relevant to our case. Failure of situational awareness is a known cause of adverse events in hospitalized patients because it causes difficulties in communication and concentration. We propose that this is warranted to recognize and minimize distraction, especially during emergence from anesthesia after interventional airway procedures. Applying the "sterile cockpit"§ rule may be useful in improving patient safety.[38] We are aware that it is very difficult to identify the absolute level of noise, distraction, or interruption that might be considered unacceptable by different team members, and common sense is inevitably required. We chose to conduct a team meeting during which data pertaining to operating room distractions and their potential for adversely affecting procedural performance and outcomes would be presented. As a result of this meeting, we concluded that an actual change in operating room practice might be needed even if it consisted of a simple reminder to physician and nonphysician staff to refrain from loud,

---

*Measurement of peak expiratory flow rate requires training to correctly use a meter; the normal expected value depends on a patient's sex, age, and height. Owing to the wide range of "normal" values and the high degree of variability, peak flow is not recommended as a diagnostic test but can be used for monitoring patients with obstructive ventilatory impairment.

*A decibel reading was taken at time zero and then subsequently at 30 second intervals during each 5 minute period.

†Common sources of such noises included slamming doors or bins, loud conversation, singing, and dropped equipment.

‡The Environmental Protection Agency has recommended that the average hospital noise level should not exceed 45 dB during the daytime and 35 dB at night.

§In aviation, the "sterile cockpit" rule prohibits nonessential activities during critical phases of flight, takeoff, and landing—phases analogous to the induction and emergence phases of anesthesia.

unnecessary, and unrelated conversations until the patient has left the operating room.*

We also acknowledged that both the bronchoscopist's and the anesthesiologist's behaviors could be perceived as unprofessional. Although interpersonal conflicts are common in the workplace because of people's different personalities, ideas, or interests, they may become more apparent in stressful settings, as when teams are needed to perform a task such as a surgical intervention.[39] Interpersonal conflict is distressing to those directly involved, and it can adversely impact patient care. Conflict often leads to miscommunication, demoralization, and poor team interaction. It is already well known that the operating room is the clinical environment where most medical accidents occur. It is interesting to note that 75% to 80% of such accidents are not caused by technical failures or incompetence, but by systemic nontechnical issues such as miscommunication. For example, one study evaluated adverse surgical events that resulted from errors of management and found that 43% of errors were actually related to a breakdown of communication between personnel.[40]

Conflict resolution is most likely to succeed in an environment built on leadership principles, clear communication skills, and flexibility. Resolution can occur only when communication is open, unemotional, and honest. Team leaders must be flexible enough to respect each individual's point of view objectively[39] and to find common ground even in cases of disagreement. The effects of unhealthy egos and narcissistic behaviors need to be minimized.[†] It is noteworthy that the day after the procedure, during an objective, friendly conversation, both the bronchoscopist and the anesthesiologist agreed that their main concern had been doing what was necessary in the patient's best interest. Literature in fact suggests that patient-centered practice can unite values and communication issues among operating room teams.[41] A mutual apology was in order; both agreed that the noise level in the operating room had been an unnecessary distraction that probably contributed to the overall sense of chaos

that day, and both agreed to do their best to control operating room noise in the future.

DISCUSSION POINTS

1. Describe the features of this lesion based on the McCaffrey and Myer-Cotton classification systems.

    These two systems are widely used for grading laryngotracheal stenosis, mainly based on literature from otorhinolaryngology.

    - *The McCaffrey system*[42]: based on the site and extent of an airway stenosis*; consists of four stages: (I) lesions confined to the subglottis or trachea that are less than 1 cm in length; (II) subglottic stenoses longer than 1 cm within the cricoid and not extending to the glottis or trachea; (III) subglottic stenoses that extend into the upper trachea but do not involve the glottis; and (IV) lesions involving the glottis. Based on this system, therefore, our patient had a stage III lesion.
    - *The Myer-Cotton system*[43]: based on the degree of narrowing; also consists of four grades: (I) lesions narrowed to maximum 50% obstruction; (II) from 51% to 70% obstruction; (III) 71% to 99% obstruction; and (IV) 100% obstruction (no lumen detected), as seen in the suprastomal region of patients with indwelling tracheostomies. Based on this system, our patient had a grade II lesion because 60% obstruction was detected by computed tomography.

2. Describe the impact of the structure on airflow limitation and symptoms in this patient.
    - A flow dynamic study assessed flow patterns and pressure drops over tracheal stenoses artificially inserted into a realistic three-dimensional upper airway model derived from computed tomography images obtained in healthy men.[17] The pressure drop over the stenosis, which correlates with the work of breathing, dramatically increased only when more than 70% of the tracheal lumen was obstructed at 15 and 30 L/min flow rates. Pressures when the stenosis was 50% were indistinguishable from pressures in the absence of stenosis, suggesting that from a physiologic perspective, lesions obstructing the trachea by 50% or less may not interfere with airflow or cause symptoms. Our patient had a stenosis index of 60%, for which a pressure drop is seen at high flow rates (30 L/min), suggesting symptoms with exertion, as was indeed the case.

3. Describe the role of impulse oscillometry in patients with tracheal stenosis.
    - Impulse oscillometry is an effort-independent technique that does not require forced expiratory maneuver. Thus it should not pose a risk of

---

*In this regard, one must acknowledge that although health care providers learn the art and science of their profession, few are exposed to leadership development or are coached in conflict resolution or behavior modification techniques. A few simple rules might be adhered to: (1) Maintain and show respect for colleagues regardless of their position; (2) use the words "please" and "thank you" often; (3) do not hesitate to provide positive reinforcement, do not hesitate to say, "You did a good job"; (4) use the word "we" often, to help instill a notion of team building, and sincerely ask, "What do you think, or what is your opinion?"; and (5) let others know why you acted in a certain way or want things done in a certain fashion. People tend to perform better when they know why they are being asked to do something; if you made a mistake, do not be afraid to say, "I admit I made a mistake, I am sorry."

†In the aviation industry, when adverse events were analyzed from a behavioral perspective, several hazardous attitudes were identified. These are the macho ("I can do it, watch me!"), antiauthority ("Don't you tell me what to do!"), impulsive ("This is an emergency, I have to do this now!"), invulnerable ("I can't do wrong, nothing can happen to me!"), and resigned attitudes ("What is the use of even trying?"). It is likely that these attitudes are also present in stressful medical and surgical environments. (Modified from Jenson RS. *Pilot Judgement and Crew Resource Management.* Burlington, VT: Ashgate Publishing; 1995.)

---

*The McCaffrey system classifies laryngotracheal stenosis based on the subsites involved and the length of the stenosis; sites of stenosis are defined as *subglottic* when the stenosis is in the region bounded superiorly by a plane 0.5 cm below the glottis and inferiorly by the lower edge of the cricoid cartilage; *tracheal* when the stenosis is below the lower edge of the cricoids; and *glottic* when stenosis of the interarytenoid space occurs.

respiratory distress in patients with critical tracheal strictures.[15]

- The procedure is more sensitive than spirometry and can be used before and after therapy to objectively document physiologic improvement, as well as for monitoring.[16]
- The procedure assists in differentiating responsible flow-limiting segments in patients with concurrent central and peripheral airway obstruction such as that caused by tracheal stenosis and COPD. Airway obstruction is revealed by an increase in R5 (respiratory system resistance at 5 Hz oscillation frequency). Increased R20 measured by IOS, however, indicates an obstruction in the central airways, thus suggesting that IOS can be helpful, in addition to body plethysmography, spirometry, and flow-volume loop, for assessing airflow obstruction.[18]

Expert Commentary

provided by Sylvia Verbanck, PhD, and Marc Noppen, MD, PhD

The Holy Grail of noninvasive diagnosis of the pulmonary system is a test, or one of its derived parameters, that can reliably ascertain small or large airway function. In this commentary, we will discuss some of the issues pertaining to distinguishing the location of airflow limitation as assessed by noninvasive physiologic testing. The ability to localize the main site of flow limitation responsible for a patient's symptoms would be helpful for the clinician treating patients with tracheal stenosis and concurrent small airway disease. The first thing to bear in mind is that until today, the most widely accepted definition of small airways (diameter <2 mm) is based on a retrograde catheter size used in pioneering work on airway resistance conducted by Macklem and Mead.[44] Several conditions define the ideal, noninvasive diagnostic test. It should be easy to perform for the patient, easy to analyze for the technician, easy to interpret for the researcher, and able to detect structural changes at an early stage in the various air spaces. The literature is littered with studies claiming to have found such tests, frequently introducing these as "reflecting" *the small* or *the large* airways. Usually, these tests do fulfill the condition that their parameters change in case of a change in particular location, but conversely, this does not unequivocally mean that the parameter's change is the result of a structural change that has occurred exclusively in that particular location and not elsewhere.

Probably overwhelmed by a sense of enthusiasm about the first condition being fulfilled, the tendency is to automatically assume that the second condition is fulfilled as well. This is when a test reported to "reflect" the small or large airways creates a "flou artistique," letting interpretation run its free course. An example is impulse oscillometry (IOS), whereby resistance can be measured at various forced oscillation frequencies, which ironically has been advocated alternatively as a "small airway" test and a "large airway" test. This is logical to the extent that both

categories of airways could be called mutually exclusive, were it not for the broad airway range in size and morphology, making either category a difficult one to pin down. Yet, the general idea is that resistance obtained at a "high" oscillation frequency preferentially reflects the large airways, based on valid models of lung mechanics that use an electrical analogy in the form of an alternating current RLC resonance circuit ("R" stands for resistor, "L" for inductor, "C" for capacitor). Hence, a change in the frequency dependence of resistance can be considered as a change in the "large" or "small" airways.

At least one other airway characteristic interferes with this interpretation of the frequency dependence of resistance: Airway resistance is distributed heterogeneously across the tracheobronchial tree (in this case modeled by parallel RLC circuits), and increased heterogeneity is predicted to affect low frequencies more than high frequencies, creating an additional source of frequency dependence, which, in principle, has nothing to do with airway size. Just like "small" and "large" airways, the terms "low" and high" frequency are being used rather liberally; in fact, in the pioneering studies, low frequency referred to frequencies in the vicinity of breathing frequency, requiring a subject to breath-hold while performing forced oscillation testing. Further complicating the interpretation of frequency dependence of IOS resistance is the fact that when a flow-limiting orifice such as a tracheal stenosis comes into play, an additional RLC compartment with different resonance characteristics may be created so as to preferentially affect low frequency resistance.[45]

For all of the reasons already discussed, the frequency dependence of resistance may well be influenced by tracheal stenosis, yet not be a unique reflection of it. The bottom line is that although it is attractive in many ways, IOS and its derived parameters should be handled with extreme caution before jumping to conclusions. In our opinion, at this point IOS is nothing more or less than a reasonable test to include in a research protocol for tracheal stenosis (exceeding, however, the status of a fishing experiment whereby you go about measuring just about anything based on the probability that eventually something will pop up). It is advised to measure several of the IOS contenders such as R5 and R25, and not to exclude one or the other just yet. A case in point is the report of a patient with recurrent tracheal stenosis in whom R5Hz was seen to increase more than R20Hz, contrary to expectations if "high" frequencies were more sensitive to "large" airway changes.[46]

When searching for a test that can diagnose a very particular structural feature and/or its location, a sensible approach is to look for a functional hallmark of that structural feature. In the case of an airway stenosis, a reflex of aerodynamic engineering is to realize that a sudden constriction will create a local pressure drop with general expression of the form $\Delta P = K.\rho.(\frac{1}{2}) v^2$, where ρ is air density and v is average air velocity. K is an empirically determined parameter that is dependent on a combination of factors: the degree of contraction (dimension of stenosis vs. airway cross-section), the shape of the contraction (sharp-edged or rounded), and the flow regime in which stenosis occurs (turbulent or laminar). A detailed simulation in a realistic model of tracheal stenosis with varying orifices predicts that the dependence of pressure drop on breathing flow rate becomes more marked with more severe stenosis. The real-life measurement of pressure drop in situ is possible[47] yet impractical: Besides being invasive for the patient, the measurement equipment may affect the local aerodynamics that it is attempting to measure. The next best thing that can be measured noninvasively is resistance (pressure drop over breathing flow rate), the trade-off being that other parts of the lung may contribute to resistance. Aerodynamics predicts that nonstenotic airways may well contribute to resistance, but they are unlikely to contribute to breathing flow dependence of resistance, which is a functional hallmark of a sudden contraction. Among existing or emerging methods of choice, we thus require the possibility to measure resistance at different breathing flows. IOS is one such method. In addition, IOS offers the possibility to separately gauge inspiratory and expiratory phases of the breathing cycle, which may be more relevant in case of a variable tracheal obstruction. Also, in case body posture plays a role in stenosis-related breathing discomfort, resistance is easier to obtain with IOS than with plethysmography, which would require a horizontal body plethysmograph.

Once it is detected by resistance, the remaining issue is the location of a stenotic lesion. Because local pressure loss is affected by whether the contraction is located in a laminar or a turbulent flow regime, this could provide a way to distinguish tracheal stenosis from that occurring more distally in the tracheobronchial airway, possibly by using heliox. In addition, we should consider that for a given degree of contraction, a stenotic constriction in a mainstem bronchus normally will have a greater impact on overall resistance measured at the mouth than a similar constriction in one of its subtending branches (summing resistance according to whether they are in series or in parallel as in an electrical circuit). Although such engineering considerations could be used to further refine resistance measurement techniques, one might bear in mind that we are dealing with the biologic variability associated with a breathing human lung. Hence, it may be wise to be satisfied with a test that detects the extent of narrowing *or* the location of narrowing, rather than trying to achieve both (at least with a simple noninvasive test). For instance, in the follow-up of a patient at risk for stricture recurrence in an established location of the trachea, a simple resistance measurement at 5 Hz could suffice. In the case of a de novo patient presenting with dyspnea, examining breathing flow dependence of resistance may be more useful in assessing how proximal the responsible airway obstruction is.

In summary, depending on how much time and effort the health care provider is willing to invest in physiologic testing, and depending on how much testing the patient is willing to accept, one or several noninvasive measurements of airway resistance can be considered. It helps if the health care provider makes an educated guess of which set of tests is best in any given clinical situation. It is our hope that this commentary helps clarify some of the issues that need to be considered in making that choice. Regardless, a noninvasive test is likely to provide only a partial answer to our questions. Isn't this typical of the human condition? After all, the Holy Grail symbolically stands for man's eternal quest for truth and wisdom. Part of that wisdom is the realization that we can't know it all.

REFERENCES

1. Murgu S, Colt HG. Morphometric bronchoscopy in adults with central airway obstruction: case illustrations and review of the literature. *Laryngoscope.* 2009;119:1318-1324.
2. Kurimoto N, Murayama M, Yoshioka S, et al. Assessment of usefulness of endobronchial ultrasonography in determination of depth of tracheobronchial tumor invasion. *Chest.* 1999;115:1500-1506.
3. Miyazu Y, Miyazawa T, Kurimoto N, et al. Endobronchial ultrasonography in the diagnosis and treatment of relapsing polychondritis with tracheobronchial malacia. *Chest.* 2003;124:2393-2395.
4. Murgu S, Kurimoto N, Colt H. Endobronchial ultrasound morphology of expiratory central airway collapse. *Respirology.* 2008;13:315-319.
5. Murgu SD, Colt HG, Mukai D, et al. Multimodal imaging guidance for laser ablation in tracheal stenosis. *Laryngoscope.* 2010;120:1840-1846.
6. Brichet A, Verkindre C, Dupont J, et al. Multidisciplinary approach to management of postintubation tracheal stenoses. *Eur Respir J.* 1999;13:888-893.
7. Mark EJ, Meng F, Kradin RL, et al. Idiopathic tracheal stenosis: a clinicopathologic study of 63 cases and comparison of the pathology with chondromalacia. *Am J Surg Pathol.* 2008;32:1138-1143.
8. Shirakawa T, Ishida A, Miyazu Y, et al. Endobronchial ultrasound for difficult airway problems. In: Bolliger CT, Herth FJF, Mayo PH, et al., eds. *Clinical Chest Ultrasound: From the ICU to the Bronchoscopy Suite.* Basel: Karger; 2009:189-201.
9. Boppart SA, Herrmann J, Pitris C, et al. High-resolution optical coherence tomography-guided laser ablation of surgical tissue. *J Surg Res.* 1999;82:275-284.
10. Imalux UCT technology. Niris Imaging System. http://www.imalux.com/products.htm. Accessed May 6, 2011.
11. Becker HD, Slawik M, Miyazawa T, et al. Vibration response imaging as a new tool for interventional-bronchoscopy outcome assessment: a prospective pilot study. *Respiration.* 2009;77:179-194.
12. Becker HD. Vibration response imaging—finally a real stethoscope. *Respiration.* 2009;77:236-239.
13. Gittoes NJ, Miller MR, Daykin J, et al. Upper airways obstruction in 153 consecutive patients presenting with thyroid enlargement. *BMJ.* 1996;312:484.
14. Melissant CF, Smith SJ, Perlberger R, et al. Lung function, CT-scan and X-ray in upper airway obstruction due to thyroid goitre. *Eur Respir J.* 1994;7:1782-1787.
15. Smith HJ, Reinhold P, Goldman MD. Forced oscillation technique and impulse oscillometry. *Eur Respir Mon.* 2005;31:72-105.
16. Verbanck S, de Keukeleire T, Schuermans D, et al. Detecting upper airway obstruction in patients with tracheal stenosis. *J Appl Physiol.* 2010;109:47-52.
17. Brouns M, Jayaraju ST, Lacor C, et al. Tracheal stenosis: a flow dynamics study. *J Appl Physiol.* 2007;102:1178-1184.
18. Pornsuriyasak P, Ploysongsang Y. Impulse oscillometry system in diagnosis of central airway obstruction in adults: comparison with spirometry and body plethysmography. *Chest.* 2009;136:123S.
19. Madsen SM, Mirza MR, Holm S, et al. Attitudes towards clinical research amongst participants and nonparticipants. *J Intern Med.* 2002;251:156-168.

20. Madsen SM, Holm S, Davidsen B, et al. Ethical aspects of clinical trials: the attitudes of participants in two non-cancer trials. *J Intern Med*. 2000;248:463-474.
21. Schaefer GO, Emanuel EJ, Wertheimer A. The obligation to participate in biomedical research. *JAMA*. 2009;302:67-72.
22. Ashiku SK, Kuzucu A, Grillo HC, et al. Idiopathic laryngotracheal stenosis: effective definitive treatment with laryngotracheal resection. *J Thorac Cardiovasc Surg*. 2004;127:99-107.
23. Valdez TA, Shapshay SM. Idiopathic subglottic stenosis revisited. *Ann Otol Rhinol Laryngol*. 2002;111:690-695.
24. Simpson GT, Strong MS, Healy GB, et al. Predictive factors of success or failure in the endoscopic management of laryngeal and tracheal stenosis. *Ann Otol Rhinol Laryngol*. 1982;91:384-388.
25. Roediger FC, Orloff LA, Courey MS. Adult subglottic stenosis: management with laser incisions and mitomycin-C. *Laryngoscope*. 2008;118:1542-1546.
26. Giudice M, Piazza C, Foccoli P, et al. Idiopathic subglottic stenosis: management by endoscopic and open-neck surgery in a series of 30 patients. *Eur Arch Otorhinolaryngol*. 2003;260:235-238.
27. Dedo HH, Catten MD. Idiopathic progressive subglottic stenosis: findings and treatment in 52 patients. *Ann Otol Rhinol Laryngol*. 2001;110:305-311.
28. Simpson CB, James JC. The efficacy of mitomycin-C in the treatment of laryngotracheal stenosis. *Laryngoscope*. 2006;116:1923-1925.
29. Marulli G, Rizzardi G, Bortolotti L, et al. Single-staged laryngotracheal resection and reconstruction for benign strictures in adults. *Interact Cardiovasc Thorac Surg*. 2008;7:227-230.
30. Ohio Surgical/Procedural Verification Protocol. http://www.ohiopatientsafety.org/surgery/Links/Ohio%20surgical%20verification%20protocol604.pdf. Accessed on March 29, 2011.
31. Mathisen DJ, Grillo HC. Endoscopic relief of malignant airway obstruction. *Ann Thorac Surg*. 1989;48:469-473.
32. Kurimoto N. Diagnosis of depth penetration in the tracheobronchial tree. In: Kurimoto N, ed. *Endobronchial Ultrasonography*. Kyoto. Japan: Kinpodo; 2001:33-38.
33. Cooper JD, Grillo HC. The evolution of tracheal injury due to ventilatory assistance through cuffed tubes: a pathologic study. *Ann Surg*. 1969;162:334-348.
34. Grillo HC, Donahue DM, Mathisen DJ, et al. Postintubation tracheal stenosis: treatment and results. *J Thorac Cardiovasc Surg*. 1995;109:486-492.
35. Couraud L, Moreau JM, Velly JF. The growth of circumferential scars of the major airways from infancy to adulthood. *Eur J Cardiothorac Surg*. 1990;4:521-525.
36. Brancatisano T, Collett PW, Engel LA. Respiratory movements of the vocal cords. *J Appl Physiol*. 1983;54:1269-1276.
37. Terra RM, de Medeiros IL, Minamoto H, et al. Idiopathic tracheal stenosis: successful outcome with antigastroesophageal reflux disease therapy. *Ann Thorac Surg*. 2008;85:1438-1439.
38. Broom MA, Capek AL, Carachi P, et al. Critical phase distractions in anaesthesia and the sterile cockpit concept. *Anaesthesia*. 2011;66:175-179.
39. Lee L, Berger DH, Awad SS, et al. Conflict resolution: practical principles for surgeons. *World J Surg*. 2008;32:2331-2335.
40. Gawande AA, Zinner MJ, Studdert DM, et al. Analysis of errors reported by surgeons at three teaching hospitals. *Surgery*. 2003;133:614-621.
41. Bleakley A. A common body of care: the ethics and politics of teamwork in the operating theater are inseparable. *J Med Philos*. 2006;31:305-322.
42. McCaffrey TV. Classification of laryngotracheal stenosis. *Laryngoscope*. 1992;102:1335-1340.
43. Myer CM, O'Connor DM, Cotton RT. Proposed grading system for subglottic stenosis based on endotracheal tube sizes. *Ann Otol Rhinol Laryngol*. 1994;103:319-323.
44. Macklem P, Mead J. Resistance of central and peripheral airways measured by a retrograde catheter. *J Appl Physiol*. 1967;22:395-401.
45. Smith HJ, Crockett AJ, Kenn K, Vogel J. New results in the differentiation of extrathoracic airway stenoses using forced oscillation technique. *Eur Respir J*. 1997;10(suppl 25):287s.
46. Vicencio AG, Bent J, Tsirilakis K, et al. Management of severe tracheal stenosis using flexible bronchoscopy and impulse oscillometry. *J Bronchol Intervent Pulmonol*. 2010;17:162-164.
47. Wassermann K, Koch A, Warschkow A, et al. Measuring in situ central airway resistance in patients with laryngotracheal stenosis. *Laryngoscope*. 1999;109:1516-1520.

Chapter 8

Post Intubation Tracheal Stenosis

> This chapter emphasizes the following elements of the Four Box Approach: physical examination, complementary tests, and functional status assessment; risk-benefit analysis and therapeutic alternatives; and techniques and instrumentation.

CASE DESCRIPTION

This patient is a 55-year-old woman with a long history of gastroesophageal reflux disease (GERD) refractory to proton pump inhibitors, who was admitted emergently to an outside hospital with stridor and respiratory distress requiring noninvasive positive-pressure ventilation (NPPV). Flexible bronchoscopy revealed a severe mid-tracheal stricture with an estimated diameter of 4 mm, based on the fact that a 5.2-mm outside diameter flexible bronchoscope could not be advanced beyond the lesion. Three months earlier, she had undergone surgical repair of a hiatal hernia, during which she was intubated for several hours. Two weeks after surgery, as she became more physically active, the patient developed wheezing and dyspnea, which did not improve with inhaled corticosteroids and bronchodilators. Stridor prompted consultation with an ear, nose, and throat physician, who made the diagnosis of tracheal stenosis and performed rigid bronchoscopy with laser and dilation. Her symptoms recurred, and 2 weeks post intervention she went to a local emergency department with respiratory distress and stridor. An emergent tracheostomy was performed. One month later, the patient was successfully decannulated, but 10 days later, she developed recurrent stridor and respiratory distress requiring hospitalization, NPPV, bronchoscopy, and subsequent transfer to our institution. She had no other medical or surgical history, lived alone, had an active lifestyle, and enjoyed hiking. Her preference was to relieve dyspnea, regain her previous lifestyle, and avoid tracheostomy if possible. Review of symptoms was unremarkable, except that she could not speak in full sentences and had obvious biphasic stridor without hoarseness. Vital signs were normal except for a heart rate of 130 (sinus rhythm). Her chest radiograph was normal. She underwent urgent rigid bronchoscopy with dilation (Figure 8-1). The stricture was circumferential, extending for 1 cm and starting 5 cm below the vocal cords.

DISCUSSION POINTS

1. Describe three favorable stenosis features for tracheal resection.
2. List five differential diagnoses of tracheal stenosis.
3. Describe three known complications of tracheal resection.

CASE RESOLUTION

Initial Evaluations

Physical Examination, Complementary Tests, and Functional Status Assessment

This patient was hospitalized for respiratory failure requiring NPPV. This is not an unusual presentation for patients with post intubation tracheal stenosis (PITS). Many patients are diagnosed when stenosis is severe enough to prompt acute respiratory failure necessitating emergency bronchoscopic dilation with or without subsequent curative surgery.[1] In one study, 54% of patients presented with acute respiratory failure requiring emergency dilation.[2] The noninvasive preoperative evaluation is limited in these emergent circumstances. For instance, the tracheal air column on chest radiograph (CXR) can be overlooked by radiologists and clinicians, and thus deserves careful inspection in any patient with symptoms of central or upper airway obstruction.[3] CXR was performed in this patient but was unrevealing (see Figure 8-1). Because CXR does not allow accurate determination of morphology, extent, or degree of narrowing, a computed tomography (CT) scan is warranted. This was not feasible in our patient, who could not lie flat and was unstable from a respiratory perspective. Inspection bronchoscopy would also allow accurate assessment of the stenosis and would provide treatment planning information, including degree of mucosal inflammation, associated cartilaginous collapse, and relative amount and location of hypertrophic fibrotic tissue,[4] but could increase respiratory compromise or cause laryngospasm and respiratory arrest. In fact, it is usually our practice to perform flexible bronchoscopy in all patients referred for rigid bronchoscopic interventions; occasionally, this examination is performed on NPPV. It is not known, however, whether such a practice should be generally applied to all cases, especially when results from a previous bronchoscopic examination are known. Indeed, in the setting of respiratory distress and need for NPPV, flexible bronchoscopy can cause airway wall edema and can trigger respiratory failure, potentially resulting in the need for emergent tracheostomy. Although bronchoscopy on NPPV in critically ill patients has been described,[5] its safety has not been studied in patients with respiratory distess resulting from tracheal stenosis. We chose to refrain from repeating a flexible bronchoscopy and proceeded directly with rigid bronchoscopic intervention to restore airway patency.

In adult patients, a tracheal diameter of 4 mm usually represents greater than 70% reduction in lumen diameter and is consistent with a severe degree of airway

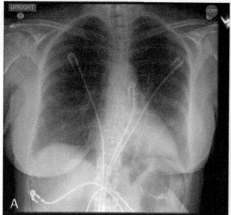
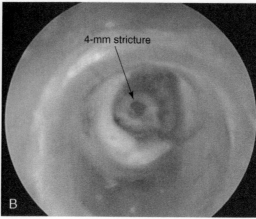

Figure 8-1 **A,** The chest radiograph performed at admission to our intensive care unit does not reveal any tracheal abnormality. **B,** The proximal aspect of the stricture is visualized through a 13 mm Efer-Dumon rigid bronchoscope. The diameter of the stricture was 4 mm—smaller than the size of the rigid telescope (5 mm).

narrowing (Myer-Cotton grade III*) and stridor.[6,7] Based on McCaffrey's system,[†] this stenosis was stage I.[8] Although PITS can be localized to the glottis or the subglottis, the most common form is seen at the site of the tube cuff (i.e., cuff stenosis). Bronchoscopically, it is usually circumferential in morphology. This patient had developed PITS 14 days after being intubated for several hours. The exact duration of intubation necessary to cause airway injury and stenosis is not known. In one study, the duration of intubation was less than 2 weeks in more than half of patients, and less than 1 month in 87%, but strictures can develop after only a few days of intubation-related mucosal and submucosal mechanical injury.[9,10] As seen in our patient, tracheal stenosis becomes symptomatic within 6 weeks after extubation in more than 50% of patients, and within 2 months after extubation in two thirds of patients.[1] Acute inflammation is the initial event that eventually leads to mucosal and submucosal ulcerations, and possibly to exposure and fragmentation of cartilaginous rings.[9] The likely pathogenesis of this process is ischemic mucosal damage when cuff-to-tracheal wall tension exceeds mucosal capillary perfusion pressure, usually 20 to 30 mm Hg.[6] Compression of the submucosa by the cuff of the tube can cause regional ischemia of the cartilaginous rings because they receive their blood supply from the submucosal plexus.[11] Subsequent inflammatory histologic changes can occur within 24 to 48 hours, and healing of the necrotic region by secondary intention occurs within 3 to 6 weeks after removal of the tube.[3]

Comorbidities

Poor general health or comorbidities may contraindicate surgery, at least temporarily. This patient had no metabolic, cardiovascular, or neurologic comorbidities that would have interfered with general anesthesia, rigid bronchoscopy, or tracheal resection and reconstruction. Her respiratory status, however, was unstable, and impending respiratory arrest was a concern.

Support System

We knew that this patient lived alone, but careful assessment of her social support was not possible because of her shortness of breath and inability to speak in full sentences.

Patient Preferences and Expectations

She clearly expressed a wish to avoid repeat tracheostomy. She was informed about available therapeutic options for her tracheal stenosis, including dilation with or without airway stent insertion, surgery, and repeat tracheostomy in case of airway emergency. After she had been informed of the risks and benefits of available therapeutic alternatives for her situation, the patient agreed to rigid bronchoscopy with dilation to improve symptoms acutely so that she might be considered for tracheal surgery afterward.

Procedural Strategies

Indications

PITS resulted in stridor and respiratory distress at rest. The bronchoscopic procedure was expected to restore airway lumen patency and improve symptoms.[1,12] During our initial encounter with the patient in the intensive care unit, we did not know the exact extent of the stricture, although we knew that its morphology was circumferential. This type of stricture would respond transiently to dilation, but the contractile scar usually recurs within several weeks, as had already happened in our patient. Published literature suggests that total loss of normal airway wall structure with replacement by fibrotic tissue permits no alternative to a concentric cicatrix, which tends to contract over time.[9] This process might explain the general failure of dilation as a method of treatment, unless lesions are not circumferential (i.e., when well-demarcated eccentric fibrotic bands are identified).[9] Surgical data support this concept, suggesting that tension at the site of anastomosis and incompletely excised fibrotic

---

*A widely used staging system for classifying tracheal stenosis based on the degree of airway narrowing.

†This system is based on the site and extent of an airway stenosis. Four stages are defined: (I) lesions confined to the subglottis or trachea that are less than 1 cm in length; (II) subglottic stenoses longer than 1 cm within the cricoid and not extending to the glottis or trachea; (III) subglottic stenoses that extend into the upper trachea but do not involve the glottis; and (IV) lesions involving the glottis.

tissue are independent risk factors for stricture recurrence after open resection of tracheal strictures.[13,14] To prevent recurrence in complex nonsurgical lesions, some experts promptly insert a silicone prosthesis at the first rigid bronchoscopic intervention rather than performing laser-assisted dilation.[1] This is not a universally accepted practice because stents themselves can cause granulation and potentially extend the degree of stenosis, making additional surgical interventions difficult or impossible. We elected, therefore, to perform dilation alone, unless significant malacia were present, which would require stent insertion.

Contraindications

This patient had no contraindications to general anesthesia or to rigid bronchoscopy.

Expected Results

Tracheal vascular anatomy* and mechanisms of tracheal wall injury in PITS highlight the transmural nature of lesions. These explain in part the limited success of purely endoluminal therapies such as laser treatment resection or dilation.[15,16] Stenotic lesions are prone to radial compressive forces and might respond favorably, albeit temporarily, to dilation. Factors negatively impacting the success rates of rigid bronchoscopic interventions include an extent longer than 1 cm and the presence of chondritis, resulting in cartilaginous collapse (malacia); in one study of patients with such complex stenoses, during a follow-up period of 28 to 72 months, only 22% of patients were treated successfully using laser-assisted mechanical dilation, whereas 78% required stent placement.[17] In another study, all patients with complex stenoses had undergone tracheal stent placement during initial rigid bronchoscopy. After 6 months of follow-up, a majority (n = 9/10) of those patients who continued to be considered inoperable eventually required permanent bronchoscopic airway stent insertion.[1]

Team Experience

The operator's experience in properly assessing the lesion and determining the most appropriate bronchoscopic intervention at a particular time is important for patients who potentially become surgical candidates once their functional status improves; preoperative bronchoscopic treatments should not result in a need to extend the length of surgical resection beyond that which would have been performed given the original length of the stenosis.[17]

Because of concerns that bronchoscopic treatment can make a lesion worse (extending its length, causing malacia, or converting a simple stricture into a complex one), therapeutic algorithms probably should be developed at each institution through collaboration between thoracic surgeons; ear, nose, and throat surgeons; and pulmonologists. Failure rates and mortality and morbidity of operative and nonoperative techniques, both in the literature and in the operators' experience, should be taken into account to establish an optimal institution-specific therapeutic algorithm.[1]

Risk-Benefit Analysis

Mechanical dilation (with or without laser assistance) provides only temporary benefit in patients with extensive (>1 cm) circumferential lesions. Repeated interventions, especially if laser is used, might increase the extent of injury in some cases, possibly resulting in damage to the cricoid posterior plate. Similarly, stent insertion could increase the length of stenosis. Some experts recommend avoiding this treatment in all patients who are candidates for surgical intervention, stating that laser or stent insertion should be performed only in patients with absolute contraindications to surgery.[18] Some believe that when one or more cartilaginous rings are involved, endoscopic treatment is contraindicated unless surgery is not a consideration.[19] However, the general applicability of such an approach has not been demonstrated. In our patient, who had an unstable respiratory status, the risks of rigid bronchoscopy were outweighed by the benefits of immediately improving airway patency, resolving respiratory distress, and avoiding respiratory failure.

Therapeutic Alternatives for Restoring Airway Patency

To optimize a patient's functional status for potentially curative open surgery, mechanical dilation with or without laser resection is often necessary. In one large reported surgical series, most patients underwent one or two preoperative rigid bronchoscopies.[1] If surgical repair is deferred for a prolonged period, or is not technically feasible, repeat dilation can be performed, but management with airway stents, laser, silicone T-tube, or tracheostomy has also been described.

1. *Self-expandable metal stents (SEMSs)* should never be used in patients who are potential candidates for resection because these are likely to cause additional airway injury and may make a potentially resectable patient unresectable.[20] Results from a surgical study suggest that all patients with tracheal and subglottic stenosis who had undergone covered or uncovered metallic stent placement developed new strictures or granulation tissue; this occurred after a short duration of stent insertion, either precluding definitive surgical treatment or requiring more extensive tracheal resection.[20] In fact, metal stents ideally should be avoided in any benign airway disorder, unless surgery and silicone stents are not a consideration.[21]

2. *Silicone stents* are helpful for splinting extensive post intubation stenoses and are appropriate for palliating airway narrowing in nonsurgical candidates.*[1,19,22] Stent-related complications, however, are not uncommon and include migration (17.5%), obstruction from secretions (6.3%), and significant granulation tissue formation at the proximal or distal extremities of the stent (6.3%).[23] Silicone

---

*The blood supply of the trachea is segmental: vessels perforate the tracheal wall at each intercartilaginous space and branch into the submucosa.

*Coexistent diseases such as coronary heart disease, severe cardiac or respiratory insufficiency, or poor general condition.

stent insertion performed using rigid bronchoscopy under general anesthesia is an acceptable alternative to surgery for inoperable patients with complex stenosis.* These stents are reported to provide long-term airway patency with minimal complications.[1] In a study of 42 patients with complex stenoses, only 9 were surgical candidates and 33 were treated with silicone stent insertion, with a success rate of 69%.[10] In general, however, the success rate of bronchoscopic treatment once stents are removed (usually after at least 6 months) in cases of complex stenosis is reportedly low (17.6%). A higher rate of airway stability after stent removal (46.8% in 22 of 47 patients) was described after stents remained in place for a mean of 11.6 months[17]; most patients (12/22) had their stents for longer than 12 months. Predictors of success of endoscopic treatments included lesions measuring less than 1 cm and those without associated malacia (chondritis). Lesion height and intubation-to-treatment latency have also been reported to independently predict the success of endoscopic intervention; 96% of patients with lesions shorter than 30 mm were successfully treated endoscopically, but the success rate fell to 20% for lesions longer than 30 mm. Patients with stenosis present for longer than 6 months since the original injury were less likely to be successfully treated endoscopically.[24]

3. *Laser-assisted mechanical dilation (LAMD)* has a failure rate of 78% to 90% for complex PITS.[17] Comparatively, failure rates for treating simple web-like PITS range from 23% to 43%.[1,25] These data are consistent with what experts stated more than 20 years ago: Only thin, web-like strictures can be removed definitively by laser resection.[15] A strong correlation between laser intensity and the magnitude of the resulting tracheal injury has been noted, especially when the laser is directed perpendicular to the airway wall.[26] Vaporization of cartilaginous structures is strictly contraindicated because it results in weakening of the tracheal framework and potentially induces restenosis to a more severe grade.[27] Despite these concerns, in a large study of patients with PITS, laser therapy did not seem to adversely affect the outcome of tracheal resection and reconstruction.[28] In a different study, however, it appeared to be responsible for most surgical complications.[18]

4. *Silicone T-tubes* (Montgomery T-tubes) or tracheostomy tubes, in this setting, should be inserted through the area of stenosis, if possible, to conserve airway not involved by the stenosis lesion. For most patients who do not require mechanical ventilatory support, a silicone T-tube provides functional capability.[3] These therapies are warranted in the few patients with critical stenoses who are candidates for neither surgery nor indwelling airway stent insertion, or who develop recurrence after such

interventions.[1] These procedures can also be used when tracheal resection and reconstruction or dilation techniques are not available or have failed, or as a solution for patients who had silicone stent placement complicated by frequent migrations.[18,23]

5. *Primary tracheal sleeve resection* is considered the treatment of choice in patients who are operable.[18,28] Proponents of open surgery believe that the transmural nature of tracheal lesions explains the limited success of purely endoluminal therapies.[16] In severe cases with airway narrowing to 5 mm diameter or less, dilation followed by tracheal resection could be performed at the same setting.[28] In our case, however, we elected to restore airway patency bronchoscopically while evaluating the patient for open surgical resection by precisely identifying the topography of the injury, the exact location and length of the stenosis, the length of tracheal involvement, and the presence of inflammation and edema at the border of stenosis. In fact, patients with severe inflammatory signs at the stenotic site should be first stabilized and re-evaluated for surgery after a period of observation.[18] We believed that although open surgery was definitive treatment indicated for our patient's mid-tracheal short stenotic lesion, her unstable respiratory status would have significantly increased the risk for postoperative complications after open surgical intervention.[29] Tracheal sleeve resection should always be considered for patients who become operable candidates after short-term successful bronchoscopic intervention, as well as when operable candidates fail bronchoscopic treatment. This open surgical procedure has a reported failure rate ranging from 5% to 15% and postoperative mortality ranging from 1.8% to 5% in expert hands.[18,28] Long-term results are satisfactory to excellent in most patients,[30] but one must recognize that most case series are reported by teams with large surgical experience. It is unclear whether these results are reproducible in a general surgical community.

Cost-Effectiveness

The most cost-effective management of PITS has not been identified, and no controlled randomized studies have been performed to evaluate the role of open surgery versus bronchoscopic treatment. Surgical series usually ignore the large number of patients not amenable to surgery, whereas bronchoscopic series exclude those undergoing open resection. To our knowledge, no cost-effectiveness evaluations of these various bronchoscopic and open surgical modalities have been published. For our patient with circumferential PITS causing respiratory failure, bronchoscopic interventions have favorable evidence-based outcomes and therefore can be offered as initial treatment to improve functional status when planes for subsequent open surgical resection are present. Many tracheal surgeons prefer rigid bronchoscopic dilation alone as compared with laser or stent insertion before tracheal resection because it is simpler and less costly, is associated with fewer side effects, and has less propensity to affect open surgical management.[12]

---

*Most studies define complex stenoses as extensive scarring ≥1 cm in vertical length, circumferential hourglass-like contraction scarring, or the presence of associated malacia.

Informed Consent

After she had been advised of the therapeutic alternatives, the patient agreed to proceed with rigid bronchoscopy under general anesthesia. She was informed of the potential risk for postoperative upper airway edema and the potential need for emergent endotracheal intubation or tracheostomy.

Techniques and Results

Anesthesia and Perioperative Care

General anesthesia using a total intravenous technique, without muscle relaxants, is our preference for rigid bronchoscopy in a patient with severe tracheal stenosis. Until control of the airway is obtained, spontaneous ventilation is maintained.[31] The anesthesia team should be ready to respond to any procedure-related complications. For example, if emergent endotracheal intubation is necessary, insertion of a No. 6 cuffless endotracheal tube can be guided bronchoscopically to avoid trauma at the stenosis level (Figure 8-2).

Instrumentation

A variety of rigid bronchoscopes were available for serial dilations (see Figure 8-2). We chose to start with a 9.5 mm external diameter rigid bronchoscope to allow gentle dilation of the stricture without damage to normal mucosa, thus avoiding the need for laser. Because the consistency of the stricture was unknown before the rigid intervention was provided, we were prepared to use potassium-titanyl-phosphate (KTP) laser for radial incisions and neodymium-doped yttrium aluminum garnet (Nd:YAG) laser if necessary in case of bleeding requiring coagulation.

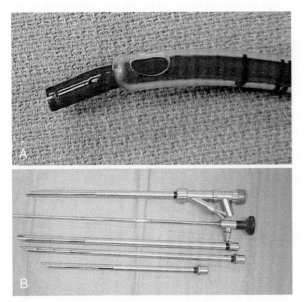

Figure 8-2 **A,** A 6 mm cuffless endotracheal tube is placed over the bronchoscope, which is ready for bronchoscopy-guided intubation in case of immediate laryngeal edema after rigid bronchoscopy. **B,** A variety of rigid bronchoscopes of different sizes should be available in case serial dilation is necessary.

Anatomic Dangers and Other Risks

When laser is used, high power density, long application times, and laser beam orientation perpendicular to the airway wall increase the risk for airway wall perforation and injury to structures adjacent to the trachea. Relevant to this patient is that an intrathoracic tracheal lesion is surrounded by the left innominate vein, the aortic arch, the innominate and left common carotid arteries, and the deep cardiac plexus. On the right, it is in relation with the pleura and the right vagus nerve, and near the root of the neck, with the innominate artery.

Results and Procedure-Related Complications

The patient was intubated with a 9.5 mm Efer-Dumon rigid bronchoscope. The circumferential stricture was noted 5 cm below the vocal cords. Its diameter was 4 mm—slightly larger than the rigid suction catheter (see Figure 8-1). Usually, if the lesion measures less than 5 mm in diameter (the size of the Hopkins lens rigid telescope), Jackson-type dilators or balloon dilators can be used to serially enlarge the stenosis. We usually proceed with gentle dilation by carefully advancing the telescope itself within the stricture. If the lesion is greater than 5 mm in diameter, dilation is achieved using the bronchoscope alone (see video on ExpertConsult.com) (Video II.8.1). Careful insertion of the tip of the bronchoscope into the stenosis, using a rotating motion and gentle forward pressure, typically advances it through the lesion. If not, one to four radial incisions are performed to release the tension in the stricture before dilation. Once the stenosis has been bypassed, assessment of the distal airway and aspiration of secretions are performed using a flexible bronchoscope introduced through the rigid tube. Most commonly, PITS injuries occur as single lesions, but given this patient's history of intubation followed by tracheostomy, other lesions may be present. A thorough evaluation of the entire upper respiratory tract, from the supraglottic structures to the carina, is therefore mandatory before surgical intervention in such patients. Serial dilation with 10.4, 12, and 13 mm rigid bronchoscopes was then performed. Measurements were taken of overall tracheal length and length of the stenosis to determine the feasibility of airway resection and reconstruction. No evidence of malacia or severe active mucosal inflammation was found and the lesion was 1 cm in length, although we noticed a mild degree of contractile retraction of the stenotic area after the rigid scope had been removed, such that after dilation, the lumen diameter was measured at 10 mm. A laser was not used because airway patency was satisfactorily restored by dilation alone and the patient was considered a good candidate for open surgical intervention. She tolerated the procedure well and was transferred to the intensive care unit (ICU) for 24 hours, during which no complications were noted. She was discharged home 2 days later.

Long-Term Management

Outcome Assessment

Post dilation, residual stenosis caused less than 50% airway lumen narrowing and the patient's symptoms

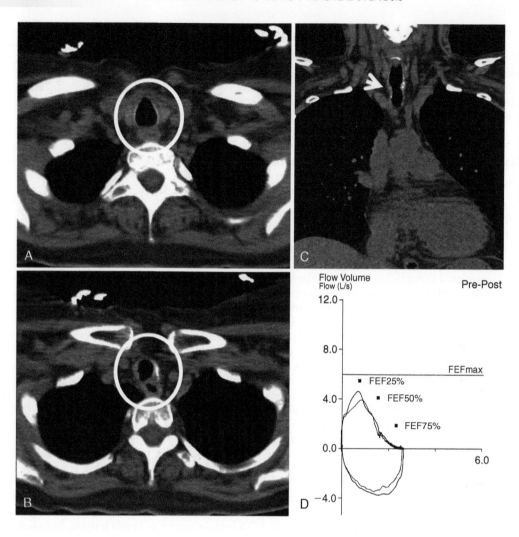

Figure 8-3 Post rigid bronchoscopic dilation, computed tomography (CT) scan showed **(A)** a normal tracheal lumen and **(B)** a mild stricture at the site of previous dilation with no evidence of extrinsic compression and no parenchymal abnormalities. **C,** Coronal CT view reveals mild stenosis and the "hourglass" morphology of the trachea at the level of stenosis *(arrow).* **D,** Flow-volume loop post dilation shows normal inspiratory and near normal expiratory curves.

improved. Stridor and respiratory distress resolved, and NPPV could be discontinued.

Referral

A thoracic surgery consultation was done during the rigid bronchoscopy so the surgeon could evaluate the lesion in real time. An outpatient consultation several days after bronchoscopic intervention was arranged to discuss tracheal sleeve resection.

Follow-up Tests and Procedures

On postoperative day 1, the patient had a CT scan of the neck and chest, as well as pulmonary function tests (PFTs). CT scan showed a mild stricture, no evidence of extrinsic compression, and no parenchymal abnormalities (Figure 8-3). Multiplanar and three-dimensional reconstruction using internal (virtual bronchoscopy) and external rendering (virtual bronchography), with excellent image quality, is achievable with low-dose techniques[32] (Figure 8-4). PFTs revealed normal forced expiratory volume in 1 second (FEV_1) and FEV_1/forced vital capacity (FVC) ratio, no flattening of the flow volume loop (FVL), and only minimal reduction in forced expiratory flow (FEF) to 69% predicted (see Figure 8-3).

Three weeks later, the patient complained of recurrent symptoms with exertion and was immediately scheduled

for surgery. She underwent a single-stage tracheal resection and reconstruction.[28] During surgery, bronchoscopic intubation was performed to reduce the risk of trauma to the airway at the stenotic level. Two centimeters of trachea was resected to ensure removal of all fibrotic tissue (Figure 8-5). The resection began just distal to the tracheal stoma site, which was not resected because it was not involved with stenosis or malacia.

The long-term outcome of this patient is expected to be good. In one of the largest series of 503 patients, 87.5% of those who underwent this procedure in an experienced tracheal surgery center had good results, and 6.2% had satisfactory results.* The overall mortality rate was 2.4%. Of the patients who died, 58% had anastomotic dehiscence, but failure occurred in 3.9% and was managed by tracheostomy, T-tube, or dilations.[28] Tracheostomy is rarely required after resection and reconstruction for PITS (in less than 5% of patients) but may

---

*Results were described as **good** if patients were functionally able to perform usual activities and if postoperative roentgenograms or bronchoscopic examinations showed an anatomically good airway. Results were considered **satisfactory** if patients could perform normal activities but were stressed on exercise, if they had abnormalities such as a paralyzed or partially paralyzed vocal cord, and if significant narrowing was evident on endoscopic or roentgenologic examination.

Figure 8-4 Computed tomography with external rendering reveals **(A)** a post intubation mid-tracheal stricture in a different patient. The extent and severity of the lesion can be measured, and these measurements correlate with **(B)** the bronchoscopic findings, but **(C)** mucosal details (hyperemia, edema) are identified only by bronchoscopic evaluation.

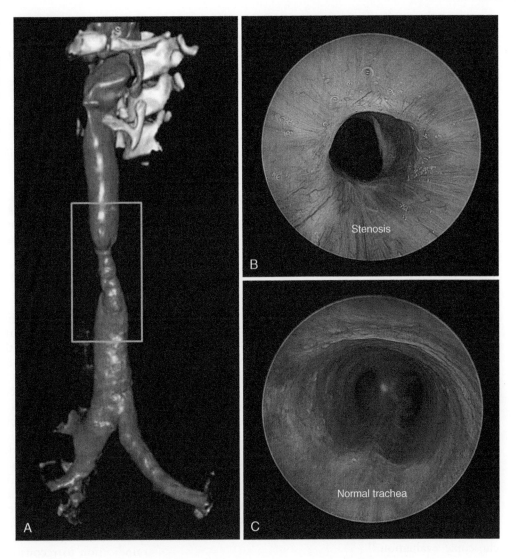

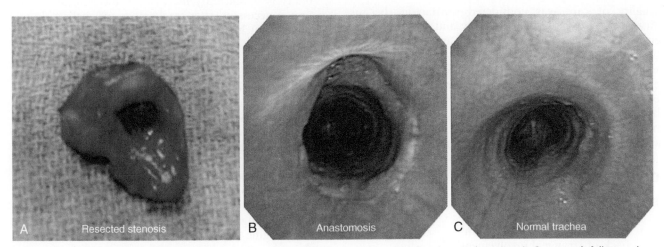

Figure 8-5 Post intubation tracheal stenosis from the patient. **(A)** Cross-section of trachea (resected specimen). One-month follow-up bronchoscopy revealed the healed anastomosis with minimal nonobstructing granulation, **(B)** no dehiscence or infection, and **(C)** a normal distal trachea.

be necessary in cases of glottis edema after laryngotracheal resection and reconstruction. Anastomotic granulation tissue is seen in only 1.6% of anastomoses performed using Vicryl suture material. Postoperative new-onset laryngeal dysfunction is seen in less than 5% of patients and is related to longer lengths of resected airway. Infectious complications are uncommon.[3] In a different study, perioperative major complications occurred in 12.3% of cases and included anastomotic dehiscence treated successfully with surgical debridement and a temporary Montgomery T-tube; vocal cord paralysis, managed with laser therapy or with cordectomy; restenosis treated with laser therapy; and deglutition dysfunction in the setting of laryngeal release, which required functional re-education. In this series, all patients with major complications received multiple preoperative laser treatments and/or endotracheal prostheses.[18]

In our patient, elective outpatient flexible bronchoscopy was scheduled 30 days after surgery to assess airway patency. She had a normal voice and denied dyspnea at rest or with exertion. During bronchoscopy, the vocal cords were mobile and symmetric, but erythema at the level of the larynx suggested uncontrolled GERD. The anastomosis line was seen 1.5 cm below the cricoid, and minimal nonobstructing granulation tissue was noted overlying the anastomosis. No dehiscence or infection was present (see Figure 8-5). Although protocols have not been universally agreed upon or studied regarding the need for or frequency of surveillance bronchoscopy, some investigators routinely perform follow-up examinations every 4 to 6 weeks during the first 6 months after intervention.[22] Others recommend bronchoscopy only in cases of new symptom development.[33] Information provided by CT scans with multiplanar reconstruction and virtual bronchoscopy may be considered a substitute for that attained by direct bronchoscopic evaluation.[34]

Quality Improvement

Quality of care was considered satisfactory because airway patency had been promptly and safely restored, emergent tracheostomy was avoided, and the patient had been discharged home 48 hours after the rigid bronchoscopic intervention. With regard to follow-up post tracheal resection, we did not perform a bronchoscopy before discharge. Some tracheal surgeons advocate early bronchoscopy to diagnose early anastomotic complications, which might be easier to manage before severe airway obstruction or infection develops.[10]

DISCUSSION POINTS

1. Describe three favorable stenosis features for tracheal resection.
   - Vertical extent less than 4 cm[12]
   - Lack of laryngeal involvement[18,28]
   - Lack of severe inflammation[18]
2. List five differential diagnoses of tracheal stenosis.
   - Post intubation/tracheostomy
   - Amyloidosis
   - Wegener's granulomatosis
   - Relapsing polychondritis

- Infectious disorders such as tuberculosis or *Klebsiella rhinoscleroma*
3. Describe three known complications of tracheal resection.
   - Anastomosis dehiscence ($\approx 6\%$) potentially requiring reoperation or permanent tracheostomy or T-tube[18,28]
   - Potentially fatal innominate artery hemorrhage (1%)[28]
   - Postoperative mortality (1.5% to 5%)[18,28]

Expert Commentary

provided by Douglas J. Mathisen, MD, and
Ashok Muniappan, MD

In the case described, a patient with post intubation stenosis was effectively managed with operative reconstruction of the trachea. Before definitive operative management, the patient had presented with acute respiratory distress requiring urgent rigid bronchoscopy and dilation for stabilization. We wholeheartedly support this strategy because patients almost never require emergent tracheal resection and reconstruction.

The decision to proceed with tracheal resection and reconstruction (TRR) is made carefully. It requires integration of clinical observations, careful review of various imaging modalities, and a thorough bronchoscopic examination of the airway. After evaluation, relatively few patients with post intubation stenoses are refused surgical management at our institution. Even patients with significant pulmonary or cardiac comorbidities may undergo tracheal resection and reconstruction safely, as long as perioperative and operative management is meticulous. An absolute contraindication to reconstruction is the patient who is ventilator dependent. We feel that postoperative morbidity is significantly increased if mechanical ventilation is necessary after tracheal reconstruction. In our opinion, such patients are best managed with a tracheostomy or a Montgomery Silastic T-tube to secure the airway. High-dose corticosteroid therapy is also a contraindication because it may impair proper healing of the anastomosis. It is prudent to wean steroids to physiologic doses or to eliminate them completely before resection. Finally, the length of trachea that may be safely resected is limited. Complex lesions of the trachea that do not leave an adequate length for reconstruction are better managed with one of the alternative techniques mentioned by the authors.

The authors emphasize the role of CT scanning and three-dimensional rendering of the airway in preoperative planning. Although many of our patients do have CT imaging preoperatively, we have not found that this enhances preoperative planning in cases of benign post intubation stenosis. We still routinely acquire conventional tracheal radiographs requiring a high kilovoltage technique that accentuates the air–soft tissue interface and softens bone shadows. CT scans are particularly deficient in evaluating the glottis and the subglottic larynx, which frequently are involved in post intubation stenosis.

Many of the limitations of current imaging techniques are overcome by flexible and rigid bronchoscopy. The rigid ventilating bronchoscope remains the best tool for properly evaluating post intubation stenosis. Although flexible bronchoscopy may be performed, it is inadvisable if rigid bronchoscopy is not available to rescue the airway. The larynx should be carefully evaluated because occasionally, laryngeal stenoses must be addressed before definitive tracheal reconstruction is undertaken. Ideally, definitive bronchoscopic examination is performed immediately before the planned surgical reconstruction, to avoid unnecessary instrumentation and additional anesthesia. For those presenting with symptoms suggestive of impending airway obstruction, such as the patient the authors present, rigid bronchoscopy and dilation are performed to manage the compromised patient before definitive reconstruction. We are wary of performing bronchoscopy while the patient is awake in cases of significant airway stenosis; we typically perform examinations under general anesthesia. Even the gentlest bronchoscopic examination can induce edema or bleeding that can lead to loss of the airway.

The authors do an excellent job of discussing the range of available treatments for post intubation tracheal stenosis. Although mechanical dilation, with or without laser incision of the scar, is often performed before definitive repair, we do not routinely prescribe it for patients at first presentation. Mechanical dilation of the typical post intubation stenosis is unlikely to have a prolonged effect, and recurrence is almost virtually ensured. We use mechanical dilation exclusively for post intubation tracheal stenosis and have not found the laser useful for managing these lesions. It is rare for us to perform a tracheostomy or to place a T-tube, because these measures may make definitive repair more complicated or even impossible. If it cannot be avoided, every effort is made to place the surgical airway through the narrowed segment of trachea, so as to avoid reducing the length of normal trachea available for reconstruction. We would echo the authors in bemoaning the use of stents in patients who are potential surgical candidates for reconstruction. Stent complications, especially induction of airway granulation tissue, may threaten the ability of the surgeon to safely reconstruct the airway. This cost cannot be justified in any way for the patient who is a reasonable surgical candidate.

Several technical concerns must be addressed before tracheal reconstruction can be performed safely. As the authors suggest, the lesion must be completely resected to ensure a satisfactory anastomosis that heals without recurrent stenosis. Given this fact, the lengths of trachea that may be resected safely are limited. Most resections are less than 4 cm in length, but occasionally longer lengths may be resected successfully. Significant kyphosis, short stature, and conditions that prevent cervical flexion may significantly limit the amount of trachea that can be resected. The prepared tracheal surgeon must be familiar with techniques such as laryngeal release that can significantly reduce tension at the anastomosis.

Anastomotic complications are the most frequent cause of mortality after tracheal reconstruction. The authors cite the 2.4% mortality in our 1995 report of 503 patients undergoing tracheal reconstruction for post intubation stenosis.[28] This greatly overestimates the expected mortality, as is seen in our most recent experience. A more recent report from us, in 2004, described 1% mortality in 901 patients undergoing tracheal reconstruction for all diagnoses at our institution.[12] The mortality rate in patients experiencing anastomotic complications was 7.4% (6/81 patients), but it was only 0.01% (5/820 patients) in patients without anastomotic complications. Of 6 deaths in the anastomotic complication group, 3 were attributed to airway obstruction, 2 occurred in patients undergoing repair of tracheoinnominate fistulas, and 1 was the result of mediastinitis. Of 5 deaths in the nonanastomotic complication group, 3 were attributed to pneumonias, 1 was the result of myocardial infarction, and 1 was caused by a pulmonary embolism. Most important, all cases of mortality occurred in the early part of the series, and no deaths were reported after 1988.

REFERENCES

1. Brichet A, Verkindre C, Dupont J, et al. Multidisciplinary approach to management of postintubation tracheal stenoses. *Eur Respir J.* 1999;13:888-893.
2. Baugnee PE, Marquette CH, Ramon P, et al. Traitement endoscopique des stenoses trachéales postintubation: a propos de 58 cas. *Rev Mal Respir.* 1995;12:585-592.
3. Wain JC Jr. Postintubation tracheal stenosis. *Semin Thorac Cardiovasc Surg.* 2009;21:284-289.
4. Colt HG. Functional evaluation before and after interventional bronchoscopy. In: Bolliger CT, Mathur PN, eds. *Interventional Bronchoscopy.* Basel, Switzerland: S. Karger; 2000:55-64.
5. Murgu SD, Pecson J, Colt HG. Bronchoscopy on noninvasive positive pressure ventilation: indications and technique. *Respir Care.* 2010;55:595-600.
6. Heffner JE, Miller KS, Sahn SA. Tracheostomy in the intensive care unit. Part 2. Complications. *Chest.* 1986;90:430-436.
7. Murgu S, Colt HG. Morphometric bronchoscopy in adults with central airway obstruction: case illustrations and review of the literature. *Laryngoscope.* 2009;119:1318-1324.
8. McCaffrey TV. Classification of laryngotracheal stenosis. *Laryngoscope.* 1992;102:1335-1340.
9. Cooper JD, Grillo HC. The evolution of tracheal injury due to ventilatory assistance through cuffed tubes: a pathologic study. *Ann Surg.* 1969;169:334-348.
10. Galluccio G, Lucantoni G, Battistoni P, et al. Interventional endoscopy in the management of benign tracheal stenoses: definitive treatment at long-term follow-up. *Eur J Cardiothorac Surg.* 2009;35:429-433; discussion 933-934.
11. Salassa JR, Pearson BW, Payne WS. Growth and microscopical blood supply of the trachea. *Ann Thorac Surg.* 1977;24:100-107.
12. Wright CD, Grillo HC, Wain JC, et al. Anastomotic complications after tracheal resection: prognostic factors and management. *J Thorac Cardiovasc Surg.* 2004;128:731-739.
13. Couraud L, Moreau JM, Velly JF. The growth of circumferential scars of the major airways from infancy to adulthood. *Eur J Cardiothorac Surg.* 1990;4:521-525.
14. Abbasidezfouli A, Akbarian E, Shadmehr MB, et al. The etiological factors of recurrence after tracheal resection and reconstruction in post-intubation stenosis. *Interact Cardiovasc Thorac Surg.* 2009;9: 446-449.

15. Shapshay SM, Beamis JF, Hybels RI, et al. Endoscopic treatment of subglottic and tracheal stenosis by radial laser incision and dilation. *Ann Otol Rhinol Laryngol.* 1987;96:661-664.

16. Grillo HC. Stents and sense. *Ann Thorac Surg.* 2000;70:1142.

17. Cavaliere S, Bezzi M, Toninelli C, et al. Management of post-intubation tracheal stenoses using the endoscopic approach. *Monaldi Arch Chest Dis.* 2007;67:73-80.

18. Rea F, Callegaro D, Loy M, et al. Benign tracheal and laryngotracheal stenosis: surgical treatment and results. *Eur J Cardiothorac Surg.* 2002;22:352-356.

19. Patelli M, Gasparini S. Post-intubation tracheal stenoses: what is the curative yield of the interventional pulmonology procedures? *Monaldi Arch Chest Dis.* 2007;67:71-72.

20. Gaissert HA, Grillo HC, Mathisen DJ, et al. Temporary and permanent restoration of airway continuity with the tracheal T-tube. *J Thorac Cardiovasc Surg.* 1994;107:600-606.

21. U.S. Food and Drug Administration. Metallic tracheal stents in patients with benign airway disorders. http://www.fda.gov/Safety/MedWatch/SafetyInformation/SafetyAlertsforHumanMedical Products/ucm153009.htm. Accessed April 15, 2011.

22. Zias N, Chroneou A, Tabba MK, et al. Post tracheostomy and post intubation tracheal stenosis: report of 31 cases and review of the literature. *BMC Pulm Med.* 2008;8:18.

23. Martinez-Ballarin JI, Diaz-Jimenez JP, Castro MJ, et al. Silicone stents in the management of benign tracheobronchial stenoses: tolerance and early results in 63 patients. *Chest.* 1996;109:626-629.

24. Nouraei SA, Ghufoor K, Patel A, et al. Outcome of endoscopic treatment of adult postintubation tracheal stenosis. *Laryngoscope.* 2007;117:1073-1079.

25. Mehta AC, Lee FYW, Cordasco EM, et al. Concentric tracheal and subglottic stenosis: management using the Nd:YAG laser for mucosal sparing followed by a gentle dilatation. *Chest.* 1993;104:673-677.

26. Goodman RL, Hulbert WC, King EG. Canine tracheal injury by neodymium-YAG laser irradiation. *Chest.* 1987;91:745-748.

27. Monnier P, George M, Monod ML, et al. The role of the CO_2 laser in the management of laryngotracheal stenosis: a survey of 100 cases. *Eur Arch Otorhinolaryngol.* 2005;262:602-608.

28. Grillo HC, Donahue DM, Mathisen DJ, et al. Postintubation tracheal stenosis: treatment and results. *J Thorac Cardiovasc Surg.* 1995;109:486-492; discussion 492-493.

29. Bisson A, Bonnette P, Ben EL, et al. Tracheal sleeve resection for iatrogenic stenoses (subglottic laryngeal and tracheal). *J Thorac Cardiovasc Surg.* 1992;104:882-887.

30. Marulli G, Rizzardi G, Bortolotti L, et al. Single-staged laryngotracheal resection and reconstruction for benign strictures in adults. *Interact Cardiovasc Thorac Surg.* 2008;7:227-230.

31. Perrin G, Colt HG, Martin C, et al. Safety of interventional rigid bronchoscopy using intravenous anesthesia and spontaneous assisted ventilation: a prospective study. *Chest.* 1992;102:1526-1530.

32. Shitrit D, Valdsislav P, Grubstein A, et al. Accuracy of virtual bronchoscopy for grading tracheobronchial stenosis: correlation with pulmonary function test and fiberoptic bronchoscopy. *Chest.* 2005;128:3545-3550.

33. Matsuo T, Colt HG. Evidence against routine scheduling of surveillance bronchoscopy after stent insertion. *Chest.* 2000;118:1455-1459.

34. Bauer TL, Steiner KV. Virtual bronchoscopy: clinical applications and limitations. *Surg Oncol Clin N Am.* 2007;16:323-328.

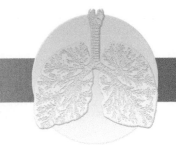

Chapter 9

Bronchoscopic Treatment of Post Tracheostomy Tracheal Stenosis with Chondritis

This chapter emphasizes the following elements of the Four Box Approach: physical examination, complementary tests, and functional status assessment; patient preferences and expectations (also includes family); and results and procedure-related complications.

CASE DESCRIPTION

This patient is an 86-year-old woman with a history of ischemic stroke and coma requiring 4 weeks of endotracheal intubation, followed by percutaneous dilational tracheostomy (PDT). She was decannulated 3 months later in the nursing home where she lived because of required assistance for daily living activities. She had been hospitalized previously for respiratory failure due to decompensated congestive heart failure (CHF). She was extubated after CHF was treated, but within minutes of extubation she developed biphasic stridor and had to be emergently reintubated. Three days later, after administration of Solu-Medrol 60 mg intravenously every 12 hours, she was successfully extubated and transferred to the medicine ward. A few days later, however, the intern on call was called to evaluate her for recurrent stridor and increased work of breathing. The chest radiograph (CXR) shown in Figure 9-1 revealed narrowing of the upper trachea, as well as cardiomegaly and pulmonary vascular congestion. Bronchoscopy confirmed radiographic findings and showed a 1.5 cm long triangular stomal stricture 4 cm below the vocal cords. During inspiration, this narrowed the lumen by 80%, but during expiration, 100% airway lumen obstruction occurred as the result of lateral cartilaginous collapse of two tracheal rings (see Figure 9-1). The rest of the airway examination was unremarkable. No evidence of mucus plugging or secretions was found distal to the stenosis. In addition to severe CHF, her medical history included hypothyroidism, hypertension, anemia, Alzheimer's dementia, and right hemiplegia from her ischemic stroke. Physical examination revealed an elderly woman in mild respiratory distress at rest who followed some simple commands and had biphasic stridor over the anterior neck auscultation. Oxygen saturation was 95% on room air. Karnofsky performance score before the episode of respiratory failure was 50, and American Society of Anesthesiologists (ASA) score at the time of the diagnostic bronchoscopy was 3. Laboratory data were normal. A two-dimensional echocardiogram performed during hospitalization revealed normal left

ventricular function, but a moderately enlarged left atrium and diastolic dysfunction were evident. The patient has one daughter, who rarely visits her in the nursing home but has been visiting her during her most recent hospitalization. According to the staff at the nursing home, the patient enjoys watching television and seems to enjoy eating a modified dysphagia diet. At baseline, she follows some simple commands but is aphasic and does not speak.

DISCUSSION POINTS

1. Describe three qualitative features of tracheal stenosis.
2. Describe three diagnostic modalities other than bronchoscopy that can be performed to assess the severity, extent, and morphology of this patient's tracheal stenosis.
3. List four therapeutic alternatives for post tracheostomy stenosis with chondritis.
4. Identify three airway stricture characteristics that determine the need for and type of treatment.

CASE RESOLUTION

Initial Evaluations

Physical Examination, Complementary Tests, and Functional Status Assessment

The initial diagnosis of tracheal stenosis occurred after a careful examination of the chest radiograph obtained post extubation. Chest radiographs are rarely diagnostic of central airway obstruction yet are often obtained as initial radiologic tests. Obvious pathology such as tracheal deviation from masses or severe tracheal stenosis similar to that seen in this case may be identified; CXR can also reveal changes that may alter the normal airway-vasculature relationship, such as skeletal deformities or mediastinal shift (Figure 9-2). In cases of post tracheostomy stenosis (PTS), the tracheal air column is easily overlooked by radiologists and clinicians alike; thus careful inspection is warranted in a patient who is symptomatic post tracheostomy.[1] The CXR does not allow accurate determination of morphology, extent, degree of narrowing, and associated findings such as chondritis (involvement of the cartilage and resulting collapse). From this perspective, standard computed tomography (CT) scans provide much more information and the ability to document airway collapse when performed during both inspiration and expiration. Multiplanar and three-dimensional reconstruction with internal (virtual

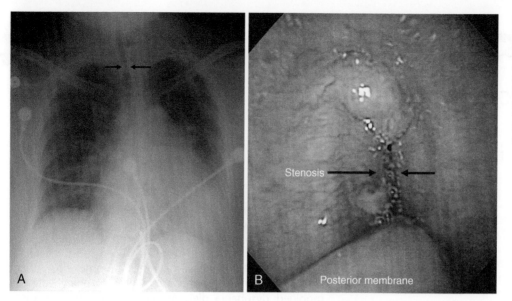

Figure 9-1 **A,** Chest radiograph revealed focal narrowing of the upper trachea, as well as cardiomegaly and pulmonary vascular congestion. **B,** Bronchoscopy showed a triangular (A-shaped, lambdoid, pseudoglottic) severe stomal stricture 4 cm below the vocal cords, which during expiration caused 100% airway lumen obstruction.

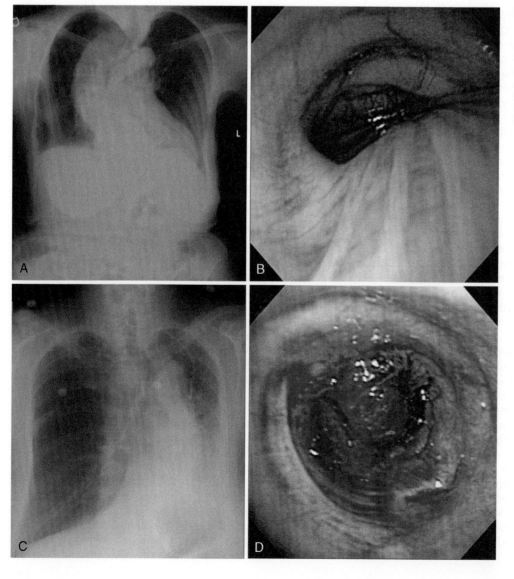

Figure 9-2 Chest x-ray (CXR) reveals **(A)** severe scoliosis resulting in **(B)** severe extrinsic compression of the posterior wall of the left main bronchus. CXR shows **(C)** left-sided mediastinal shift in a patient with **(D)** hemoptysis from a bleeding tumor completely occluding the distal left main bronchus.

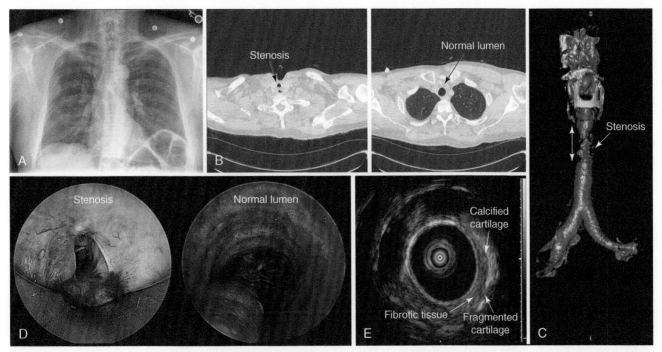

Figure 9-3 **A,** Chest x-ray in a patient with post tracheostomy stenosis fails to reveal tracheal narrowing. **B,** Axial computed tomography (CT) images reveal focal airway narrowing. **C,** External three-dimensional (3D) rendering reveals the complex stenosis 4 cm in length. **D,** Bronchoscopy confirmed the results of 3D CT imaging and showed patency distal to the stenosis. **E,** High-resolution endobronchial ultrasound shows fragmentation of the cartilage.

bronchoscopy) and external rendering (virtual bronchography), with excellent image quality, is achievable with the use of low-dose techniques (Figure 9-3). Analysis using these newer imaging protocols better characterizes whether the lesion is intraluminal, extrinsic, or mixed, and whether the airway distal to the obstruction is patent.[2,3] In addition, the length and diameter of the lesions and their relationship to adjacent vascular structures are assessed with a higher degree of accuracy. These features may assist physicians in determining appropriate therapy.[4]

Magnetic resonance imaging (MRI) has been used in small case series of tracheal stenosis.[5-7] Results of these studies show that MRI can be used to identify the relationship of the trachea to adjacent vascular structures, and to determine the degree and length of tracheal stenosis, without the use of ionizing radiation or intravenous contrast medium (Figure 9-4). Following percutaneous dilational tracheostomy, MRI provides an excellent noninvasive method of assessing the integrity of the tracheal lumen.[8] Neither MRI nor CT provides information about mucosal changes, and neither can reliably image the integrity of the cartilaginous framework of the airway. Although investigators are exploring the use of high-resolution endobronchial ultrasonography (see Figure 9-3), it appears as of this writing that optical imaging using flexible bronchoscopy remains a procedure of choice to diagnose and identify the type, location, and severity of an airway stricture before therapeutic interventions are proposed.[9,10]

This patient had developed a postsurgical tracheostomy–related stricture 90 days after an indwelling size 8 cuffed tracheostomy tube with 11 mm outside diameter was inserted. The true incidence of PTS is difficult to determine accurately from the published literature because of inconsistent follow-up, but it is estimated to be 1% to 2%.[11] The mean onset of strictures seems to be earlier after PDT than after open surgical tracheostomy: 5.0 weeks versus 28.5 weeks ($P = .009$).[12]

PTS appears in three locations:

1. *Suprastomal stenosis:* When defined as involving more than 50% of the lumen, this type of stricture was noted in 23.8% of PDT patients and in 7.3% of surgical tracheostomies in one study.[13] The superior level (proximal) of the stenosis was located at a mean distance of 1.6 cm from the vocal cords in PDT patients, and at 3.4 cm from the cords in surgical tracheostomy patients ($P = .04$). This might be secondary to the use of incorrect needle puncture sites during PDT.

2. *Stenoses at the level of the tracheostomy tube cuff:* These are caused by ischemic mucosal damage when cuff-to-tracheal wall tension exceeds the mucosa capillary perfusion pressure, usually 20 to 30 mm Hg; subsequent inflammatory histologic changes may occur as soon as within 24 to 48 hours. The incidence of these lesions has been reduced 10-fold after transition to high-volume–low-pressure cuffs. It is therefore warranted that when patients have indwelling endotracheal or tracheostomy tubes, peak inspiratory and expiratory cuff pressures should be kept below 15 mm Hg, and definitely below 25 mm Hg.[14]

3. *Stomal strictures:* This is the type of stenosis described in our patient. These stenoses account for more than 85% of cases of PTS.[10] They may be secondary to inadequate tracheal incisions, ongoing stomal infection, or a rigid tube-connecting system

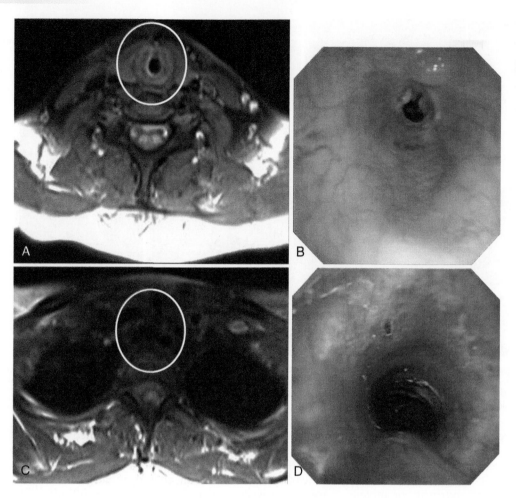

Figure 9-4 Axial T1 magnetic resonance imaging (MRI) of the neck clearly reveals **(A)** subglottic stenosis **(B)** identified on flexible bronchoscopy. The distal normal tracheal lumen is less clearly seen on **(C)** MRI than on **(D)** bronchoscopy.

that generates excess tube motion within the trachea. In one review paper, stomal wound infection was a causative factor in 42% of stomal stenoses following open tracheostomy.[15] Strictures may result from abnormal wound healing and excess granulation tissue formation around the tracheal stoma site; excess granulation tissue can also develop over cartilage fractured during tracheostomy.[16] Cartilage damage can result from mechanical leverage of the tracheal tube at the stoma site from the unsupported weight of ventilator attachments. This can cause pressure necrosis of tracheal mucosa and the underlying cartilaginous frame. Because risk is high if the tracheostomy tube is too large for the airway, recommendations are to consider a size 8 tube with an 11 mm outer diameter as an upper limit in men, and a size 7 tube with a 10 mm outer diameter in women.[14] We presume that the 11 mm external diameter tube used in our patient was probably too large and may have contributed to the development of her PTS.

Symptoms (at rest) in tracheal stenosis usually are not present until a 70% reduction in lumen diameter occurs, but stridor, as seen in our patient, occurs when the tracheal lumen is less than 5 mm in diameter.[10] The presence of stridor on neck auscultation is consistent with a bronchoscopic classification of severe airway narrowing

signaling greater than 70% airway lumen narrowing.[9,17,18] Indeed, based on the Myer-Cotton classification system* for laryngotracheal stenosis, this patient has a grade III lesion because her stenotic index† was 80%.[19]

In addition to an accurate assessment of airway lumen, the functional status of the tracheal stenosis patient should be part of a multidimensional evaluation. On this note, the Medical Research Council (MRC) dyspnea scale was found to be highly sensitive to the presence of varying degrees of tracheal stenosis. Strong correlation was noted between the severity of the stenosis and the MRC grade. The MRC scale furthermore was found to be responsive to changes in a patient's effort tolerance resulting from treating the obstructive lesion.[20]

Comorbidities

This patient had significant comorbidities, including CHF and a history of ischemic stroke. When surgical or bronchoscopic interventions are provided under general

---

*A widely used staging system for classifying tracheal stenosis based on the degree of airway narrowing.

†The stenotic index (SI) represents the cross-sectional area (CSA) of the obstructed area relative to that of a normal airway lumen proximal or distal to the stenosis. $SI = (CSA_{normal} - CSA_{abnormal})/(CSA_{normal} \times 100\%)$; the greater the SI, the greater the degree of airway narrowing and the more severe the obstruction.

anesthesia, comorbidities could significantly increase the risks for perioperative adverse events such as decompensated CHF or new cerebral ischemia.[21] Preoperative decompensated CHF, as seen in our patient, has been identified as a risk factor for other cardiac complications after surgery and often requires postponing elective surgery for a week after resolution of symptoms.[22] Although a therapeutic bronchoscopic intervention in this patient is not considered a high–cardiac risk procedure (contrary to vascular, intraperitoneal, or intrathoracic procedures), her age greater than 70 years and her previous history of CHF and cerebrovascular disease are independent risk factors for major cardiac complications that need to be seriously considered.[23] The presence of cerebrovascular disease is a particularly important finding in elderly patients undergoing general anesthesia. In general, at least 2 weeks should elapse after a stroke before elective surgery is attempted. Furthermore, if recurrent transient ischemic attacks (TIAs) have occurred, an evaluation for carotid artery disease is warranted. Our patient had her stroke several years before her tracheal stricture. No signs of recurrent TIAs were noted, and her CHF had been stabilized for a week before our evaluation.

Support System

The patient was a resident of a nursing home and had poor family support. The quality of social relationships for nursing home residents was shown to have a significant effect on older people's self-perceived quality of life, life satisfaction, and well-being. Residents of nursing homes consistently report that they experience limited meaningful interaction with others and may feel socially isolated, despite the busyness of a long-term care home.[24] Social interaction in these institutions can be difficult and is not always well supported by the environment or the staff. In addition, as noted in our patient, individual factors such as restricted mobility and diminished cognitive ability can further limit interaction with other people.[24]

Patient Preferences and Expectations

Because of her dementia and post stroke aphasia, the patient was unable to clearly express a desire for treatment. Her daughter, as the next of kin, had durable power of attorney and was the designated health care decision maker. She was informed about available therapeutic options for her mother's tracheal stenosis, including dilation with airway stent insertion, surgery, and even repeated tracheostomy. Because it was believed that tracheostomy would further compromise her quality of life, this was considered a less optimal alternative. The likelihood of complications resulting from tracheal resection was felt to outweigh the benefits in this particular case because of her cardiac and neurologic comorbidities; in addition, from a surgical standpoint, the risk for anastomotic complications was increased in view of a previous tracheostomy and the high likelihood of peritracheal fibrosis, which limits tracheal mobility and increases tension, potentially leading to catastrophic failure of the anastomosis.[25] Thus rigid bronchoscopy under general anesthesia with stent placement was

offered to this patient as the therapeutic alternative of choice.

Procedural Strategies

Indications

This was a symptomatic PTS that resulted in stridor and respiratory distress at rest. A bronchoscopic procedure or open surgery may be offered to improve dyspnea, restore satisfactory airway lumen patency, and improve symptoms.[9,26] Symptoms in tracheal stenosis are related mainly to the degree of airway narrowing and flow velocity through the stenosis, and to a lesser degree to the extent or morphology of the stricture. The drop in airway pressure along the stenotic area increases significantly at rest when more than 70% of the tracheal lumen is obliterated. Our patient's inactive lifestyle caused routinely low-flow velocity through her stenotic airway. This explains why she developed symptoms only when a severe degree of airway narrowing was present. Improving airway patency to a lesser (mild) degree of narrowing (<50%) would partially or completely alleviate this patient's shortness of breath.[27] Palliation of her airway narrowing was therefore warranted.

The stricture was 1.5 cm in extent. Although this length is considered of moderate degree and may impact surgical decisions or choice of stent type and length, long stenoses show a modest difference in pressure profile with a slightly smaller magnitude of total pressure drop than the simple shorter and less than 1 cm stenosis of comparable diameter.[27] It appears that in terms of flow dynamics and symptoms, the degree of airway narrowing is more important than the extent of stenosis.

Tracheal stricture morphology in this case was triangular. Triangular stenoses have been described as lambdoid, pseudoglottic, or A-shaped strictures. Experimental flow dynamic studies show that this morphologic type of stenosis results in slightly less pressure drop than an elliptical morphology of similar degree of airway narrowing,[28] suggesting that an accurate description of the morphologic type (i.e., triangular, circumferential, or elliptical) may impact symptoms and eventually decisions about treatment. To our knowledge, however, no common language or nomenclature has been universally accepted for tracheal strictures.

Contraindications

No absolute contraindications to rigid bronchoscopy were known in our patient. However, the risk for perioperative cardiac complications is almost doubled when clinical signs of CHF are present preoperatively.[29] Our patient had no clinical signs of CHF at the time of our evaluation. She was therefore continued on her medicines, which included angiotensin-converting enzyme (ACE) inhibitors, diuretics, and beta blockers. Decompensated CHF (New York Heart Association [NYHA] class IV), if present, should be treated to the extent possible before surgery, and postponement of surgery is often appropriate.[30] Regarding her history of cerebrovascular disease, perioperative stroke is an infrequent but serious complication, occurring at a rate of 0.3% to 3.5%, with most cases occurring during the postoperative period.[31]

Expected Results

Rigid intubation was planned using a large (13 mm)-diameter Efer-Dumon nonventilating rigid bronchoscope (Bryan Corp., Woburn, Mass) to dilate the lesion and allow deployment of a large silicone stent. The scope would be introduced through the mouth and then between the vocal cords under direct visualization so as to ensure a secure airway at all times. Careful attention would be necessary to maintain airway patency because the patient was edentulous and may develop a difficult airway during anesthesia, when a collapsed upper airway might limit the field of view during intubation.

In patients with PTS, therapeutic success of rigid bronchoscopic interventions is variable. Factors influencing the success rate include the presence or absence of chondritis resulting in cartilaginous collapse (malacia), a characteristic of complex stenosis. This triangular stenosis, due to loss of varying amounts of anterior and lateral cartilaginous wall, will accept various sizes of dilating instruments, such as rigid bronchoscopes, but generally will not respond more than transiently with an increase in airway cross-sectional area.[1] For instance, in one study of patients with complex stenosis, including those with PTS, during a follow-up period of 28 to 72 months, only 22% of patients (n = 13) were treated successfully with laser-assisted mechanical dilation, whereas 47 patients (78%) required stent placement; 22 had their stent removed after 1 year and did not require further therapy. Thirteen inoperable patients required permanent stent insertion, and 12 others were referred to surgery after failure despite numerous repeated endoscopic treatments.[32] In another study, all patients with complex stenosis including PTS had undergone tracheal stent placement during an initial rigid bronchoscopy. After 6 months of follow-up, of those patients who continued to be considered inoperable (n = 10), most (n = 9) eventually required permanent bronchoscopic airway stent insertion.[9]

Team Experience

Experience and expediency might result in reduced complications in this patient with cardiac and neurologic comorbidities. Team experience and an available multidisciplinary airway disease program, including thoracic and ear, nose, and throat surgeons, anesthesiologists, and pulmonologists, can result in the elaboration of specific therapeutic algorithms for patients with this disease. Failure rates, mortality, and morbidity of operative and nonoperative techniques in the published literature and in the operators' experience should be taken into account to establish a specific therapeutic approach.[9]

Risk-Benefit Analysis

The risks of postoperative decompensated CHF and postoperative stroke were outweighed by the benefit of improving airway patency to relieve this patient's respiratory distress and avoid recurrent respiratory failure caused by severe tracheal stenosis. Although tracheal sleeve resection is considered the definitive treatment for this type of lesion, this patient's poor general health, previous tracheostomy, and cardiac and cerebrovascular comorbidities would significantly increase the risk for postoperative complications after open surgical interventions.[33] Therefore, other techniques have been proposed in the literature as alternatives to open surgery.

Therapeutic Alternatives for Restoring Airway Patency

- *Dilation using balloon, bougies, or dilators* (e.g., Jackson dilators): These tools are usually used if the stenosis shows stenotic hypertrophic fibrotic tissue in a circumferential pattern, which was not seen in our patient. Simple dilation would not be appropriate because cartilage would collapse again once the dilating instruments were removed from the stricture.[34]
- *Laser resection using neodymium-doped yttrium aluminum garnet (Nd:YAG) lasers*[35]: This approach can be successfully used in conjunction with dilation to release the tension of the stricture by performing radial incisions onto the hypertrophic stenotic tissues; because these were not present in our patient, this modality was not a consideration.
- *Carbon dioxide (CO_2) laser resection of the collapsed tracheal cartilage, with sparing of the posterior membrane to prevent circumferential restenosis (endoscopic tracheoplasty)*[36]: This procedure is done under general anesthesia, often with muscle relaxants, high-frequency supraglottic jet ventilation, and suspension microlaryngotracheoscopy. In one study, this recently proposed technique achieved a successful outcome (decreased MRC dyspnea scale) and lack of need for repeated intervention after 6 months of symptom-free follow-up, thus avoiding the operative risks, prolonged hospitalization, and morbidity associated with open surgical tracheal resection. More experience, reproducible evidence, and longer follow-up are necessary before this treatment modality can be recommended routinely.
- *Covered and uncovered metal stent insertion using flexible bronchoscopy:* These techniques have been reported to be successful in series of tracheal stenoses including complex PTS.[37,38] However, recurrent obstruction from granulation can occur in up to 36% of patients as the result of tissue growth through the spaces in a stent's wire mesh. Metal stents are associated with significant complications, especially when placed in the subglottic region, prompting statements that this location should ideally be avoided,[38] especially in cases of histologically proven benign airway disorders.[39] A study published in the surgical literature suggests that all patients with tracheal and subglottic stenosis who had undergone covered or uncovered metallic stent placement developed new strictures or granulation tissue.[40] Injuries were severe, occurred after a short duration of stent insertion, and either precluded definitive surgical treatment or required more extensive tracheal resection. Metal stents, therefore, should not be used in patients who are potential candidates for resection because these are highly likely to cause additional airway injury and to make a potentially resectable patient inoperable.[41]
- *Self-expandable silicone stents:* Unlike metal stents, silicone stents have the advantage of being easily removable. They are placed under rigid bronchoscopy

or suspension laryngoscopy, and therefore require expertise in these techniques. Some silicone stents have been studied in benign airway obstruction, including tracheal stenosis and malacia.[42] Although immediate symptom palliation was established in most cases, the incidence of complications was high (75%), with stent migration occurring in 69% of cases.[42,43]

- *Silicone stent insertion* is an acceptable alternative to surgery for many inoperable patients with complex stenosis. It is reported to maintain airway patency over the long term with minimal complications.[9] However, the success rate of bronchoscopic treatment after stent removal (after 6 months) in cases of complex stenosis, as in patients with chondritis (as in our case), is reportedly low (17.6%). This low definitive curative yield of bronchoscopic procedures in cases of complex stenosis and the reported risk that a stent might lengthen the tracheal segment to be resected suggest that a tracheal sleeve resection should be the first option in cases of complex stenosis with chondritis if the patient is suitable for surgery.[44] In fact, national societies such as the Interventional Pulmonology Study Group of the Italian Association of Pulmonologists (AIPO) recommend that when one or more cartilaginous rings are involved, endoscopic treatment is usually contraindicated unless surgery is not feasible (Level of Recommendation B).[44] Other investigators have noted a high rate of airway stability and good results following stent insertion, with definitive and curative success described in 22 of 47 patients (46.8 %) after stent removal.[32] In this study, airway stents had remained in place for a mean of 11.6 months, but most patients (12/22) had their stent placed for longer than 12 months. A more recent study showed that of 42 patients with complex stenoses, only 9 were surgical candidates and 33 were treated with silicone stent insertion, with a success rate of 69%.[45] It is noteworthy, however, that studies evaluating complex stenoses do not specifically report separate results for post intubation and post tracheostomy subgroups. The pathogenesis and treatment approach for these stenoses, therefore, may indeed differ significantly.[10]

- *Montgomery T-tube:* This tube can be used when tracheal repair and reconstruction or dilation techniques are not available or have failed, or occasionally as an initial therapy or as a solution for patients who had silicone stent placement complicated by frequent migrations.[46,47] For most patients who do not require mechanical ventilatory support, a silicone T-tube provides greater functional capability and comfort.[1] In a large case series consisting of 53 patients with complex tracheal stenoses (24 post tracheostomy), silicone T-tube insertion was effective in 70% of patients with limited complications. Concurrent cardiopulmonary disease and intractable infection were the two major causes of failure after T-tube placement.[48] Granulation tissue formation at the proximal end of the T-tube has also been noted. Chronic airway irritation incites infection and promotes or aggravates granulation tissue formation. The sharper edge of the proximal aspect of the T-tube (when it has to be cut) and its placement within 0.5 cm of the vocal cords are known risk factors for granulation tissue development.[48] If the T-tube is not properly capped, allowing the patient to breathe through the mouth, airway secretions become dry and may cause obstruction. Patients, families, and referring health care providers probably benefit from diligent instruction on how to care for and monitor T-tubes. Frequent bronchoscopies may be necessary to remove extremely thick and sticky mucous plaques; some investigators perform three to four biweekly bronchoscopies, followed by procedures once every 4 weeks, once good stent patency has been documented.[48]

- *Open surgical interventions* such as tracheal sleeve resection or airway reconstruction are preferred initial therapies and are considered for patients who become operable candidates after short-term successful bronchoscopic intervention, as well as for operable candidates who have failed bronchoscopic treatment. Surgical tracheal sleeve resection has a failure rate ranging from 5% to 15% and a postoperative mortality ranging from 1.8% to 5%.[49,50] More recently, single-stage laryngotracheal resection was performed successfully with what has been considered acceptable morbidity in specialized centers, with 3 patients (8.1%) developing major complications (2 fistulas and 1 early stenosis) that required a second surgical procedure. Long-term results were excellent to satisfactory in 36 patients (97.3%) and unsatisfactory in 1 (2.7%).[51] Proponents of open surgery as the treatment of choice believe that the unique tracheal vascular anatomy and the mechanism of injury underscore the transmural nature of airway lesions, which also explains the limited success of purely endoluminal therapies (e.g., laser treatments) in the management of tracheal strictures.[52]

- Permanent tracheostomy is warranted in the few patients with critical stenoses who neither are candidates for surgery or stent insertion nor develop recurrence after such interventions[9] and, of course, in regions where airway expertise may not be available. Referral to tertiary care centers in these instances can be beneficial for patients and caregivers.

Cost-Effectiveness

No formal cost-effectiveness evaluations of the various bronchoscopic and open surgical modalities have yet been published. For this type of PTS with chondritis, however, bronchoscopic interventions seem to have less-favorable evidence-based outcomes and therefore should be offered if definitive surgical resection is not feasible.

Informed Consent

The purposes of informed consent are to promote autonomy, to protect a patient from undesired treatment, and to help patients make appropriate medical care decisions that correlate with their personal values. Elderly patients are particularly vulnerable in the informed consent process. Not only are they more likely to suffer from medical conditions that can impair cognition by virtue of age or disease morbidity, they may also suffer from physical disabilities (such as hearing loss or aphasia) that impair communication even when cognition is intact.

Obtaining an informed consent supports the principle of autonomy by providing information in a context that allows voluntary choice to potential participants who are competent to decide, to affirm their understanding, and to agree to participate. Because of their cognitive impairment, persons with dementia (similar to our patient) not only are vulnerable but often are incapable (to varying degrees) of protecting their own interests during the informed consent process.[53] The National Bioethics Advisory Commission specifically identified Alzheimer's dementia as a disorder that can affect decision-making capacity. The American Geriatrics Society, however, took the position that "a diagnosis of dementia does not automatically confer decisional incapacity on affected individuals," and that because decision making is task specific, some persons with cognitive impairment will be able to provide a valid informed consent. Establishing capacity for decision making, therefore, was an important aspect of the consent process for our patient.

The capacity to consent is usually determined by assessing specific decision-making abilities; this involves asking patients narrative questions that provide information about their understanding, appreciation, reasoning, and ability to express a choice. One must also be able to understand the consequences of one's decision to undergo or refuse a therapeutic course of action. Expressing a choice is described as having the ability to communicate a desire to participate or not participate in a certain intervention and is considered a threshold ability: If the patient is unable to express a choice, assessment of other abilities is not necessary. Establishing decision-making capacity does not require specific subspecialty consultation. When a patient lacks decision-making capacity, of course, the clinician must document the finding, state the cause, and search for a reliable surrogate to make decisions considered to be in the best interests of the patient and/or according to what would have been the patient's desires had he or she been able to make the decision. If the patient has an advance directive that identifies a surrogate, this choice should be respected.[54] Fortunately, our patient had an advance directive that delegated her daughter as the health care decision maker. Advance directives are legally and ethically binding tools by which patients can express their own decisions regarding medical care before they actually lose the capacity to do so.

After she had been advised of all the therapeutic alternatives, the patient's daughter elected to proceed with rigid bronchoscopy under general anesthesia. She was informed of the potential risks for postoperative development of decompensated CHF, stroke, myocardial infarction, cardiac arrhythmias, and death. She was also told about potential upper airway edema and the subsequent potential need for emergent intubation or even tracheostomy.

Techniques and Results

Anesthesia and Perioperative Care

The anesthesiologist should be informed about the procedure plan, and the bronchoscopist should describe the patient's airway anatomy (severe upper tracheal stenosis) to the anesthesia team, so that team members can be ready to respond to any procedure-related complications. For example, if emergent endotracheal intubation is necessary, the tube can be guided bronchoscopically to avoid trauma at the stenosis level. Given the fact that our patient is edentulous, she could develop a difficult airway during and after induction, so the team should be ready to promptly perform a chin lift maneuver, insert an oral airway, and apply positive-pressure ventilation by mask. Upper airway muscle relaxation after induction can make rigid intubation more difficult because normal airway landmarks are obliterated by redundant or collapsing soft tissues.

With regard to her comorbidities, in general, patients with a history of CHF who are asymptomatic at the time of surgery should continue their current medical regimen. ACE inhibitors are considered safe during the perioperative period, despite concern for postoperative hypotension. It is noteworthy that hypotension was a frequently noted adverse event during rigid bronchoscopic procedures in one series of octogenarians.[55] Diuretics are safe as long as attention is paid to fluid status and electrolytes. Patients with CHF already receiving beta blockers should be continued on these medications perioperatively.[56] With regard to the need for invasive intraoperative monitoring, randomized controlled studies do not support the use of pulmonary artery catheters over standard care in the elderly, high-risk surgical patient.[57] If postoperative pulmonary edema develops, however, the patient should be evaluated for new myocardial ischemia. Physicians should also pay close attention to volume infusion perioperatively, examining records from both the operating room and the immediate postoperative period, because excessive fluid administration is a common cause of postoperative pulmonary edema.

Instrumentation

We chose a 13 mm Efer rigid nonventilating bronchoscope to allow deployment of a large tracheal stent. This bronchoscope is an open tube in which the telescope resides freely. This type of rigid bronchoscope has a uniform diameter from proximal to distal end and a beveled tip, which facilitates lifting of the epiglottis and gentle passage of the scope through the vocal cords, but also assists with dilation and removal of exophytic endoluminal lesions. This particular model of the Efer-Dumon bronchoscope does not have a stopper for the stent introducer. Newer models by Efer and by the Karl Storz Company (Tuttlingen, Germany) provide such instruments. Regardless, operators should be familiar with the length of the scope (in this case, 10 inches) and should be able to decide how far the stent introducer should be inserted inside the scope to avoid deployment of the stent too distally (beyond the stenosis) or too proximally (inside the rigid bronchoscope). Of course, several techniques of stent insertion may be used because one can expulse the stent beyond or within the stricture itself. Accessory instruments include grasping forceps and suction tubing that are readily available to assist with stent unfolding and positioning in the desired location. Vaseline petroleum gauze packing strip and a Kerlex gauze roll can be used to pack the nose and the mouth, respectively, in cases of significant air leak and subsequent impaired ventilation and oxygenation.

Anatomic Dangers and Other Risks

Major structures neighboring the larynx include the carotid arteries, jugular veins, superior and inferior thyroid veins and arteries, and superior and recurrent laryngeal nerves. Theoretically, these should not be injured during a bronchoscopic procedure with stent placement, especially when laser resection is not performed. Excessive tension on the larynx from a large rigid bronchoscope may cause laryngeal edema or arytenoid cartilage dislocation, resulting in postoperative stridor and respiratory distress. Care should be taken to avoid excessive pressure of the rigid tube on the larynx.

Results and Procedure-Related Complications

This patient was atraumatically intubated with the rigid bronchoscope, and the stricture was reassessed in terms of precise location, extent, and associated mucosal changes. The stricture indeed extended for 1.5 cm, starting at 4 cm below the vocal cords, with its distal aspect located 7 cm above the main carina. Following this evaluation, the 13 mm rigid bronchoscope was gently advanced, and the stricture was dilated. A 16 mm wide by 40 mm long straight studded silicone stent was inserted into the stricture. The stent had to be grasped using forceps, twisted, and pulled proximally so that the proximal aspect of the stent sat 1 cm above the stricture. This resulted in satisfactory positioning, with the stent's proximal aspect located 2.5 cm below the cords, specifically, 0.5 cm below the cricoids (see video on ExpertConsult.com) (Video II.9.1). Airway patency was restored and the stenotic index was estimated at less than 50%, which was later confirmed by morphometric bronchoscopic analysis.[18] The case lasted 20 minutes. The patient tolerated the procedure well, and extubation was uneventful. The patient was transferred to the postanesthesia care unit for 24 hours, during which no complications were noted. She was discharged to her nursing home 2 days later.

Long-Term Management

Outcome Assessment

Improving this patient's stenosis so that stenosis involves less than 50% of the airway lumen should enhance a patient's exercise capacity. Because of limited mobility caused by her neurologic deficits, we were unable to objectively document improvement using the MRC dyspnea scale validated for laryngotracheal stenosis,[58] but airway patency palliation resulted in resolution of stridor and respiratory distress.

Referral

In this case, multidisciplinary assessment involved thoracic and ear nose and throat surgeons, respiratory physicians, and radiologists. It was decided that given her comorbidities, a surgical intervention would not be feasible, and that if she failed stent insertion, Montgomery T-tube placement or tracheostomy would be recommended after the goals of care were discussed with the patient's daughter. Because provision of high-quality, yet fiscally responsible, care is necessary, a palliative care consultation was warranted in this patient. Because the literature shows that providing such a service can result in reduced daily costs and length of stay, a referral to palliative care medicine was requested.[59]

Follow-up Tests and Procedures

In our patient, elective outpatient flexible bronchoscopy was scheduled at 30 days after the procedure to reassess stent patency and consider the need for additional therapies in case of stent-related complications. Although definitive protocols have not been universally agreed upon or studied regarding the need for or frequency of follow-up bronchoscopy, some investigators routinely perform a follow-up bronchoscopy every 4 to 6 weeks during the first 6 months after intervention.[10] Others recommend bronchoscopy only in cases of new symptom development.[60] Information provided by spiral CT scans with multiplanar reconstruction and virtual bronchoscopy may allow them to be considered a substitute for direct bronchoscopic examination.[61]

With regard to potential future interventions in case the patient does not tolerate the stent, the literature shows that most patients with complex stenoses who are considered inoperable at the initial encounter remain inoperable at 6-month follow-up.[9] According to these data, it is unlikely that our patient would become a surgical candidate; however, a Montgomery T-tube and a tracheostomy could be feasible and safe alternatives to stent insertion in cases of stent failure.

Quality Improvement

A team meeting took place after the procedure. For this patient, quality of care was considered satisfactory because airway patency had been safely restored and the patient had been discharged back to her nursing home within 48 hours. We discussed whether the patient should have undergone CT or MRI after her tracheostomy tube had been decannulated, with the intention to detect earlier the development of stenosis. One study using CT scanning, for instance, in 48 patients followed for 30 months after PDT found that only 1 patient (2%) developed severe tracheal stenosis, and mild to moderate stenosis was detected in 14 patients (29.3%).[62] We also discussed whether the patient should be prescribed antireflux medications, because a history of gastroesophageal reflux is often present in patients with PTS.[10] We decided to prescribe proton pump inhibitors twice daily, in addition to saline nebulization, which is necessary for stent humidification.

DISCUSSION POINTS

1. Describe three qualitative features of tracheal stenosis.
   - From a qualitative standpoint, tracheal stenosis can be classified on the basis of the following:
     - *Histology:* benign or malignant
     - *Mechanism:* extrinsic, intraluminal, or mixed
     - *Dynamics:* fixed or dynamic[63,64]

- This patient had a benign intraluminal fixed stricture. We considered this lesion fixed because even though worsening of obstruction occurred during expiration, severe airway lumen narrowing was seen during inspiration as well (80%). Therefore, airflow was limited during both respiratory phases. This is contrary to dynamic obstruction, in which the lumen limits flow only during one respiratory phase (i.e., tracheobronchomalacia).

2. Describe three diagnostic modalities other than bronchoscopy that can be performed to assess the severity, extent, and morphology of this patient's tracheal stenosis.
   - *Conventional axial view* CT: may miss simple, focal lesions
   - *CT with three-dimensional reconstruction:* can evaluate airways distal to the stenosis in cases of very severe airway narrowing when the bronchoscope cannot and should not be advanced beyond the stricture; allows for noninvasive follow-up post stent insertion[65,66]
   - *MRI:* limited evidence but does avoid radiation exposure[8]

3. List four therapeutic alternatives for PTS with chondritis.
   - *Open surgical resection:* In experienced centers, it is the treatment of choice in patients who are operable.[49,50]
   - *Silicone stent insertion:* appropriate for palliating airway narrowing in nonsurgical candidates[9,10,44]
   - *Montgomery T-tubes:* can be used if surgery or insertion of airway silicone stents is not available or has failed[46,47]
   - *Tracheostomy:* used if the previously mentioned alternatives are not possible or have failed[9]

4. Identify three airway stricture characteristics that determine the need for and type of treatment.
   - *Extent of the lesion:* determines the length of the stent (usually selected to be 2 cm longer than the stricture, extending 1 cm above and 1 cm below the stricture itself)
   - *Severity of airway narrowing:* degree of airway narrowing influences flow dynamics and symptoms; more than 70% stenosis is usually required to cause symptoms at rest
   - *Functional status:* as assessed by MRC dyspnea scale may be more sensitive to the presence of varying degrees of tracheal stenosis than peak expiratory flow and forced expiratory volume in 1 second[20]

Expert Commentary

provided by Lutz Freitag, MD, FCCP

This is a case of a post tracheostomy stenosis localized in the upper third of the trachea. The patient was symptomatic, so treatment was required. Although in general, the gold standard for treating benign tracheal stenosis remains sleeve resection, this woman was certainly not a surgical candidate. The stenosis had a dominantly malacic component, ruling out any endoscopic resection techniques. It was decided to place a silicone stent via rigid bronchoscopy. For an experienced team, this can be considered a safe and effective procedure. In contrast to metallic stents, self-expanding polymeric stents provide relief with acceptable risks of long-term complications. Diagnostic and therapeutic approaches such as those described in the text are consistent and patient centered. Although I fully agree with the therapeutic decision, I would like to discuss several biomechanical issues that are pertinent to the disease process and to the therapeutic procedures described.

Most acquired benign stenoses result from a mucosal trauma such as tracheostomy or long-term intubation. After a symptom-free period of several weeks, patients usually notice increasing shortness of breath on exertion. Eventually, they present with stridor or impaired cough clearance. In the text, the authors discuss the three typical levels of tracheal narrowing. One aspect that I will elaborate on is stricture shape, also known as *morphology.* Tracheas are not round in the first place. The horseshoe type is most common but changes with age. Sakai has shown that aging results in increased tracheal area and in distortion of the roundness.[67] Traditionally, all commercially available tracheal cannulas and tubes, however, are round. This mismatch between the shape of the cannula and the shape of the trachea, especially when devices are slightly oversized, as discussed in the text, can lead to critically high localized pressures on the tracheal mucosa. In combination with impaired blood supply and hypoxia, this can easily result in permanent tissue damage. Modern low-pressure, high-volume cuffs have lowered the incidence of stenosis in the cuff region, but stomal stenoses remain a problem. In addition, as a result of irreversible damage to airway cartilage, the airway morphology may become tent shaped (also known as the **A**-type, or the triangular form, of benign tracheal stenosis). Now, we are forced to deal with an even worse mismatch between the actual shape of the stricture and the devices available in our therapeutic toolbox.

The following estimations are based on experimental results obtained from my laboratory.[68] To compress a typical silicone stent such as a 50 mm long, 16 mm diameter, studded silicone Dumon-type stent, or a Polyflex stent down to half its diameter, a force of roughly 5 Newtons is required (weight, 500 g). Pressure is force divided by contact area. The outer surface area ($2r \times \pi \times$ length) of this stent is approximately 25 cm^2. If the expansion force of this stent would be distributed equally over its complete outer surface, this would result in a contact pressure of 2 kPa. However, if the stent wall would touch only a fifth of the inner tracheal wall, as illustrated in Figure 9-5, local pressure at that contact zone would be 10 kPa. Because the normal tracheal blood vessel pressure is in the range of 4 to 5 kPa, such high-contact pressure would result in considerable impairment of mucosal blood flow, promoting further tissue damage.

Figure 9-5 Chest computed tomography (CT) axial image shows *(left)* the triangular morphology of the trachea, and *(right)* the discrepancy in morphology (shape) between the trachea and a round prosthesis.

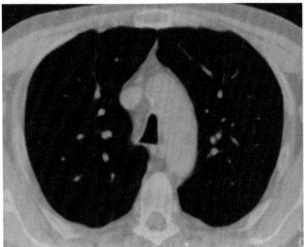 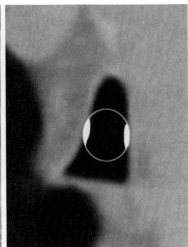

Figure 9-5 Chest computed tomography (CT) axial image shows *(left)* the triangular morphology of the trachea, and *(right)* the discrepancy in morphology (shape) between the trachea and a round prosthesis.

It is already problematic to deal with the normal horseshoe shape of a trachea; however, none of the existing polymeric devices has enough shape adaptability to cope with the variety of stricture morphologies that we find in pathologically altered airways. The situation gets even worse if a self-expanding wire mesh stent is used. Although such a stent may have the same overall expansion force as a silicone stent, it can completely shut down the mucosal blood flow at spots where the thin wires come in contact with the tissue. We should not be surprised that the formerly ciliated epithelium is replaced by less demanding fibroblasts and granulation tissue.

Indwelling stents are held in place by friction. If the wall pressure is insufficient, stents will migrate. After all, their hoop stress (expansion force) must be sufficiently high to counteract the force of the stricture to maintain airway patency. Attempts have been made by our group to measure the constricting force of stenoses in individual patients. The idea was to select a stent that has just the necessary recoil force to maintain airway patency. We experimented with strain gauges and compared results with stress-strain curves of airway stents. However, no company was prepared to develop such an instrument to the stage that it could be used reliably in patients. Even so, if the question of necessary hoop stress could have been answered, meaning that we would be able to select a stent that will keep the airway open, will not overstretch the tissues, and will not migrate, the shape problem would still remain. Unfortunately, as of this writing, no commercially available stent can really adapt to irregular shapes, such as the tent (A-type) shape that is most commonly seen in cases of chondritis. For the time being, therefore, we must admit that (necessary) treatment with a stent can be a cause of further damage, potentially requiring additional treatments with potentially more side effects. It cannot be overemphasized that for such benign central airway disease, surgery is the first option, and a stent should be used only when all other options have been exhausted or are unavailable.

Other options, such as Montgomery T-tubes and bifurcated stents, cannot migrate. They stabilize an airway without exerting high pressure on the tissues. However, they can irritate the mucosa in a different way. During the breathing cycle, the trachea changes its length by 15%, and neck movement (bending, turning) causes another 20% change in length. Coughing results in changes in cross-sectional area greater than 50% (dynamic compression). Because stents cannot adequately follow these movements, their sometimes sharp edges permanently scratch the mucosa. These movements of the trachea are poorly recognized by many practitioners. Older stents were even worse because they changed their length with compression. The once popular Wallstent had an extreme foreshortening. Owing to its zigzag design, it increased its length by several millimeters when it was squeezed to 50% of its nominal diameter with every cough. Microtrauma caused by the sharp wires promotes the development of granulation tissue, tissue shrinking, and the development of secondary web stenoses.

The ideal stent should stay in place, should not scratch the mucosa, should exert just enough force to keep the airway open, and should distribute its expansion force evenly over its contact surface with the tissue, irrespective of the altered geometric shape of the narrowed airway. It might take a while before such a magical device is on the market.

Another biomechanical aspect relates to the special location of the stenosis and the malacic component. The authors discuss the often noticed mismatch between the measurable degree of narrowing and patients' symptoms. We have developed a technique to superimpose signals of wall pressure, pressure drops, or flows in the airway over the endoscopic image in real time. This is accomplished by obtaining physiologic data with the use of slightly modified standard instruments such as a pneumotachograph, by feeding the output signal into a computer, and by mixing the curve with the video signal from the endoscope. Using this *endospirometry* technique, we can study dynamic changes

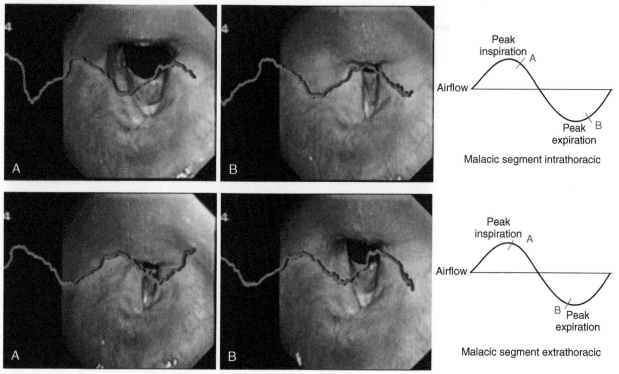

Figure 9-6   Endospirometry in a patient with a triangular stomal stricture located at the level of the thoracic inlet. Top panel: Malacic segment intrathoracic. Bottom panel: Malacic segment extrathoracic. **A,** Peak inspiration. **B,** Peak expiration.

that occur, for example, during quiet breathing and rapid forced breathing maneuvers. Especially interesting are patients with malacic segments at the level of the thoracic inlet, such as the patient described in this chapter. Figure 9-6 shows the different cross-sectional areas of such a malacic segment in one of my own patients. During bronchoscopy, this patient was breathing through a flow transducer (pneumotachograph with mouthpiece). Superimposed over the bronchoscopic image is the airflow curve. In the upper panel of Figure 9-6, it is clearly visible that the collapse occurs during expiration, but the trachea is almost normal during inspiration. The images in the lower panel of the figure were taken from the same patient. The conditions are just the opposite—open during expiration, collapsed during inspiration. All I did was ask the patient to extend his neck. Stretching and extending his neck let the choke point migrate proximally, above the thoracic inlet, where the pressure vectors are reversed. In a certain position, this patient was almost asymptomatic, but he became stridorous when flexing his head.

In this commentary, I discussed the impact of airway morphology on stent-tissue interactions and described how endospirometry can provide new insights into airway flow dynamics in patients with central airway obstruction. Interventional bronchoscopy, in my opinion, involves more than acquiring technical skills. As procedures evolve and interventional bronchoscopists find themselves treating patients with increasingly complex airway disorders, understanding airflow pathophysiology and biomechanics becomes essential for selecting optimal treatment strategies.

REFERENCES

1. Wain JC Jr. Postintubation tracheal stenosis. *Semin Thorac Cardiovasc Surg.* 2009;21:284-289.
2. Remy-Jardin M, Remy J, Artaud D, et al. Volume rendering of the tracheobronchial tree: clinical evaluation of bronchographic images. *Radiology.* 1998;208:761-770.
3. Shitrit D, Valdsislav P, Grubstein A, et al. Accuracy of virtual bronchoscopy for grading tracheobronchial stenosis: correlation with pulmonary function test and fiberoptic bronchoscopy. *Chest.* 2005;128:3545-3550.
4. Boiselle PM, Feller-Kopman D, Ashiku S, et al. Tracheobronchomalacia: evolving role of dynamic multislice helical CT. *Radiol Clin North Am.* 2003;41:627-636.
5. Hofmann U, Hofmann D, Vogl T, et al. Magnetic resonance imaging as a new diagnostic criterion in paediatric airway obstruction. *Prog Pediatr Surg.* 1991;27:221-230.
6. Vogl TJ, Diebold T, Bergman C, et al. MRI in pre- and postoperative assessment of tracheal stenosis due to pulmonary artery sling. *J Comput Assist Tomogr.* 1993;17:878-886.
7. Lebovics RS, Hoffman GS, Leavitt RY, et al. The management of subglottic stenosis in patients with Wegener's granulomatosis. *Laryngoscope.* 1992;102:1341-1345.
8. Carney AS. The use of magnetic resonance imaging to assess tracheal stenosis following percutaneous dilatational tracheostomy. *J Laryngol Otol.* 1998;112:599.
9. Brichet A, Verkindre C, Dupont J, et al. Multidisciplinary approach to management of postintubation tracheal stenoses. *Eur Respir J.* 1999;13:888-893.
10. Zias N, Chroneou A, Tabba MK, et al. Post tracheostomy and post intubation tracheal stenosis: report of 31 cases and review of the literature. *BMC Pulm Med.* 2008;8:18.
11. De Leyn P, Bedert L, Delcroix M, et al. Belgian Association of Pneumology and Belgian Association of Cardiothoracic Surgery. Tracheotomy: clinical review and guidelines. *Eur J Cardiothorac Surg.* 2007;32:412-421.
12. Raghuraman G, Rajan S, Marzouk JK, et al. Is tracheal stenosis caused by percutaneous tracheostomy different from that by surgical tracheostomy? *Chest.* 2005;127:879-885.

13. Koitschev A, Simon C, Blumenstock G, et al. Suprastomal tracheal stenosis after dilational and surgical tracheostomy in critically ill patients. *Anaesthesia.* 2006;61:832-837.

14. Heffner JE, Miller KS, Sahn SA. Tracheostomy in the intensive care unit. Part 2. Complications. *Chest.* 1986;90:430-436.

15. Sarper A, Ayten A, Eser I, et al. Tracheal stenosis after tracheostomy or intubation: review with special regard to cause and management. *Tex Heart Inst J.* 2005;32:154-158.

16. Pearson FG, Andrews MJ. Detection and management of tracheal stenosis following cuffed tube tracheostomy. *Ann Thorac Surg.* 1971;12:359-374.

17. Hollingsworth HM. Wheezing and stridor. *Clin Chest Med.* 1987;8:231-240.

18. Murgu S, Colt HG. Morphometric bronchoscopy in adults with central airway obstruction: case illustrations and review of the literature. *Laryngoscope.* 2009;119:1318-1324.

19. Myer CM, O'Connor DM, Cotton RT. Proposed grading system for subglottic stenosis based on endotracheal tube sizes. *Ann Otol Rhinol Laryngol.* 1994;103:319-323.

20. Nouraei SA, Nouraei SM, Randhawa PS, et al. Sensitivity and responsiveness of the Medical Research Council dyspnoea scale to the presence and treatment of adult laryngotracheal stenosis. *Clin Otolaryngol.* 2008;33:575-580.

21. Mittnacht AJ, Fanshawe M, Konstadt S. Anesthetic considerations in the patient with valvular heart disease undergoing noncardiac surgery. *Semin Cardiothorac Vasc Anesth.* 2008;12:33-59.

22. Detsky AS, Abrams HB, Forbath N, et al. Cardiac assessment for patients undergoing noncardiac surgery: a multifactorial clinical risk index. *Arch Intern Med.* 1986;146:2131-2134.

23. Lee TH, Marcantonio ER, Mangione CM, et al. Derivation and prospective validation of a simple index for prediction of cardiac risk of major noncardiac surgery. *Circulation.* 1999;100:1043-1049.

24. Berry L. Pledges on dementia care. *Nurs Older People.* 2010;22:3.

25. Wright CD, Grillo HC, Wain JC, et al. Anastomotic complications after tracheal resection: prognostic factors and management. *J Thorac Cardiovasc Surg.* 2004;128:731-739.

26. Simpson GT, Strong MS, Healy GB, et al. Predictive factors of success or failure in the endoscopic management of laryngeal and tracheal stenosis. *Ann Otol Rhinol Laryngol.* 1982;91:384-388.

27. Brouns M, Jayaraju ST, Lacor C, et al. Tracheal stenosis: a flow dynamics study. *J Appl Physiol.* 2007;102:1178-1184.

28. Brouns M, Verbanck S, Lacor C. Influence of glottic aperture on the tracheal flow. *J Biomech.* 2007;40:165-172.

29. Detsky AS, Abrams HB, Forbath N, et al. Cardiac assessment for patients undergoing noncardiac surgery: a multifactorial clinical risk index. *Arch Intern Med.* 1986;146:2131-2134.

30. Fleisher LA, Beckman JA, Brown KA, et al. 2009 ACCF/AHA focused update on perioperative beta blockade incorporated into the ACC/AHA 2007 guidelines on perioperative cardiovascular evaluation and care for noncardiac surgery: a report of the American College of Cardiology Foundation/American Heart Association Task Force on Practice Guidelines. *Circulation.* 2009;120:e169-e276.

31. Hart R, Hindman B. Mechanisms of perioperative cerebral infarction. *Stroke.* 1982;13:766-773.

32. Cavaliere S, Bezzi M, Toninelli C, et al. Management of postintubation tracheal stenoses using the endoscopic approach. *Monaldi Arch Chest Dis.* 2007;67:73-80.

33. Bisson A, Bonnette P, Ben EL, et al. Tracheal sleeve resection for iatrogenic stenoses (subglottic laryngeal and tracheal). *J Thorac Cardiovasc Surg.* 1992;104:882-887.

34. Rahman NA, Fruchter O, Shitrit D, et al. Flexible bronchoscopic management of benign tracheal stenosis: long term follow-up of 115 patients. *J Cardiothorac Surg.* 2010;5:2.

35. Mehta AC, Lee FY, Cordasco EM, et al. Concentric tracheal and subglottic stenosis: management using the Nd-YAG laser for mucosal sparing followed by gentle dilatation. *Chest.* 1993;104:673-677.

36. Nouraei SA, Kapoor KV, Nouraei SM, et al. Results of endoscopic tracheoplasty for treating tracheostomy-related airway stenosis. *Clin Otolaryngol.* 2007;32:471-475.

37. Dasgupta A, Dolmatch BL, Abi-Saleh WJ, et al. Self-expandable metallic airway stent insertion employing flexible bronchoscopy: preliminary results. *Chest.* 1998;114:106-109.

38. Saad CP, Murthy S, Krizmanich G, et al. Self-expandable metallic airway stents and flexible bronchoscopy: long-term outcomes analysis. *Chest.* 2003;124:1993-1999.

39. U.S. Food and Drug Administration. Metallic tracheal stents in patients with benign airway disorders. http://www.fda.gov/Safety/MedWatch/SafetyInformation/SafetyAlertsforHumanMedicalProducts/ucm153009.htm. Accessed July 20, 2011.

40. Gaissert HA, Grillo HC, Wright CD, et al. Complication of benign tracheobronchial strictures by self-expanding metal stents. *J Thorac Cardiovasc Surg.* 2003;126:744-747.

41. Gaissert HA, Grillo HC, Mathisen DJ, et al: Temporary and permanent restoration of airway continuity with the tracheal T-tube. *J Thorac Cardiovasc Surg.* 1994;107:600-606.

42. Gildea TR, Murthy SC, Sahoo D, et al. Performance of a self-expanding silicone stent in palliation of benign airway conditions. *Chest.* 2006;130:1419-1423.

43. Jog M, Anderson DE, McGarry GW. Polyflex stent: is it radiopaque enough? *J Laryngol Otol.* 2003;117:83-84.

44. Patelli M, Gasparini S. Post-intubation tracheal stenoses: what is the curative yield of the interventional pulmonology procedures? *Monaldi Arch Chest Dis.* 2007;67:71-72.

45. Galluccio G, Lucantoni G, Battistoni P, et al. Interventional endoscopy in the management of benign tracheal stenoses: definitive treatment at long-term follow-up. *Eur J Cardiothorac Surg.* 2009;35:429-433; discussion 933-934.

46. Martinez-Ballarin JI, Diaz-Jimenez JP, Castro MJ, et al. Silicone stents in the management of benign tracheobronchial stenoses: tolerance and early results in 63 patients. *Chest.* 1996;109:626-629.

47. Liu HC, Lee KS, Huang CJ, et al. Silicone T-tube for complex laryngotracheal problems. *Eur J Cardiothorac Surg.* 2002;21:326-330.

48. Liu HC, Lee KS, Huang CJ, et al. Silicone T-tube for complex laryngotracheal problems. *Eur J Cardiothorac Surg.* 2002;21:326-330.

49. Rea F, Callegaro D, Loy M, et al. Benign tracheal and laryngotracheal stenosis: surgical treatment and results. *Eur J Cardiothorac Surg.* 2002;22:352-356.

50. Grillo HC, Donahue DM, Mathisen DJ, et al. Postintubation tracheal stenosis: treatment and results. *J Thorac Cardiovasc Surg.* 1995;109:486-492; discussion 492-493.

51. Marulli G, Rizzardi G, Bortolotti L, et al. Single-staged laryngotracheal resection and reconstruction for benign strictures in adults. *Interact Cardiovasc Thorac Surg.* 2008;7:227-230.

52. Grillo HC. Stents and sense. *Ann Thorac Surg.* 2000;70:1139.

53. Mayo AM, Wallhagen MI. Considerations of informed consent and decision-making competence in older adults with cognitive impairment. *Res Gerontol Nurs.* 2009;2:103-111.

54. American College of Physicians. Ethics Manual. 4th ed. *Ann Intern Med.* 1998;128:576-594.

55. Davoudi M, Shakkottai S, Colt HG. Safety of therapeutic rigid bronchoscopy in people aged 80 and older: a retrospective cohort analysis. *J Am Geriatr Soc.* 2008;56:943-944.

56. Fleisher LA, Beckman JA, Brown KA, et al. 2009 ACCF/AHA focused update on perioperative beta blockade incorporated into the ACC/AHA 2007 guidelines on perioperative cardiovascular evaluation and care for noncardiac surgery: a report of the American College of Cardiology Foundation/American Heart Association Task Force on Practice Guidelines. *Circulation.* 2009;120:e169-e276.

57. Sandham JD, Hull RD, Brant RF, et al. Canadian Critical Care Clinical Trials Group. A randomized, controlled trial of the use of pulmonary-artery catheters in high-risk surgical patients. *N Engl J Med.* 2003;348:5-14.

58. Nouraei SA, Nouraei SM, Randhawa PS, et al. Sensitivity and responsiveness of the Medical Research Council dyspnoea scale to the presence and treatment of adult laryngotracheal stenosis. *Clin Otolaryngol.* 2008;33:575-580.

59. Ciemins EL, Blum L, Nunley M, et al. The economic and clinical impact of an inpatient palliative care consultation service: a multifaceted approach. *J Palliat Med.* 2007;10:1347-1355.

60. Matsuo T, Colt HG. Evidence against routine scheduling of surveillance bronchoscopy after stent insertion. *Chest.* 2000;118:1455-1459.

61. Bauer TL, Steiner KV. Virtual bronchoscopy: clinical applications and limitations. *Surg Oncol Clin N Am.* 2007;16:323-328.

62. Norwood S, Vallina VL, Short K, et al. Incidence of tracheal stenosis and other late complications after percutaneous tracheostomy. *Ann Surg.* 2000;232:233-241.

63. Murgu SD, Colt HG. Interventional bronchoscopy from bench to bedside: new techniques for central and peripheral airway obstruction. *Clin Chest Med.* 2010;31:101-115.

64. Freitag L, Ernst A, Unger M, et al. A proposed classification system of central airway stenosis. *Eur Respir J.* 2007;30:7-12.

65. Dialani V, Ernst A, Sun M, et al. MDCT detection of airway stent complications: comparison with bronchoscopy. *AJR Am J Roentgenol.* 2008;191:1576-1580.

66. Boiselle PM, Ernst A. Recent advances in central airway imaging. *Chest.* 2002;121:1651-1660.

67. Sakai H, Nakano Y, Muro S, et al. Age-related changes in the trachea in healthy adults. *Adv Exp Med Biol.* 2010;662: 115-120.

68. Freitag L. Airway stents. In: Strausz J, Bolliger CT, eds. *Interventional Pulomonology.* Sheffield, UK: European Respiratory Society; 2010:190-217.

Chapter 10

Bronchoscopic Treatment of Wegener's Granulomatosis–Related Subglottic Stenosis

This chapter emphasizes the following elements of the Four Box Approach: physical examination, complementary tests, and functional status assessment; patient's support system (also includes family), anesthesia and other perioperative care; and follow-up tests, visits, and procedures.

CASE DESCRIPTION

A 49-year-old woman with a 20 year history of Wegener's granulomatosis (WG) now presents with cough and limited exercise capacity. Disease had been limited to her sinuses and had been treated in years past with prednisone and cyclophosphamide (CYC). CYC was switched to methotrexate owing to hematuria. Her last relapse occurred 18 months earlier. She was active and routinely swam 10 laps in her pool until 2 months ago, when she developed a dry cough and shortness of breath. Her primary care physician ordered a two-dimensional echocardiogram, which was normal. Physical examination was unremarkable except for her cushingoid face. Chest radiograph, complete blood count, urine analysis, and liver function test results were normal. Diagnostic flexible bronchoscopy revealed a circumferential subglottic stenosis (SGS) extending 0.5 cm and starting 1.5 cm below the vocal cords. The cross-sectional area at the level of the stricture was reduced by 53% when compared with the normal tracheal lumen distal to the stricture, as measured by morphometric analysis of the bronchoscopic images (Figure 10-1).

DISCUSSION POINTS

1. Describe five central airway abnormalities seen in Wegener's granulomatosis.
2. Discuss the role of antineutrophil cytoplasmic antibody (ANCA) in monitoring this patient's disease activity.
3. Describe two adjuvant treatments to laser-assisted dilation of WG-related stenosis.
4. Discuss the prognosis of patients with WG and subglottic stenosis.

CASE RESOLUTION

Initial Evaluations

Physical Examination, Complementary Tests, and Functional Status Assessment

In our patient, the diagnosis of subglottic stenosis occurred in the absence of other features of active disease.

Tracheobronchial manifestations of WG may take place after remission has been achieved with appropriate immunosuppressive therapy, and airway disease may proceed to airway scarring and stenosis.[1] In the absence of persistent active inflammation, however, the development of SGS does not necessarily indicate failure of immunosuppressive therapy. As in our patient, published and anecdotal evidence suggests that when airway obstruction is caused by fibrotic scarring rather than by active inflammation, strictures develop independently of other features of WG and are unresponsive to systemic immunosuppressive therapy.[2] SGS, seen in approximately 8.5% to 23% of patients, is considered the most common central airway manifestation of WG. It may be the initial presenting feature in 1% to 6% of patients.[3] Isolated SGS is observed in approximately 50% of patients with strictures; in the other half, strictures occur while patients are receiving systemic immunosuppressive therapy for disease activity involving other sites.[4]

This patient had no stridor on neck auscultation. This finding is consistent with the bronchoscopic classification of moderate airway narrowing based on a stenotic index of 53%. Indeed, stridor is usually a sign of severe laryngeal or tracheal obstruction, signaling more than 70% airway lumen narrowing.[5-7] Anatomically fixed obstruction of moderate degree such as that seen in our patient usually causes symptoms with exertion but not at rest.

The absence of ANCA in our patient was not unexpected. In fact, the presence or absence of ANCA neither confirms nor excludes a diagnosis of systemic vasculitis, and both negative and positive predictive values will be strongly influenced by clinical presentation. Most patients with generalized WG have glomerulonephritis and are ANCA positive (90%), whereas those without renal involvement have a lower incidence of ANCA (70%). Among patients with limited forms of the disease, such as those without significant renal involvement and in whom upper respiratory tract symptoms predominate, only 60% are ANCA positive.[8]

Comorbidities

Lack of cardiac involvement by two-dimensional echocardiography (2D echo) was reassuring because WG disease relapse is often associated with heart involvement, less intensive initial treatment in terms of lower CYC doses, and shorter length of time on prednisone >20 mg/day.[9] No evidence of renal or hepatic dysfunction was found; if surgical or bronchoscopic interventions were to be provided under general anesthesia, such dysfunction

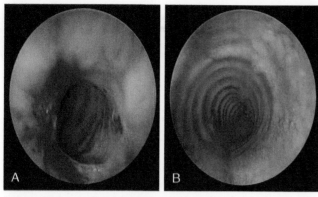

Figure 10-1 **A,** Circumferential subglottic stenosis with the most prominent hypertrophic tissue on the left lateral wall. **B,** Normal trachea distal to the stenosis. The stenotic index was 53%, as calculated by morphometric bronchoscopy analysis.

could adversely affect perioperative fluid management, increase risks for bleeding, and cause postoperative changes in neurologic status.

Support System

Our patient was married and had a good social support system. As with other chronic conditions, considerable evidence suggests that vasculitis negatively affects patients' health-related quality of life (HRQL),[10] which usually includes general health, physical functioning, emotional role limitations, physical role limitations, social functioning, mental health, and energy/vitality. Contrary to cancer, which is often considered a "family affair" with significant psychological and emotional impact on family members,[11] results of recent studies show that spouses of patients with ANCA-associated vasculitis (AAV), including WG, scored similarly to national norms. Patients with AAV, however, scored lower than normal on all HRQL subscales with the exception of bodily pain. When age, education, race, illness duration, and disease severity were controlled, no significant sex differences in HRQL were noted for patients or spouses.[12]

Patient Preferences and Expectations

This patient had a very active lifestyle and had clearly expressed a desire for treatment. She was prepared to consider all available therapeutic options, including dilation, laser, surgery, and even airway stent insertion if necessary. She agreed to our request that alternatives be discussed with her husband, so they could participate together in medical decision making. Health care provider investment in patient-centered conversations with family members is usually justified because management of chronic illness is a dyadic process that often involves spouses.[13]

Procedural Strategies

Indications

Symptomatic WG-related subglottic stenosis is often part of the spectrum of a multisystem inflammatory process that warrants administration of immunosuppressive agents. Some patients, however, develop or continue to

have symptoms of airway obstruction after clinical remission induced by standard therapeutic regimens. Although airway manipulation during periods of active WG should be minimized, other treatment modalities may be warranted[14] after disease has first been controlled in collaboration with a rheumatologist. A bronchoscopic procedure or open laryngotracheoplasty may be offered to improve dyspnea and restore satisfactory airway lumen patency by mechanical dilation with or without laser.

In patients with tracheal obstruction, dyspnea depends on the degree of airway narrowing, as well as on flow velocity. Airway pressures increase dramatically at rest when well over 70% of the tracheal lumen is obliterated. Our patient's active lifestyle caused high flow velocity through her stenotic airway. This further increased the pressure drop through the stricture, increasing the work of breathing.[15] Improving airway patency to a lesser (mild) degree of narrowing (<50%) would allow our patient to improve exercise capacity and shortness of breath. In one physiology study, the effect of the normal glottis on airway pressure drop is, in fact, of the same order as that of 50% airway narrowing.[16] Thus when airway narrowing is treated, symptoms and exercise tolerance may be dramatically improved by small changes in airway caliber, and perfect normalization of airway lumen patency may not be necessary.

Contraindications

No contraindications to rigid bronchoscopy were known in this patient. However, although this patient had normal dentition without loose teeth, a crown recently placed on the right upper first premolar could potentially be damaged during rigid intubation. The cervical spine range of motion was normal, but her mouth opening measured only two fingerbreadths. This could also increase the risk for tooth damage during rigid bronchoscopy. A plastic tooth guard, rather than a gauze pad, used to protect the teeth would further diminish mouth opening.

Expected Results

Rigid intubation was planned using a small (9.5 mm)-diameter rigid bronchoscope. The scope would be introduced through the vocal cords under direct visualization so as to ensure a secure airway at all times. Careful attention would be necessary to avoid trauma to the teeth given her limited mouth opening and her recently placed dental crown.

In patients with subglottic strictures, the therapeutic success of rigid bronchoscopic dilation is variable. In one study (follow-up after the first dilation of 25.4 ± 14.1 months), two of nine patients never recurred after the initial dilation, and seven required more than one dilation, with one patient requiring permanent tracheostomy.[17] In another study, three patients required repeated treatment using neodymium-doped yttrium aluminum garnet (Nd:YAG) or carbon dioxide (CO_2) laser–guided resection to control airway narrowing.[14]

Team Experience

Experience and expediency might result in reduced complications, a greater chance to restore airway patency, and earlier discharge from the hospital, although studies are needed to support this hypothesis. Prospective and ongoing data analysis for bronchoscopic procedures, both feasible and ongoing, might answer these questions in the future.[18]

Risk-Benefit Analysis

The risk of further airway injury, resulting in scarring and consequent recurrence of stenosis, is outweighed by the benefit of improving airway patency to improve this patient's exercise capacity and quality of life. Recurrence, however, may be related to the disease process or to the bronchoscopic treatment itself.

Therapeutic Alternatives for Restoring Airway Patency

Therapeutic alternatives include systemic, bronchoscopic, and open surgical therapies. If disease severity is judged to be life threatening or to be putting an affected organ at risk for irreversible damage, such as airway or renal disease, glucocorticoids in combination with CYC remain the treatment of choice. In less severe cases, methotrexate is the preferred alternative to CYC. Regardless of the severity of other organ manifestations, severe tracheobronchial disease should initially be treated with a combination of oral glucocorticoids and CYC. For patients with documented tracheobronchial disease, some experts use high-dose inhaled glucocorticoids, such as fluticasone 440 to 880 mg twice daily, which is usually initiated when oral glucocorticoids have been tapered to daily doses less than 30 mg.[19] Because our patient had failed two immunosuppressive drugs (glucocorticoids and methotrexate) and was intolerant to CYC, one might consider her as having refractory disease. A monoclonal anti-CD20 antibody, rituximab, was shown to be successful in inducing remission in patients with refractory but limited WG manifestations, including chronic sinusitis, pulmonary nodules, orbital pseudotumor, and subglottic stenosis.[20] Others, however, report systemic therapy–induced cures at all disease locations except the subglottis.[21]

Because isolated airway lesions secondary to scarring may improve only after interventional procedures, the decision to use concomitant immunosuppressive medications depends on clinical and laboratory features that may suggest active disease.[3] Overall, only 20% to 26% of subglottic strictures caused by Wegener's granulomatosis respond to glucocorticoids alone or in combination with another immunosuppressant. The remaining 74% to 80% of patients usually require interventional therapies to improve symptoms. In our patient, without clinical or laboratory evidence of other organ involvement, the isolated SGS was considered a manifestation of the scarring process, and she was offered an interventional procedure.

- Balloon or bougie dilation (e.g., Maloney bougies, Fogarty catheter balloon) can be used to increase the airway lumen to facilitate the atraumatic passage of a rigid bronchoscope, or as a sole treatment modality. Balloon dilation can be performed by using flexible bronchoscopy with a balloon catheter threaded over a guidewire and positioned across the stenosis, or by inserting the balloon catheter through the working channel of the bronchoscope. Under direct visualization, the balloon is inflated for 30 to 120 seconds. Repeat inflation-deflation cycles are done if airway narrowing persists after the initial attempt.[22]

- Adjuvant therapies such as intralesional corticosteroid injection have been reported to reduce the rate of recurrence after bronchoscopic dilation of WG-related SGS. Methylprednisolone acetate is injected directly into the stenotic segment, followed by lysis of the stenotic tissue and serial dilation.[4,23,24] In a series with 21 patients (no control group) followed for a mean of 40.6 months, patients who did not have scarring from previous procedures required a mean of 2.4 procedures at mean intervals of 11.6 months to maintain subglottic patency. Patients with established laryngotracheal scarring required a mean of 4.1 procedures at mean intervals of 6.8 months to maintain patency. None of the 21 patients required a new tracheostomy.[24] Older studies with a larger number of patients (n = 43) also showed that this approach provides safe and effective treatment for WG-associated subglottic strictures, and that in the absence of major organ disease activity, it can be performed without concomitant administration of systemic immunosuppressive agents.[4] Topical application of mitomycin C, an alkylating agent that inhibits fibroblast proliferation and extracellular matrix protein synthesis, can be performed after intralesional corticosteroid injection, dilation, or laser resection with the intent of reducing fibrosis and restenoses. Some authors, however, recommend its use only in patients with active inflammatory lesions.[17] A randomized, placebo-controlled trial of patients with laryngotracheal stenosis, including 2 patients with WG, compared restenosis rates with two applications of mitomycin C (0.5 mg/mL for 5 minutes on a 1 × 1 inch cottonoid) given 3 to 4 weeks apart versus one application immediately after surgery.[25] Although relapses occurred at a slower rate in the two-application group during the first 3 years, recurrence of laryngotracheal stenosis 5 years after surgery was similarly high (70%) in both groups.

- Laser resection using CO_2 or Nd:YAG lasers in Wegener's granulomatosis patients has shown conflicting results.[2,14,26,27] Two studies showed good outcomes in 5 patients after repeated sessions with both lasers[14] and in 12 patients with a combination of CO_2 laser and dilation.[27] In another study, 8 patients developed rapid restenosis after treatment with a CO_2 laser.[26] Favorable results have been described for avoiding laser intervention when disease is active, prompting investigators to recommend minimizing airway manipulation during periods of systemic disease activity.[27]

- Silicone and covered metal stent insertion have been used successfully in WG-related subglottic strictures when the glottis is not involved (diseased segment starting at least 1 cm below the vocal cords).[28] Covered metal stents are associated with significant complications, especially when in the subglottic region,[29] however, and probably should be avoided for histologically proven benign airway disorders.[30] Silicone stents seem to provide long-lasting symptomatic relief[31] but should be considered only when more conservative treatment modalities fail to restore or maintain airway patency. Stents of any type are a last resort in WG-related subglottic stenosis; some experts consider subglottic stent insertion, without first-line medical and conservative therapy, to be a simple but wrong solution for a complex problem.[29]

- Open surgical resection such as laryngotracheoplasty or other reconstructive techniques are alternatives for patients who fail bronchoscopic intervention. In one study, 3 of 5 patients underwent primary thyrotracheal anastomosis while disease was in clinical remission, without postoperative compromise of anastomotic integrity or wound healing despite concurrent use of prednisone and CYC.[32] Extensive surgical resection is not recommended in patients with active disease because reactivation in the remaining subglottis may cause dehiscence of anastomotic sites and recurrent stenosis.[33] Following surgical resection, patients may require dilations or stent placement.[34] Results from an older, larger study of thoracic surgery in patients with WG showed that among 47 patients followed over 16 years, only 3 had subglottic strictures. Each was treated by dilation, not by surgical resection.[35]
- Tracheostomy is warranted in patients with critical airway stenosis unresponsive to medical and dilational therapies. This procedure can be lifesaving and can provide long-term relief. In one series of 27 patients with WG and subglottic strictures, 11 (41%) underwent tracheotomy. Eventual decannulation was possible in a variable percentage of patients.[27]

Cost-Effectiveness

No formal cost-effectiveness evaluations of these various modalities have yet been published. Bronchoscopic interventions seem to have favorable evidence-based outcomes and therefore should be offered before surgical resection or definitive tracheostomy.

Informed Consent

After they had been advised of all of the alternatives, the patient and her husband elected to proceed with rigid bronchoscopy under general anesthesia. They were informed of our potential failure to restore airway patency and were told about the risks for tooth injury, bleeding, airway perforation, upper airway edema, and temporary and prolonged mechanical ventilation; the potential need for tracheostomy; and the potential risk of procedure-related recurrence. They were informed of our more than 25 years' combined experience in treating patients with this disorder, and of our inclination to minimize airway manipulations. Feedback communication techniques were used, the patient showed good understanding of her disease, and both she and her spouse were able to accurately describe the proposed procedure, alternatives, and

potential complications. Studies demonstrate a correlation between effective physician–patient communication and improved patient health outcomes.[36] Respect for patient autonomy and shared decision making, the process by which a health care choice is made jointly by the practitioner and the patient, are considered to be core values of patient-centered care.[37]

Techniques and Results

Anesthesia and Perioperative Care

Discussion with the anesthesiologist should take place before induction. The anesthesiologist should understand the procedure plan, and the bronchoscopist should describe the patient's airway anatomy to the anesthesia team so that they can be ready to respond to any procedure-related complications. For example, laryngospasm may occur during laryngotracheal analgesia with lidocaine. Although self-limited by prolonged hypoxia or hypercarbia, laryngospasm can result in negative-pressure pulmonary edema and even cardiac arrest.[38] The team should be ready to promptly perform a chin lift maneuver, apply positive-pressure ventilation by mask (continuous positive airway pressure [CPAP] at approximately 10 cm H_2O) with 100% oxygen, and, if refractory, administer succinylcholine (0.1 mg/kg).[39] Upper airway muscle relaxation, however, can make rigid intubation more difficult because normal airway landmarks are obliterated by redundant or collapsing soft tissues.

When laser is used, fire safety precautions are implemented. The fraction of inspired oxygen (FiO_2) should be reduced to less than 0.4 before laser activation. During rigid scope removal, risk for laryngospasm is again present, so the tube should be removed atraumatically and not while the patient is coughing.[39] After removal of the rigid bronchoscope, transient but potentially fatal laryngeal or subglottic edema can occur. Laryngoscopically guided endotracheal reintubation can be difficult; therefore a fiberoptic bronchoscope should be readily available. Results from clinical trials suggest that prophylactic corticosteroid therapy (methylprednisolone 20 to 40 mg every 4 to 6 hours, 12 to 24 hours before the planned extubation) reduces the incidence of laryngeal edema and the subsequent need for reintubation in patients requiring mechanical ventilation for longer than 6 days,[40] but no clear evidence indicates that perioperative administration of corticosteroids prevents laryngeal edema in patients undergoing rigid bronchoscopy. In animals with induced laryngeal injury, dexamethasone before extubation resulted in reduced submucosal edema.[41] Anecdotally, laryngeal edema after rigid bronchoscopic treatment of subglottic stenosis is rare. Only 1 of 56 patients developed this complication after rigid bronchoscopy for malignant airway obstruction.[42] Extrapolating from this information, we administer dexamethasone 8 to 10 mg intravenously after bronchoscopic interventions lasting longer than 1 hour. Furthermore, given that procedure-related laryngeal and subglottic edema can occur within 2 to 24 hours after extubation, patients are carefully monitored during this period.

Instrumentation

We chose a 9.5 mm Efer rigid nonventilating broncho-scope and a potassium-titanyl-phosphate (KTP) laser in a near contact mode for performing radial incisions into the fibrotic tissue constituting the stenosis. High power density (contact or near contact mode) minimizes col-lateral injury to normal mucosa and cartilage. In canine experiments, surrounding tissue damage was least when contact Nd:YAG laser was used as compared with CO_2 and noncontact Nd:YAG lasers, and laser-induced injury was the fastest healing, with only minimal damage to cartilage and soft tissue.[43] We chose the KTP laser because its delivery fiber can be inserted through the rigid bron-choscope; it has stronger tissue absorption than Nd:YAG but less than CO_2, resulting in more shallow tissue pen-etration (≈ 2 mm) than Nd:YAG but deeper than CO_2; and its visible green light allows accurate beam placement for incisions, minimizing collateral injury.[44]

Anatomic Dangers and Other Risks

Major structures neighboring the larynx include the carotid arteries, jugular veins, superior and inferior thyroid veins and arteries, and superior and recurrent laryngeal nerves. Resection of high tracheal/subglottic lesions may injure the thyroid veins that drain into the left brachiocephalic vein above the sternal notch. Exces-sive tension on the larynx from a large rigid broncho-scope may cause laryngeal edema or arytenoid cartilage dislocation.

Results and Procedure-Related Complications

Subglottic stenotic lesions in WG are typically circum-ferential with friable mucosa. Histologic section typically shows a nonspecific pattern of inflammation as opposed to biopsies from other sites. Biopsy yield is low, with only 5% sensitivity.[4] Our patient was atraumatically intubated, and the stricture was assessed in terms of precise location, extent, and associated mucosal changes (see video on ExpertConsult.com) (Video II.10.1). KTP laser at 6 W power, 1 second pulses, for a total energy of 105 Joules and a total duration of 17 seconds allowed radial incisions at the 11 o'clock (left antero-lateral) and 7 o'clock (left posterolateral) positions. The yellowish discoloration frequently seen in active Wegener's granulomatosis stricture was absent. High absorption of laser energy by the dark charred tissue accumulating on the tip of the bare laser fiber creates a fire hazard, and the tissue should be removed (see video on ExpertConsult.com) (Video II.10.2). Follow-ing this, the 9.5 mm rigid bronchoscope was gently advanced and the stricture was dilated. After approxi-mately 2 minutes, the scope was removed, and the patient was promptly reintubated with a 10.5 mm Efer rigid bronchoscope. Airway patency was restored and the stenotic index was estimated at less than 50%; this was later confirmed by morphometric bronchoscopic analysis (Figure 10-2). The surgery lasted less than 1 hour. Extubation was uneventful, and the patient was transferred to the postanesthesia care unit for 24 hours, during which no complications were noted. She was discharged home the following morning.

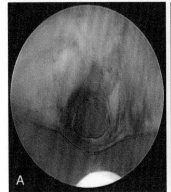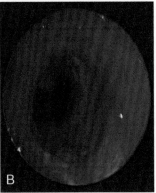

Figure 10-2 Rigid bronchoscopic images with telescope placed 1 cm proximal to the stenosis **(A)** before and **(B)** after laser and dila-tion. The stenotic index post dilation was 30%.

Long-Term Management

Outcome Assessment

Airway patency was restored. Stenosis of less than 50% should improve the patient's exercise capacity and can be objectively documented using the MRC dyspnea scale validated for laryngotracheal stenosis during follow-up clinic visits.[45]

Referral

The multidisciplinary assessment involved thoracic and ear, nose, and throat surgeons; respiratory physicians; radiologists; and a vasculitis specialist.[46] The decision was made to continue systemic therapy on an outpatient basis because no other signs of active disease were noted.

Follow-up Tests and Procedures

Serial ANCA titers are not of great benefit for monitor-ing individual disease activity. The sensitivity of an increase in ANCA titer for the diagnosis of relapse appears to be as low as 24% or as high as 100%. Continuation of ANCA positivity, however, predicts a likelihood of relapse. Our patient had negative ANCA. Furthermore, the stricture was considered to be an end result of previous inflammation, not a relapse of active WG. In addition, although ANCA is monitored during treatment, modifications to immunosuppression are based on clinical evidence of recurrent disease. It is clear that treatment decisions should never be based solely on ANCA results, but rather should be based on careful assessment of clinical and histologic findings.[47]

Results of recent studies in Northern Europe show that the overall 1 year survival rate for WG was 83.3%, and the 5 year survival rate was 74.2%. The standardized mortality ratio for all WG patients was 3.43 (95% con-fidence interval [CI], 2.98 to 3.94); for women, it was 4.38 (95% CI, 3.59 to 5.61), and for men, 2.80 (95% CI, 2.28 to 3.41). The most frequent causes of death were WG or another connective tissue disease, cardiovascular events, and cancer. Prognosis did not change markedly over the 20 year period. Older age and elevated creatinine level at presentation were associated with poorer prognosis, whereas primary ear, nose, and throat involvement, in addition to prompt treatment with CYC, predicted longer survival.[48]

In our patient, follow-up appointments were arranged for 2 weeks after the procedure to ensure involvement of subspecialty physicians as part of a multidisciplinary approach to WG. Elective outpatient flexible bronchoscopy was scheduled for 30 days after the procedure to reassess the degree of airway obstruction and to consider the need for additional therapies in case of stricture recurrence.

Quality Improvement

A team meeting each week provides an opportunity to discuss patient-related management decisions and outcomes, as well as to reflect on quality practice. In this patient, quality of care was considered satisfactory because airway patency had been safely restored, and the patient had been discharged home within 24 hours. We discussed whether follow-up flexible bronchoscopy was necessary and concluded that the indication would be triggered by the presence of symptoms after the first surveillance procedure, scheduled at 30 days. Because this patient had a very active lifestyle and was symptomatic only on exertion, we chose a validated dyspnea assessment instrument (Medical Research Council scale) to evaluate response to treatment, rather than static pulmonary function studies, imaging studies, or repeat routine flexible bronchoscopy.[49]

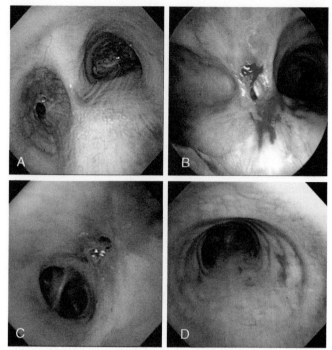

Figure 10-3 **A,** Circumferential proximal left main bronchial stenosis and complete (100%) stenosis of the proximal bronchus intermedius. **B,** Submucosal tunnel at the level of the main carina. **C,** Circumferential left upper bronchial stenosis with associated edema and erythema. **D,** Mucosal plaques with patchy distribution in the trachea of a patient with active Wegener's granulomatosis.

DISCUSSION POINTS

1. Describe five central airway abnormalities seen in Wegener's granulomatosis.
   - Subglottic stenosis is the most frequent manifestation, seen in 10% to 20% of all cases.[26]
   - Bronchial stenosis is usually circumferential and may be bilateral involving lobar or mainstem bronchi (Figure 10-3).
   - Submucosal tunnels are usually present in the trachea and the mainstem bronchi, presumably formed by excessive mucosal pseudomembrane formation, which becomes incorporated into the normal mucosa by epithelialization (see Figure 10-3).
   - Mucosal edema and erythema are the most common mucosal abnormalities in WG[19] (see Figure 10-3).
   - Yellow mucosal plaques are noted (see Figure 10-3) **(see video on ExpertConsult.com)** (Video II.10.3).
2. Discuss the role of ANCA in monitoring this patient's disease activity.
   - In limited WG (including SGS), only 60% of cases are ANCA positive.[8]
   - The reappearance of ANCA in a patient rendered ANCA negative following treatment may indicate relapse (sensitivity, 24% to 100%). ANCA titers may fall during treatment and often rise before relapse.[47]
   - Modifications to immunosuppression often are based on clinical evidence of recurrent disease, not solely on ANCA titers.

3. Describe two adjuvant treatments to laser-assisted dilation of WG-related stenosis.
   - Intralesional corticosteroid injection may reduce the rate of recurrence after bronchoscopic dilation of WG-related subglottic stenosis.[4,23,24]
   - Mitomycin C topical application is associated with less relapse over the short term, but recurrence at 5 years is not affected.[25]
4. Discuss the prognosis of patients with WG and subglottic stenosis.
   - Stenosis often occurs or progresses independently of other features of active disease. Only 20% to 26% of WG-related subglottic strictures respond to glucocorticoids alone or in combination with another immunosuppressant. The remaining 74% to 80% of patients (with stenosis due to scarring, not to active inflammation) usually require interventional therapies to improve their symptoms.[3,46]
   - Patients require multiple mechanical dilations and laser therapy to restore airway patency. Despite the need for repeated interventions, these should be offered before surgical resection or tracheostomy is considered.[32,33,46]
   - Overall 10 year survival is 75%. Primary ear, nose, and throat involvement and prompt treatment with CYC predict longer survival. Older age and elevated creatinine levels at the time of presentation are associated with poorer prognosis.[48]

Expert Commentary

provided by Eric Edell, MD

This is a case of limited Wegener's granulomatosis with symptomatic subglottic stenosis and no evidence of active disease. I agree that ANCA serologies are not reliable indicators of active disease, but nonspecific inflammatory markers such as erythrocyte sedimentation rate (ESR) and C-reactive protein (CRP) might be used to follow disease activity and may have provided, if negative, further evidence of disease quiescence.

The lesion identified at bronchoscopy appears relatively bland with little evidence of active inflammation. Because no evidence of active inflammation was found, I agree that direct treatment of the subglottic stenosis would be an appropriate next step. Several approaches have been described in the literature and are nicely outlined by the authors. Regardless of the cause of the subglottic stenosis, the basic principles of treatment remain the same. These include the following:

- Maximizing airway lumen diameter with minimal insult to the airway epithelium
- Managing other sources of inflammation that could accelerate or induce recurrence
- Developing a strategy for early detection of recurrence

The authors chose to treat this patient's subglottic stenosis with a 9.5 Efer-Dumon rigid bronchoscope and a KTP laser in near contact mode. Radial laser incisions were made at the 11 o'clock and 7 o'clock positions. Following laser treatment, the stenosis was dilated sequentially to 10.5 mm with the use of a rigid bronchoscope. Systemic therapy was continued, and elective bronchoscopy was scheduled 30 days after the procedure to reassess the degree of obstruction and to consider the need for additional therapies. This approach is quite reasonable. Management strategies should be developed after consideration of local expertise, equipment availability, and the best evidence for such treatments. I would like to describe an alternative approach for managing this patient according to the basic principles listed earlier.

The first principle is to maximize luminal diameter with minimal insult to airway epithelium. This can be accomplished by using the various techniques described in the text. The author's use of a sequential dilation strategy after radial incisions is well described. Our experience suggests that the most important step in maximizing luminal diameter is, in fact, treatment of the scar band using radial cuts. We have not found that eventual luminal diameter depends on dilation at the time of treatment; in fact, it may be in direct opposition to minimizing mucosal insult and may potentially accelerate recurrence.

To address this issue of minimal mucosal insult, we use suspension laryngoscopy rather than rigid bronchoscopy. Suspension laryngoscopy provides stable access to the subglottic trachea and may be less traumatic than rigid bronchoscopy. First, the patient is ventilated via a 5.0 endotracheal tube that is gently removed and reinserted during the procedure by the bronchoscopist. Second, we pretreat the area of the stenosis with an injection of corticosteroids. I realize that the data supporting this approach are weak, but as noted by the authors, some reports have described better outcomes with its use. Third, we use a carbon dioxide laser rather than a KTP or Nd:YAG laser. As the authors point out, evidence for this practice is also limited; however, the CO_2 laser is a very precise "cutting" laser and thus theoretically is less likely to cause collateral damage to adjacent mucosa. The final step in our protocol is the application of mitomycin C to the treated area (I realize the paucity of data for this as well). I need to point out that the second, third, and final steps of our approach are more difficult with a rigid bronchoscope, in my opinion, but are quite straightforward when a suspension laryngoscope is used.

The second principle of our management protocol is to manage other sources of inflammation. We know in this case that the stenosis is the direct result of this patient's underlying Wegener's granulomatosis. In addition to the systemic medications she is taking, we would add a single dose of trimethoprim-sulfamethoxazole. Evidence suggests that use of this medication improves outcomes for patients with limited Wegener's granulomatosis.[50] We would also prescribe high-dose inhaled corticosteroids. Their use in the management of airway complications resulting from Wegener's is supported by our experience. Finally, we would advise that the patient use antireflux precautions, including nothing to eat or drink 2 hours before bedtime and, with symptoms suggestive of gastroesophageal reflux disease (GERD), use of proton pump inhibitors.

The third and final principle is to develop a strategy for early detection of recurrence. We do not routinely schedule a post procedure bronchoscopy, but patients may return for direct flexible laryngoscopy in the outpatient setting. It is important to follow the patient's symptoms and intervene as soon as symptoms recur. Our theory is that by detecting recurrence early and proceeding to subsequent repeated treatment, we may create less mucosal trauma and thus less scarring over the long term. We also use a peak flow meter to monitor for recurrence. Patients are instructed on its use and are encouraged to maintain a log of their measurements starting 1 month after surgical intervention, and to continue measuring peak flow 2 to 3 times per week.[51] If their maximum peak flow becomes reduced by 20% or greater, they are to contact us for an appointment. Patients undergo spirometry with maximum voluntary ventilation (MVV), flexible laryngoscopy, and laboratory testing to assess for disease activity. If objective findings of recurrence are noted, with no evidence of disease activity, the procedure already described is repeated.

Patients with airway involvement from Wegener's granulomatosis need a multidisciplinary team that should include a rheumatologist, a pulmonologist, and an otorhinolaryngologist. A team approach that uses standardized evidence-based protocols, when available, will ensure optimal treatment and outcomes for these patients.

REFERENCES

1. Gluth MB, Shinners PA, Kasperbauer JL. Subglottic stenosis associated with Wegener's granulomatosis. *Laryngoscope*. 2003;113:1304-1307.
2. Strange C, Halstead L, Baumann M, et al. Subglottic stenosis in Wegener's granulomatosis: development during cyclophosphamide treatment with response to carbon dioxide laser therapy. *Thorax*. 1990;45:300-301.
3. Hernández-Rodríguez J, Hoffman GS, Koening CL. Surgical interventions and local therapy for Wegener's granulomatosis. *Curr Opin Rheumatol*. 2010;22:29-36.
4. Langford CA, Sneller MC, Hallahan CW, et al. Clinical features and therapeutic management of subglottic stenosis in patients with Wegener's granulomatosis. *Arthritis Rheum*. 1996;39:1754-1760.
5. Hollingsworth HM. Wheezing and stridor. *Clin Chest Med*. 1987;8:231-240.
6. Brichet A, Verkindre C, Dupont J, et al. Multidisciplinary approach to management of postintubation tracheal stenoses. *Eur Respir J*. 1999;13:888-893.
7. Murgu S, Colt HG. Morphometric bronchoscopy in adults with central airway obstruction: case illustrations and review of the literature. *Laryngoscope*. 2009;119:1318-1324.
8. Hoffman GS, Specks U. Antineutrophil cytoplasmic antibodies. *Arthritis Rheum*. 1998;41:1521-1537.
9. Koldingsnes W, Nossent JC. Baseline features and initial treatment as predictors of remission and relapse in Wegener's granulomatosis. *J Rheumatol*. 2003;30:80-88.
10. Boomsma MM, Bijl M, Stegeman CA, et al. Patients' perceptions of the effects of systemic lupus erythematosus on health, function, income, and interpersonal relationships: a comparison with Wegener's granulomatosis. *Arthritis Rheum*. 2002;47:196-201.
11. Duhamel F, Dupuis F. Guaranteed returns: investing in conversations with families of patients with cancer. *Clin J Oncol Nurs*. 2004;8:68-71.
12. Carpenter DM, Thorpe CT, Lewis M, et al. Health-related quality of life for patients with vasculitis and their spouses. *Arthritis Rheum*. 2009;61:259-265.
13. Lewis MA, McBride CM, Pollak KI, et al. Understanding health behavior change among couples: an interdependence and communal coping approach. *Soc Sci Med*. 2006;62:1369-1380.
14. Shvero J, Shitrit D, Koren R, et al. Endoscopic laser surgery for subglottic stenosis in Wegener's granulomatosis. *Yonsei Med J*. 2007;48:748-753.
15. Murgu SD, Colt HG. Interventional bronchoscopy from bench to bedside: new techniques for central and peripheral airway obstruction. *Clin Chest Med*. 2010;31:101-115.
16. Brouns M, Jayaraju ST, Lacor C, et al. Tracheal stenosis: a flow dynamics study. *J Appl Physiol*. 2007;102:1178-1184.
17. Schokkenbroek AA, Franssen CF, Dikkers FG. Dilatation tracheoscopy for laryngeal and tracheal stenosis in patients with Wegener's granulomatosis. *Eur Arch Otorhinolaryngol*. 2008;265:549-555.
18. Ernst A, Simoff M, Ost D, et al. A multicenter, prospective, advanced diagnostic bronchoscopy outcomes registry. *Chest*. 2010;138:165-170.
19. Polychronopoulos VS, Prakash UB, Golbin JM, et al. Airway involvement in Wegener's granulomatosis. *Rheum Dis Clin N Am*. 2007;33:755-775.
20. Seo P, Specks U, Keogh KA. Efficacy of rituximab in limited Wegener's granulomatosis with refractory granulomatous manifestations. *J Rheumatol*. 2008;35:2017-2023.
21. Bakhos D, Lescanne E, Diot E, et al. Subglottic stenosis in Wegener's granulomatosis. *Ann Otolaryngol Chir Cervicofac*. 2008;125:35-39.
22. Sheski FD, Mathur PN. Long-term results of fiberoptic bronchoscopic balloon dilation in the management of benign tracheobronchial stenosis. *Chest*. 1998;114:796-800.
23. Stappaerts I, Van Laer C, Deschepper K, et al. Endoscopic management of severe subglottic stenosis in Wegener's granulomatosis. *Clin Rheumatol*. 2000;19:315-317.
24. Hoffman GS, Thomas-Golbanov CK, Chan J, et al. Treatment of subglottic stenosis, due to Wegener's granulomatosis, with intralesional corticosteroids and dilation. *J Rheumatol*. 2003;30:1017-1021.
25. Smith ME, Elstad M. Mitomycin C and the endoscopic treatment of laryngotracheal stenosis: are two applications better than one? *Laryngoscope*. 2009;119:272-283.

26. Lebovics RS, Hoffman GS, Leavitt RY, et al. The management of subglottic stenosis in patients with Wegener's granulomatosis. *Laryngoscope*. 1992;102:1341-1345.
27. Gluth MB, Shinners PA, Kasperbauer JL. Subglottic stenosis associated with Wegener's granulomatosis. *Laryngoscope*. 2003;113:1304-1307.
28. Watters K, Russell J. Subglottic stenosis in Wegener's granulomatosis and the Nitinol stent. *Laryngoscope*. 2003;113:2222-2224.
29. Mair EA. Caution in using subglottic stents for Wegener's granulomatosis. *Laryngoscope*. 2004;114:2060-2061.
30. U.S. Food and Drug Administration. Metallic tracheal stents in patients with benign airway disorders. http://www.fda.gov/Safety/MedWatch/SafetyInformation/SafetyAlertsforHumanMedicalProducts/ucm153009.htm. Accessed February 20, 2011.
31. Daum TE, Specks U, Colby TV, et al. Tracheobronchial involvement in Wegener's granulomatosis. *Am J Respir Crit Care Med*. 1995;151:522-526.
32. Herridge MS, Pearson FG, Downey GP. Subglottic stenosis complicating Wegener's granulomatosis: surgical repair as a viable treatment option. *J Thorac Cardiovasc Surg*. 1996;111:961-966.
33. McDonald TJ, Neel HB, 3rd, DeRemee RA. Wegener's granulomatosis of the subglottis and the upper portion of the trachea. *Ann Otol Rhinol Laryngol*. 1982;91:588-592.
34. Utzig MJ, Warzelhan J, Wertzel H, et al. Role of thoracic surgery and interventional bronchoscopy in Wegener's granulomatosis. *Ann Thorac Surg*. 2002;74:1948-1952.
35. Flye MW, Mundinger Jr GH, Fauci AS. Diagnostic and therapeutic aspects of the surgical approach to Wegener's granulomatosis. *J Thorac Cardiovasc Surg*. 1979;77:331-337.
36. Stewart MA. Effective physician-patient communication and health outcomes: a review. *CMAJ*. 1995;152:1423-1433.
37. Légaré F, Ratté S, Stacey D, et al. Interventions for improving the adoption of shared decision making by healthcare professionals. *Cochrane Database Syst Rev*. 2010;5:CD006732.
38. Deepika K, Kenaan CA, Barrocas AM, et al. Negative pressure pulmonary edema after acute upper airway obstruction. *J Clin Anesth*. 1997;9:403-408.
39. Hobaika AB, Lorentz MN. Laryngospasm. *Rev Bras Anestesiol*. 2009;59:487-495.
40. Roberts RJ, Welch SM, Devlin JW. Corticosteroids for prevention of postextubation laryngeal edema in adults. *Ann Pharmacother*. 2008;42:686-691.
41. Kil HK, Kim WO, Koh SO. Effects of dexamethasone on laryngeal edema following short-term intubation. *Yonsei Med J*. 1995;36:515-520.
42. Mathisen DJ, Grillo HC. Endoscopic relief of malignant airway obstruction. *Ann Thorac Surg*. 1989;48:469-473.
43. Shapshay SM. Laser applications in the trachea and bronchi: a comparative study of the soft tissue effects using contact and noncontact delivery systems. *Laryngoscope*. 1987;97:1-26.
44. Ishman SL, Kerschner JE, Rudolph CD. The KTP laser: an emerging tool in pediatric otolaryngology. *Int J Pediatr Otorhinolaryngol*. 2006;70:677-682.
45. Nouraei SAR, Winterborn C, Nouraei SM, et al. Quantifying the physiology of laryngotracheal stenosis: changes in pulmonary dynamics in response to graded extrathoracic resistive loading. *Laryngoscope*. 2007;117:581-588.
46. Solans-Laqué R, Bosch-Gil J, Canela M, et al. Clinical features and therapeutic management of subglottic stenosis in patients with Wegener's granulomatosis. *Lupus*. 2008;17:832-836.
47. Sinclair D, Stevens JM. Role of antineutrophil cytoplasmic antibodies and glomerular basement membrane antibodies in the diagnosis and monitoring of systemic vasculitides. *Ann Clin Biochem*. 2007;44:432-442.
48. Takala JH, Kautiainen H, Leirisalo-Repo M. Survival of patients with Wegener's granulomatosis diagnosed in Finland in 1981-2000. *Scand J Rheumatol*. 2010;39:71-76.
49. Nouraei SA, Nouraei SM, Randhawa PS, et al. Sensitivity and responsiveness of the Medical Research Council dyspnoea scale to the presence and treatment of adult laryngotracheal stenosis. *Clin Otolaryngol*. 2008;33:575-580.
50. Stegeman CA, Cohen Tervaert JW, de Jong PE, et al. Trimethoprim-sulfamethoxazole (co-trimoxazole) for the prevention of relapses of Wegener's granulomatosis. *N Engl J Med*. 1996;335:16-20.
51. Alon EE, Edell ES, Kasperbauer JL. Monitoring recurrent subglottic stenosis via peak flowmeter. *Otolaryngol Head Neck Surg*. 2007;137:237-238.

SECTION 3

Practical Approach to Expiratory Central Airway Collapse

Silicone Stent Insertion for Focal Crescent–Type Tracheomalacia in a Patient with Sarcoidosis

> This chapter emphasizes the following elements of the Four Box Approach: physical examination, complementary tests, and functional status assessment; patient's support system (also includes family); anesthesia and other perioperative care; and follow-up tests, visits, and procedures.

CASE DESCRIPTION

A 62-year-old man with a history of pulmonary sarcoidosis diagnosed 10 years earlier presented with chronic cough and inability to clear secretions. He described his cough as "seal barking." He had also noted increasing dyspnea with normal physical activities. For the past month, his primary care physician had treated him with short- and long-acting bronchodilators, as well as inhaled and systemic steroids (prednisone 20 mg/day) for suspected adult-onset asthma. He was a nonsmoker, worked as an electrician, and had a history of hypertension and supraventricular tachycardia controlled by diltiazem. Electrocardiogram (ECG) and two-dimensional (2D) echocardiogram were unremarkable. Pulmonary function testing (PFT) revealed moderate obstructive ventilatory impairment without improvement after bronchodilators. Flow volume loop (FVL) showed an airway collapse pattern on the expiratory curve (Figure 11-1). Paired inspiratory/expiratory dynamic computed tomography showed bilateral upper lobe fibrosis, tracheomegaly, and localized narrowing of the lower trachea during dynamic expiration (see Figure 11-1). Flexible bronchoscopy revealed fibrotic closure of the right and left upper lobar bronchi and complete expiratory collapse of the anterior cartilaginous structures in the lower trachea, giving the airway lumen the shape of a crescent (see Figure 11-1).

DISCUSSION POINTS

1. Describe five criteria used in classifying expiratory central airway collapse.
2. List three imaging modalities used to diagnose expiratory central airway collapse.
3. List three indications for treatment in this patient.

CASE RESOLUTION

Initial Evaluations

Physical Examination, Complementary Tests, and Functional Status Assessment

This patient presented with dyspnea, cough, and mucus retention. These nonspecific symptoms of pulmonary disorders are seen primarily in patients suffering from asthma, chronic obstructive pulmonary disorder (COPD), or bronchiectasis. His cough, however, was described as "seal barking." This pattern is suggestive of expiratory central airway collapse (ECAC) and presumably is caused by vibration of the floppy membranous posterior wall against the anterior airway wall during expiration.[1] As in our patient, symptoms are usually refractory to corticosteroids and bronchodilators.[2] In addition, patients with ECAC may have recurrent bronchitis, pneumonia, and even respiratory failure.[3] Some patients experience cough-syncope, presumably as a result of a significant rise in intrathoracic pressure and a sudden drop in venous return and cardiac output[4] during violent coughing episodes.

Spirometry showed obstructive ventilatory impairment. In ECAC, spirometry usually demonstrates obstruction that is proportionate to the severity of the disease.[5] The expiratory FVL seen in this patient suggested compression of the central airways (see Figure 11-1). This "airway collapse" pattern occurs when maximal flow is quickly reached after expiration of a small volume of air. Following maximal flow, a large fall in flow occurs, although only a small volume is exhaled. Subsequently, the flow rate falls very little during the remainder of expiration. This phase is responsible for the long plateau seen on the FVL (see Figure 11-1).[6] However, the FVL is neither sensitive nor specific; it can be seen in almost 40% of patients with severe COPD.[7] Flow oscillations on the FVL have also been described. These take on a sawtooth appearance, defined as a reproducible sequence of alternating decelerations and accelerations of flow. This pattern is nonspecific because it can be seen in patients with obstructive sleep apnea, structural or functional disorders of the upper airway, and neuromuscular diseases.[8] Lack of clinical and spirometric improvement after bronchodilator administration might be explained by the effects of bronchodilators on central airways. Bronchodilators cause smooth muscle relaxation, further decreasing tracheobronchial wall stiffness and worsening airway obstruction. Bronchodilators increase airway wall compliance. The resulting increased airway compressibility will cause the choke point to be localized to a point closer to the thoracic outlet. The increased length of the upstream segment (from the alveoli to the choke point) and the decreased cross-sectional area at the choke point offset any advantages gained by bronchodilator-induced caliber increase in upstream airways with respect to maximal expiratory flow.[9] In fact, although this effect has not been studied in adults, a dramatic fall in peak flow in response

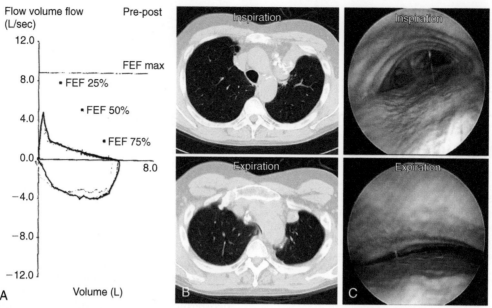

Figure 11-1 A, Flow-volume loop shows a sudden drop in expiratory flow followed by a plateau phase; these findings characterize the "airway collapse" pattern. **B,** Paired inspiratory/expiratory computed tomography shows complete collapse of the lower trachea during expiration. **C,** Dynamic bronchoscopy reveals similar findings and confirms that the collapse is caused by flattening of the anterior tracheal wall, which characterizes the crescent type of tracheomalacia.

to bronchodilators has been described in pediatric cases of tracheobronchomalacia (TBM).[10]*

In our patient, a diagnosis of expiratory central airway collapse was made bronchoscopically and on paired dynamic inspiratory/expiratory computed tomography (CT) scanning. Because of the obvious weakness of the lower anterior tracheal cartilaginous wall, this patient had focal crescent tracheomalacia.[11] The disorder was characterized by a severe (100%) degree of airway narrowing. During dynamic (functional) bronchoscopy, the airways were visualized by moving the patient into supine, upright, and lateral decubitus positions during spontaneous breathing, as well as during cough, forced expiration, and deep inspiration. During these bronchoscopic assessments, changes in airway lumen can be measured and the extent of collapse noted, and narrowing can be classified as being of the crescent, saber-sheath, or circumferential type. Regions of cartilaginous weakness (tracheomalacia)

can be differentiated from areas of excessive dynamic airway collapse (EDAC) or normal physiologic dynamic airway collapse (DAC) (Figure 11-2).

Among radiologic studies, fluoroscopy was used to diagnose tracheomalacia in the past. During fluoroscopy, one can visualize the airway collapse, but it is difficult to appreciate whether it is due to softening of the cartilage or to excessive bulging of the posterior membrane (Figure 11-3).[12] Today, with the use of dynamic CT, one more easily distinguishes cartilaginous from posterior wall collapse (see Figure 11-3). Results from studies show that dynamic CT correlates well with bronchoscopy findings,[13] offers excellent display of anatomic details of the airway and adjacent structures,[14] and allows objective interpretation and quantitative measurements of the degree of airway wall collapse before and after airway splinting interventions.[14,15] Dynamic magnetic resonance imaging (MRI) has been insufficiently studied, but small case series support its use for quantifying the degree of airway collapse[16] (see Figure 11-3). Its main advantage over CT is that radiation is avoided and contrast materials used are not nephrotoxic.

We quantified this patient's functional impairment on the basis of World Health Organization (WHO) functional class criteria.[17] He had WHO class II functional impairment defined as mild limitation of physical activity without discomfort at rest, but with normal physical activity causing increased symptoms.[18] The use of other dyspnea or quality of life (QOL) instruments (St. George's Respiratory Questionnaire [SGRQ], American Thoracic Society [ATS] Dyspnea Scale, Baseline Dyspnea Index [BDI]/Transitional Dyspnea Index [TDI], Karnofsky Performance Scale [KPS], and a 6-minute walk test [6MWT]) in these patients to objectively determine response to interventions has been studied.[19]

---

*In children, the primary or congenital form of malacia is believed to be a consequence of the inadequate maturity of tracheobronchial cartilage, resulting from premature delivery or from an innate immaturity despite normal gestation. It also could be caused by disease processes that result in the formation of an abnormal cartilaginous matrix of the trachea, as is seen with several genetic syndromes. Most infants outgrow the condition by the age of 2 years because the cartilage strengthens and stiffens, but the disease often persists in children with connective tissue disorders and congenital syndromes. Current management following diagnosis includes medical approaches aimed at reducing associated symptoms of tracheomalacia, ventilation modalities of continuous positive airway pressure (CPAP) and bilateral positive airway pressure (BiPAP), and, in the most severe forms of malacia, surgical approaches aimed at improving the caliber of the airway, such as airway stenting, aortopexy, or tracheopexy. For comprehensive reviews of pediatric malacia, interested readers may wish to refer to articles by I.B. Masters (*Cochrane Database Syst Rev.* 2005;[4]:CD005304), K. Carden (*Chest.* 2005;127:984-1005), R.D. Jaquiss (*Semin Thorac Cardiovasc Surg.* 2004;16:220-224), and J. Austin (*Paediatr Anaesth.* 2003;13:3-11).

Figure 11-2 A, Normal dynamic airway collapse characterized by bulging of the posterior membrane inside the airway lumen. The cartilage is intact, and airway narrowing during expiration *(bottom)* is less than 50% as compared with inspiration *(top).* **B,** Excessive dynamic airway collapse is caused by excessive bulging of the posterior membrane, which leads to greater than 50% reduction in the airway lumen during expiration. **C,** In crescent-type tracheomalacia, airway collapse is caused by weakness of the anterior wall, which leads to airway narrowing during expiration.

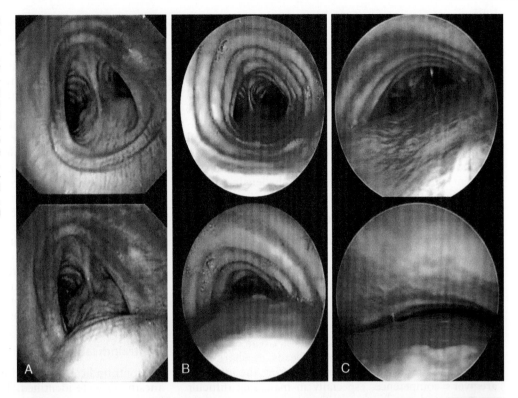

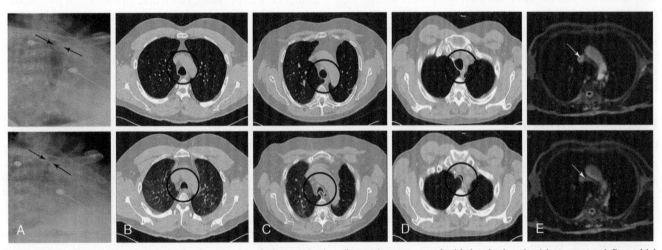

Figure 11-3   Fluoroscopy reveals tracheal narrowing during expiration *(bottom)* as compared with inspiration *(top)* but cannot define which airway wall is abnormal, nor can it detect adjacent structures **(A).** Dynamic computed tomography shows **(B)** normal, physiologic dynamic airway collapse, **(C)** excessive dynamic airway collapse, and **(D)** crescent-type tracheomalacia. **E,** Dynamic magnetic resonance imaging reveals normal dynamic airway collapse during expiration without exposure to ionizing radiation.

Comorbidities

The patient had controlled cardiac arrhythmia and no evidence of systolic or diastolic dysfunction on 2D echocardiogram. Although moderate obstructive ventilatory impairment was noted, clinical evaluation and the 2D echocardiogram showed no evidence of pulmonary hypertension, which might prompt hemodynamic instability in case of general anesthesia.[20]

The patient had been on prednisone 20 mg/day for 4 weeks. Traditionally, any patient who has received the equivalent of 15 mg/day of prednisone for longer than 3 weeks should be suspected of having hypothalamic-adrenal axis suppression.[21] As a general rule, any patient who has received glucocorticoids in doses equivalent to at least 20 mg/day of prednisone for longer than 5 days is at risk for hypothalamic-pituitary-adrenal (HPA) axis suppression.[22] Furthermore, this patient had been on high-dose inhaled fluticasone (440 mcg twice daily) for several years. The development of adrenal suppression from inhaled steroids is known to be related to dose, duration of therapy, and use of a potent agent (such as fluticasone).[23]

Support System

The patient is married, but his wife suffers from severe COPD and is on continuous home oxygen supplementation. He is her caregiver. Investigators have found that informal caregivers (defined as untrained and unpaid persons who provide care to an ill person) have needs that go largely unmet, and that they usually receive insufficient help from services with regard to daily physical caring and emotional issues, as well as regarding information about available health and social services. Caring for a patient with dyspnea is particularly challenging and is most difficult to cope with.[24]

Patient Preferences and Expectations

Similar to other people caring for patients with dyspnea, this patient expressed uncertainty about the future and feared there would come a time when he could no longer help his spouse, or that helping her would be done at the expense of his own health. Active participation and availability of health care professionals are needed to assist informal caregivers with coping strategies they are already using and to address future challenges. Greater involvement of health care professionals leads to sharing of information and advice, thereby enhancing the informal caregiver's competence, especially in managing difficult symptoms such as dyspnea.[24] This patient was particularly motivated to improve his own symptoms so that he could maintain and improve his caregiving role for his wife. He had clearly expressed his willingness for treatment and was ready to consider all available treatment options, including noninvasive positive-pressure ventilation, airway stent insertion, and open surgical resection if necessary.

Procedural Strategies

Indications

Focal Tracheomalacia Resulting in Functional Impairment

The treatment of severe malacia often involves the use of minimally invasive or open surgical procedures.[25,26] The exact degree of expiratory airway narrowing responsible for symptoms and requiring intervention remains unknown. Many investigators use 50% or greater reduction in airway caliber between inspiration and expiration to identify abnormal central airway collapse on dynamic CT or bronchoscopy.[27-29] This criterion, however, is applied during coughing or forced exhalation, and its use may lead to false-positive results: 78% of normal individuals exceed the current diagnostic criterion for tracheomalacia in the upper and/or lower trachea.[30] Furthermore, patients with other airway disorders such as bronchiolitis, COPD, or cystic fibrosis have peripheral airway obstruction, and the expiratory airway collapse seen in the central airways represents normal physiology.[31-33] Indeed, during flow-limited breathing, the central airways become severely compressed, particularly during forced expiration and cough—maneuvers often used in diagnosing this entity on dynamic imaging studies. The Starling resistor

model* shows that the pressure drop occurs across a very short length of airway, and that proximal airway (downstream from the choke point, mouth ward) resistance should not affect airflow. Pressure catheter measurements demonstrate this flow-limiting choke point and lack of further pressure drop in airways between the mouth and the flow-limiting segment.[34] Because the choke point in adult humans is often located at the level of the lobar bronchi and is even more peripheral in patients with COPD,[35] central airway collapsibility should not impede airflow.[32]

Our patient had severe (100%) collapse, resulting not just in exertional dyspnea but also in refractory cough and inability to raise secretions. For these reasons, after taking into account the patient's goals of care, we elected to proceed with rigid bronchoscopy under general anesthesia to place an indwelling silicone stent that would splint open the lower trachea. Our goal was to improve airway lumen patency to less than 50% collapse during exhalation, which, by convention, is currently considered by most investigators to be within normal limits.[17]

Contraindications

No contraindications to rigid bronchoscopy under general anesthesia were identified. The patient had no abnormal head or neck anatomy that would limit ability to intubate, nor was evidence of cardiac involvement by sarcoidosis noted on ECG and 2D echocardiogram; this would increase the risk for arrhythmia. No evidence of pulmonary artery hypertension was found; this would increase the risks of right ventricular failure and hemodynamic collapse during general anesthesia.

Expected Results

We intended to insert a large silicone stent at the site of severe airway collapse localized in the lower trachea. Therefore, rigid intubation was planned using a large (13 mm)-diameter open ventilating rigid bronchoscope. Careful attention would be necessary to avoid trauma to the teeth, arytenoid cartilage, and vocal cords, given the large diameter of the rigid scope. Also, airway perforation and spinal cord injury can theoretically occur, especially if intubation is performed when the patient is not fully asleep.

In the short term (up to 10 to 14 days), airway stabilization with silicone stents in patients with various forms of expiratory central airway collapse was shown to improve respiratory symptoms, quality of life, and functional status.[18,19] In one large study evaluating stent insertion for this disease, 45 of 58 patients (77%) reported symptomatic improvement; quality of life scores improved in 19 of 27 patients (70%) ($P = .002$), dyspnea scores improved in 22 of 24 patients (91%) ($P = .001$), and functional status scores improved in 18 of 26 patients (70%) ($P = .002$).[19]

---

*The Starling resistor is a simple model of the lung that comprises an elastic tube mounted between two rigid tubes inside a chamber filled with air; airflow is driven through the system. This model has been used to explain expiratory flow limitations.

Team Experience

Silicone stent insertion requires rigid bronchoscopy—a skill possessed by a minority of pulmonologists.[36] Even for those who have undergone training, the technique of gentle, atraumatic rigid intubation and stent insertion is one that is gradually perfected over time.

Risk-Benefit Analysis

The rare risk of airway injury is outweighed by the benefit of improving airway patency to improve the patient's exercise capacity, cough, and quality of life.

Therapeutic Alternatives for Restoring Airway Patency

These include conservative, minimally invasive, and open surgical therapies.

- *Continuous positive airway pressure (CPAP):* Excessive airway narrowing and the resulting turbulent flow result in increased airway resistance, which requires greater transpulmonary pressures to maintain expiratory airflow. This will increase the work of breathing and will result in dyspnea. Adjunctive noninvasive positive-pressure ventilation decreases pulmonary resistance and can be used to maintain airway patency, facilitate secretion drainage, and improve expiratory flow. Small studies have showed that the addition of nasal CPAP improves spirometry values, sputum production, atelectasis, and exercise tolerance, but its long-term efficiency has not been clearly demonstrated.[37,38]
- *Metal stent insertion:* This approach has been used in the past with variable success.[11] Advantages include placement by flexible bronchoscopy, dynamic expansion, and preservation of airway mucociliary function with uncovered stents. In some studies, however, metal stents had to be removed because of stent failure, or because of stent-related complications. Stent fracture and fatal hemorrhage from perforation, for example, have been reported.[39] The Food and Drug Administration (FDA) recommends against the use of metallic stents for histologically benign forms of airway obstruction, as in the case described herein.[40]
- *Open surgical interventions:* Airway splinting has been used to consolidate and reshape the airway wall. Before an open surgical intervention is proposed, a stent trial has been recommended to identify those patients who are likely to benefit from surgery over the long term. Among surgical interventions, membranous tracheoplasty seems to provide a favorable outcome in uncontrolled studies. This procedure reinforces the membranous portion of the trachea in severe diffuse expiratory central airway collapse.[41,42] However, our patient had mild functional impairment and focal disease limited to the lower trachea, probably warranting a more conservative approach.
- *Tracheostomy:* This technique may be used to splint the malacic airway and provide invasive ventilatory support if necessary; because it can be complicated by secondary tracheomalacia and stenosis at the stoma site, it should not be considered a first-line treatment in elective cases. In our case, the malacic segment would not have been bypassed by tracheostomy because it was localized in the lower trachea.
- Tracheal resection has been proposed for focal tracheomalacia with good outcome and low mortality in experienced centers.[43] This procedure, however, has been performed for post-tracheostomy–related malacia, not for lesions localized in the lower trachea.

Cost-Effectiveness

Therapeutic alternatives offered to patients depend on the extent, type, and severity of airway collapse; the degree of functional impairment; and access to and the level of medical or surgical expertise available.[11] Although no formal cost-effectiveness evaluations of these various modalities have yet been published, future studies may examine this topic if a consensus is reached regarding classification of this syndrome. Such an assessment would provide clinicians and researchers with an objective tool that can be used in designing outcome studies.[17]

Informed Consent

With the shift toward a more "consumer-centric" health care system as part of an overall effort to improve the quality of health care and to reduce costs, people need to take an even more active role in health care–related decisions. To accomplish this in an age of shared responsibility between physician and patient, patients must display strong decision-making skills.[44] Although the impact of health literacy levels and outcomes has not been addressed for this patient population, it is known that poor health literacy is "a stronger predictor of a person's health than age, income, employment status, education level, and race."[45]

This patient was informed of the risks and benefits of the procedure. He demonstrated an understanding of the indications and potential-associated complications. He was able to understand treatment alternatives and consent forms and asked pertinent questions. After he had been advised of all the alternatives, he chose to proceed with rigid bronchoscopy and silicone stent insertion under general anesthesia.

Techniques and Results

Anesthesia and Perioperative Care

Upper airway instrumentation such as intubation and inhalation of irritants (e.g., desflurane) may trigger vagally mediated bronchospasm, thereby promoting expiratory collapse of the peripheral airways with incomplete lung alveolar emptying (air trapping).[46] This can potentially lead to hypercarbia, hypoxemia, and hemodynamic instability from high intrathoracic pressures and reduced cardiac output.

Also of concern is the uncommon event of perioperative hypotension and death in patients treated on a long-term basis with glucocorticoids. Although it is well known that patients with adrenal suppression require perioperative glucocorticoid supplementation therapy, serious omissions can occur as a result of inadequate or unclear instructions from the treating team. Therefore, it is important to clearly document and institute an appropriate perioperative glucocorticoid management plan.[21] Current recommendations address the need for increased glucocorticoid supplementation in patients with adrenal suppression during medical and surgical stress without exposing patients to excessive or prolonged steroid dosing. Although the level of physiologic stress has not been studied for rigid bronchoscopy, by extrapolating from available guidelines, this can be considered a minor to moderate surgical stress. The recommended glucocorticoid dosage for such situations is intravenous hydrocortisone 75 mg/day on the day of the procedure (e.g., 25 mg every 8 hours) with taper over the next 1 to 2 days to the usual replacement dose in uncomplicated cases (for minor stress), and intravenous hydrocortisone 150 mg/day (e.g., 50 mg every 8 hours) with taper over the next 2 to 3 days to the usual replacement dose in uncomplicated cases (for moderate stress). Short courses (<48 hours) of increased glucocorticoid therapy rarely cause significant complications. Our patient was treated with a moderate stress dose of hydrocortisone (150 mg divided in three doses).

The anesthesiologist should be made aware of the patient's adrenal suppression, so that safe drugs are used for induction. Etomidate, for instance, is a parenteral hypnotic agent that decreases cortisol synthesis by inhibiting 11-beta hydroxylase, a mitochondrial enzyme in the final step of cortisol synthesis. Single-dose etomidate is common for induction of anesthesia, especially for hemodynamically unstable patients and patients who may not tolerate wide variance in heart rate or blood pressure. A single bolus dose of etomidate has been shown to cause adrenal insufficiency in elective cardiopulmonary bypass patients and may induce postoperative vasopressor dependency.[47,48] Use of etomidate is a modifiable risk factor for the development of adrenal insufficiency that should be avoided because safer alternatives are available.

The anesthesiologist should also be aware that worsening airway obstruction may occur during induction. This phenomenon has been reported with the use of both intravenous and inhalational induction.[49] The use of neuromuscular blocking agents should be avoided because these drugs may eliminate the only muscle tone that keeps the airway open. Spontaneous assisted ventilation is in fact preferred because of its safety profile.[50] Patients with ECAC may not tolerate the supine position after induction; therefore the bronchoscopist should be stationed at the head of the bed throughout induction of anesthesia in case emergent bronchoscopic intervention is required to secure and control the airway.

Instrumentation

We used a 13 mm Efer-Dumon rigid nonventilating bronchoscope (Bryan Corp., Woburn, Mass). This large-diameter scope allows insertion of a silicone stent larger than 12 mm. Based on bronchoscopy and CT scanning, the patient had secondary tracheomegaly caused by bilateral upper lobe fibrosis (see Figure 11-1). Because of this, we intended to use a 20 mm diameter stent. Based on

measurements performed during flexible bronchoscopy, the extent of the collapse was 4 cm in the lower trachea. We therefore chose a 20 × 60 mm straight studded silicone stent to properly cover the abnormal collapsing airway (1 cm above and 1 cm below).

Anatomic Dangers and Other Risks

No anatomic dangers, other than those present in cases of airway wall perforation, have been noted during stent insertion in the trachea. In the absence of tumor or an incredibly thin posterior airway wall, it is unlikely that the tracheal airway will be perforated and a stent deployed into the mediastinum (although this is a risk, particularly in left main bronchus insertions, because of the angles and curvatures of the bronchus). One should make sure that the rigid scope is aligned with the airway. Older models of the 13 mm Efer-Dumon bronchoscope do not have a stopper at the distal aspect of the tube, so the bronchoscopist must know and recall its length (10 inches) during advancement of the stent introducer. Use of large stents does pose the risk of lack of unfolding and consequent inability to ventilate or oxygenate the patient. Furthermore, excessive pressure on the larynx from a large rigid bronchoscope may increase risk for laryngeal edema and arytenoid dislocation.

Results and Procedure-Related Complications

The patient was atraumatically intubated, and airway collapse could be accurately assessed in terms of exact location, type, extent, and severity. It was indeed noted that the patient had severe airway collapse in the lower trachea, characterized by flattening of the anterior cartilaginous wall, giving the trachea the shape of a crescent. The collapsing airway segment ended 2 cm above the main carina. The rigid bronchoscope was gently advanced distal to the obstruction, and the 20 × 60 mm stent was deployed with the distal extremity placed 1 cm above the main carina (see video on ExpertConsult.com) (Video III.11.1). Airway patency was restored and the collapsing index was estimated at less than 50%; this was later confirmed by morphometric bronchoscopic analysis (Figure 11-4). The case lasted 20 minutes. The patient was extubated without difficulty and was transferred to the postanesthesia care unit (PACU) for 24 hours, during which no postoperative stridor or hypotension was noticed. He was kept NPO until the following day in case immediate stent migration might prompt urgent rigid bronchoscopy for stent revision. This did not occur, so the next day the patient was discharged home after stent instructions were provided to the patient and his daughter.

No immediate anesthesia- or stent-related complications were reported. Because the dynamic features of expiratory central airway collapse continuously alter the shape of the central airways, as well as the contact between a stent and the airway walls, stent-related complications may occur more frequently in this setting than in other benign disorders or malignancy. Indeed, 26 stent-related complications (12 mucus plugs, 8 migrations, and 6 granulation tissues) were seen in 10 of the 12 patients (83%) who underwent silicone stent

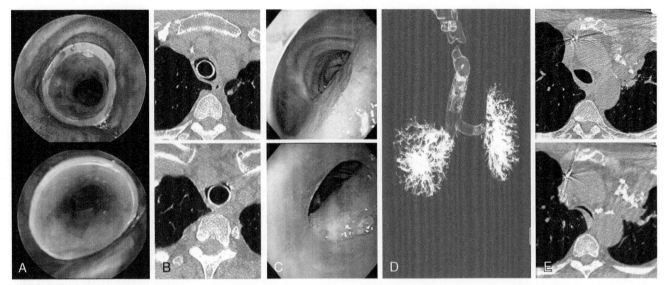

Figure 11-4 **A,** Rigid bronchoscopy images during inspiration *(top)* and expiration *(bottom)* performed immediately after stent insertion show less than 50% collapse during expiration. **B,** Dynamic computed tomography shows similar findings at 8 weeks post intervention. **C,** Flexible bronchoscopy 3 years later shows collapse of the posterior membrane distal to the stent during expiration *(bottom),* consistent with distal choke point migration. **D,** Three-dimensional external computed tomography (CT) reconstruction shows no evidence of stent migration. **E,** Dynamic CT confirms choke point migration distal to the stent.

insertion for ECAC.[18] In another study with 57 patients, authors had 21 partial stent obstructions, 14 infections, and 10 stent migrations.[19] These complications usually are not life threatening, but they do require repeated bronchoscopic interventions.

Long-Term Management

Outcome Assessment

Relief of airway obstruction was successfully achieved, as assessed bronchoscopically. The patient had noticed immediate improvement in his ability to raise secretions, and his seal barking cough had subsided. A less than 50% airway collapse should have also improved the patient's exercise capacity. His exercise capacity and QOL scores can be objectively documented at follow-up clinic visits by using one of the previously applied scales for tracheobronchomalacia, such as the ATS Dyspnea Scale, BDI/TDI, SGRQ, KPS, or WHO functional class impairment.[17-19]

Referral

A multidisciplinary approach to management of tracheomalacia, involving thoracic surgeons, respiratory physicians, and radiologists, is warranted. After discussion in our multidisciplinary chest conference, the patient was tapered off corticosteroids during the following weeks and received a prescription for nebulized saline 3 times a day to maintain stent patency.

Follow-up Tests and Procedures

Follow up bronchoscopy is warranted for at least two reasons:
1. It may detect the evolution of the disease process. The prognosis of pure malacia is not completely understood, in part because previous studies did not differentiate dynamic abnormalities of the posterior membrane from abnormalities of the cartilaginous airway wall. Results of older studies demonstrate that expiratory central airway collapse is progressive in most patients.[2,29] In one study of 17 patients, 76% of patients had worse airway narrowing detected on repeat bronchoscopy.[2] A larger study followed 94 patients with tracheomalacia (TM), TBM, or bronchomalacia for an average of 5.2 years. Among those who underwent repeat bronchoscopy, most had worsening disease, some had stable disease, and none improved spontaneously. Six of the nine patients (66%) with what was called tracheomalacia progressed to diffuse tracheobronchomalacia.[5]
2. It may detect possible stent-related complications or migrated choke points requiring further intervention.[11] In one study, stent-related adverse events were common and usually occurred within the first few weeks after stent insertion (median of 29 days).[18] Another study showed that complications occurred within the first 3 months after stent insertion (median time, 26 days; range, 3 to 865 days).[19] These results certainly seem to justify follow-up bronchoscopy 4 weeks after stent insertion.

Our patient had a surveillance bronchoscopy 4 weeks after stent insertion. This showed no evidence of stent-related complications. The airway lumen had remained patent, and less than 50% collapse occurred during expiration. These findings were also seen on follow-up dynamic CT scanning 8 weeks later (see Figure 11-4), confirming preliminary results suggesting a potentially important role for CT in preintervention and postintervention assessments of patients with tracheobronchomalacia.[15]

Two years after initial presentation to our department, this patient developed newly recurrent dyspnea and an inability to raise secretions. Bronchoscopy revealed that the stent had migrated 1 centimeter proximally and that a small amount of associated granulation tissue was evident (see video on ExpertConsult.com) (Video III.11.2). Rigid bronchoscopy with stent revision was performed, and the stent was repositioned in its original location. Surveillance bronchoscopy and dynamic CT 1 year later showed that the patient had no stent-related complications, but the choke point migrated distal to the stent with evidence of a moderate degree of airway narrowing (see Figure 11-4), which was associated with exertional dyspnea. After readdressing the treatment alternatives, we decided to place the patient on CPAP 10 cm H_2O as an adjuvant treatment to splint open residual collapsing airway in the distal trachea.

Quality Improvement

Airway patency was restored and symptoms improved, but during the 3 year follow-up, our patient developed both stent-related complications and choke point migration requiring further therapy.[11] We discussed whether follow-up flexible bronchoscopy would be performed on CPAP to determine an optimal pressure level that would maintain airway patency.[51] We concluded that this will be performed if the patient does not tolerate the current CPAP pressure, and/or if no symptomatic improvement is noted.

DISCUSSION POINTS

1. Describe five criteria used in classifying expiratory central airway collapse.

    No classification system for this disease has been universally accepted. After synthesizing various criteria proposed in the literature in a multidimensional classification system,[17] we use the following parameters:

    - *Morphology:* refers to the abnormal collapsing airway wall—cartilaginous wall (TBM with three subtypes depending on the shape of the airway lumen during expiration: crescent, saber sheath, or circumferential) or posterior wall (EDAC)
    - *Origin (etiology):* idiopathic and secondary to other disease entities
    - *Extent:* describes the location and distribution of the abnormal airway tracheobronchial segment as assessed by bronchoscopy or radiographic studies:
        - *Normal:* No airway abnormality has been identified.
        - *Focal:* Abnormality is present in one main or lobar bronchus or one tracheal region (upper, middle, or lower).
        - *Multifocal:* Abnormality is present in two contiguous or at least two noncontiguous regions.
        - *Diffuse:* Abnormality is present in more than two contiguous regions.
    - *Severity of airway collapse:* describes the degree of airway collapse during expiration as assessed by bronchoscopy or radiographic studies. These cutoff values may change because studies will clarify the

exact degree of physiologically significant narrowing in a specific patient.
    - *Normal:* expiratory collapse of less than 50%
    - *Mild:* expiratory airway collapse of 50% to 75%
    - *Moderate:* expiratory airway collapse of 75% to 100%
    - *Severe:* expiratory airway collapse of 100%; the airway walls make contact
    - *Functional impairment:* describes the severity of symptoms as assessed by a modified WHO functional status classification (other scales can be used)
        - *Normal:* no limitation of usual physical activity; ordinary physical activity does not cause symptoms
        - *Mild:* limitation of physical activity; no discomfort at rest is reported, but normal physical activity causes increased symptoms
        - *Moderate:* marked limitation of physical activity; no discomfort at rest is reported, but less than ordinary activity causes increased symptoms
        - *Severe:* unable to perform any physical activity at rest; symptoms may be present at rest, and symptoms are increased by almost any physical activity

2. List three imaging modalities used to diagnose expiratory central airway collapse.
    - *Fluoroscopy:* poorly displays anatomic details of tracheal and paratracheal structures and is unable to display simultaneously the anteroposterior and lateral walls of the airway; it is operator dependent and airway visualization is difficult in obese patients[52]
    - *Paired inspiratory/expiratory dynamic CT:* in a standard or low-dose protocol, allows excellent display of anatomic detail of the airway and quantification of airway collapse[53]
    - *Dynamic MRI:* limited experience, but advantages include documentation of the effects of pulsating vessels on adjacent airways and airway collapsibility without exposing patients to ionizing radiation or iodinated contrast media[16]

3. List three indications for treatment in this patient.

    Because the criteria used to define the exact degree of airway narrowing that leads to symptoms remain vague at this time, physicians should treat only patients who are functionally impaired. Patients with incidental abnormal airway collapse on bronchoscopy or CT scanning performed for other reasons probably should not undergo treatment.[25,26] Functional impairment may result from at least three causes:
    - Dyspnea
    - Cough
    - Mucus retention

    Dyspnea and cough are the main presenting complaints in TBM in at least three older studies.[2,5,52] More recent evidence shows that almost all patients have dyspnea as a main symptom or in combination with cough or mucus retention.[17,19] Therefore as for other pulmonary disorders, QOL and functional impairment scales may be appropriate to measure the impact of respiratory symptoms on overall health, daily life, and perceived well-being in patients suffering from malacia.

Expert Commentary

provided by Armin Ernst, MD

Tracheomalacia (TM) and tracheobronchomalacia (TBM) have been described already in the 1970s, but the area of symptomatic dynamic airway collapse has received significant widespread interest only in the last few years. It is a complicated issue: Symptoms of shortness of breath and recurrent infections are common problems in pulmonary practice, and unexplained extubation failures in critical care units can be frustrating. If examined and investigated, increasingly often the question is raised of whether observed expiratory collapse in a patient may be responsible for or may be contributing to the problem, and whether airway stabilization is indicated.

Tracheomalacia in adults seems to be common and has been reported to be present in up to a quarter of patients with COPD who undergo bronchoscopy. The advent and increased use of CT imaging and use of dynamic airway protocols also contribute to the increasing frequency of the finding. It is interesting to note that a certain amount of collapse is normal, and the frequently used cutoff of 50% reduction in cross-sectional area is arbitrary. Exhalation maneuvers used to elicit collapse are not standardized. Emerging evidence supports that this level is not uncommonly reached by healthy volunteers. In our practice, no interventions are performed if near total occlusion is not present AND if the patient has symptoms that are likely related.

In our experience, TBM may be associated with other entities such as emphysema, but it also occurs in idiopathic forms. Most important, not everyone with airway collapse is symptomatic from it, and not every airway collapse in a patient with symptoms is responsible for the problem. Pulmonary function tests have proved to have limited value in the assessment of patients, and even bronchoscopy performed with esophageal balloons in place is not always helpful and is difficult to perform routinely.

If sufficient collapse is present and the patient has symptoms, the next step is a trial of central airway stabilization. It serves diagnostic/confirmatory purposes as much as providing therapeutic relief. Even in a tracheomalacia specialty clinic, only about 75% of patients do improve with interventions. In our practice, we do not distinguish different TBM types, because this does not influence decision making or outcomes. For example, our patients with or without underlying COPD undergoing stent insertion have similar chances of improvement. Stent-related complications are frequent, often limiting the quality of life gains attained through airway stabilization. Therefore in experienced centers, surgical intervention should be considered.

The case presented here is typical. Secretion retention due to inability to effectively cough often paired with recurrent infections is the main symptom. Exercise-related dynamic occlusion and airflow obstruction cause dyspnea on exertion. Patients are treated empirically for obstructive pulmonary airway disorders for prolonged periods of time without clinical improvement. Pulmonary function tests generally are not helpful but here offer a lead followed by confirmatory CT imaging. CT is performed more easily than bronchoscopy for screening purposes, and dynamic protocols are superior to simple paired in/expiratory images but do require a more experienced technician who can coach the patient through the procedure.

As is appropriate, bronchoscopy was also performed. As pointed out earlier, maneuvers are not standardized and are performed differently at different institutions. Even coaching for forced exhalation may differ from operator to operator. At our institution, functional or dynamic bronchoscopy implies that physiologic measures must be obtained, such as pressure through an esophageal balloon, which often adds to the baseline evaluation. Philosophically, we would not call something "normal physiologic collapse" because "collapse" implies something bad or abnormal.

After evaluation, this patient had a high likelihood of benefiting from stent placement. Before proceeding, a full baseline performance evaluation must be established because the goal is to affect QOL and functional improvement. It would be our suggestion to include such baseline studies in the evaluation protocol, for example, by performing a St. George Respiratory Questionnaire and a 6-minute walk test to help evaluate treatment success.

Airway stent insertion is indicated as the next step, and metal stents must be avoided, as the authors suggest. Concerns about the use of muscle relaxants during general anesthesia in this patient population are of historic interest, as shown by the age of the reference. Use of muscle relaxants, in our experience, is safe, and we prefer standard intravenous induction for the procedure. Also, we prefer the placement of silicone Y-stents in the setting of adult TBM. Migration is a factor to consider, and it is effectively prevented with the use of a bifurcated stent. Placement technique or postprocedural management does not change significantly compared with straight stent insertion.

This patient appears to have improved, and management is fairly standard. Migration had to be addressed, and surgery could have been discussed with the patient, taking into account the limited comorbidities presented by the patient. Because the patient did not have significant stent-related problems, however, conservative management is certainly a viable option. Tapering of long-term respiratory medications should be attempted in all patients experiencing improvement after therapeutic bronchoscopy, as was done in this case. We were not told about measured improvements in his QOL or functional performance, nor were results of a 6MWT provided.

Of high importance and reflecting assessment by the authors that the disease is poorly understood, patients should be treated on protocols and prospective data obtained to enhance our knowledge. Patients with TBM should therefore be referred to centers that employ such protocols and record patient data and outcomes. Only through this increase in available data will we be able to design trials aimed at improving diagnostic standards and treatment approaches for this disease.

REFERENCES

1. Wright CD. Tracheomalacia. *Chest Surg Clin North Am.* 2003; 13:349-357.
2. Jokinen K, Palva T, Sutinen S, et al. Acquired tracheobronchomalacia. *Ann Clin Res.* 1977;9:52-57.
3. Collard P, Freitag L, Reynaert MS, et al. Respiratory failure due to tracheobronchomalacia. *Thorax.* 1996;51:224-226.
4. Koziej M, Górecka D. Cough-syncope syndrome in tracheobronchomalacia. *Pneumonol Alergol Pol.* 1992;60:89-91.
5. Nuutinen J. Acquired tracheobronchomalacia: a clinical study with bronchological correlations. *Ann Clin Res.* 1977;9:350-355.
6. Campbell AH, Faulks LW. Expiratory air-flow pattern in tracheobronchial collapse. *Am Rev Respir Dis.* 1965;92:781-791.
7. Healy F, Wilson AF, Fairshter RD. Physiologic correlates of airway collapse in chronic airflow obstruction. *Chest.* 1984;85:476-481.
8. Vincken WG, Cosio MG. Flow oscillations on the flow-volume loop: clinical and physiological implications. *Eur Respir J.* 1989;2: 543-549.
9. Bouhuys A, van de Woestijne KP. Mechanical consequences of airway smooth muscle relaxation. *J Appl Physiol.* 1971;30: 670-676.
10. Finder JD. Primary bronchomalacia in infants and children. *J Pediatr.* 1997;130:59-66.
11. Murgu SD, Colt HG. Treatment of adult tracheobronchomalacia and excessive dynamic airway collapse: an update. *Treat Respir Med.* 2006;5:103-115.
12. Murgu SD, Colt HG. A 68-year-old man with intractable dyspnea and wheezing 45 years after a pneumonectomy. *Chest.* 2006;129: 1107-1111.
13. Lee KS, Sun MR, Ernst A, et al. Comparison of dynamic expiratory CT with bronchoscopy for diagnosing airway malacia: a pilot evaluation. *Chest.* 2007;131:758-764.
14. Boiselle PM, Feller-Kopman D, Ashiku S, et al. Tracheobronchomalacia: evolving role of dynamic multislice helical CT. *Radiol Clin North Am.* 2003;41:627-636.
15. Baroni RH, Ashiku S, Boiselle PM. Dynamic CT evaluation of the central airways in patients undergoing tracheoplasty for tracheobronchomalacia. *AJR Am J Roentgenol.* 2005;184:1444-1449.
16. Suto Y, Tanabe Y. Evaluation of tracheal collapsibility in patients with tracheomalacia using dynamic MR imaging during coughing. *AJR Am J Roentgenol.* 1998;171:393-394.
17. Murgu SD, Colt HG. Description of a multidimensional classification system for patients with expiratory central airway collapse. *Respirology.* 2007;12:543-550.
18. Murgu SD, Colt HG. Complications of silicone stent insertion in patients with expiratory central airway collapse. *Ann Thorac Surg.* 2007;84:1870-1877.
19. Ernst A, Majid A, Feller-Kopman D, et al. Airway stabilization with silicone stents for treating adult tracheobronchomalacia: a prospective observational study. *Chest.* 2007;132:609-616.
20. Mercer M. Anesthesia for the patient with respiratory disease. *Update in Anaesthesia.* 2000;12:1-3.
21. Jung C, Inder JW. Management of adrenal insufficiency during the stress of medical illness and surgery. *Med J Aust.* 2008;188: 409-413.
22. Axelrod L. Perioperative management of patients treated with glucocorticoids. *Endocrinol Metab Clin N Am.* 2003;32:367-383.
23. Lipworth BJ. Systemic adverse effects of inhaled corticosteroid therapy: a systematic review and meta-analysis. *Arch Intern Med.* 1999;159:941-955.
24. Gysels MH, Higginson IJ. Caring for a person in advanced illness and suffering from breathlessness at home: threats and resources. *Palliat Support Care.* 2009;7:153-162.
25. Murgu SD, Colt HG. Tracheobronchomalacia and excessive dynamic airway collapse. *Respirology.* 2006;11:388-406.
26. Carden KA, Boiselle PM, Waltz DA, Ernst A. Tracheomalacia and tracheobronchomalacia in children and adults: an in-depth review. *Chest.* 2005;127:984-1005.
27. Zhang J, Hasegawa I, Feller-Kopman D, Boiselle PM. 2003 AUR Memorial Award. Dynamic expiratory volumetric CT imaging of the central airways: comparison of standard-dose and low-dose techniques. *Acad Radiol.* 2003;10:719-724.
28. Gilkeson RC, Ciancibello LM, Hejal RB, et al. Tracheobronchomalacia: dynamic airway evaluation with multidetector CT. *AJR Am J Roentgenol.* 2001;176:205-210.
29. Nuutinen J. Acquired tracheobronchomalacia. *Eur J Respir Dis.* 1982;63:380-387.
30. Boiselle PM, O'Donnell CR, Bankier AA, et al. Tracheal collapsibility in healthy volunteers during forced expiration: assessment with multidetector CT. *Radiology.* 2009;252:255-262.
31. Park JG, Edell ES. Dynamic airway collapse: different from tracheomalacia. *Rev Port Pneumol.* 2005;11:600-602.
32. Baram D, Smaldone G. Tracheal collapse versus tracheobronchomalacia: normal function versus disease. *Am J Respir Crit Care Med.* 2006;174:724; author reply 724-725.
33. Park J, Edell E. It's in the definition. *Chest.* 2006;129:497; author reply 497-498.
34. Smaldone GC, Smith PL. Location of flow-limiting segments via airway catheters near residual volume in humans. *J Appl Physiol.* 1985;59:502-508.
35. Hogg JC, Macklem PT, Thurlbeck WM. Site and nature of airway obstruction in chronic obstructive lung disease. *N Engl J Med.* 1968;278:1355-1360.
36. Colt H, Prakash U, Offord K. Bronchoscopy in North America: survey by the American Association for Bronchology. *J Bronchol.* 1999;2000:8-25.
37. Ferguson GT, Benoist J. Nasal continuous positive airway pressure in the treatment of tracheobronchomalacia. *Am Rev Respir Dis.* 1993;147:457-461.
38. Adliff M, Ngato D, Keshavjee S, et al. Treatment of diffuse tracheomalacia secondary to relapsing polychondritis with continuous positive airway pressure. *Chest.* 1997;112:1701-1704.
39. Bolot G, Poupart M, Pignat JC, et al. Self-expanding metal stents for the management of bronchial stenosis and bronchomalacia after lung transplantation. *Laryngoscope.* 1998;108: 1230-1233.
40. FDA Public Health Notification. Complications from metallic tracheal stents in patients with benign airway disorders. 2005; Available at: http://www.fda.gov/MedicalDevices/Safety/Alertsand Notices/PublicHealthNotifications/ucm062115.htm. Accessed February 21, 2011.
41. Wright CD, Grillo HC, Hammoud ZT, et al. Tracheoplasty for expiratory collapse of central airways. *Ann Thorac Surg.* 2005;80: 259-267.
42. Majid A, Guerrero J, Gangadharan S, et al. Tracheobronchoplasty for severe tracheobronchomalacia: a prospective outcome analysis. *Chest.* 2008;134:801-807.
43. Grillo HC. Surgical treatment of postintubation tracheal injuries. *J Thorac Cardiovasc Surg.* 1979;78:860-875.
44. National Network of Libraries of Medicine. Health literacy. Available at: http://nnlm.gov/outreach/consumer/hlthlit.html#A1. Accessed February 21, 2011.
45. Ad Hoc Committee on Health Literacy for the Council on Scientific Affairs, American Medical Association. Health literacy: report of the Council on Scientific Affairs. *JAMA.* 1999;281: 552-557.
46. Licker M, Schweizer A, Ellenberger C, et al. Perioperative medical management of patients with COPD. *Int J Chron Obstruct Pulmon Dis.* 2007;2:493-515.
47. Iribarren JL, Jiménez JJ, Hernández D, et al. Relative adrenal insufficiency and hemodynamic status in cardiopulmonary bypass surgery patients: a prospective cohort study. *J Cardiothorac Surg.* 2010;5:26.
48. Seravalli L, Pralong F, Revelly JP, et al. Adrenal function after induction of cardiac surgery patients with an etomidate bolus: a retrospective study. *Ann Fr Anesth Reanim.* 2009;28:743-747.
49. McMahon CC, Rainey L, Fulton B, Conacher ID. Central airway compression: anaesthetic and intensive care consequences. *Anaesthesia.* 1997;52:158-162.
50. Perrin G, Colt HG, Martin C, et al. Safety of interventional rigid bronchoscopy using intravenous anesthesia and spontaneous assisted ventilation: a prospective study. *Chest.* 1992;102:1526-1530.
51. Murgu SD, Pecson J, Colt HG. Bronchoscopy on noninvasive positive pressure ventilation: indications and technique. *Respir Care.* 2010;55:595-600.
52. Johnson TH, Mikita JJ, Wilson RJ, Feist JH. Acquired tracheomalacia. *Radiology.* 1973;109:576-580.
53. Boiselle PM, Reynolds KF, Ernst A. Multiplanar and three-dimensional imaging of the central airways with multidetector CT. *AJR Am J Roentgenol.* 2002;179:301-308.

Chapter 12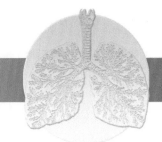

Stent Insertion for Diffuse Circumferential Tracheobronchomalacia Caused by Relapsing Polychondritis

This chapter emphasizes the following elements of the Four Box Approach: physical examination, complementary tests, and functional status assessment; risk-benefits analysis and therapeutic alternatives; techniques and instrumentation; and follow-up tests, visits, and procedures.

CASE DESCRIPTION

The patient was a 58-year-old woman who had respiratory arrest while playing golf. She was intubated by paramedics and was brought to the hospital, where she was found to be in hypercapnic respiratory failure despite being mechanically ventilated. Arterial blood gas analysis showed the following: pH 7.16/PCO_2 70 mm Hg/PaO_2 300 mm Hg/HCO_3 24 mm Hg, consistent with acute respiratory acidosis. Peak airway pressures were consistently high ($\approx$60 cm H_2O), but plateau pressure was normal on mechanical ventilation in assist control volume control mode: TV 500 mL, RR 16, PEEP 5 cm H_2O, and FiO_2 of 1. According to her husband, shortness of breath and wheezing several days earlier had prompted a visit to the emergency department at an outside hospital. There, she was treated with systemic corticosteroids. Apparently her symptoms improved quickly, and she was discharged home within 48 hours. She had in fact been diagnosed with adult-onset asthma several years ago, for which she was taking albuterol inhalers as needed, fluticasone/salmeterol, Singulair, and prednisone 10 mg every other day. Several months before this admission, however, the patient had developed stridor. A working diagnosis of relapsing polychondritis was made on the basis of tracheal wall thickening noted on computed tomography of her neck. Her past medical history included a nonmalignant thyroid goiter, which had been removed because it was presumptively contributing to her shortness of breath. She had an office job, had never smoked, and had no occupational exposure to toxins or fumes. Her basic metabolic panel and electrocardiogram were normal. Complete blood count revealed hemoglobin of 10.5 g/dL. On arrival, flexible bronchoscopy showed complete collapse of the airway distal to the No. 7 endotracheal tube. Emergent rigid bronchoscopy showed a severe subglottic stricture and diffuse collapse of the entire cartilaginous structure from the subglottis to the distal mainstem bronchi (Figure 12-1).

DISCUSSION POINTS

1. Describe the relationship between airway stents and respiratory tract infections.
2. Describe two strategies used to prevent stent-related infections and mucus plugging.
3. Describe two alternative treatments to silicone stent insertion in patients with tracheobronchomalacia resulting from relapsing polychondritis.

CASE RESOLUTION

Initial Evaluations

Physical Examination, Complementary Tests, and Functional Status Assessment

This patient had bronchoscopic evidence of diffuse collapse of the cartilaginous wall of the trachea and mainstem bronchi with sparing of the posterior membrane—findings consistent with a diagnosis of circumferential tracheobronchomalacia (TBM), and classic for relapsing polychondritis (RP). RP is a multisystem disease,* and it is incapacitating and life threatening because of its airway involvement.[1] Auricular chondritis, the most common initial presentation, is seen in 85% to 95% of patients with RP. This patient, however, had no evidence of RP in the eyes, nose, or external ears. Isolated pulmonary presentation, as seen in this case, is not that unusual, and because of its often episodic nature, may result in a significant delay in diagnosis. In a review of 66 patients, the elapsed time from patient presentation for medical care for RP-related symptoms† to diagnosis was reportedly 2.9 years.[1] In a small case series of five patients with RP and severe airway involvement requiring stent insertion, all patients were given the diagnosis of asthma before RP was diagnosed.[2]

Malacia, identified as loss of supportive cartilaginous structures, is a chronic consequence of RP and is probably due to recurrent extensive inflammation. It may be asymptomatic in earlier stages and detected only on pulmonary function testing, but it becomes symptomatic when it involves the upper airways.[3] Similar to this case, dynamic tracheal collapse might occur suddenly, causing

---

*It is characterized by recurrent and potentially severe episodes of inflammation of cartilaginous structures of the external ear, nose, peripheral joints, larynx, and tracheobronchial tree. Other proteoglycan-rich structures can become involved, including the eyes, heart, blood vessels, and inner ear.

†Systemic symptoms include fever, lethargy, and weight loss; common organ-specific symptoms include external ear pain, nasal pain, hoarseness, throat pain, difficulty talking, and arthralgias.

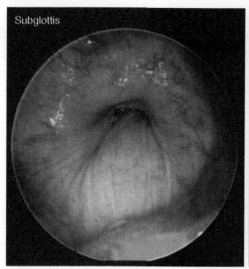
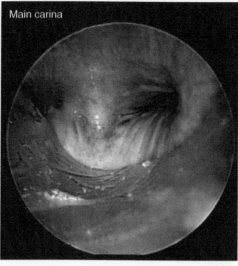

Figure 12-1 The subglottis and the lower trachea at the level of the main carina show complete collapse of the cartilaginous structures and severe airway wall edema—findings consistent with severe, diffuse, circumferential tracheobronchomalacia.

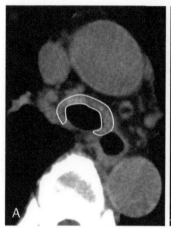
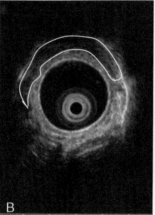
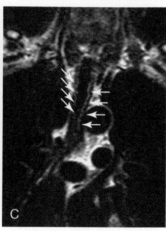

Figure 12-2 **A,** Axial computed tomography view shows thickened cartilage. **B,** High-frequency ultrasound (20 MHz) shows thickened cartilage. **C,** Coronal T2 magnetic resonance imaging reveals diffusely thickened cartilage *(white arrows).* Images are obtained from a different patient. *(Courtesy Teruomi Miyazawa and Noriaki Kurimoto, St. Mariana University, Kawasaki, Japan.)*

dyspnea, respiratory arrest, and death.[4] On histology, the airway cartilage shows empty lacunae (empty spaces within the cartilage), a mixed population of inflammatory cells,[5] and abundant inflammatory exudates that are often noted to invade the periphery of necrotic cartilaginous tissues. An immunologic mechanism is likely responsible for this disease because RP is often associated with rheumatic or autoimmune disease, although the presence of autoantibodies* is inconsistent. Various studies have found circulating antibodies to cartilage-specific collagen types II, IX, and XI to be present in 30% to 70% of patients with RP, with antibodies to type II collagen[†] noted and correlating with the severity of acute RP episodes.[6] Airway wall structural abnormalities in RP are detected by histopathology but can be identified using high-frequency (20 MHz) radial probe endobronchial ultrasonography (EBUS).[7] EBUS reveals thickened and

irregular cartilage, but the posterior membrane is normal (Figure 12-2).[8] A definitive diagnosis of RP usually is based on the following criteria set by MacAdam et al.[*5] and Damiani and Levine[†9]: (1) bilateral auricular chondritis; (2) nonerosive seronegative inflammatory polyarthritis; (3) nasal chondritis; (4) ocular inflammation; (5) respiratory tract chondritis; and (6) audiovestibular damage.

In one case series, the tracheobronchial tree was involved in about 56% of patients, and respiratory symptoms were responsible for the initial presentation in about 14%.[5] In a larger case series of 145 patients suffering from RP, 31 patients had airway involvement, making the prevalence 21%.[10] In many of these patients, similar to our patient, complaints of respiratory symptoms led to the diagnosis of RP, underscoring the fact that clinically significant airway compromise does not necessarily

---

*Evidence suggesting an autoimmune cause includes pathologic findings of infiltrating T cells, the presence of antigen-antibody complexes in affected cartilage, cellular and humoral responses against collagen type II and other collagen (i.e., types IX and XI) antigens, and the observation that immunosuppressive regimens most often suppress the disease.

†Also seen in rheumatoid arthritis.

---

*Three of six clinical features necessary for diagnosis.

†One of three conditions necessary for diagnosis: three McAdam et al. criteria; one McAdam et al. criterion plus positive histology results; or two McAdam et al. criteria plus therapeutic response to corticosteroid or dapsone therapy.

Figure 12-3 End-inspiratory axial computed tomography in **(A)** mediastinal window and **(B)** lung window, showing thickening of the tracheal wall and consequent airway narrowing.

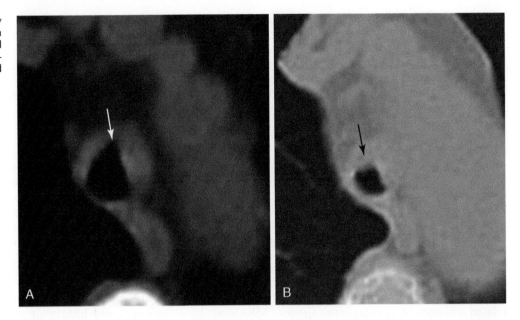

present late in the course of the disease. RP-related airway disease is more common among women and in patients between 11 and 61 years of age (median age, 42 years) at the time of first symptoms.* In this particular study, respiratory symptoms were the first manifestation of disease in 17 patients (54%), and dyspnea was the most common symptom in 20 patients (64%), followed by cough, stridor, and hoarseness. Airway involvement in remaining patients included subglottic stenosis (n = 8; 26%), focal and diffuse malacia (n = 15; 48%), and focal stenosis in different areas of the bronchial tree.[10]

In addition to a thorough review of systems during initial evaluation of a patient suffering from this disease, the treating team should set up realistic expectations, because it is known that the 5 year survival rate associated with RP is reported to be 66% to 74% but could be as low as 45% if RP occurs with systemic vasculitis. Other studies report a survival rate of 94% at 8 years, but these data may represent RP in patients with less severe disease than was observed in patients studied in earlier reports.[1]

Dynamic (aka functional) bronchoscopy with dynamic breathing and coughing maneuvers is usually performed to visualize and quantify the airway collapse when patients are evaluated for TBM. The degree of dynamic collapse is estimated by visual inspection but can be objectively quantified using morphometric bronchoscopy.† If TBM is present, the amount of collapse during passive and forced exhalation, as well as cough, is documented. In our case, complete collapse was clearly seen on bronchoscopy, making other quantifying methods unnecessary (see Figure 12-1).

Paired inspiratory/expiratory dynamic computed tomography (CT) scanning can reveal the degree, and

potentially the cause, of expiratory central airway collapse.[11] The boundary between normal physiologic dynamic airway compression and abnormal collapse is far from established, however, and disagreement continues regarding how much of a decrease in cross-sectional area actually signals clinically and physiologically significant airway narrowing.[12] Although many investigators use 50% or greater reduction in airway cross-sectional area between inspiration and expiration to identify malacia, recent studies suggest that this definition leads to overdiagnosis, given that 78% of normal people reportedly exceed this criterion.[13] However, it is noteworthy that in RP, thickened airway wall is noted, and even during inspiration, the lumen caliber is not normal (Figure 12-3) (see video on ExpertConsult.com) (Video III.12.1). In view of this, the use of absolute cutoff values to define abnormal collapse is less relevant, and what matters most when evaluating these patients is the impact on flow dynamics and symptoms. One disadvantage of dynamic CT scanning is that expiratory images can be technically unsatisfactory when patients are unable to cooperate with dynamic breathing instructions, thus failing to coordinate breathing with the timing of the scan. This is particularly the case in patients with respiratory distress or respiratory failure on mechanical ventilation. In these cases, CT is inadequate to evaluate for malacia.[12] Given our patient's unstable respiratory status, CT scanning was not performed preoperatively.

When feasible, however, CT should be performed and may show tracheobronchial wall thickening (see Figure 12-2) with or without calcification (seen in ≈40 % of patients). These findings are not very sensitive (seen in 17 of 30 patients in one study); however, all patients will have sparing of the posterior membrane—a characteristic finding in RP.[10] CT may also reveal varying degrees of tracheal narrowing, often involving multiple segments of the trachea. In addition to its ability to reveal malacia, expiratory images may reveal consequent air trapping. The CT scan is also sensitive in detecting lower airway disease manifested by concentric narrowing in lobar and

---

*Among patients with serious airway manifestations, females predominate (female-to-male ratio, 2.6:1).

†A software processing method whereby bronchoscopic digital images are analyzed to measure airway lumen diameter can be used to objectively quantify the degree of airway narrowing.

segmental bronchi and subsegmental bronchi.[14] Dynamic CT scanning should be done according to the institution's central airways CT investigation protocol, usually without intravenous contrast administration. Images are initially obtained using a standard radiation dose technique at end inspiration (170 mAs, 120 kVp, 2.5 mm collimation, high-speed mode, and pitch equivalent of 1.5). This is followed by a low-dose examination (40 mAs, 120 kVp, 2.5 mm collimation, high-speed mode, and pitch equivalent of 1.5) during the dynamic expiratory phase of respiration. Axial CT data are subsequently used to create a series of multiplanar and three-dimensional (3D) images, which are reviewed in conjunction with the axial images.

Magnetic resonance imaging (MRI) is also a useful adjunct in clinical diagnosis. MRI is better than CT in distinguishing between edema, fibrosis, and inflammation. T1-weighted images, T2-weighted images (see Figure 12-2), and T1-weighted images with gadolinium contrast provide characterization of relapsing polychondritis-related changes in cartilaginous tissues. MRI may be useful in detecting other potential RP-related problems such as thickening of the thoracic aorta before dilation occurs. Because of its lack of ionizing radiation, MRI may be a useful noninvasive test for monitoring the effects of treatment.

Pulmonary function testing (PFT) with flow-volume loop studies were not feasible in our patient but are recommended in patients with RP who present with respiratory symptoms. PFTs may assist in differential diagnoses and provide information about the severity of airway obstruction. PFTs can also be used to monitor disease activity. PFTs in patients with RP who have respiratory involvement demonstrate a nonreversible obstructive pattern with the decrease in forced expiratory volume in 1 second correlating with the degree of dyspnea.[15] In general, both in normal people and in patients with obstructive ventilatory impairment, the flow-limiting segment, called the *choke point,* tends to be located in a region of minimum cross-sectional area and minimum side pressure within the airway when maximal flow is reached.[16] Because maximum expiratory flow is airway compliance dependent, increased compliance, as is seen in patients with TBM, results in increased airway resistance and decreased maximum expiratory flow. Studies of airflow limitation in experimental models demonstrate that when the collapsing trachea is supported by a rigid tube, airflow improves and the flow-limiting segment migrates from the central airway toward the periphery.[17]

In this regard, studies in patients with RP have evaluated dynamic intrathoracic obstruction using a combination of physiologic and imaging modalities consisting of PFT, airway measurements with 3D-CT, and radial probe EBUS. To properly assess the location of the choke point, investigators measured intra-airway pressure and cross-sectional areas of the airway from bronchi to trachea.[18] For seven patients who underwent self-expandable metallic stent insertion, choke points were detected in the trachea, mainstem bronchi, or lobar bronchi. After stent insertion, the flow-volume curves displayed significant improvements in flow limitation. Intraluminal catheter measurements of pressure differences decreased significantly, suggesting that stents had been inserted appropriately at the flow-limiting segments. Expiratory CT scanning revealed mosaic patterns, indicating air trapping due to migration of the choke points to smaller bronchi, as had been demonstrated in previous experimental studies.[17,18]

Comorbidities

This patient had no evidence of other organ involvement from RP. The clinical relevance of RP is not limited to airflow obstruction but extends to other systems and may include heart block and vasculitis of both small and larger vessels. Making a prompt diagnosis of heart involvement is essential, especially if patients are scheduled to undergo general anesthesia.[19] The cardiovascular system is reportedly affected in 24% of patients with RP. When possible, a thorough history and physical examination should be performed to evaluate for chest pain, abdominal pain, history of pericarditis, abnormal heart rate or rhythm, syncope, and history of subacute myocardial infarction (found on electrocardiogram [ECG]). Aortic and mitral valve regurgitation, aortic aneurysm, aortitis, aortic thrombosis, pericarditis, first- to third-degree heart block, and myocardial infarction, at times mediated through ostial stenosis of a coronary artery or arteries, have been reported.[20] Furthermore, although the life expectancy in all patients with RP is decreased compared with age- and sex-matched healthy individuals, patients with RP and renal involvement have a significantly lower age-adjusted life expectancy. Among those with renal disease (glomerulonephritis* diagnosed on the basis of a diagnostic renal biopsy or the presence of microhematuria and proteinuria), uremia is a common cause of death.[21]

A high prevalence of other autoimmune disorders has been found in patients with RP. These may include systemic vasculitis ($\approx$13%), cutaneous leukocytoclastic vasculitis ($\approx$7%), thyroid disease ($\approx$6%), rheumatoid arthritis ($\approx$5%), and systemic lupus erythematosus ($\approx$4%).[20] Association with complex immunologic conditions such as a combination of Crohn's disease ($\approx$2%), ulcerative colitis ($\approx$2%), and epidermolysis bullosa acquisita has also been described.[22]

Support System

The husband was very supportive. He requested more information about her diagnosis and searched Internet support sites for patients with RP and their families. Although we do not take responsibility for quality, the website from the Relapsing Polychondritis Support and Awareness Foundation may be helpful.[23]

Patient Preferences and Expectations

For patients with TBM, the need for intervention is determined on a per-patient basis and involves consideration of the identified abnormality, the severity of symptoms, and patient preferences. In this case, the patient's malacia

---

*A proposed mechanism in the pathogenesis of renal involvement in relapsing polychondritis derives from the deposition of immune complexes leading to glomerular damage.

resulted in respiratory failure. On the basis of previous conversations between the patient and her husband, she desired to undergo further tests and procedures to improve her breathing, and had not selected comfort care in case of respiratory failure or risk of death.

Procedural Strategies

Indications

In general, treatment for patients with expiratory central airway collapse caused by TBM depends on the severity of functional impairment, the cause, the severity of airway narrowing, and the extent of airway collapse. This patient had severe, diffuse circumferential tracheobronchomalacia resulting from RP. She presented with respiratory insufficiency requiring prompt intervention. Weaning from the ventilator without intervention was not feasible in view of central airway obstruction distal to the endotracheal tube, resulting in persistent respiratory acidosis despite positive-pressure ventilation.

Contraindications

No contraindications to rigid bronchoscopy were noted.

Expected Results

Study results show that many patients with severe TBM requiring airway stabilization who are not surgical candidates can benefit immediately from airway stent insertion in terms of improvement in functional status, decreased extent of airway narrowing, and reduced severity of airway collapse.[24] In one series, adverse effects from silicone stent insertion were very common; however, a total of 26 stent-related adverse events were noted in 10 of 12 patients (83%) a median of 29 days after intervention, including 6 cases of granulation tissue formation, 8 stent migrations, and 12 cases of partial obstruction from mucus plugs. Five emergent flexible bronchoscopies were necessary, of which 1 prompted an emergent rigid bronchoscopy to manage granulation tissue and post obstructive pneumonia; the other 4 emergent flexible bronchoscopies were done to remove mucus plugging. Six rigid bronchoscopies were performed emergently because of new respiratory symptoms.[24] In a different series evaluating only patients with RP and airway involvement, 12 patients (40%) required intervention, including balloon dilation alone (n = 5), stent placement (n = 3), tracheotomy (n = 1), balloon dilation with stent insertion (n = 1), balloon dilation with tracheostomy (n = 1), and tracheostomy with stent insertion (n = 1). Most patients experienced improvement in airway symptoms after intervention, although 1 patient died of progression of airway disease during the follow-up period.[10] Most of the patients treated in this study had stenosis, not malacia; in fact, of 8 patients with bronchoscopically detected TBM in the study, only 3 were treated (2 by stent insertion and 1 by tracheostomy and removal of previously placed stents).[10]

Team Experience

Rigid bronchoscopy is performed on a weekly basis at this institution, and TBM is a major focus of the operators' clinical research. However, such a severe form of

diffuse, circumferential TBM resulting in respiratory failure is rarely seen, making it impossible to predict success or failure of the procedure in terms of ability to remove the patient from mechanical ventilation.

Therapeutic Alternatives

As of this writing, no medical, minimally invasive, or surgical treatment that cures RP is available, especially once cartilage destruction and malacia are established. Stents are reserved for patients with airway involvement (stenosis or malacia) and severe functional impairment.[2] In milder forms of airway involvement, treatment should be optimized before invasive therapies are considered. Continuous prednisone therapy has been shown to decrease the severity, frequency, and duration of relapses but does not stop disease progression.[5] Prednisone (20 to 60 mg/day) is administered in the acute phase and is tapered to 5 to 25 mg/day for maintenance. Severe relapses may require 80 to 100 mg/day.[5] Newer immuno-modulating agents such as tumor necrosis factor receptor blockers may have a role in treating the inflammatory destruction of cartilaginous structures and can also be used as steroid-sparing agents.[25] Despite aggressive medical therapy (prednisone, mycophenolate mofetil, etanercept, and methotrexate), many patients experience symptom progression warranting invasive interventions.

1. *Tracheostomy:* may not fully palliate airway collapse owing to malacia of the more distal airways beyond the tracheotomy site.[26,27] Tracheostomy is useful when it stents or bypasses the malacic airway or a subglottic stenosis, as is noted in this video from a different patient with RP and subglottic stenosis (see video on ExpertConsult.com) (Video III.12.2); tracheostomy also allows invasive ventilatory support when necessary and offers a secured airway in cases of acute airway obstruction.[12] However, tracheostomy can be complicated by secondary tracheomalacia and stenosis at the stoma site.[28] From a physiologic standpoint, tracheostomy may be inadequate and may exacerbate diffuse malacia because it bypasses the physiologic function of the glottis to maintain positive transmural pressure that keeps the airway lumen patent.[12]

2. *Membranous tracheoplasty:* not an option for patients with true malacia from cartilaginous destruction[24]; surgical cases of tracheoplasty excluded RP. In the largest case series reported of patients with RP and airway involvement, none of the 30 patients underwent tracheoplasty.[10] This procedure is advocated for some patients with tracheomalacia. The procedure attempts to restore a normal anatomic configuration of the airway, so that cartilaginous structures are brought into a more normal C shape from their flattened pattern.[29] This procedure is associated with significant complications* and does not apply to patients with circumferential

---

*Complications included a new respiratory infection in 14 patients, pulmonary embolism in 2, and atrial fibrillation in 6. Six patients required reintubation, and 9 received a postoperative tracheotomy; 47 patients required postoperative aspiration bronchoscopy.

diffuse TBM from RP, but only to carefully selected patients with crescent-type TBM.[30]

3. *Other surgical interventions:* External airway splinting using other tissues of the body or Gore-Tex (A. L. Gore, Flagstaff, Ariz) reportedly prevents collapse in cases of severe upper airway disease.[27] The success of laryngotracheal reconstruction has been anecdotally reported when tracheal or subglottic stenosis occurs in isolated segments.[31]

4. *Other types of straight airway stents* (Figure 12-4): Proper sizing of the stent (length and diameter) in relation to the dimensions of the trachea or bronchus is important to avoid stent-related complications such as migration, mucus plugging, granulation, and tumor ingrowth. Both self-expandable metallic stents and silicone stents have been used in patients with malacia from RP.[2,4,18] Sometimes, more than one stent may be required if symptoms persist after stent insertion, presumably because of distally migrated choke points.[18,32] With regard to stent selection for this disease, the bronchoscopist should consider the biomechanical properties of the airway stents: Silicone stents have excellent force compression characteristics and are readily removable in case of complications[33]; metal stents on the other hand, have been associated with severe complications including stent fracture, rupture, and excessive mucosal ingrowth and epithelialization in patients with malacia.[34]

5. *The dynamic stent (Rusch Y stent, Rusch AG, Duluth, Ga) is a bifurcated silicone stent that is designed to simulate tracheal morphology:* It is reinforced anteriorly by horseshoe-shaped metal rings that resemble tracheal cartilages and a soft posterior wall that behaves like the membranous trachea by allowing inward bulging during cough. Stent fracture from fatigue and retained secretions are rarely encountered,* and the stent is used for strictures of the trachea, main carina, and/or main bronchi; tracheobronchomalacia; tracheobronchomegaly with excessive dynamic airway collapse; and esophago-respiratory fistula.[35]

6. The Polyflex stent (Boston Scientific, Natick, Mass) is a self-expanding stent made of cross-woven polyester threads embedded in silicone. Its wall to inner diameter is thinner than that of Dumon (Novatech, Grasse, France) or Noppen (Reynder Medical Supplies, Lennik, Belgium) stents. Its expansile force is stronger than that seen with the Dumon or Ultraflex stent (Boston Scientific).[36] This stent can be used to treat benign and malignant strictures, esophago-respiratory fistula, and tracheomalacia (Figure 12-5); stents of different lengths and diameters and tapered models are available for sealing stump fistulas. Incorporation of tungsten into the stent makes it radiopaque and easier to identify on chest radiograph. The stent's outer surface, however, is smooth, which increases the risk for migration. In a small series of 12 patients in whom 16 Polyflex stents were used for benign airway disorders including TBM, the reported complication rate was 75% even though immediate palliation was achieved in most cases (90%). Stent migration was the most common complication that occurred between 24 hours and 7 months after deployment with all 4 patients with lung transplant–related anastomotic stenoses encountering complications: 2 had significant mucus plugging requiring emergent bronchoscopy, whereas the stents migrated in the other 2 patients.[37]

7. *Laser treatment:* Yttrium aluminum pevroskyte (YAP) laser treatment was anecdotally reported to improve lung function and symptoms in excessive dynamic airway collapse due to Mounier-Kuhn syndrome; this was done, however, with the intention of stiffening the posterior membrane by devascularization and subsequent retraction of tissues.[38] The YAP laser has been used for treatment of a variety of disease processes involving the central airways.

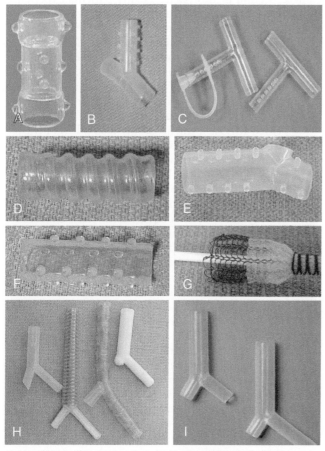

Figure 12-4 Types of stents. **A,** Tracheobronxane (aka Vergnon) stent. **B,** Y-shaped custom-made stent with studded bronchial arm. **C,** Montgomery T-tubes. **D,** Noppen stent. **E,** L-shaped studded silicone stent. **F,** Dumon-type studded straight silicone stent. **G,** Ultraflex partially covered self-expanding metallic stent. **H,** Various types of Y stents. From left to right: the Hood Y stent, the Dynamic (Rusch) stent, the Orlowski stent, and the custom bifurcated stent with blind bronchial limb. **I,** Hood Y stents with different left bronchial arm lengths.

---

*Other disadvantages include its small airway diameter, danger of bilateral obstruction from secretions, and potential loss of airway when the stent is inserted by rigid laryngoscopy.

Figure 12-5 A, Severe crescent-type tracheomalacia in a patient with tracheomegaly. **B,** Airway patency is restored by a 22 × 60 mm Polyflex stent.

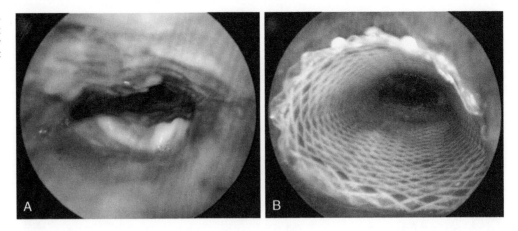

Its wavelength is double that of the yttrium aluminum garnet (YAG) laser, allowing for tissue devascularization and coagulation at low power (15 to 20 W) in a discontinuous mode.[39] The depth of penetration using the YAP laser is estimated at 3 mm, and it may reach the submucosal tissues, triggering a retractile fibrotic process that rigidifies the posterior membrane. This effect has been studied in humans to reduce palatal flutter in an attempt to reduce snoring.[40]

8. Noninvasive positive-pressure ventilation can be used to maintain airway patency, facilitate secretion drainage, and improve expiratory flow. Continuous positive airway pressure (CPAP) acts as a pneumatic stent, decreases pulmonary resistance, and improves expiratory airflow obstruction. It has been used successfully in patients with tracheomalacia due to RP.[41] The response to CPAP can be documented by performing CPAP-assisted bronchoscopy[42] or CPAP-assisted computed tomography.[43]

Cost-Effectiveness

No guidelines or randomized controlled studies have compared the different treatment alternatives for malacia due to RP. In an airway emergency, as was seen in our case, our responsibility was to attempt to restore airway patency and therefore emergent rigid bronchoscopy with performance of silicone stent placement.

Informed Consent

Informed consent was obtained from the husband because the patient was mildly sedated and was on mechanical ventilation and unable to speak. Although she was able to follow commands, we considered that her relative state of alertness was misleading, and that she was not able to make an autonomous decision. From a bioethics perspective, autonomy is often viewed as "self-governing." Physicians may presume that any decision coming from a competent individual is autonomous. It is suggested, however, to focus on the "governing" aspect, which emphasizes controlling, directing, and influencing. This means that someone's choice is insightful and is directed or controlled by adequate information, a clear perspective on values, and an appreciation of options.[44] The patient should also be able to appreciate alternatives and

understand the consequences of removing treatment or selecting certain alternative diagnostic or therapeutic modalities. In our judgment, our patient was not able to do so reliably, thus the need to obtain consent from her husband, who acted in his wife's best interests.

Techniques and Results

Anesthesia and Perioperative Care

In a patient with severe TBM, worsening intrathoracic airway obstruction may occur during induction of anesthesia despite the presence of the indwelling endotracheal tube. We do not use neuromuscular blocking agents. We believe that these agents should probably be avoided because they may eliminate airway muscle and chest wall tone, which normally provides extrinsic support for the critically narrowed airway during spontaneous ventilation.[45] In addition, patients with TBM may not tolerate the supine position after induction.

Instrumentation

We used a 12 mm Efer-Dumon rigid ventilating bronchoscope (Bryan Corp., Woburn, Mass). The dynamic features of TBM can make selection of the type and size of the stent being inserted problematic. For example, we use Y-shaped stents infrequently because we try to preserve as much normal mucosa as possible, thereby decreasing the likelihood of stent obstruction by tenacious mucous secretions, a common complication, especially in patients with chronically inflamed airways. Y-shaped or L-shaped stents do not usually migrate, but from a technical standpoint, insertion in a patient with complete airway collapse is not always straightforward. Insertion of Y- and L-shaped stents can be more problematic than straight stent insertion, especially if the patient's airway mucosa is severely inflamed and friable. In this patient, we decided to insert three separate straight studded silicone stents: a 12 × 30 mm in the right main bronchus (RMB), a 12 × 40 mm in the left main bronchus (LMB), and a 12 × 50 mm in the upper trachea.

Anatomic Dangers and Other Risks

The risk of airway perforation during intubation with the rigid bronchoscope and stent insertion is small in the absence of tumor, necrosis, fistula, or a very thin posterior

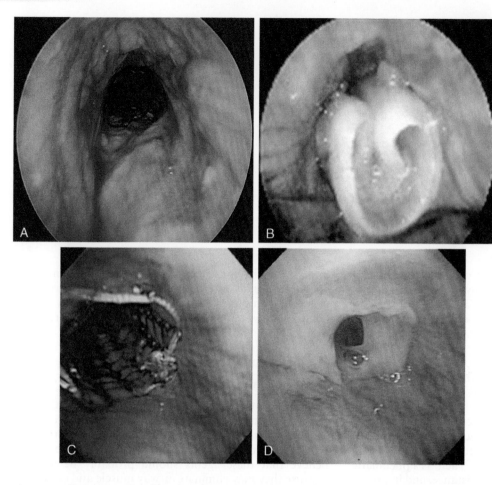

Figure 12-6 A, A patient with "hourglass"-shaped tracheal stenosis with malacia underwent a 14 × 40 mm straight studded silicone stent after dilation with a 12 mm Efer-Dumon rigid bronchoscope. **B,** The stent, however, failed to unfold, causing tracheal obstruction and prompting its immediate manipulation. **C,** A different patient with distal left main bronchial tumor and cartilaginous destruction underwent stent insertion with a 12 × 30 mm partially covered self-expandable metallic stent. **D,** Three weeks later, on follow-up bronchoscopy, the patient had near complete obstruction of the stent by thick yellow-green mucoid secretions, despite using saline nebulization 3 times daily.

airway wall. In a patient like this, however, with virtually no airway lumen, the operator should ascertain that the rigid scope is properly aligned with the airway, "feeling the airway" while advancing the rigid bronchoscope, noting, as taught by Chevalier Jackson, that "bronchoscopists must have eyes on the tips of their fingers." Once the rigid scope is in position, unfolding silicone stents may be difficult once deployed (Figure 12-6), especially because the exact expansile force needed to restore airway patency is not known. In theory, one could optimize therapeutic outcome by matching the stent's expansile force with the stress-strain properties of the stenosis.[46] Details of these biomechanical properties of airway stents,* however, were not available to the operators at the time of this case, and intraoperative measurements of airway wall tension were not performed.

Results and Procedure-Related Complications

The patient was intubated with a 12 mm Efer-Dumon rigid bronchoscope after the endotracheal tube was removed under direct bronchoscopic visualization. Severe

airway narrowing started in the subglottis and extended to the mainstem bronchi. Complete cartilaginous collapse occurred, consistent with a diagnosis of relapsing polychondritis (see video on ExpertConsult.com) (Video III.12.3). The airway lumen was slightly increased by administration of positive-pressure ventilation through the rigid bronchoscope. We placed three separate straight studded silicone stents in the following order: first, the 12 × 40 mm in the LMB, overriding the main carina and customized onsite to allow ventilation to the RMB; then the 12 × 30 mm in the RMB, cut obliquely at the distal aspect to allow ventilation to the right upper lobe; and last, the 12 × 50 mm in the trachea to ensure patency of the middle and upper trachea with the proximal aspect 2 cm below the cords. Patency of the trachea and mainstem bronchi was restored, but the choke points had migrated distal to the bronchial stents (see video on ExpertConsult.com) (Video III.12.4).

We did not perform biopsies of the airway wall for the following reasons: (1) Biopsy of the cartilage is a potential source of infection in a patient who is already immunosuppressed from long-term steroid use; (2) biopsies of the cartilage are indicated only if histopathologic data are required to meet the diagnostic criteria for RP; and (3) in a patient with respiratory failure and airway compromise, the risk of bleeding from deep biopsy outweighs the benefit of having histologic confirmation. Once the stents were in place, the anesthetic drugs were stopped. The patient was extubated several minutes later, when she

---

*Biomechanical properties of an airway stent may influence the operator's decision regarding stent selection. For instance, a very tortuous left main bronchus may benefit from a stent that has high resistance to angulation (i.e., a self-expanding metallic stent), and a critical tracheal stenosis due to severe extrinsic compression may benefit from a stent with high expansile force (i.e., a straight studded silicone stent). Manufacturers should be asked to make this information public.

showed signs of awakening (coughing and bucking). She was transferred to the intensive care unit for monitoring.

Long-Term Management

Outcome Assessment

The patient continued to be hospitalized for 5 more days. On postoperative day 5, she had a repeat flexible bronchoscopy, and a minimal amount of necrotic tissue was present in the subglottis just proximal to the tracheal stent. This was removed with the flexible bronchoscope. She was discharged home on oral prednisone 20 mg daily. At a follow-up visit 3 weeks later, her breathing had improved, and she was able to resume a regular treadmill exercise program. Without his wife present, her husband asked us to reiterate that airway involvement by RP, especially in the setting of malacia, is generally considered ominous and portends a poor prognosis.[3] At his request, we informed him that reported death from respiratory tract involvement varies from 10% (4 of 41) to 59% (17 of 29) of total deaths.[3,5] As it turns out, he had already discovered this information from his own reading of the literature.

Referrals

RP is a complex condition that requires a team approach to provide optimal medical care. Rheumatologists may need to become the primary care providers and should be involved early on in the patient's care. Often, they will attempt to taper steroids before significant side effects occur, and they will determine which long-term medications might prevent further cartilage inflammation. Medications may include high-dose methotrexate, cyclosporine, cellcept, or etanarcept.* Dermatologists or specialists in infectious diseases are also involved early in the course of the disease in patients with cellulitis or perichondritis to exclude infectious causes of these processes. Ophthalmologists, cardiologists, neurologists, nephrologists, and otolaryngologists may be asked to manage other aspects of RP, when present.[20]

Follow-up Tests and Procedures

No laboratory findings are specific for RP. Anemia, as seen in this patient, is typically normochromic and normocytic and by itself is also associated with a poor prognosis.[20] Nonspecific indicators of inflammation (e.g., elevated erythrocyte sedimentation rate, elevated levels of C-reactive protein) are often present, but they were not checked in our patient preoperatively. Because RP is associated with many systemic diseases, once the patient is stabilized, a laboratory evaluation† is indicated to

---

*A purified protein derivative (PPD) should be checked before this therapy is initiated, given its association with reactivation of tuberculosis.

†Use an antinuclear antibody reflexive panel, rheumatoid factor, and antiphospholipid antibodies (if a history of thrombosis is found) to evaluate for other autoimmune connective tissue diseases. For a vasculitis workup, perform a complete blood count (CBC) with differential; a metabolic panel; creatinine, liver transaminase, and serum alkaline phosphatase studies; urinalysis dipstick and microscopic evaluation of sediment; cryoglobulins; a viral hepatitis panel; and antinuclear antibody (ANA) and antineutrophil cytoplasmic antibody (ANCA) tests.

ascertain the presence of complicating conditions. Use of the purified protein derivative test to evaluate for exposure to tuberculosis is warranted not only in view of initiating immunosuppressive therapy, but also because tuberculosis is a recognized infectious cause of chondritis and malacia.[47]

With regard to bronchoscopic follow-up, after stent insertion at the choke point, expected migration of the choke points occurs distal to the stented airways. Lehman et al. stated that placing a stent at the site of maximal collapse during exhalation might result in migration of the choke point toward the periphery of the lung.[48] This issue has been addressed in patients with central airway obstruction due to lung cancer and also in patients with malacia from RP. Additional stents may be required if patients are still symptomatic and the choke points are still in the central airways. In one series after stent insertion, bilevel positive airway pressure (BiPAP) was used for all patients whose choke points had migrated to the small bronchi, as documented on computed tomography (CT).[18]

If stent insertion does not improve patient symptoms and no migration of the choke points occurs, then stent removal is warranted to avoid complications. Stent migration, obstruction by mucus and granulation tissue, infection, fracture, and airway perforation are well described in the literature.[12] The distinction between stent-related adverse events and symptoms related to TBM may be difficult to assess based on clinical grounds, so the new onset of symptoms should prompt inspection bronchoscopy.[12]

Quality Improvement

We wondered whether a silicone Y stent would have been a better choice in this patient. Indeed, patients with diffuse, severe tracheobronchomalacia can benefit from such devices[49]; in this patient, however, we considered that three separate stents constituted a reasonable first attempt at restoring airway patency for two reasons: (1) The straight stents are easier to remove should one or all of them prove to be unsuccessful or poorly tolerated; and (2) the patient would have required a Y stent with a very long tracheal arm, thereby increasing the risk for severe mucus plugging.

Because stent-related adverse events are common and usually occur within the first few weeks after stent insertion in patients with TBM,[24,49] the practice of early surveillance bronchoscopy is potentially warranted. Indeed, the overall frequency of stent-related adverse events in patients with malacia is higher than the frequency reported for patients with fixed airway obstruction.[24] This is likely because of the dynamic features of the airway and the inflamed airway mucosa. In view of the high rate of stent-related complications in this population, stent insertion should be reserved for patients with significant functional impairment, which certainly was the case in our patient with acute respiratory failure.

DISCUSSION POINTS

1. Describe the relationship between airway stents and respiratory tract infections.

Colonization of the airway with potentially pathogenic organisms is common after stent insertion[50] and is likely related to the actual presence of the indwelling airway stent. Initial colonization improves after relief of stenosis by rigid bronchoscopy without stent placement.[51] Stent-associated respiratory tract infections (SARTIs) have been documented in the literature. After accumulating data from 501 patients with airway stents (polymeric, metallic, or hybrid), the authors of a systematic review suggested that the frequency of SARTI* was as high as 20%.[52] The most common type of airway stent–related infection was pneumonia, and the pathogens most frequently implicated were *Staphylococcus aureus* and *Pseudomonas aeruginosa*; although only an association rather than a pathogenic correlation between stent insertion and respiratory tract infection could be confirmed, evidence potentially explains why insertion of an airway stent may increase susceptibility to infection or may complicate an already present infectious process. SARTI may present in two different patterns:

- As a postoperative complication in patients with or without previous respiratory tract infection. This category also includes patients in whom the stent complicated the clinical course of a respiratory tract infection that was active before stent insertion.
- As a condition that becomes manifest at various time intervals following stent insertion in patients with or without previous respiratory tract infection

No conclusive studies suggest that inhaled antibiotics play a role in managing airway colonization or infection after stenting. In one survey, a single respondent (of 62) used inhaled antibiotics as part of a maintenance strategy, and 12.9% of respondents used inhaled antibiotics in the setting of clinical decompensation.[53]

2. Describe two strategies used to prevent stent-related infections and mucus plugging.

Mucus plugging is probably the most common adverse event noted in patients with indwelling airway stents (see Figure 12-6). To prevent obstruction from secretions, several strategies have been proposed:

- *Surveillance bronchoscopy:* In general, for all patients with indwelling airway stents, routine use of surveillance bronchoscopy was not found to be helpful in detecting asymptomatic stent-related complications.[54] In patients with TBM, most complications occur early (within 4 to 6 weeks) after stent insertion[24,49]; therefore surveillance bronchoscopy in

this patient population may be warranted. This is not common practice, however, and in fact, a survey of 62 members of the American Association of Bronchology and Interventional Pulmonology showed that only 17.7% of respondents performed scheduled flexible bronchoscopy in patients with airway stents, and that less than 50% of respondents protocolized management after stent insertion.[53] The most common time frame for scheduled evaluation occurred 3 months after stent placement, but this was performed by only 53% of respondents. Methods used included physical examination (42.9%), chest radiograph (25.8%), and bronchoscopy (17.7%).[53]

- *Medications:* Considerable variability has been reported among physicians in terms of medications used for maintenance after stent insertion. In the same survey, bronchodilators, saline humidification, and mucolytics were used in some combination by almost half of respondents. Bronchodilators were the most commonly used medications (59.8%), followed by humidification (46.8%) or mucolytics (46.8%). Fifteen percent of respondents did not prescribe inhaled medications of any type.[53]

3. Describe two alternative treatments to silicone stent insertion in patients with tracheobronchomalacia from relapsing polychondritis.

- *Noninvasive positive-pressure ventilation:* This approach may be useful as stand-alone therapy for patients with milder forms of airway collapse,[41] or as an adjunct in patients with stents who remain symptomatic and have distally migrated choke points.[18]
- *Self-expandable metal stent (SEMS):* Although not advocated for patients with histologically proven benign disease, these stents were shown to restore airway patency and improve symptoms in patients with TBM from RP.[2,18] In a small case series, use of a SEMS (Wallstent, Schneider, Minneapolis, Minn) facilitated extubation in three patients with respiratory failure requiring mechanical ventilation. One patient, however, died a week later from suspected persistent malacia distal to the stent. Careful monitoring is necessary in these patients, not only to detect choke point migration, but also to evaluate for possible stent-related adverse events such as mucus plugging, granulation, migration, or fracture.[36]

Expert Commentary

provided by Teruomi Miyazawa, MD, PhD, FCCP, and Noriaki Kurimoto, MD, PhD, FCCP

This case is illustrative of many of the concerns faced by physicians caring for patients with airway compromise resulting from relapsing polychondritis (RP) and other forms of expiratory central airway collapse. In this commentary, rather than address any of the issues outlined in the Four Box Approach of a procedure-related consultation, we will focus on physiology issues related to stent insertion at the level of the choke point.

---

*Stent-associated respiratory tract infection (SARTI) is most often diagnosed when the following criteria are fulfilled: (1) Radiologic and/or bronchoscopic findings involve predominantly the stent, the stented airway, or the anatomic region it drains; (2) the patient presents with symptoms attributable to infection (namely, fever, increased sputum volume and purulence, fatigue) with or without deterioration in dyspnea scores or lung function tests; and (3) the condition necessitates antimicrobial treatment and/or stent replacement/removal.

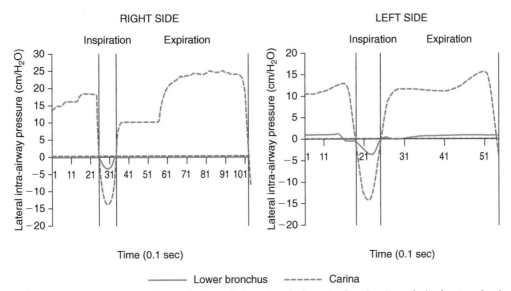

Figure 12-7 Lateral pressure measurements using catheter technique for choke point location in malacia due to relapsing polychondritis. A patient with malacia from relapsing polychondritis (RP) was anesthetized by intravenous injection using propofol. After intubation with a rigid bronchoscope, a double lumen airway catheter was inserted into the working channel during bronchoscopy. A catheter constructed of nylon elastomer with two holes premanufactured into the side at 5 cm intervals was then inserted. Lateral pressure (P_{lat}) was measured simultaneously at two points during tidal breathing using the double lumen airway catheter. The tidal flow–limiting segment was evaluated using the pressure difference between the two points. Pressure differences are noted between the lower bronchus and the carina. The tidal flow–limiting segment was located in both mainstem bronchi. The pressure difference during expiration was larger than during inspiration.

Wave speed theory suggests that airway flow limitation occurs when flow velocity equals the speed of propagation of pressure-pulse waves at some point within the airway. This flow-limiting segment, called the *choke point,* tends to be located in a region of minimum cross-sectional area and minimum side pressure within the airway when maximal flow is reached. Because maximum expiratory flow is airway compliance dependent, increased compliance, such as that seen in patients with expiratory central airway collapse, results in increased airway resistance and decreased maximum expiratory flow.

Although both malacia and excessive dynamic airway collapse (EDAC) are forms of expiratory central airway collapse, choke point considerations may be different and, in malacia, choke points may be located in the central airways, whereas in EDAC, they may be located more peripherally. For patients with RP, however, airway collapse may be severe and present during both inspiration and expiration (Figure 12-7). Stent insertion palliates airway obstruction and increases airway wall stiffness, but is vulnerable to distal migration of the choke point after the initial stent placement is performed. We believe that investigation of this process is important, because the repercussions of choke point migration on physiologic function can still adversely affect the patient's quality of life, making additional stent insertion and/or non-invasive ventilatory support a consideration.

One noninvasive physiologic test that might be used to identify airflow dynamics and the effect of choke point migration on ventilatory function in patients with malacia and RP before and after stent insertion is impulse oscillometry (IOS). This is an effort-independent test during which brief random pressure pulses of 5 to 35 Hz generated by a small loudspeaker mounted in series with a pneumotachygraph are applied during tidal breathing. Pressure-flow oscillations are superimposed on the subject's tidal breaths, and real-time recordings are used to provide an estimate of total respiratory system impedance, including measurements of resistance (R) and reactance (X)* at different frequencies that might differentiate between central and peripheral components of airway obstruction. Increased R at a low oscillation frequency (5 Hz) reflects an increase in total respiratory resistance suggestive of airway obstruction such as that found in patients with chronic obstructive pulmonary disease (COPD), but an increase at a higher frequency (20 Hz) may reflect more specifically increased central airway resistance, such as that found in patients with malacia or stenosis (Figure 12-8). This is because the 5 Hz signal has a slower cycle timer and a larger wavelength, so it reaches the periphery of the lungs and gives information about the entire respiratory tract. The 20 Hz signal, on the other hand, has a faster cycle timer and a shorter wavelength; these signals penetrate only the larger airways and therefore provide information about proximal, large airway processes. Changes in IOS values have been documented after

---

*Reactance refers to rebound resistance from the distensible airways and lung. X5 (lung reactance at 5 Hz) is supposed to reflect the elasticity of the lung and thorax and distention of the ventilated airways; thus it is an indirect measure of peripheral airway obstruction. The worse the peripheral resistance, the more negative the X5 values.

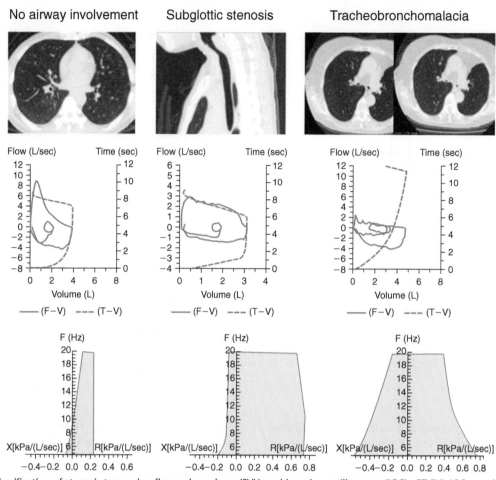

Figure 12-8 Classification of stenosis type using flow-volume loop (FVL) and impulse oscillometry (IOS): CT-FVL-IOS correlations. In tracheo-bronchomalacia, FVL shows the "airway collapse" pattern with a sudden drop in peak expiratory flow during a forced expiratory maneuver; in subglottic stenosis, classic flattening of inspiratory and expiratory curves of the FVL is evident. IOS findings reveal that respiratory resistance in malacia showed frequency dependence, whereas it was nearly consistent for all frequencies in the fixed subglottic stenosis. Reactance components are mainly determined by lung compliance and central airway inertance; however, reactance components in malacia are determined by airway compliance instead of lung compliance, resulting in a decrease in X5.

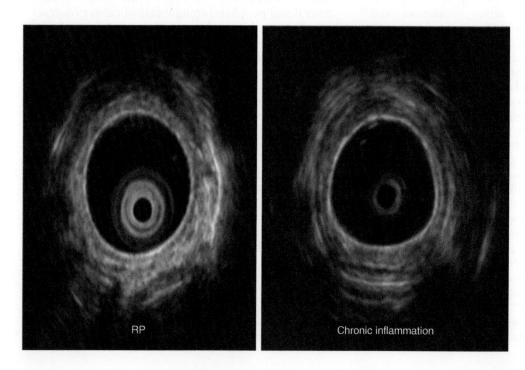

Figure 12-9 High-frequency endobronchial ultrasonography (EBUS) imaging patterns in relapsing polychondritis (RP) and in chronic inflammation. Note that in RP, the posterior membrane is spared, but in chronic inflammation, the airway is involved circumferentially.

administration of bronchodilators; in addition, relevant to the case presented herein, after stent insertion at the level of the choke point, both the flow-volume loop and IOS can display significant improvement in flow limitation.

Another way to assess central airway function and structure in patients with RP is by using the endobronchial ultrasonography (EBUS) radial probe (20 MHz). In our experience, thickening of the submucosa and the tracheobronchial cartilage, calcifications, and the degree of integrity of the membranous portion of the airway can be ascertained. In patients with chronic inflammatory conditions such as post-tracheotomy inflammation, Wegener's granulomatosis, or ulcerative colitis, the inflammatory process involves the entire circumference of the trachea, and thickening of cartilaginous and membranous portions of the tracheal and main bronchial walls can be seen on EBUS radial probe images. This, we believe, helps distinguish these conditions from RP, in which the membranous portion appears to be spared (Figure 12-9).

We conclude that a combination of novel diagnostic imaging and physiologic assessment technologies can be applied to elucidate the characteristics of choke point physiology and airway wall structure in patients with tracheobronchomalacia. The central airway location of flow-limiting segments can be precisely localized, and choke point analysis may be concordant with physiologic models predicted by wave-speed theory of expiratory flow limitation.

REFERENCES

1. Trentham DE, Le CH. Relapsing polychondritis. *Ann Intern Med.* 1998;129:114-122.
2. Sarodia BD, Dasgupta A, Mehta AC. Management of airway manifestations of relapsing polychondritis: case reports and review of literature. *Chest.* 1999;116:1669-1675.
3. Michet CJ, McKenna CH, Luthra HS, et al. Relapsing polychondritis: survival and predictive role of early disease manifestations. *Ann Intern Med.* 1986;104:74-78.
4. Dunne JA, Sabanathan S. Use of metallic stents in relapsing polychondritis. *Chest.* 1994;105:864-867.
5. McAdam LP, O'Hanlan MA, Bluestone R, et al. Relapsing polychondritis: prospective study of 23 patients and a review of the literature. *Medicine.* 1976;55:193-215.
6. Foidart JM, Abe S, Martin GR, et al. Antibodies to type II collagen in relapsing polychondritis. *N Engl J Med.* 1978;299:1203-1207.
7. Miyazu Y, Miyazawa T, Kurimoto N, et al. Endobronchial ultrasonography in the diagnosis and treatment of relapsing polychondritis with tracheobronchial malacia. *Chest.* 2003;124:2393-2295.
8. Murgu S, Kurimoto N, Colt H. Endobronchial ultrasound morphology of expiratory central airway collapse. *Respirology.* 2008;13:315-319.
9. Damiani JM, Levine HL. Relapsing polychondritis. *Laryngoscope.* 1979;89:929-946.
10. Ernst A, Rafeq S, Boiselle P, et al. Relapsing polychondritis and airway involvement. *Chest.* 2009;135:1024-1030.
11. Gilkeson RC, Ciancibello LM, Hejal RB, et al. Tracheobronchomalacia: dynamic airway evaluation with multidetector CT. *AJR Am J Roentgenol.* 2001;176:205-210.
12. Murgu SD, Colt HG. Tracheobronchomalacia and excessive dynamic airway collapse. *Respirology.* 2006;11:388-406.
13. Boiselle PM, O'Donnell CR, Bankier AA, et al. Tracheal collapsibility in healthy volunteers during forced expiration: assessment with multidetector CT. *Radiology.* 2009;252:255-262.
14. Davis SD, Berkmen YM, King T. Peripheral bronchial involvement in relapsing polychondritis: demonstration by thin section CT. *Am J Roentgenol.* 1989;153:953-954.
15. Mohsenifar Z, Tashkin DP, Carson SA, et al. Pulmonary function in patients with relapsing polychondritis. *Chest.* 1982;81:711-717.
16. Dawson SV, Elliott EA. Wave-speed limitation on expiratory flow a unifying concept. *J Appl Physiol.* 1977;43:498-515.
17. Pedersen OF, Ingram Jr RH. Configuration of maximum expiratory flow volume curve: model experiments with physiological implications. *J Appl Physiol.* 1985;58:1305-1313.
18. Miyazawa T, Nishine H, Handa H, et al. Migration of the choke point in relapsing polychondritis after stenting. *Chest.* 2009;136:81S.
19. Hojaili B, Keiser HD. Relapsing polychondritis presenting with complete heart block. *J Clin Rheumatol.* 2008;14:24-26.
20. Compton N. Polychondritis. Available at: http://emedicine.medscape.com/article/331475-overview. Accessed March 31, 2011.
21. Chang-Miller A, Okamura M, Torres VE, et al. Renal involvement in relapsing polychondritis. *Medicine.* 1987;66:202-217.
22. Vicente EF, Hernández-Núñez A, Aspa J, et al. Crohn's disease, relapsing polychondritis and epidermolysis bullosa acquisita: an immune-mediated inflammatory syndrome. *Rheumatology.* 2008;47:380-381.
23. Relapsing Polychondritis Support and Awareness Foundation. Available at: http://www.wecaretoo.com/Organizations/OR/relapsing polychondritis.html. Accessed May 7, 2011.
24. Murgu SD, Colt HG. Complications of silicone stent insertion in patients with expiratory central airway collapse. *Ann Thorac Surg.* 2007;84:1870-1877.
25. Cazabon S, Over K, Butcher J. The successful use of infliximab in resistant relapsing polychondritis and associated scleritis. *Eye.* 2005;19:222-224.
26. Behar JV, Choi YW, Hartman TA, et al. Relapsing polychondritis affecting the lower respiratory tract. *AJR Am J Roentgenol.* 2002;178:173-177.
27. Eng J, Sabanathan S. Airway complications in relapsing polychondritis. *Ann Thorac Surg.* 1991;51:686-692.
28. Greenholz SK, Karrer FM, Lilly JR. Contemporary surgery of tracheomalacia. *J Pediatr Surg.* 1986;21:511-514.
29. Wright CD, Grillo HC, Hammoud ZT, et al. Tracheoplasty for expiratory collapse of central airways. *Ann Thorac Surg.* 2005;80:259-266.
30. Gangadharan SP, Bakhos CT, Majid A, et al. Technical aspects and outcomes of tracheobronchoplasty for severe tracheobronchomalacia. *Ann Thorac Surg.* 2011 Mar 4. [Epub ahead of print]
31. Spraggs PDR, Tostevin PMJ, Howard DJ. Management of laryngotracheobronchial sequelae and complications of relapsing polychondritis. *Laryngoscope.* 1997;107:936-941.
32. Miyazawa T, Miyazu Y, Iwamoto Y, et al. Stenting at the flow-limiting segment in tracheobronchial stenosis due to lung cancer. *Am J Respir Crit Care Med.* 2004;169:1096-1102.
33. Freitag L, Eicker K, Donovan TJ, et al. Mechanical properties of airway stents. *J Bronchol.* 1995;2: 270-278.
34. Hramiec JE, Haasler GB. Tracheal wire stent complications in malacia: implications of position and design. *Ann Thorac Surg.* 1997;63:209-212.
35. Lee P, Kupeli E, Mehta AC. Airway stents. *Clin Chest Med.* 2010;31:141-150.
36. Freitag L. Airway stents. In: Strausz J, Bolliger CT, eds. *Interventional Pulmonology.* Sheffield, UK: European Respiratory Society; 2010:190-217.
37. Gildea TR, Murthy SC, Sahoo D, et al. Performance of a self-expanding silicone stent in palliation of benign airway conditions. *Chest.* 2006;130:1419-1423.
38. Dutau H, Maldonado F, Breen DP, et al. Endoscopic successful management of tracheobronchomalacia with laser: apropos of a Mounier-Kuhn syndrome. *Eur J Cardiothorac Surg.* 2011 Mar 5. [Epub ahead of print]
39. Dumon MC, Cavaliere S, Vergnon JM. Bronchial laser: techniques, indications, and results. *Rev Mal Respir.* 1999;16:601-608.
40. Ellis PD. Laser palatoplasty for snoring due to palatal flutter: a further report. *Clin Otolaryngol Allied Sci.* 1994;19:350-351.

41. Adliff M, Ngato D, Keshavjee S, et al. Treatment of diffuse tracheomalacia secondary to relapsing polychondritis with continuous positive airway pressure. *Chest.* 1997;112:1701-1704.

42. Murgu SD, Pecson J, Colt HG. Bronchoscopy on noninvasive positive pressure ventilation: indications and technique. *Respir Care.* 2010;55:595-600.

43. Joosten S, Macdonald M, Lau KK, et al. Excessive dynamic airway collapse co-morbid with COPD diagnosed using 320-slice dynamic CT scanning technology. *Thorax.* 2010 Jul 7. [Epub ahead of print]

44. Hawkins J. Making autonomous decisions: million dollar baby. In: Colt HG, Quadrelli S, Friedman L, eds. *The Picture of Health: Medical Ethics and the Movies.* New York: Oxford University Press; 2011.

45. Mackie AM, Watson CB. Anesthesia and mediastinal masses. *Anesthesia.* 1984;39:899-903.

46. Venhaus M, Behn C, Freitag L, et al. Simulations and experiments of the balloon dilatation of airway stenoses. *Biomed Tech.* 2009; 54:187-195.

47. Iwamoto Y, Miyazawa T, Kurimoto N, et al. Interventional bronchoscopy in the management of airway stenosis due to tracheobronchial tuberculosis. *Chest.* 2004;126:1344-1352.

48. Lehman JD, Gordon RL, Kerlan Jr RK, et al. Expandable metallic stents in benign tracheobronchial obstruction. *J Thorac Imaging.* 1998;13:105-115.

49. Ernst A, Majid A, Feller-Kopman D, et al. Airway stabilization with silicone stents for treating adult tracheobronchomalacia: a prospective observational study. *Chest.* 2007;132:609-616.

50. Noppen M, Pierard D, Meysman M, et al. Bacterial colonization of central airways after stenting. *Am J Respir Crit Care Med.* 1999;160:672-677.

51. Noppen M, Pierard D, Meysman M, et al. Absence of bacterial colonization of the airways after therapeutic rigid bronchoscopy without stenting. *Eur Respir J.* 2000;16:1147-1151.

52. Agrafiotis M, Siempos II, Falagas ME. Infections related to airway stenting: a systematic review. *Respiration.* 2009;78:69-74.

53. Hoag J, Sherman M, Lund M. Practice patterns for maintaining airway stents deployed for malignant airway obstruction. *J Bronchol Intervent Pulmonol.* 2010;17:131-135.

54. Matsuo T, Colt HG. Evidence against routine scheduling of surveillance bronchoscopy after stent insertion. *Chest.* 2000;118: 1455-1459.

Chapter 13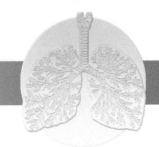

CPAP Treatment for Moderate Diffuse Excessive Dynamic Airway Collapse Caused by Mounier-Kuhn Syndrome

This chapter emphasizes the following elements of the Four Box Approach: indications, contraindications, and expected results; anesthesia and other perioperative care; and techniques and instrumentation.

CASE DESCRIPTION

The patient was a 70-year-old man with "seal barking" cough for longer than a year. His cough was associated with congestion and was worse at night and in the supine position. He had dyspnea on exertion (World Health Organization [WHO] class II). His past medical history was significant for asthma and frequent hospitalizations for pneumonia and "bronchitis." At the time of our evaluation, his medications included fluticasone/salmeterol 250/50 mg twice daily, tiotropium one inhalation daily, prednisone 10 mg/day, mometasone nasal spray, Mucinex, loratadine, and inhaled tobramycin for recurrent lower respiratory tract *Pseudomonas aeruginosa* infection. In addition, he was using omeprazole 20 mg daily for gastroesophageal reflux disease (GERD) and albuterol 2.5 mg nebulization 3 times daily, followed by application of high-frequency chest oscillation (i.e., percussion vest). He was not a smoker and had no occupational exposure to fumes and toxins. On examination, wheezing over the trachea and bilateral rhonchi could be heard early during expiration. His oxygen saturation was 92% on 4 L/min of oxygen. Pulmonary function testing (PFT) revealed the following: forced expiratory volume in 1 second (FEV$_1$) 1.93 L (51% predicted), which increased to 2.26 L (60% predicted), resulting in 17% improvement after bronchodilators; and forced vital capacity (FVC) 2.62 L (52% predicted) increased to 3.19 L (63% predicted)—a 22% improvement after bronchodilators. Total lung capacity (TLC) was 98% predicted, residual volume (RV) 171% predicted, and diffusing capacity of the lung for carbon monoxide (DLCO) 89% predicted. A paired inspiratory-expiratory dynamic computed tomography (CT) scan of the chest showed tracheobronchomegaly, expiratory bulging of the posterior membrane inside the airway lumen, narrowing the cross-sectional area of the trachea and mainstem bronchi by 67%, and bronchiectasis (Figure 13-1). A review of his old records revealed that several sputum and bronchioloalveolar lavage (BAL) cultures showed multiple bacteria, including *Stenotrophomonas*, *Nocardia*, *Escherichia coli*, *Pseudomonas*, and *Aspergillus*.

DISCUSSION POINTS

1. Provide two indications for bronchoscopy on continuous positive airway pressure (CPAP) in this patient.
2. List two differential diagnoses for excessive dynamic airway collapse (EDAC).
3. Provide two reasons why CPAP might help a patient with expiratory central airway collapse.

CASE RESOLUTION

Initial Evaluations

Physical Examination, Complementary Tests, and Functional Status Assessment

This patient's PFTs showed moderate obstructive ventilatory impairment responsive to bronchodilators, a normal DLCO, and evidence of air trapping. These findings were consistent with his diagnosis of asthma. The CT scan, however, showed tracheobronchomegaly, moderate EDAC on expiratory images, bronchiectasis, bronchial thickening, and bronchiolitis in the lower lobes (see Figure 13-1). During the initial evaluation of a patient with bronchiectasis, the presumed cause of this patient's recurrent episodes of bronchitis and pneumonia, the clinician must select diagnostic studies to determine the cause of the disorder. If bronchiectasis is truly focal (i.e., confined to one lobe), then it is highly unlikely that inherited or systemic causes are responsible, and investigations can be tailored appropriately,[1] for example, bronchoscopy might be performed to identify possible obstruction by foreign body, tumor, or stricture (Figure 13-2).

In a patient with bilateral bronchiectasis, such as that noted in our patient, a battery of immunologic and genetic tests can be tailored on the basis of clinical suspicions.[1] Our patient had no evidence of autoimmune disease, immunodeficiency, or genetic disorders such as alpha 1-antitrypsin deficiency or cystic fibrosis: The autoantibody screen that comprised antinuclear antibodies (ANAs), antineutrophil cytoplasmic antibodies (ANCAs), anti-SSA, anti-SSB, and rheumatoid factor, along with cystic fibrosis (CF) testing for 97 mutations, was negative; the alpha 1-antitrypsin level and immunoglobulin (Ig)G, IgM, IgA, and IgE were normal; and the erythrocyte sedimentation rate (ESR) was slightly elevated at 25 (normal <20). Because chronic aspiration is another cause of bilateral bronchiectasis, an esophagogram and a hypopharyngogram were performed, revealing no evidence of

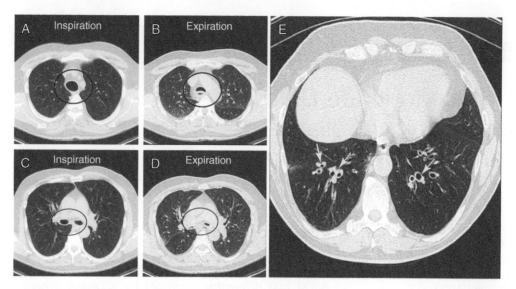

Figure 13-1 Paired inspiratory and expiratory dynamic computed tomography (CT) scans show (**A** and **C**) tracheobronchomegaly during inspiration and (**B** and **D**) excessive dynamic airway collapse during exhalation. **E,** Inspiratory images also show bronchial wall thickening and bronchiectasis *(arrows)*.

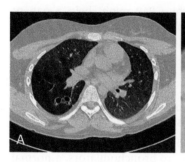
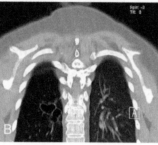
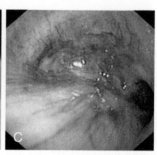

Figure 13-2 Focal right lower lobe bronchiectasis on (**A**) axial and (**B**) coronal computed tomography (CT) images resulting from (**C**) bronchus intermedius stricture caused by Wegener's granulomatosis.

aspiration or obstruction. However, high-grade reflux, which in fact can be seen in almost a fourth of patients with bronchiectasis, is usually asymptomatic. One study showed that only 27% of patients with bronchiectasis and coexisting GERD have typical reflux symptoms such as heartburn, regurgitation, or dyspepsia.[2]

Today, chest high-resolution computed tomography (HRCT) scans are performed in almost anyone suspected of having bronchiectasis. A classic finding of bronchiectasis is the "signet ring" sign (this was present in our patient), characterized by a diameter of the bronchus greater than the adjacent artery (broncho-arterial ratio >1)* (see Figure 13-1). Bronchial wall thickening,[†] bronchi filled with mucus, and mosaic perfusion (air trapping on expiration) are indirect HRCT signs that assist in diagnosis (Figure 13-3; see also Figure 13-1). HRCT also narrows the differential diagnosis by revealing specific disease processes such as situs inversus in Kartagener syndrome[‡] (see Figure 13-3), or by revealing a specific distribution of the abnormalities. For instance, in allergic

bronchopulmonary aspergillosis (ABPA),* the distribution of bronchiectasis is usually central (see Figure 13-3), but in tuberculosis, it is usually unilateral and upper lobe predominant. In our patient, the distribution was in the lower lobes, suggesting impaired mucociliary mechanisms or postinfectious causes. In addition, HRCT, when performed with a dynamic protocol,[†] can detect and quantify the degree of central airway collapse.[3] Very high resolution images and three-dimensional (3D) reconstruction using 320-slice CT have been reported for diagnosis of EDAC.[‡4]

The patient's "seal barking" cough, nocturnal congestion in the supine position, and wheezing were suggestive of expiratory central airway collapse. The paired inspiratory-expiratory dynamic CT showed

---

*Other direct signs of bronchiectasis include tram tracks, string of pearls, lack of tapering, and visualization of the airway within 1 cm of coastal/adjacent mediastinal pleura.

[†]Bronchial wall thickening is defined as thickness of the bronchial wall that is >0.5 times the diameter of the adjacent vertical pulmonary artery.

[‡]Usually an autosomal recessive disorder characterized by mirror image organ arrangement, bronchiectasis, and sinusitis due to congenital reduction or absence of ciliary function.

*ABPA is characterized by a history of asthma, immediate skin test reactivity to *Aspergillus* antigens, precipitating serum antibodies to *Aspergillus fumigatus,* serum total IgE concentration greater than 1000 ng/mL, peripheral blood eosinophilia >500/mm³, lung infiltrates on chest x-ray or chest HRCT, central bronchiectasis on chest CT, and elevated specific serum IgE and IgG to *A. fumigatus.*

[†]Images are initially obtained using a standard radiation dose technique at end inspiration (170 mAs, 120 kVp, 2.5-mm collimation, high-speed mode, and pitch equivalent of 1.5). This is followed by a low-dose examination (40 mAs, 120 kVp, 2.5-mm collimation, high-speed mode, and pitch equivalent of 1.5) during the dynamic expiratory phase of respiration.

[‡]Images obtained during this study were conducted at a dose of 7.2 mSv, which is comparable with the dose received during a standard CT chest.

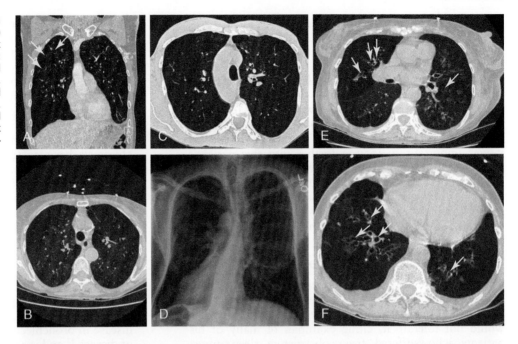

Figure 13-3 High-resolution computed tomography (HRCT) signs of bronchiectasis in a patient with Kartagener's syndrome: **A,** Lack of tapering and **(B)** mosaic perfusion are noted. **C,** Right-sided aortic arch and **(D)** situs inversus can be seen. **E,** Central bronchiectasis and **(F)** mosaic perfusion are evident in a patient with allergic bronchopulmonary aspergillosis.

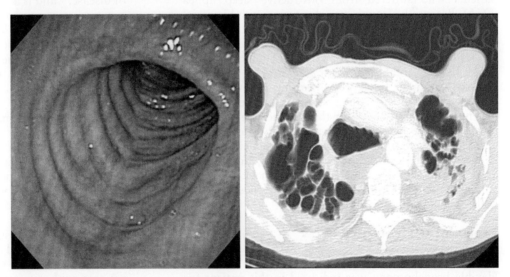

Figure 13-4 Secondary tracheomegaly in a patient with bilateral upper lobe fibrosis and bronchiectasis related to prior tuberculosis.

tracheobronchomegaly, mild tracheal collapse (67%), and moderate collapse in the mainstem bronchi, with near complete closure of the lumen during exhalation (90%)* (see Figure 13-1). Tracheobronchomegaly is usually secondary to bilateral upper lobe fibrosis as a sequel of pulmonary fibrosis, tuberculosis, cystic fibrosis, or sarcoidosis (Figure 13-4), but our patient had other parenchymal/interstitial lung findings on HRCT.

In the absence of alternative explanations, we believed that our patient had primary tracheobronchomegaly in association with bronchiectasis—findings known as

Mounier-Kuhn syndrome. This syndrome is characterized by atrophy or absence of elastic fibers and smooth muscle cells. These structural alterations may lead to collapse of the airway during exhalation, making expectoration by cough inefficient. Although considered to be a congenital condition, 50% of patients have no symptoms until the third decade of life, when frequent lower respiratory tract infections and sputum production become manifest, probably as a result of bronchiectasis.[5]

Comorbidities

This patient had asthma and was already on maximum medical therapy, including systemic corticosteroids. Despite this, he had chronic early expiratory wheezing. Therefore, we did not consider that asthma was the sole explanation for his wheezing (especially in view of EDAC as seen on dynamic CT), and we did not consider his chronic wheezing a contraindication to bronchoscopy.

---

*The severity of airway narrowing in expiratory central airway collapse describes the degree of airway collapse during expiration, as assessed by bronchoscopy or radiographic studies, and can be classified as follows: 1, Normal: expiratory collapse of less than 50%; 2, Mild: expiratory airway collapse of 50% to 75%; 3, Moderate: expiratory airway collapse of 75% to 100%; and 4, Severe: expiratory airway collapse of 100% (the airway walls make contact).

Support System

The patient was married, but separated. He told us that he spent occasional holidays with his wife, but that he was alone often and occasionally felt depressed. He felt isolated and lonely, in part because of his symptoms. Jokingly he told us that no woman would want to bear a man who barked all the time. Once the suspicion for EDAC had been raised by the CT findings, we believed it was important to inquire further into this patient's social support environment, and we took the liberty to ask about his home situation. Published evidence suggests that one's living situation and potential resolution of marital conflicts may be targeted by interventions leading to improved CPAP adherence—one of the conservative treatments for EDAC.*[6,7]

Patient Preferences and Expectations

The patient was a retired physician who showed good understanding of his disease process. He was willing to try wearing a CPAP mask but was concerned that he would not tolerate it, citing examples of many of his patients who suffered from obstructive sleep apnea (OSA). Because his cough was interfering with his social life and his frequent lower respiratory tract infections required multiple hospitalizations, he was determined to try his best to wear CPAP apparatus, if indicated, provided that a notable symptomatic benefit would be derived. Although he expressed strong motivation initially, we were not certain about the long-term health benefits of wearing CPAP for this disease. We explained to him that the immediate benefit of CPAP for patients with EDAC (in terms of severity of airway collapse) could be detected at the time of bronchoscopy, and that in general, with regard to adherence to treatment, data from patients with OSA show increased adherence to CPAP with time in continuous users.[8]

Procedural Strategies

Indications

Flexible bronchoscopy was indicated in this patient for several reasons: (1) to obtain specimens for microbiologic assessment of the chronically infected lower airways; (2) to perform dynamic bronchoscopy to diagnose and determine the severity of EDAC suggested by the dynamic CT scan; and (3) to apply CPAP assistance during bronchoscopy to determine precise CPAP pressures that maintain airway patency and prevent excessive collapse. These three aspects of the procedure were discussed with the patient and his spouse, who had accompanied him to the consultation.

1. *Bronchoscopic diagnosis of infection:* Infections play an important role in exacerbation of bronchiectasis and baseline symptoms. Our patient's main reason for chronic infections and exacerbations was his anatomic airway abnormality. Excessive collapse of the trachea and mainstem bronchi leads to inability to raise secretions, infections, damage to the bronchial walls, and progressive airway dilation (bronchiectasis). This further reduces one's ability to clear secretions from the distal airways, setting up a repetitive cycle of purulent drainage and tissue damage.[9] Studies using techniques that have avoided contamination by upper airway flora (such as bronchoscopic protected brush specimens and BAL) show that more than 50% of patients with bronchiectasis have potentially pathogenic bacteria in their lower airways. Although the presence of pathogenic bacteria in the lower airways in these patients has often been termed *colonization,* the spectrum of pathogenic bacteria isolated in patients at baseline and during exacerbations is remarkably similar.* Furthermore, improvement in baseline symptoms after long-term antibiotics suggests that bacteria may be causing inflammation.[10-12] Some pathogens have a definite role in long-term prognosis. Relevant to this patient, the isolation of *Pseudomonas aeruginosa* correlates with severe clinical disease in bronchiectasis, occurs later in the course of disease,[13] and is associated with a decline in lung function as measured by FEV_1 (50 mL/yr).[14]

2. One indication† for dynamic bronchoscopy (aka functional bronchoscopy) is the evaluation of EDAC. This technique allows for real-time observations of changes in the airways in response to various maneuvers. It is performed using flexible bronchoscopy with minimal or moderate (conscious) sedation so that the patient can cooperate and obey commands during the procedure.[15] With the flexible bronchoscope at the midline, the patient is asked to inhale and exhale deeply, hyperflex and hyperextend the neck, and cough. These maneuvers are done while the patient is placed in upright, supine, and lateral decubitus positions (Figure 13-5).

3. CPAP (or BiPAP) assistance during flexible bronchoscopy can be used to confirm the possible effectiveness of conservative management in symptomatic patients with expiratory central airway collapse (EDAC or malacia), as well as to prevent respiratory distress and intubation in high-risk patients requiring flexible bronchoscopy.[16,17] Bronchoscopy allows removal of mucus plugs and improves ventilation and oxygen exchange, but by occupying 10% to 15% of the normal tracheal lumen, the bronchoscope can decrease PaO_2 (partial pressure of oxygen in arterial blood) by 10 to 20 mm Hg, which may contribute to respiratory complications and cardiac arrhythmias. Hypoxemia is worsened when local anesthetics or saline solution is instilled

---

*Of note, this was studied in patients suffering from obstructive sleep apnea (OSA), not from EDAC.

*In non–cystic fibrosis bronchiectasis, *Haemophilus influenzae* has been the most common pathogen isolated, followed by *Streptococcus pneumoniae* and *Pseudomonas aeruginosa.* Less common pathogens include *Enterobacter, Nocardia, Staphylococcus,* and nontuberculous mycobacteria.

†This bronchoscopic technique can also be used to explore tracheoesophageal or bronchoesophageal fistulas, as well as tracheobronchomalacia.

Figure 13-5 Dynamic bronchoscopy performed in the upright *(top panel)*, supine *(middle panel)*, and lateral decubitus *(bottom panel)* positions in a patient with tracheomalacia and an indwelling lower tracheal stent.

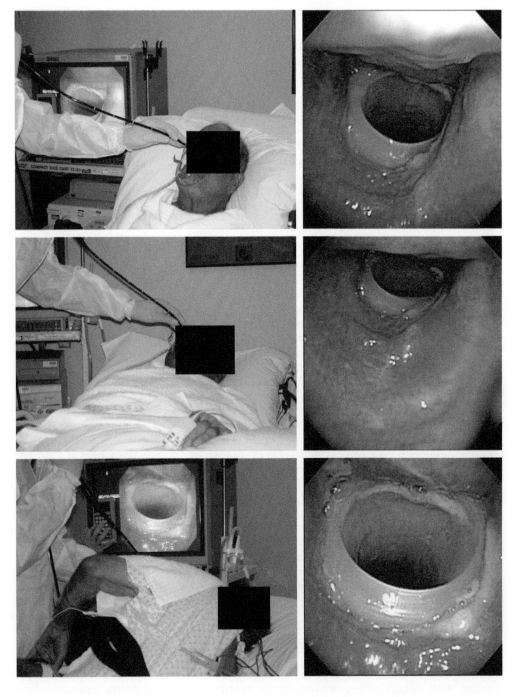

into the lower airways. The American Thoracic Society recommends avoiding flexible bronchoscopy and lavage in patients with hypoxemia that cannot be corrected to at least a PaO_2 of 75 mm Hg or an SaO_2 (saturated oxygen level in hemoglobin) greater than 90%.[18,19] In patients with severe obstructive ventilatory impairment, bronchoscopy can lead to air trapping because functional residual capacity (FRC) increases when the scope is inserted nasally; and in children and in patients with OSA or obesity hypoventilation syndrome (OHS) who already have awake hypercapnia, bronchoscopy can exacerbate hypoxemia and hypercapnia because of sedation-related increased collapsibility of the central and upper airways. In these settings, bronchoscopy can be performed with CPAP or BiPAP assistance, potentially sparing patients the discomfort and risks of refractory hypoxemia, intubation, and mechanical ventilation.[20,21] However, CPAP can thwart an accurate evaluation of dynamic airway obstruction by preventing airway collapse. For this reason, dynamic airway lesions within extrathoracic and intrathoracic airways (e.g., laryngomalacia, tracheobronchomalacia [TBM], EDAC) should be bronchoscopically visualized with and without CPAP to assess collapsibility.[22]

Contraindications

Contraindications to performing flexible bronchoscopy on CPAP include respiratory insufficiency requiring endotracheal intubation (e.g., cardiopulmonary resuscitation for respiratory arrest), severe hemodynamic instability (i.e., systolic blood pressure <80 mm Hg), encephalopathy, recent (within 1 week) myocardial infarction, respiratory failure caused by neurologic disease or status asthmaticus, and the presence of facial deformities. Another contraindication is recent oral, esophageal, or gastric surgery that prohibits the use of a face mask or increases the risk of gastric insufflation and aspiration.[23] Our patient had no such contraindications.

Expected Results

CPAP can be used in patients with EDAC or TBM to ameliorate airway collapse. The exact CPAP settings that maintain airway patency in expiratory central airway collapse of various degrees of severity have not been systematically studied. If an evaluation of central airway collapse is performed, digital imaging documentation is obtained in upright and supine positions both on and off CPAP so the degree of airway narrowing and the response to positive pressure can be evaluated. The pressure requirements are individualized and determined during CPAP-assisted bronchoscopy, or, alternatively, with CPAP-assisted CT scanning.[4] A recent case study reported that a pressure of 10 cm H_2O abolished a patient's symptoms and ameliorated EDAC, as evaluated by 320-slice CT scanning with 3D reconstruction.*[4] In EDAC or TBM, a CPAP of 7 to 10 cm H_2O usually ensures airway patency.[24,25] Overall, noninvasive positive-pressure ventilation (CPAP or BiPAP) assistance helps ensure an uncomplicated bronchoscopy in hypercapnic chronic obstructive pulmonary disease (COPD) patients with pneumonia,[26] compensates for the hypotonicity of the upper airway muscles in patients with OSA,[27] and improves tidal volume and respiratory flow in spontaneously breathing children with easily collapsible upper airways.[22]

Team Experience

CPAP-assisted bronchoscopies can be performed by a bronchoscopist (i.e., intensivist, pulmonologist, thoracic or trauma surgeon) with the help of a bronchoscopy assistant and respiratory therapists or nurses who are familiar with noninvasive positive-pressure ventilation. These nonphysician health care providers are thus actively involved in preparation for and performance of this procedure, form a relationship with the patient, and are involved in or responsible for postprocedure surveillance,[28] including telephone follow-up to troubleshoot and to ensure compliance.

Diagnostic Alternatives

1. *CPAP-assisted computed tomography:* Noninvasive methods of assessing the degree of collapse and response to CPAP can be offered by CPAP-assisted computed tomography.[4] Evaluation of the lung parenchyma may be necessary during CPAP application, especially in patients with COPD. Results from one study showed that a CPAP of 5 cm H_2O caused little increase in lung aeration in healthy volunteers and COPD patients, but in a couple of patients with COPD (2 out of 11), CPAP deflated some regions of the lungs. CPAP levels of 10 cm H_2O and 15 cm H_2O increased the emphysematous zones in all sectors of the lungs, including dorsal and apical regions, in patients with COPD, but caused little hyperaeration predominantly in the ventral areas in healthy volunteers.[29] This is potentially harmful, given the already hyperinflated status of a COPD patient's lungs. Optimal CPAP levels should counteract the increased effort of breathing while improving expiratory airflow to its maximum without causing further hyperinflation.[30] Thin HRCT scan slices may better estimate CPAP-induced lung hyperinflation, provided that an appropriate radiologic density threshold is used for quantification of hyperinflated zones.[31] This method is useful for EDAC assessment, but not for collecting specimens for microbiologic analysis.

2. *Polysomnography:* This technique was reportedly useful in a case of EDAC due to tracheobronchomegaly; evidence of both obstructive apnea and hypopnea was found with an apnea-hypopnea index (AHI) of 11, no snoring, and associated oxygen desaturation of 75%. During a second overnight study with nasal CPAP at a pressure of 8 cm, the AHI decreased to 3 and no drop in oxygen saturation was noted.[32] This raises the yet unstudied issue of a possible role for polysomnography in patients with expiratory central airway collapse.

3. *Endotracheal intubation–assisted bronchoscopy:* This approach should be used instead of CPAP-assisted bronchoscopy when it is not possible to maintain SaO_2 above 85% despite the use of a high fraction of inspired oxygen (FiO_2),[33] or when a patient has copious secretions that cannot be cleared or are associated with acidosis or changes in mental status.[34] Mechanical ventilation through an indwelling endotracheal tube offers the benefit of a secure airway, facilitates carbon dioxide clearance, improves gas exchange, unloads respiratory muscles, and reduces the risk for massive aspiration during bronchoscopy. It also allows repeated insertions of the bronchoscope to remove obstructing mucus plugs or blood clots. Obviously, proper assessment of airway dynamics is impaired by the indwelling endotracheal tube and the need for sedation in intubated patients.

Therapeutic Alternatives

With regard to bronchiectasis, large population-based, long-term studies of efficacy are lacking. Still, loosening of secretions combined with enhanced removal using standard pulmonary hygiene measures is probably warranted, regardless of the cause. Approaches include administration of bronchodilators, chest physiotherapy (postural drainage, hand or mechanical chest clapping, incentive spirometry, and high-frequency chest wall compression),

---

*Clinicians, when performing these types of studies, should take into account the potential effects of radiation exposure in a given individual.

hypertonic saline,* and mucolytics and anti-inflammatory medications (i.e., inhaled glucocorticosteroids).[35]

With regard to EDAC, laser application on the posterior membrane to stiffen the airway and prevent collapse, although it has been described,[36] has not been systematically studied, and its safety profile is unknown. Therefore, this approach cannot be recommended as of this writing. Stent insertion and membranous tracheoplasty are indicated for severely symptomatic patients with severe and diffuse collapse of the central airways, usually caused by cartilaginous weakness in the setting of crescent-type TBM and rarely EDAC.[37,38]

Cost-Effectiveness

No cost-effectiveness or risk-benefit analyses have been performed to evaluate the role of CPAP-assisted bronchoscopy in evaluating patients with EDAC; in addition, no studies have compared the application of noninvasive positive-pressure ventilation versus semi-invasive or open surgical treatments (e.g., airway stent insertion, laser application, membranous tracheoplasty) for patients with tracheobronchomegaly and EDAC.

Informed Consent

The patient had good understanding of the indications, contraindications, and alternatives of the procedure. He agreed to proceed with CPAP-assisted bronchoscopy under moderate sedation.

Techniques and Results

Anesthesia and Perioperative Care

Intravenous sedation is usually necessary to ensure patient comfort, but it can compromise ventilatory status, especially in children and in patients with awake hypercapnia, OSA, or OHS who are at risk for sedation-related increased collapsibility of the upper or central airways.[39] In our experience, it is helpful for one designated team member to continuously observe the patient and monitors, and to be ready to reposition the patient or suction the mouth in case of aspiration of gastric contents. Reassurance is provided continuously because patient cooperation is essential, even when sedation is being administered. The choice of sedative agent and its dose generally depend on age, underlying medical comorbidities, concomitant medications, and operator preference. Careful monitoring and adherence to sedation guidelines help to ensure a safe outcome.[33] Monitoring helps prevent procedure-related morbidity and assists the clinician in applying appropriate ventilatory settings and detecting early signs of respiratory or hemodynamic compromise.[40] These may occur as a result of performing bronchoscopy in an already frail patient (i.e., extensive pulmonary infiltrates, SaO_2 <90%, PaO_2 <75 mm Hg, FEV_1 <1 L),[41] but may also be caused by aspiration, which is more likely with CPAP owing to gastric distention.[42] Electrocardiography and pulse oximetry are continuously monitored. If the oxygen saturation drops below 80% for

longer than 1 minute, or if poor clinical tolerance is observed, the nurse or respiratory therapist should increase the FiO_2 to keep the SaO_2 above 90%.[21]

Technique and Instrumentation

A full face mask is secured to the patient's face with elastic straps (Figure 13-6). The patient is then connected to the ventilator with a dual-axis swivel adapter (T-adapter) attached to the face mask. CPAP (or BiPAP) is delivered at parameters that depend on clinical indications. We start at a pressure of 0 cm H_2O and titrate upward according to the indications. For instance, in cases of refractory hypoxemia or hypercarbia from COPD, ventilator parameters are set at CPAP of 5 cm H_2O and pressure support ventilation at 15 to 17 cm H_2O. During bronchoscopy, FiO_2 is kept at 1 and is decreased to prebronchoscopy levels after the procedure if the patient is able to maintain SpO_2 (pulse oximeter oxygen saturation) greater than 92%. The bronchoscope is advanced to the nares through the swivel adapter and face mask (see video on ExpertConsult.com) (Video III.13.1). If necessary, as in evaluation of central airway collapse, procedures are performed in the upright and supine positions, as well as on and off CPAP, to evaluate the degree of airway narrowing and response to CPAP (see Figure 13-6). In EDAC, CPAP pressures of 7 to 10 cm H_2O usually ensure airway patency, but pressures can be raised incrementally by 3 cm H_2O until airway caliber during exhalation is at least 50% of that noted during inspiration* (see video on ExpertConsult.com) (Video III.13.2). When CPAP is used for bronchoscopy in severely hypoxemic patients, positive-pressure ventilation is maintained for at least 30 minutes after the procedure, after which CPAP is discontinued if SpO_2 is greater than 92% and no evidence of respiratory insufficiency is noted.

Anatomic Dangers and Other Risks

The flexible bronchoscope occupies 10% to 15% of a normal tracheal lumen;[43] this may result in hypoventilation and hypoxemia. Bronchoscopy may induce or exacerbate bronchospasm, especially in patients with known asthma.[44] The risk for respiratory insufficiency or cardiac arrhythmias[45-47] is increased in hypoxemic patients.†

Topical anesthetics such as lidocaine or tetracaine, saline washes, and bronchoalveolar lavage (BAL) fluid administered during the procedure may induce bronchospasm and allergic reactions. Furthermore, gas exchange is impaired through a process of alveolar filling, especially after BAL, and even in relatively normal patients, hypoxemia may persist for up to 6 hours.[40]

---

*This is usually a subjective assessment during bronchoscopy; a more accurate analysis of the still images obtained during bronchoscopy and quantification of the degree of airway narrowing (aka morphometric bronchoscopy) can be performed post procedure with the use of image processing software.

†Procedure-related hypoxemia occurs after insertion of the bronchoscope through the glottis, which causes partial tracheal obstruction and ventilation-perfusion mismatch. It is also caused by excessive suctioning, which reduces end-expiratory volume and promotes alveolar closure.

---

*The mechanism of action probably is the result of improved mucus flow, increased ciliary motility, and enhanced cough.

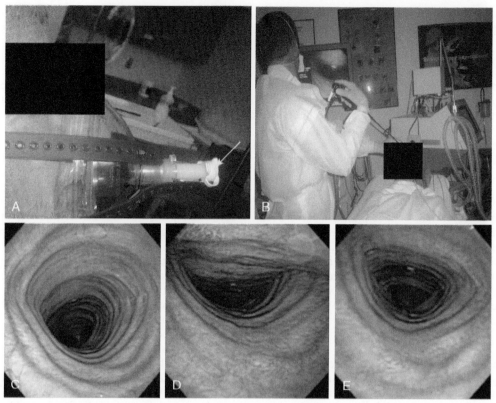

Figure 13-6 **A,** A full face mask is secured to the patient's head with elastic straps and is connected to the ventilator through the airway swivel adapter *(arrow)*. **B,** Bronchoscopy in supine position on and off continuous positive airway pressure (CPAP). **C,** Tracheal lumen in upright position during inspiration off CPAP. **D,** Tracheal lumen in supine position during expiration off CPAP. **E,** Tracheal lumen in supine position during expiration on CPAP of 10 cm H_2O.

If excessive cough is noted before the procedure, as was the case in our patient, the bronchoscopist may be tempted to use higher doses of lidocaine for local laryngeal analgesia. The major toxic side effect of lidocaine for local anesthesia is seizures (also seen with tetracaine). Concern for this is increased when plasma levels are greater than 5 mg/L. The dose of lidocaine should therefore be limited to 400 mg or 3 to 4 mg/kg.[48] Vigilance is warranted in elderly patients with liver or cardiac involvement because lidocaine is metabolized mainly in the liver, and low cardiac output delays its metabolism. The bronchoscopy team should continuously monitor the patient's mental status because seizures may present in a nonconvulsive pattern. Adverse reactions to lidocaine during bronchoscopy are, in fact, primarily related to toxicity rather than to allergy,[49] but true allergic reactions to local anesthetics are rare and account for less than 1% of adverse reactions to these anesthetic preparations.* In our practice, we do not use nebulized lidocaine. Studies have shown that the addition of nebulized lidocaine for

airway analgesia before the start of flexible bronchoscopy offered no benefit when flexible bronchoscopy was performed using combined topical analgesia and moderate (conscious) sedation.[50] Peak lidocaine plasma levels occur 15 minutes after direct topical application to the larynx and trachea, and 5 minutes after ultrasonic or other nebulization, but the maximum duration of the anesthetic effect of lidocaine, regardless of the mode of administration, is between 20 and 30 minutes.[51] These pharmacodynamic properties of lidocaine should be taken into account when patients cough excessively during bronchoscopy, because the cough can be solely related to inadequate laryngeal analgesia and often improves after the bronchoscope is removed from the patient's airway.

Results and Procedure-Related Complications

Bronchoscopy on CPAP was performed with minimal sedation (midazolam 2 mg intravenously) and with 300 mg of 1% lidocaine for laryngeal analgesia. We evaluated central airway dynamics during upright and supine positions at CPAP pressures of 0, 5, 7, 10, and 12 cm H_2O. The airway lumen was evaluated first in the upright position during tidal respiration, then during forced expiration and cough. We observed that the degree of airway compression was normal during tidal respiration but became abnormal with forced exhalation and cough (**see video on ExpertConsult.com**) (Video III.13.3). These findings were worse in the supine position when collapse in the mainstem bronchi was near complete. Findings

---

*With the exception of the gastrointestinal system, side effects are primarily dose related. Most lidocaine-related side effects involve the central nervous system—seizures, tremors, dysarthria, ataxia, hallucinations, nystagmus, and memory impairment; the cardiovascular system—sinus slowing, asystole, hypotension, and shock; and the gastrointestinal tract—nausea, vomiting, and anorexia. If an allergy to a local anesthetic belonging to the ester class is found, then generally speaking, an anesthetic from the amide class may be used, and vice versa.

were consistent with the patient's worsened symptoms at night. The degree of collapse improved with application of CPAP of 12 cm H_2O (see video on ExpertConsult. com) (Video III.13.4). After airway dynamics had been evaluated, BAL was performed by sequential instillation and aspiration of 3 aliquots of 30 mL of physiologic saline solution, with the tip of the bronchoscope wedged in the right lower lobe bronchus. After BAL was completed, positive-pressure ventilation could have been maintained for at least 30 minutes after the procedure and discontinued if SaO_2 were greater than 92% and the patient was without evidence of respiratory insufficiency.[20] In our patient, however, CPAP was discontinued immediately after removal of the bronchoscope because we used CPAP assistance to determine the optimal pressure that maintained airway patency for EDAC, not for severe refractory hypoxemia. Monitoring continued until the effects of intravenous sedation had subsided and the gag reflex had returned. Nursing staff who monitored the patient during this period were aware that respiratory distress from hypoxemia or bronchospasm can occur after the scope is removed from the airway.

Long-Term Management

Outcome Assessment

The patient was discharged home after he had been monitored for 30 minutes. He continued treatment with bronchodilators and pulmonary hygiene (postural drainage and percussion vest). Based on bronchoscopy findings and in light of evidence of improved airflow, symptoms, and atelectasis with the use of CPAP,[24,25] CPAP 12 cm H_2O was prescribed at night and intermittently during the day as conservative management of his EDAC.

Follow-up Tests and Procedures

The patient's BAL culture showed 3+ *Pseudomonas aeruginosa* (multidrug resistant) and a few colonies of *Aspergillus fumigatus*. On a follow-up clinic visit 3 weeks later, the patient stated that although subjectively he had improved with regard to cough and ability to raise secretions, he could not tolerate the CPAP mask and had decided to discontinue its use.

Referrals

He was referred to an infectious disease specialist to determine whether his chronic *Pseudomonas aeruginosa* infection should be treated. He was also referred to a sleep center to further explore and potentially resolve issues of CPAP noncompliance.* A gastroenterologist was asked to readdress his GERD.

Quality Improvement

We considered that despite this patient's inability to use CPAP over the long term, our procedure improved his care because it offered a microbiologic diagnosis, identified the severity of airway collapse, and determined its response

to CPAP. We used this case at an in-service for our department to discuss the feasibility and safety of bronchoscopy on CPAP for patients with EDAC, with TBM, and in the intensive care unit, especially if bronchoscopy is warranted in patients at high risk for respiratory failure, in whom intubation or reintubation is avoided.

DISCUSSION POINTS

1. Provide two indications for bronchoscopy on CPAP in this patient.
   - *To avoid bronchoscopy-induced hypoxemia:* Noninvasive positive-pressure ventilation was shown to improve oxygenation compared with high-flow oxygen alone in patients at high risk for respiratory complications during bronchoscopy due to severe hypoxemia.*[20,21]
   - *To evaluate EDAC and its response to CPAP:* Dynamic bronchoscopy with the patient in upright and supine positions and performed during various respiratory maneuvers can reveal central airway collapse. Evaluation of response to CPAP in terms of airway collapsibility can be performed at the same time to determine the optimal pressure necessary to improve expiratory airway collapse to an accepted normal of less than 50% as compared with the inspiratory phase. Prospective studies are needed to objectively document whether CPAP results in improvements in dyspnea scale and functional status.
2. List two differential diagnoses for excessive dynamic airway collapse (EDAC).
   - *Congenital tracheobronchomegaly (Mounier-Kuhn syndrome):* In this syndrome, EDAC is likely due to congenital atrophy or absence of elastic fibers and smooth muscle cells, resulting in a redundant posterior tracheobronchial wall.
   - *COPD:* EDAC is likely due to the basic pathophysiology of COPD, including decreased elastic recoil and increased peripheral airway resistance. The determinants of maximal expiratory flow have been modeled using equations that relate pressure drop (Bernoulli forces) to local airway wall compliance. In COPD, significant loss of pressures in the periphery results in reduced intraluminal pressures in the central airways during exhalation; this phenomenon causes compression of the tracheobronchial wall at its weakest portion (i.e., the posterior membrane), leading to EDAC.[52]
3. Provide two reasons why CPAP might help a patient with expiratory central airway collapse.
   - *Pneumatic splinting:* CPAP influences factors involved in dynamic airway compression. Wave speed theories explain the phenomenon of expiratory airflow limitation. CPAP can decrease the

---

*Reasons for CPAP noncompliance may include true anatomic reasons (beards, mustaches, or facial irregularities), as well as poor mask fit, leaks, humidifier problems, high flow impeding exhalation, and nasal congestion.

---

*It should be noted, however, that oxygen supplementation alone is not the standard of practice in severe respiratory conditions with severe hypoxemia. This population might be better served by invasive or noninvasive positive-pressure ventilation (NPPV), regardless of their need for bronchoscopy. To our knowledge, no head-to-head trials have compared NPPV versus endotracheal intubation for severely hypoxemic patients requiring bronchoscopy.

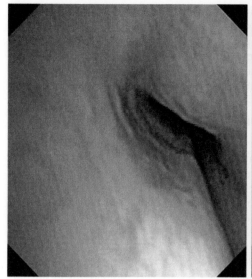 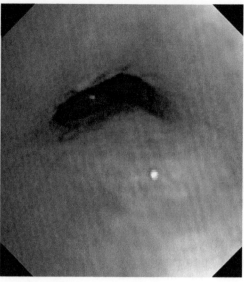

Figure 13-7 This figure shows how the image/perception changes with angulation of the scope, repositioning of the scope, and repositioning of the patient. All these maneuvers may have the same effect (i.e., change in the image perspective), even though no anatomic/structural change is seen in the actual airway lumen.

resistance of collapsible airways and prevent critical airway closure.[53-55] It also increases cross-sectional area and airway elastance, making them stiffer and increasing wave velocity along the airway wall. In addition, CPAP can act as an expiratory retard agent,[56] preventing the development of flow-limiting segments in the bronchial tree and in the upper airways early during expiration, thereby facilitating lung emptying.

- *Improved lung volumes:* This provides an alternative explanation for symptomatic improvement on CPAP.[57] Because the measured flow and the shape of the flow-volume curve depend on the lung volume at which they are measured, expiratory flow is greater at higher lung volumes than at lower lung volumes. In one report of healthy infants and infants with tracheomalacia, application of CPAP significantly increased maximal expiratory flow at FRC. This increase was secondary to the increase in lung volume found with CPAP, because maximal expiratory flows measured at different levels of CPAP were not different when compared at the same lung volumes. This suggests that the optimal level of CPAP may be attained by increasing lung volumes to a level at which patients are not flow-limited during tidal breathing.*

Expert Commentary

provided by Ian Brent Masters, MB BS, FRACP, PhD

In this case, a 70-year-old male with Mounier-Kuhn syndrome, asthma-like illness, bronchiectasis, and GERD is presented, and the functional implications of cough, as well as the chronic disorders themselves, are described. Controversial management issues raised by

the authors include indications for bronchoscopy and use of CPAP and functional bronchoscopy to assess EDAC and CPAP pressure settings in structural airway disease. Overall, this case highlights the need for improved morphometric bronchoscopy techniques, which will be the focus of my commentary.

In my opinion, the indications for bronchoscopy in this patient could be extended to visual inspection of the entire airway, because Mounier-Kuhn syndrome is often associated with malacia and dilated bronchi; indeed, the bronchoscope will often pass through many generations of the airways beyond those expected. In addition, the orifices of lobar and segmental bronchi may function unpredictably and may appear as aberrant shapes. Chest CT poorly defines bronchomalacia, let alone shapes of lobar bronchi. Bronchoscopy could thus enhance diagnostic accuracy and the understanding of the extent of changes in large to medium airways to a substantially greater extent compared with CT.

The belief that real-time bronchoscopy can determine the severity of EDAC is based on visual perspectives and perceptions of changes in size or cross-sectional area across the respiratory cycle. This is a controversial concept. In clinical terms, it could be regarded as being "good enough." However, this type of assessment has many limitations.[58] Short excerpts of the patient's bronchoscopy display many of the issues that will be raised in the following paragraphs.

It is worthwhile remembering that the airway does lengthen and dilate with inspiration and then progressively contracts to its original position by the end of expiration. Bronchoscopic appreciation of this change is gained by holding the scope in a fixed position, but as the object of interest moves away from the tip of the scope, it actually moves to a lower magnification power; thus perceptions of change are gained through unknown but lower values of magnification, distortion effects, unknown distance traveled by the point of interest, and perspective change (Figure 13-7). In addition, effects on cross-sectional area change are due to

---

*This is possible if no associated increased work of breathing is seen to result from decreased pulmonary compliance at increased lung volumes.

uncontrolled changes in lung volume associated with the depth of anesthesia/sedation effects on respiratory system mechanics, resistance effects of the broncho-scope, and effects of movement of mucus on ventilation distribution and regional lung volumes (Figure 13-8). These effects are not readily perceived or appreciated despite the use of modern digital imaging techniques, television screens, or computer display panels. Memory function and the level of experience of the bronchoscopist are also likely to change these perceptions.[59] Thus perceived change in airway size should be treated cautiously, or at its best should be regarded as an appreciable underestimate.

Planar quantitative or morphometric bronchoscopy, which enables assessment of airway lumen size, is available with techniques such as color histogram mode techniques,[58,60,61] but precise measurement is limited to the expiratory position because the peak inspiratory position may be difficult to define in complex lesions (Figure 13-9). The expiratory position is chosen because it can be touched by the broncho-scope (the zero position), and because airway collapse may be present across both inspiration and expiration (see video on ExpertConsult.com) (Video III.13.2), and it may be available over long distances. Thus, the bronchoscope can be entrapped by collapsed tissue, or perspective may be lost by angulation changes (see video on ExpertConsult.com) (Video III.13.3). Change in airway size at the point of interest cannot be measured without knowledge of the distance traveled during the respiratory cycle and without placement of calibration objects in the airways.*

---

*To correct for these distortions, calibration of images requires insertion of bodies of known diameter (e.g., biopsy forceps, marker bodies).

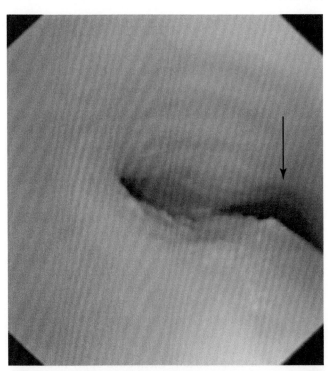

Figure 13-8 Bilateral proximal mainstem malacia: In this case, the view is "off center" because the airway is distorted; therefore, the right mainstem bronchus is off to the periphery *(right lower corner of the image)*. Correction of this view is impossible short of advancing the scope. This type of image negates measurement. In the pediatric setting, with the use of general anesthesia techniques (gaseous or propofol), tidal volumes are relatively small, so the airways do not necessarily open on inspiration even when bagged, but the scope is pushed through these malacic lesions relatively easily. Often, the scope cannot be positioned to accurately define the end point of the lesion, and if it is long enough, one can see only the mucosa until the scope is actually out of the lesion. In the pediatric setting, these lesions may occur over 1 mm to 2 cm only, so the actual hand movements required to gain a clear view are very subtle to say the least.

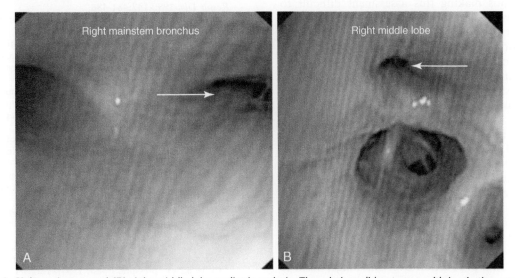

Figure 13-9 **A,** Right mainstem and **(B)** right middle lobe pediatric malacia. These lesions did not open with inspiration, except for the very slight opening seen at the proximal end of the bronchus, but they could be opened with the scope. Although the pediatric setting is vastly different from the adult setting, the principles of measurement are the same.

In addition, this method does require quantification of magnification characteristics and power of the particular bronchoscope selected. Post hoc analyses are necessary to attain quantitative measurements with strong intraobserver and interobserver agreement.[60,61] Three-dimensional (3D) bronchoscopic reconstruction of the airways and morphometry across both phases of respiration represent an advance in determining precise relative change, but accurate distance measurements are still needed to allow quantitative measurements. Computing power will have to be substantial to enable real-time in vivo measurements.

Reference points are required for comparative quantitative bronchoscopy assessments. Because the cricoid is a complete ring and a relatively rigid structure, reproducibility of measurement is high. Measurements in this region have strong relationships to lower airway measurements. However, the weak point of this technique is that intersubject variability is relatively high.[62] This potentially makes grading of severity relatively weak, but it does provide a quantifiable comparative approach.

All of the issues already mentioned apply to assessments with CPAP as well. Just how far upstream the CPAP effect is seen is not known, and how these respiratory mechanical characteristics correlate with awake and sleep states is also unknown. The infant's larynx is markedly different from that of the adult in terms of position and structural composition; thus extrapolation to the adult and justification of decisions on these grounds are fraught with potential errors. In addition, evidence suggests that bronchoscopically assessed cross-sectional area of airway lesions in pediatric disease does not necessarily correlate with severity of illness. The addition of endobronchial lesions or changes in mucosal patterns associated with bronchiectasis and mucus sleeves, plaques, and plugs to the scenario of a rather transient period of time for assessment enhances negative arguments, thus making this assessment difficult to justify. In my opinion, quantitative bronchoscopy, in whatever form, would improve this situation, but standardization of the whole bronchoscopic approach, its timing, control of anesthetic depth, and control of the adjustments required after coughing or during periods of supported ventilation will need to be considered and accounted for if accuracy is to be maximized.

Just what effect long-term nocturnal CPAP has on surrogates of Mounier-Kuhn syndrome such as tracheobronchomalacia and on airway clearance of sputum in non-CF bronchiectasis and CF bronchiectasis is not clearly known. For short-term use, benefit in terms of airway patency, mucus clearance, gas exchange, and sleep quality is apparent. Whether this will result in improved airway tone or worsening of dilation/malacia due to overstretching and reduced or increased sputum production over the longer term is open to conjecture.

REFERENCES

1. Bilton D. Update on non-cystic fibrosis bronchiectasis. *Curr Opin Pulm Med.* 2008;14:595-599.
2. Koh WJ, Lee JH, Kwon YS, et al. Prevalence of gastroesophageal reflux disease in patients with nontuberculous mycobacterial lung disease. *Chest.* 2007;131:1825-1830.
3. Boiselle PM, Feller-Kopman D, Ashiku S, et al. Tracheobronchomalacia: evolving role of dynamic multislice helical CT. *Radiol Clin North Am.* 2003;41:627-636.
4. Joosten S, Macdonald M, Lau KK, et al. Excessive dynamic airway collapse co-morbid with COPD diagnosed using 320-slice dynamic CT scanning technology. *Thorax.* 2010 Jul 7. [Epub ahead of print]
5. Bateson EM, Woo-Ming M. Tracheo-bronchomegaly. *Clin Radiol.* 1973;24:345-358.
6. Baron KG, Smith TW, Czajkowski LA, et al. Relationship quality and CPAP adherence in patients with obstructive sleep apnea. *Behav Sleep Med.* 2009;7:22-36.
7. Murgu SD, Colt HG. Tracheobronchomalacia and excessive dynamic airway collapse. *Respirology.* 2006;11:388-406.
8. Sucena M, Liistro G, Aubert G, et al. Continuous positive airway pressure treatment for sleep apnoea: compliance increases with time in continuing users. *Eur Respir J.* 2006;27:761-766.
9. Barker AF. Bronchiectasis. *N Engl J Med.* 2002;346:1383-1393.
10. Pang JA, Cheng A, Chan HS, et al. The bacteriology of bronchiectasis in Hong Kong investigated by protected catheter brush and bronchoalveolar lavage. *Am Rev Respir Dis.* 1989;139:14-17.
11. Tsang KW, Ho PI, Chan KN, et al. A pilot study of low-dose erythromycin in bronchiectasis. *Eur Respir J.* 1999;13:361-364.
12. Angrill J, Agustí C, de Celis R, et al. Bacterial colonisation in patients with bronchiectasis: microbiological pattern and risk factors. *Thorax.* 2002;57:15-19.
13. Ho PL, Chan KN, Ip MS, et al. The effect of *Pseudomonas aeruginosa* infection on clinical parameters in steady-state bronchiectasis. *Chest.* 1998;114:1594-1598.
14. Martínez-García MA, Soler-Cataluña JJ, Perpiñá-Tordera M, et al. Factors associated with lung function decline in adult patients with stable non-cystic fibrosis bronchiectasis. *Chest.* 2007;132: 1565-1572.
15. Cortese DA, Prakash UBS, Stubbs SE. Technical solutions to common problems in bronchoscopy. In: Prakash UBS, ed. *Bronchoscopy.* New York: Raven Press; 1994:111-133.
16. Benditt JO. Novel uses of noninvasive ventilation. *Respir Care.* 2009;54:212-219.
17. Murgu SD, Colt HG. Treatment of adult tracheobronchomalacia and excessive dynamic airway collapse: an update. *Treat Respir Med.* 2006;5:103-115.
18. Goldstein RA, Rohatgi PK, Bergofsky EH, et al. Clinical role of bronchoalveolar lavage in adults with pulmonary disease. *Am Rev Respir Dis.* 1990;142:481-486.
19. Dellinger RP. Fiberoptic bronchoscopy in adult airway management. *Crit Care Med.* 1990;18:882-887.
20. Antonelli M, Conti G, Rocco M, et al. Noninvasive positive-pressure ventilation versus conventional oxygen supplementation in hypoxemic patients undergoing diagnostic bronchoscopy. *Chest.* 2002;121:1149-1154.
21. Maitre B, Jaber S, Maggiore SM, et al. Continuous positive airway pressure during fiberoptic bronchoscopy in hypoxemic patients: a randomized double-blind study using a new device. *Am J Respir Crit Care Med.* 2000;162:1063-1067.
22. Trachsel D, Erb TO, Frei FJ, et al. Use of continuous positive airway pressure during flexible bronchoscopy in young children. *Eur Respir J.* 2005;26:773-777.
23. Antonelli M, Pennisi M, Conti G, et al. Fiberoptic bronchoscopy during noninvasive positive pressure ventilation delivered by helmet. *Intensive Care Med.* 2003;29:126-129.
24. Wiseman NE, Duncan PG, Cameron CB. Management of tracheobronchomalacia with continuous positive airway pressure. *J Pediatr Surg.* 1985;20:489-493.
25. Adliff M, Ngato D, Keshavjee S, et al. Treatment of diffuse tracheomalacia secondary to relapsing polychondritis with continuous positive airway pressure. *Chest.* 1997;112:1701-1704.
26. Da Conceicao M, Genco G, Favier JC, et al. Fiberoptic bronchoscopy during non-invasive positive pressure ventilation in patients

with chronic obstructive lung disease with hypoxemia and hypercapnia. *Ann Fr Anesth Reanim.* 2000;19:231-233.

27. Borowiecki B, Pollack CP, Weitzman ED, et al. Fibro-optic study of pharyngeal airway during sleep in patients with hypersomnia obstructive sleep-apnea syndrome. *Laryngoscope.* 1978;88:1310-1313.

28. Murgu SD, Pecson J, Colt HG. Bronchoscopy on noninvasive positive pressure ventilation: indications and technique. *Respir Care.* 2010;55:595-600.

29. Holanda MA, Fortaleza SC, Alves-de-Almeida M, et al. Continuous positive airway pressure effects on regional lung aeration in patients with COPD: a high-resolution CT scan study. *Chest.* 2010;138:305-314.

30. Khirani S, Biot L, Eberhard A, et al. Positive end expiratory pressure and expiratory flow limitation: a model study. *Acta Biotheor.* 2001;49:277-290.

31. Parr DG, Stoel BC, Stolk J, et al. Influence of calibration on densitometric studies of emphysema progression using computed tomography. *Am J Respir Crit Care Med.* 2004;170:883-890.

32. Sundaram P, Joshi JM. Tracheobronchomegaly associated tracheomalacia: analysis by sleep study. *Indian J Chest Dis Allied Sci.* 2004;46:47-49.

33. Martin J. Preparing and supporting patients undergoing a bronchoscopy. *Nurse Times.* 2003;99:52-55.

34. Esteban A, Frutos-Vivar F, Ferguson ND, et al. Noninvasive positive-pressure ventilation for respiratory failure after extubation. *N Engl J Med.* 2004;350:2452-2460.

35. McCool FD, Rosen MJ. Nonpharmacologic airway clearance therapies: ACCP evidence-based clinical practice guidelines. *Chest.* 2006;129:250S.

36. Dutau H, Maldonado F, Breen DP, et al. Endoscopic successful management of tracheobronchomalacia with laser: apropos of a Mounier-Kuhn syndrome. *Eur J Cardiothorac Surg.* 2011 Mar 5. [Epub ahead of print]

37. Murgu SD, Colt HG. Complications of silicone stent insertion in patients with expiratory central airway collapse. *Ann Thorac Surg.* 2007;84:1870-1877.

38. Wright CD, Grillo HC, Hammoud ZT, et al. Tracheoplasty for expiratory collapse of central airways. *Ann Thorac Surg.* 2005;80:259-267.

39. Chhajed PN, Aboyoun C, Malouf MA, et al. Management of acute hypoxemia during flexible bronchoscopy with insertion of a nasopharyngeal tube in lung transplant recipients. *Chest.* 2002;121:1350-1354.

40. Matsushima Y, Jones RL, King EG, et al. Alterations in pulmonary mechanics and gas exchange during routine fiberoptic bronchoscopy. *Chest.* 1984;86:184-188.

41. Klech J, Pohl W. Technical recommendations and guidelines for bronchoalveolar lavage (BAL). Report of the European Society of Pneumology Task Group. *Eur Respir J.* 1989;2:561-585.

42. Aoyama K, Yasunaga E, Takenaka I, et al. Positive pressure ventilation during fibreoptic intubation: comparison of the laryngeal mask airway, intubating laryngeal mask and endoscopy mask techniques. *Br J Anaesth.* 2002;88:246-254.

43. Lindholm CE, Ollman B, Snyder GV, et al. Cardiorespiratory effects of flexible fiberoptic bronchoscopy in critically ill patients. *Chest.* 1978;74:362-368.

44. Pue CA, Pacht ER. Complications of fiberoptic bronchoscopy at a university hospital. *Chest.* 1995;107:430-432.

45. Payne CB Jr, Goyal PC, Gupta SC. Effects of transoral and transnasal fiberoptic bronchoscopy on oxygenation and cardiac rhythm. *Endoscopy.* 1986;18:1-3.

46. Katz AS, Michelson EL, Stawicki J, et al. Cardiac arrhythmias, frequency during fiberoptic bronchoscopy and correlation with hypoxemia. *Arch Intern Med.* 1981;141:603-606.

47. Albertini R, Harrel JH, Moser KM. Hypoxemia during fiberoptic bronchoscopy. *Chest.* 1974;65:117-118.

48. Langmarc EL. Serum lidocaine concentration in asthmatics undergoing research bronchoscopy. *Chest.* 2000;117:1055-1060.

49. Gall H, Kaufman CM. Adverse reactions to local anesthetics: analysis 7 of 179 cases. *J Allergy Clin Immunol.* 1996;97;933-937.

50. Stolz D, Chhajed P, Leuppi J, et al. Nebulized lidocaine for flexible bronchoscopy. *Chest.* 2005;128:1756-1760.

51. Reed A. Preparation of the patient for awake flexible fiberoptic bronchoscopy. *Chest.* 1992;101:244.

52. Baram D, Smaldone G. Tracheal collapse versus tracheobronchomalacia: normal function versus disease. *Am J Respir Crit Care Med.* 2006;174:724.

53. Guerin C, LeMasson S, de Varax R, et al. Small airway closure and positive end-expiratory pressure in mechanically ventilated patients with chronic obstructive pulmonary disease. *Am J Respir Crit Care Med.* 1997;155:1949-1956.

54. Schwab RJ, Pack AI, Gupta KB, et al. Upper airway and soft tissue structural changes induced by CPAP in normal subjects. *Am J Respir Crit Care Med.* 1996;154(4 Pt 1):1106-1116.

55. Dellacà RL, Rotger M, Aliverti A, et al. Noninvasive detection of expiratory flow limitation in COPD patients during nasal CPAP. *Eur Respir J.* 2006;27:983-991.

56. Lourens MS, van den Berg B, Verbraak AFM, et al. Effect of series of resistance levels on flow limitation in mechanically ventilated COPD patients. *Respir Physiol.* 2001;127:39-52.

57. Davis S, Jones M, Kisling J, et al. Effect of continuous positive airway pressure on forced expiratory flows in infants with tracheomalacia. *Am J Respir Crit Care Med.* 1998;158:148-152.

58. Murgu S, Colt HG. Morphometric bronchoscopy in adults with central airway obstruction: case illustrations and review of the literature. *Laryngoscope.* 2009;119:1318-1324.

59. Masters IB, Chang AB. Tracheobronchomalacia in children. *Expert Rev Respir Med.* 2009;3:425-439.

60. Masters IB, Eastburn MM, Francis PW, et al. Quantification of the magnification and distortion effects of a pediatric flexible video-bronchoscope. *Respir Res.* 2005;6:16.

61. Masters IB, Eastburn MM, Wootton R, et al. A new method for objective identification and measurement of airway lumen in paediatric flexible videobronchoscopy. *Thorax.* 2005;60:652-658.

62. Masters IB, Ware RS, Zimmerman PV, et al. Airway sizes and proportions in children quantified by a video-bronchoscopic technique. *BMC Pulm Med.* 2006;6:5.

Chapter 14

Stent Insertion for Severe Diffuse Excessive Dynamic Airway Collapse Caused by COPD

This chapter emphasizes the following elements of the Four Box Approach: risk-benefit analysis and therapeutic alternatives; anesthesia and other perioperative care; and follow-up tests, visits, and procedures.

CASE DESCRIPTION

The patient was a 64-year-old obese female with a body mass index (BMI) of 45, a 5-month history of progressive shortness of breath, and recent dyspnea at rest. Complaints included mucus production and inability to raise secretions. Recent hospitalization for pneumonia prompted treatment with systemic antibiotics. Comorbidities included obstructive sleep apnea (OSA) treated with 12 cm H_2O of continuous positive airway pressure (CPAP), severe chronic obstructive pulmonary disease (COPD) requiring home oxygen (3 L via nasal cannula), recurrent bronchitis, usually treated in the ambulatory setting, diabetes, and gastroesophageal reflux disease (GERD). She lived in a nursing facility and had no close family members or friends. During the physical examination, the patient expressed her frustration that she was often ignored by nursing home staff. Bilateral diffuse rhonchi with early expiratory wheezing were noted on lung examination. Trace pedal edema was observed bilaterally. The arterial blood gas revealed pH of 7.46, PCO_2 (partial pressure of carbon dioxide) of 38, and PO_2 (partial pressure of oxygen) of 60 on 3 L of oxygen. Complete blood count showed a white blood cell (WBC) count of 18,000 and hemoglobin of 16.6. Chest radiograph showed bibasilar atelectasis, a right infrahilar infiltrate suggestive of pneumonia, and mild pulmonary vascular congestion. Echocardiography showed normal left and right ventricular function, but the right ventricular systolic pressure was calculated at 52 mm Hg. Chest computed

tomography (CT) revealed bulging of the posterior membrane inside the airway lumen and 75% narrowing of the upper trachea associated with complete collapse of the lower trachea and mainstem bronchi during expiration, consistent with excessive dynamic airway collapse (EDAC) (Figure 14-1). Bronchoscopy confirmed CT findings (see video on ExpertConsult.com) (Video III.14.1).

DISCUSSION POINTS

1. Explain the impact of EDAC on expiratory flow limitation in COPD.
2. List three considerations pertaining to the administration of anesthesia during rigid bronchoscopy for this patient with severe EDAC.
3. Which two alternative treatments to stent insertion might be considered in this patient?
4. Describe three potential complications from stent insertion in this particular patient.

CASE RESOLUTION

Initial Evaluations

Physical Examination, Complementary Tests, and Functional Status Assessment

Dyspnea, recurrent pneumonia, and inability to raise secretions are nonspecific but common findings in patients with expiratory central airway collapse.[1,2] Symptoms are usually refractory to conventional treatments such as corticosteroids and bronchodilators for suspected asthma and COPD.[3] Occasionally, hypercarbic respiratory failure can occur. Once intubated, patients may be difficult to wean from mechanical ventilation.[4,5] In nonintubated patients, spirometry often shows obstructive ventilatory impairment that is proportionate to the severity of the disease.[6] The expiratory flow-volume loop (FVL) often reveals an airway collapse pattern* (Figure 14-2). Expiratory airway collapse is also seen during dynamic bronchoscopy,†[7] and in fact has been reported in up to 40% of patients with severe COPD.[7,8]

In our patient, a diagnosis of diffuse, severe expiratory central airway collapse was made bronchoscopically and on paired dynamic inspiratory-expiratory CT scanning. This was characterized by weakness of the posterior membranous wall, resulting in excessive bulging of the posterior membrane within the airway lumen and causing 100% airway narrowing in the mainstem bronchi and lower trachea (see Figure 14-1).[2,9] No evidence of

---

*This pattern occurs when maximal flow is quickly reached after expiration of a small volume of air. Following maximal flow is a large fall in flow, although only a small volume is exhaled. Subsequently, the flow rate falls very little during the remainder of expiration. This phase is responsible for the long plateau seen on the FVL.

†During dynamic (functional) bronchoscopy, the airways were visualized by moving the patient into the supine, upright, and lateral decubitus positions during spontaneous breathing, as well as during cough, forced expiration, and deep inspiration. During these bronchoscopic assessments, changes in the airway lumen can be measured, the extent of collapse noted, and narrowing classified as being of the crescent, saber-sheath, or circumferential type. Regions of cartilaginous weakness (tracheomalacia) can be differentiated from areas of excessive dynamic airway collapse (EDAC) or normal physiologic dynamic airway collapse (DAC).

Figure 14-1 Paired inspiratory-expiratory dynamic computed tomography images *(upper panel)* and corresponding bronchoscopic images *(lower panel)* show narrowing of the lower trachea caused by excessive bulging of the posterior membrane within the airway lumen in the absence of cartilaginous abnormalities—findings consistent with excessive dynamic airway collapse.

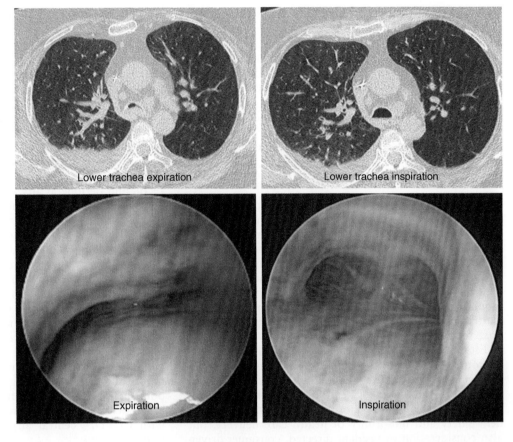

Figure 14-2 A, This flow-volume loop shows a sudden decrease in peak expiratory flow, defined as a 50% drop within 10% of forced vital capacity. This *airway collapse pattern* is commonly seen in patients with severe chronic obstructive pulmonary disease (COPD). **B,** The corresponding bronchoscopic image during inspiration shows normal tracheal lumen. **C,** During expiration, evidence of excessive dynamic airway collapse is found (the flow-volume loop and the bronchoscopic images are from the same patient).

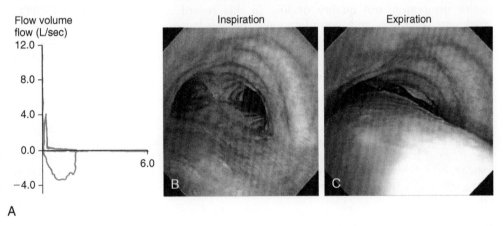

cartilaginous weakness was noted. Results from studies show that dynamic CT correlates well with bronchoscopy findings in patients with central airway collapse.[10] CT scanning offers complementary information by revealing structures adjacent to the airway and by allowing quantitative measurements of the degree of airway narrowing before and after airway splinting procedures.[11,12] No evidence of extrinsic compression was observed resulting from mediastinal masses or vascular structures (e.g., double aortic arch, aortic aneurysm); also, on expiratory images, no evidence of air trapping and mosaic attenuation suggested bronchiolitis. The patient's severe limitation of physical activity at rest was consistent with functional impairment class IV based on World Health Organization (WHO) criteria.[13] Other dyspnea or quality of life (QOL) instruments (St. George's Respiratory Questionnaire [SGRQ], American Thoracic Society Dyspnea Scale [ATS], Baseline Dyspnea Index [BDI]/Transitional Dyspnea Index [TDI], Karnofsky Performance Scale [KPS], and 6-Minute Walk Test [6MWT]) have been studied in these patients to objectively determine response to interventions.[14]

Comorbidities

This patient had no evidence of systolic or diastolic dysfunction on echocardiogram, but evidence revealed moderate pulmonary hypertension, which could result in hemodynamic instability during general anesthesia.[15]

She suffered from obesity and GERD, both of which increase the risk for aspiration of gastric contents during general anesthesia,[16] which might be required for any form of bronchoscopic or surgical treatment of EDAC. Additionally, OSA raised concerns regarding difficult mask ventilation, difficult tracheal intubation, hypoxemia, postprocedure airway obstruction, cardiac arrhythmias, and myocardial infarction. The presence of both obesity and hypoventilation perioperatively has been shown to be associated with worse outcomes and higher mortality.[17]

Support System

The patient was a resident of a nursing home. Published literature focusing on patient safety in the nursing home environment states that clinical assessments are frequently absent or unsatisfactory at critical points during a nursing home resident's stay (to ensure prevention and timely treatment of potentially dangerous conditions).[18] Pertinent to this patient's case is her history of recurrent pneumonias and refractory COPD, both of which should have alerted physicians to a potential alternative diagnosis (i.e., central airway obstruction).

Establishing a differential diagnosis when therapeutic outcomes are not in line with expectations is essential to ensure early diagnosis and treatment for a variety of disorders, including EDAC. In the setting of a long-term care facility, this requires not only an emphasis on resident safety and uniformity of health care delivery, but also consideration of resident-directed, consumer-driven health promotion and quality of life. In this regard, workforce redesign and considerations for resident-centered care are key elements of culture change to ensure a person's well-being in these institutions.[19]

Patient Preferences and Expectations

This patient was motivated to improve her symptoms so that she could increase her mobility and potentially leave the nursing home. She clearly expressed her dissatisfaction with her current care environment, a willingness to consider all available treatment options, including airway stent insertion or open surgical resection if necessary, which might help her regain independent living conditions.

Procedural Strategies

Indications

Treatment of severe diffuse EDAC includes minimally invasive or open surgical procedures.[1,2] Some central airway narrowing during expiration is normal, however, and it has been suggested that airway splinting procedures should be considered only when excessive narrowing results in symptomatic airflow limitation.[20] From both anatomic and physiologic perspectives, the boundary between normal and abnormal narrowing of the central airways is far from being established, and the exact degree of expiratory airway narrowing responsible for symptoms and requiring intervention remains unknown. For example, even an 80% reduction in tracheal lumen cross-section at the end of a "forced" expiration, when the flow in central airways physiologically

nears zero, may well be within normal limits.* Some authors propose 30%[21] and others 40%,[22] but most investigators use 50% or greater reduction in airway caliber between inspiration and expiration to identify abnormal central airway collapse on dynamic CT or bronchoscopy.[23-25] Upon application of these criteria when a patient is asked to cough or perform a forced expiration, false positives may be noted; in one study, investigators reported that nearly 80% of normal people exceeded the diagnostic criteria of 50% or greater obstruction in the upper and/or lower trachea.[26]

Patients with concurrent COPD have reduced elastic recoil and peripheral airway obstruction. The expiratory airway collapse seen in the central airways thus represents normal physiology,[20,27,28] because during flow-limited breathing, the central airways become severely compressed, particularly during forced expiration and cough. Both of these maneuvers are routinely used to detect this entity on dynamic imaging studies. The Starling resistor model† shows that a pressure drop occurs across a very short length of airway, and that proximal airway resistance, downstream from the choke point, mouthward, should not affect airflow. Pressure catheter measurements demonstrate the flow-limiting choke point and lack of further pressure drop in airways between the mouth and the flow-limiting segment.[29] Because the choke point in adult humans is often located at the level of the lobar bronchi, and is even more peripheral in patients with COPD,[30] central airway collapsibility should not impede airflow.[20,29]

Patients with COPD and EDAC, however, may still improve their symptoms and functional status after central airway stabilization with stents or tracheoplasty despite lack of improvement in forced expiratory volume in 1 second (FEV_1).[31] By stabilizing and reducing central airway flow turbulence, in addition to improving secretion management and preventing excessive cough from chronic airway inflammation, these procedures might result in improved quality of life and dyspnea improvement with exertion caused by a reduction in hyperinflation.[14,31] Our patient had severe (100%) collapse resulting in dyspnea at rest, inability to raise secretions, and recurrent pneumonia. These symptoms were not responding to optimal COPD treatment and CPAP for OSA. For these reasons, after taking into account the patient's wishes, we elected to perform rigid bronchoscopy under general anesthesia to place an indwelling silicone stent that would splint open the lower trachea and mainstem bronchi. Our goal was to improve airway lumen patency to less than 50% collapse during exhalation, which, by

---

*The choke points (flow-limiting segments) in humans are often located in the lobar bronchi, so mainstem bronchial or tracheal collapsibility should not result in any pressure drop between the mouth and the choke point and therefore should not affect expiratory airflow. Physiologists suggest that bronchoscopic or radiologic detection of expiratory tracheal or mainstem bronchial compression should trigger a search for causes of airflow obstruction within the lung, not in the central airways.[20]

†The Starling resistor is a simple model of the lung that comprises an elastic tube mounted between two rigid tubes inside a chamber filled with air; airflow is driven through the system. This model has been used to explain expiratory flow limitation.

convention, is currently considered within normal limits by most investigators.[13]

Contraindications

No absolute contraindications to rigid bronchoscopy were noted. Evidence of pulmonary artery hypertension was likely due to her COPD and OSA, which could increase the risk of right ventricular dysfunction and hemodynamic instability during general anesthesia.

Expected Results

In the short term (up to 10 to 14 days), airway stabilization with silicone stents in patients with expiratory central airway collapse (malacia and EDAC) improves symptoms, quality of life, and functional status.[4,14] In one study, quality of life and functional status scores improved in 70% of patients and dyspnea scores improved in 91% of patients after stent insertion.[14] Stent-related complications included obstruction from mucus plugging and migration, and almost 10% of patients (5 of 52 patients) had complications related to the bronchoscopic procedure itself. Because the dynamic features of expiratory central airway collapse continuously alter the shape of the central airways, as well as the surface contact between a stent and the airway wall, stent-related complications may occur more frequently in dynamic forms of airway obstruction than in fixed benign obstruction or malignancy.[4] In one study of 57 patients, 21 partial stent obstructions, 14 infections, and 10 stent migrations were noted.[14] Although not life threatening, these stent-related adverse events required multiple repeat bronchoscopies.

Team Experience

As of this writing, silicone stent insertion requires rigid bronchoscopy. The technique of atraumatic rigid intubation, single stent insertion, or Y stent insertion using the "push" or "pullback" technique* is one that is gradually perfected with practice and experience.

Risk-Benefit Analysis

The rare potential risks of airway injury during rigid bronchoscopy, hemodynamic instability during general anesthesia in the setting of pulmonary hypertension, and postoperative complications from OSA were considered to be outweighed by the potential benefits of improved airway patency, diminished shortness of breath, restored ability to clear secretions, and an enhanced quality of life.

Therapeutic Alternatives for Restoring Airway Patency

Other than silicone stent insertion, therapeutic alternatives for EDAC include noninvasive positive-pressure ventilation, metal stent insertion, and open surgical treatment.

---

*In the "push" technique, the stent is ejected from the bronchoscope above the carina and then is pushed distally with an open rigid grasping forceps placed at the stent bifurcation, so that each limb of the stent enters the appropriate bronchus. In the "pullback" technique, the bronchoscope is placed into one main bronchus (usually the one involved with the most disease). As both bronchial limbs are expulsed, the bronchoscope is pulled slowly proximally toward the carina until the shorter limb extends toward and into the contralateral bronchus.

- *Continuous positive airway pressure (CPAP):* This patient was symptomatic despite already being on CPAP 12 cm H_2O. Bronchoscopy on CPAP could have been performed to assess the optimal pressure needed to maintain patency of the central airways. This was not done however, because 24-hour continuous CPAP was not desirable (this patient's symptoms were not only positional or presented only during sleep).[32] CPAP decreases pulmonary resistance and can be used to restore and maintain airway patency, facilitate secretion drainage, and improve expiratory flow. Small studies showed that the addition of nasal CPAP improves spirometry values, sputum production, atelectasis, and exercise tolerance, but its long-term efficacy has not been clearly demonstrated.[33,34]

- *Metal stent insertion* was used in the past for central airway collapse with variable success.[9] Advantages include placement by flexible bronchoscopy, dynamic expansion, and preservation of airway mucociliary function with uncovered stents. In some studies, however, metal stents had to be removed because of stent failure or because of stent-related complications. Cases of stent fracture and fatal hemorrhage from perforation have prompted the Food and Drug Administration (FDA) to recommend against the use of metallic stents for histologically benign forms of airway obstruction.[35]

- *Membranous tracheoplasty* has been proposed to consolidate and reshape the airway wall. Before open surgical intervention, a stent trial is recommended to identify patients most likely to benefit from surgery in the long term.[14] Tracheoplasty reinforces the membranous portion of the trachea and seemed to provide favorable outcomes in uncontrolled studies.[31,36]

- *Indwelling tracheostomy tubes* may splint the collapsible airway, ensure airway access and patency, and allow invasive ventilatory support if necessary. In this patient, however, airway compromise extended into both mainstem bronchi. The obstruction would not have been bypassed by a simple tracheostomy tube; a long, bifurcated Montgomery T-tube would have been required, making clearance of spontaneous or cough-induced secretions difficult, and creating a risk for subglottic granulation tissue formation and further airway obstruction.

Cost-Effectiveness

No published studies have evaluated the cost-effectiveness of stent insertion or surgery for severe diffuse EDAC. Based on available literature, operable patients with severe diffuse disease refractory to conservative treatment for the underlying disorders (e.g., COPD) and severe functional impairments attributable to this process probably should be evaluated for membranous tracheoplasty. If the condition is not operable, then permanent stent insertion with or without adjuvant noninvasive positive-pressure ventilation can be offered as long as objective improvement in the patient's functional status is observed after stent insertion.[9]

Informed Consent

Risks, benefits, and alternatives to rigid bronchoscopy with stent insertion were discussed with the patient. When feedback techniques were used, she demonstrated good understanding of the indications, expected results, and potential complications associated with rigid bronchoscopy and silicone stent insertion under general anesthesia. She understood that she had to be compliant with stent care measures, including the use of saline nebulization three to four times per day and huffing breathing techniques and deep breathing exercises to help clear secretions. We asked whether she had any specific concerns about the procedure and invited her to provide us with informational needs that she might have and that were not obvious to us. On this note, she voiced concern about the nursing home staff and shared with us her perception that they would not help her with saline nebulization if help were needed. We assured her that we would provide learning materials to the nursing home staff.

We felt confident that we had provided this patient with complete and truthful information about the proposed therapy, its risks and benefits, and its alternatives, including the alternative of no additional therapy. It is unclear whether differences in stress levels occur in patients who receive detailed information about treatment considerations compared with those who receive little or no information. We were thorough in our description of risks and benefits of the proposed intervention.

Techniques and Results

Anesthesia and Perioperative Care

In addition to the possibility of upper airway obstruction related to this patient's OSA (worsened by diminished upper airway muscle activity), risk for collapse of an already weakened upper (extrathoracic) tracheal wall is present owing to large negative pressures generated by inspiration against a closed glottis or an obstructing tongue.[37] The anesthesiologist should be aware of the potential for worsening intrathoracic airway obstruction during induction of anesthesia (see video on ExpertConsult.com) (Video III.14.2). This occurrence has been reported with both intravenous and inhalational agents.[38] Use of neuromuscular blocking agents should probably be avoided because these drugs may eliminate airway muscle tone and chest wall tone, which normally provide extrinsic support for the critically narrowed airway during spontaneous ventilation.[39] Patients may not tolerate the supine position after induction. Therefore, the bronchoscopist should be stationed at the head of the bed throughout induction of anesthesia, in case emergent bronchoscopic intubation is required to secure and control the airway. To avoid potential complications resulting from excessive muscle relaxation or paralysis, we prefer to use spontaneous assisted ventilation for rigid bronchoscopy (with an open, ventilating rigid tube rather than jet ventilation) in the setting of severe central airway obstruction.[40]

General anesthesia in patients with obesity and OSA may be associated with worsening hypoventilation and hypoxemia. In patients with known or suspected right heart failure, acute hypoxia should be avoided because it can cause pulmonary vasoconstriction, leading to further increases in pulmonary artery pressure and potentially precipitating acute cor pulmonale. Furthermore, the reduction in functional residual capacity (FRC) associated with obesity decreases lung gas reserves. Thus, any change in alveolar ventilation results in more rapid changes in blood gas values. Changes in body position may improve these abnormalities. Under general anesthesia, lowering the head of the bed by 15 degrees was shown to reduce PaO_2 (partial pressure of oxygen in arterial blood) levels to below 80 mm Hg on 40% inspired oxygen.[41] Hence, a complete supine position should be avoided when possible if hypoxemia develops during the procedure. In contrast to normal people, little difference in FRC is noted between supine and seated positions in those who are obese, probably because the mass of the abdomen is pushed against the diaphragm.[42] A supine but tilted position may reduce intra-abdominal pressure more effectively than an upright position.

Some experts recommend extubation of patients with OSA after they are fully awake. This should be performed in the reverse Trendelenburg (semi-upright) position. Sedatives, even those used preoperatively, may increase the arousal threshold, thus increasing the likelihood and duration of apnea and the severity of hypoxemia during each apneic episode in patients with OSA during the perioperative period.[43] Drugs that may cause central nervous system depression should be administered sparingly. Close monitoring for signs of hypoventilation is crucial to help ensure patient safety during the hours following the bronchoscopic intervention.

Instrumentation

We used a 13-mm Efer-Dumon rigid nonventilating bronchoscope (Bryan Corp., Woburn, Mass). This bronchoscope is a stainless steel tube with an exterior diameter of 13.2 mm, an internal diameter of 12.2 mm, and a length of 26.98 cm. The beveled tip of the tube allows for easy spreading of the vocal cords during intubation. This tracheal tube may be used for placement of stents 16 to 20 mm in diameter, including Y silicone stents. Based on bronchoscopy and CT scanning, this patient had EDAC without evidence of tracheomegaly, so we intended to use a Y stent with a 16-mm diameter for the tracheal arm and a 12-mm diameter for the bronchial arm to properly cover the full extent of the collapsing central airways.

Anatomic Dangers and Other Risks

The risk of airway perforation during stent insertion is rare in the absence of tumor, necrosis, fistula, or a very thin posterior airway wall. The operator should ascertain that the rigid scope is aligned with the airway. Our model of the 13-mm Efer-Dumon bronchoscope does not have a stopper at the tube's distal aspect, so the bronchoscopist must know and recall its length (10 inches) during advancement of the stent introducer into the rigid tube. Large stents can be more difficult to unfold, so forceps should be available with which to grasp and rotate the stent as needed.

Results and Procedure-Related Complications

With the rigid bronchoscope in the lower trachea, flexible bronchoscopy was performed through the rigid scope to remove bilateral thick tenacious secretions. The patient had severe airway collapse in the lower trachea and mainstem bronchi, characterized by protrusion of the posterior wall, giving the trachea the shape of a crescent. The stent was deployed using a "push" technique (see video on ExpertConsult.com) (Video III.14.3) and had a 2-cm-long right bronchial limb, a 3.5-cm-long left bronchial limb, and a 4-cm-long tracheal limb. Airway patency was restored, but migration of the collapsible airway segments was obvious distal to the bronchial limbs of the Y stent. The patient was extubated and was transferred to the postanesthesia care unit (PACU) for 2 hours, during which no complications occurred. Stent instructions were provided on the following day, after which the patient was discharged to the nursing home with plans to perform follow-up bronchoscopy 2 weeks later to assess for possible stent-related complications.

Long-Term Management

Outcome Assessment

Relief of this form of dynamic airway obstruction was successfully achieved as assessed by bronchoscopy. The patient noticed immediate improvement in her ability to raise secretions. Airway collapse of less than 50% should have improved the patient's exercise capacity, but this was not assessed during her short hospitalization at our facility. Exercise capacity and QOL scores can be objectively documented at follow-up visits by using one of the applied scales for tracheobronchomalacia, such as the ATS dyspnea scale, the BDI/TDI, the SGRQ, the KPS, or the WHO functional class impairment scale.[13,14]

Referral

A multidisciplinary approach to managing these patients involves thoracic surgeons, pulmonary physicians, and radiologists to best ascertain whether symptoms are related to EDAC, or whether they simply reflect the effects of small airway disease, often identified by pulmonary function tests or dynamic CT scanning (e.g., COPD, bronchiolitis). We believed that our patient's significant comorbidities precluded her from open surgery; therefore her condition was discussed with our thoracic surgery team, but formal consultation was not requested.

Follow-up Tests and Procedures

In addition to its role in detecting stent-related complications, follow-up bronchoscopy allows monitoring of the evolution of the disease process.[4,9] Results from older studies demonstrate that EDAC is progressive in most patients.[3,25] Approximately 66% to 75% of patients who do not undergo stent insertion or surgery have worse airway narrowing on follow-up bronchoscopy.[3,6] Our patient's referring physician performed surveillance bronchoscopies at 2 and 4 weeks after stent insertion; these showed satisfactory airway patency and no evidence of stent-related complications.

Quality Improvement

We discussed whether follow-up flexible bronchoscopy on CPAP was needed to identify an optimal pressure level that would maintain airway patency distal to the bronchial arms of the Y stent.[32] We decided that this would have been performed had the patient developed worsening symptoms.[9] Choke point migration distal to the stent could be detected on follow-up bronchoscopy or dynamic CT scanning.[9] In this case, one could insert another stent at the new choke point or, less invasively, could initiate adjuvant CPAP. The amount of airway pressure necessary to maintain airway patency could be determined by performing bronchoscopy on noninvasive positive-pressure ventilation.[32]

DISCUSSION POINTS

1. Explain the impact of EDAC on expiratory flow limitation in COPD.
   - EDAC is not uncommon in patients with COPD, symptomatic asthma, and obesity[44] and is seen in the absence of cartilage abnormalities.[2] EDAC affects outcomes among elderly patients undergoing sleeve resections and was an independent risk factor for increased morbidity and mortality in this patient population.[45]
   - The impact on expiratory flow limitation, however, is not entirely clear. Narrowing of the central airways is usually exaggerated in patients with small airway disease, in part because of loss of intraluminal pressure in the periphery (friction losses in small airways). The resulting negative transmural pressure gradient causes excessive invagination of the posterior wall. In these situations, pressure catheter measurements demonstrate no pressure drop along the trachea and mainstem bronchi, thus predicting no improvement in airflow after central airway stabilization procedures;[20] in fact, studies evaluating these procedures showed improvement in health-related QOL scores, but not in expiratory flow rates.[14,31]
   - In COPD, two pathophysiologic abnormalities coexist: (1) decreased elastic recoil at all lung volumes (emphysema), and (2) inflammatory narrowing of small airways (bronchitis); these determine the major site of increased resistance in the peripheral airways (less than 2 mm in diameter).[30] The severity of expiratory flow limitation is not closely related to tracheal collapsibility assessed bronchoscopically in patients with EDAC.[46] Physiologists believe that bronchoscopic or radiologic detection of EDAC should trigger a search for causes of airflow obstruction within the lung, not in the central airways.[20]

2. List three considerations pertaining to the administration of anesthesia during rigid bronchoscopy for this patient with severe EDAC.

- *Loss of airway control* has been reported using both intravenous and inhalational induction: Intravenous induction is faster and smoother and causes less airway irritation. If induction is too rapid, however, the airway may be lost.[47] Patients in respiratory distress may not tolerate the supine position. Neuromuscular blocking drugs may eliminate the only muscular tone that keeps the airway patent.
- *ASA grade* should be assessed preoperatively. Most patients with central airway obstruction are American Society of Anesthesiologists (ASA) class 3 or 4.[48] Respiratory complications occur more frequently in patients with ASA class 3 and 4 and Karnofsky Performance Scale scores less than 70.[40]
- *Spontaneous assisted ventilation* has a relatively good cardiac safety profile in patients with central airway obstruction who are undergoing therapeutic rigid bronchoscopy.[40] Even among octogenarians, although intraoperative hypotension was found to be common during spontaneous assisted ventilation (39%), no mortality or reintubation was necessary with the use of this anesthesia technique.[49] One alternative to spontaneous assisted ventilation is neuromuscular blockade with jet ventilation, but this may increase the risk for postoperative respiratory depression, leading to reintubation in approximately 10% of patients.[50]

3. Which two alternative treatments to stent insertion might be considered in this patient?

- Continuous positive airway pressure may act as a "pneumatic stent."[51] CPAP also affects airflow by increasing lung volumes because expiratory flows measured at the same lung volumes do not differ for the different levels of CPAP.
- Membranous tracheoplasty was believed to cause subjective improvement in all patients (N = 14) in one post intervention study, as noted by decreased dyspnea, cough, and secretion retention.[36]

4. Describe three potential complications from stent insertion in this particular patient.

- Mucus plugging
- Granulation tissue formation
- Stent migration

Most patients with expiratory central airway collapse develop stent-related nonfatal complications; in one case series, 26 stent-related complications (12 mucus plugs, 8 migrations, and 6 granulation tissues) were seen in 10 of 12 patients (83%), and they usually occurred within the first few weeks after stent insertion (median, 29 days). This high rate of adverse effects increased the need for repeat bronchoscopic interventions.[4] In a larger study of patients with EDAC, similar stent complications occurred within the first 3 months post intervention (median, 26 days; range, 3 to 865 days).[14] These findings probably justify surveillance flexible bronchoscopy within the first few weeks following stent insertion in this patient population.

Expert Commentary

provided by Cameron D. Wright, MD

The patient under discussion is certainly at high risk, and I agree that she was not a surgical candidate. I would not have recommended a stent insertion in this case, for fear of late complications given that it would be a long-term stent. Sometimes the best treatment is supportive care rather than an invasive intervention. Two forms of tracheobronchomalacia (TBM) have been identified and are often grouped together in reports or discussions about this topic, which can confuse the issues. In this patient, EDAC was present. In this case, the cartilage of the trachea is normal, and the membranous wall is seen to invaginate into the airway during expiration to a greater extent than is normal. My personal belief is that this finding is incidental, does not represent tracheal disease, and probably is overdiagnosed (especially with increased use of CT scans) and therefore overtreated. The other form of TBM is seen when the cartilage of the trachea is weak, leading to loss of the normally D-shaped trachea. This is a true tracheal disease in that at rest the trachea can be seen to be abnormally flattened. Both forms lead to a narrowed central airway. Whether this narrowed central airway has anything to do with a patient's symptoms is problematic and difficult to discern. As Baram and Smaldone point out,[20] it is well documented that essentially all flow limitation with lung disease occurs in the peripheral airways, not in the large airways. They point out the classic example of a collapsible Penrose drain as a surrogate for a collapsible trachea, with experiments confirming no flow limitation.

Given that lung physiologists seem to agree on this point, I am unclear why there is such enthusiasm for stenting airways in this essentially physiologic condition of membranous wall invagination. This seems to me similar to the early days of percutaneous coronary intervention, when moderate stenoses were treated even though they were not the culprit lesion, and no survival advantage was demonstrated. The pictures are indeed dramatic, leading one to be urged to do something. We must remember, however, that a placebo effect has been associated not only with pills but also with procedures. It makes no physiologic sense to me that a stent would improve dyspnea, mucus production, or clearance of secretions. Furthermore, most of these patients have intrinsic lung disease, most often COPD that remains after stent insertion. In my experience, most of these patients are obese as well, which leads to further pulmonary limitation. I believe we need to study these two disease entities much more thoroughly and should involve lung physiologists in the evaluation process to document what happens after stent insertion, because most of the reported results reflect subjective improvement. I also think a randomized sham-controlled trial (with a cross-over option) with at least 1 year of follow-up needs to be done, so we can learn whether stents should be inserted.

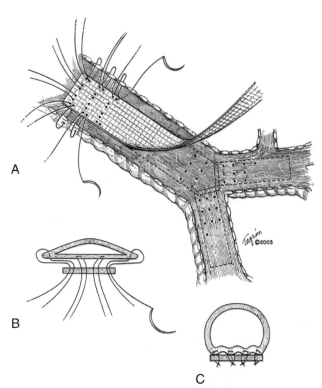

Figure 14-3 Illustration of posterior splinting procedure for expiratory tracheobronchial collapse. **A,** Polypropylene strip of appropriate width is sutured to the posterior membranous tracheal wall from the apex of the thorax to the carina. Successive rows of sutures are placed to reef the posterior membranous wall to the mesh. Dots indicate general placement of sutures. Dashed lines indicate placement of Marlex strips. **B,** Cross-sectional diagram showing placement and spacing of sutures. **C,** When tied, sutures pull the cartilage into more nearly normal C configurations and quilt the widened membranous wall to the polypropylene. *(Reproduced with permission of the artist, Edith Tagrin. From Grillo HC. Surgery of the Trachea and Bronchi. Hamilton, Canada: BC Decker; 2004:647.)*

I would like to make a few comments pertaining to membranous wall tracheobronchoplasty. Some patients with cartilaginous TBM—those who are relatively fit—are candidates for this open surgical procedure. The posterior membranous wall of the trachea is reefed and sutured to a strip of polypropylene mesh to stabilize the membranous wall and reconfigure the trachea back to a more normal shape (Figure 14-3). Wright and colleagues reported a retrospective series of membranous tracheobronchoplasty for cartilaginous TBM in 14 patients.[36] Presenting symptoms included dyspnea (79%), severe cough (36%), recurrent infections (36%), and difficulty clearing secretions (36%). Percent predicted FEV_1 improved from 51% to 73%, and peak expiratory flow rate improved from 49% to 70%. Ten patients were available for long-term follow-up: 6 were judged to have an excellent result, 2 good, and 2 poor. Two (14%) early complications were reported (1 pneumonia, 1 ileus). No postoperative deaths occurred. The mean length of hospital stay was 8.8 days.

Majid and colleagues reported a prospective series of 35 patients with TBM (it is not clear what

proportion of patients had EDAC or TBM) who underwent tracheobronchoplasty.[31] Presenting symptoms included dyspnea (94%), severe cough (74%), and recurrent pulmonary infection (51%). Important selection criteria included trial placement of a temporary silicone stent to see whether patients improved (37 of 57 improved). If significant improvement was noted and patients were medically fit, they were then referred for open surgical intervention. After surgery, QOL scores improved in 25 of 31 patients, dyspnea scores improved in 19 of 26 patients, and functional status improved in 20 of 31 patients. The median length of hospital stay was 8 days. However, surgical complications occurred in 15 patients (43%) (7 mechanical ventilation >24 hours, 4 pneumonia, 4 subcutaneous emphysema, 3 atrial fibrillation, 1 hemothorax, 1 transverse myelitis), and 2 patients died (6% mortality).

Because of uncertainty about the indications for intervention, patients who present with TBM must be carefully evaluated when treatment is considered; treatment results are somewhat unpredictable. Patients with COPD, who represent the majority of evaluated patients, are the most difficult to evaluate because their symptoms overlap with symptoms of TBM. Use of a temporary silicone stent as part of the diagnostic evaluation has much to recommend it. I remain concerned, however, about the long-term therapeutic use of silicone stents for TBM because of very frequent late complications. I have seen mucus plugging cause cardiopulmonary arrest, and I have encountered problematic granulation tissue formation in patients who have had their stents for only short periods of time. Because of these and other complications, I rarely recommend stent insertion as definitive treatment for patients with TBM, regardless of how symptomatic they may be. Patients who are fit, respond well to temporary stent insertion, have true TBM (as opposed to EDAC), and are surgically minded are seriously considered for open surgical membranous wall tracheobronchomalacia. In this regard, it is my opinion that patients with disease limited to the trachea are better candidates than those with distal involvement. I remain guarded in recommending this procedure because it is a major operation with unpredictable results.

REFERENCES

1. Carden KA, Boiselle PM, Waltz DA, et al. Tracheomalacia and tracheobronchomalacia in children and adults: an in-depth review. *Chest.* 2005;127:984-1005.
2. Murgu SD, Colt HG. Tracheobronchomalacia and excessive dynamic airway collapse. *Respirology.* 2006;11:388-406.
3. Jokinen K, Palva T, Sutinen S, et al. Acquired tracheobronchomalacia. *Ann Clin Res.* 1977;9:52-57.
4. Murgu SD, Colt HG. Complications of silicone stent insertion in patients with expiratory central airway collapse. *Ann Thorac Surg.* 2007;84:1870-1877.
5. Murgu SD, Cherrison LJ, Colt HG. Respiratory failure due to expiratory central airway collapse. *Respir Care.* 2007;52: 752-754.

6. Nuutinen J. Acquired tracheobronchomalacia: a clinical study with bronchological correlations. *Ann Clin Res.* 1977;9:350-355.
7. Campbell AH, Faulks LW. Expiratory air-flow pattern in tracheobronchial collapse. *Am Rev Respir Dis.* 1965;92:781-791.
8. Healy F, Wilson AF, Fairshter RD. Physiologic correlates of airway collapse in chronic airflow obstruction. *Chest.* 1984;85:476-481.
9. Murgu SD, Colt HG. Treatment of adult tracheobronchomalacia and excessive dynamic airway collapse: an update. *Treat Respir Med.* 2006;5:103-115.
10. Lee KS, Sun MR, Ernst A, et al. Comparison of dynamic expiratory CT with bronchoscopy for diagnosing airway malacia: a pilot evaluation. *Chest.* 2007;131:758-764.
11. Boiselle PM, Feller-Kopman D, Ashiku S, et al. Tracheobronchomalacia: evolving role of dynamic multislice helical CT. *Radiol Clin North Am.* 2003;41:627-636.
12. Baroni RH, Ashiku S, Boiselle PM. Dynamic CT evaluation of the central airways in patients undergoing tracheoplasty for tracheobronchomalacia. *AJR Am J Roentgenol.* 2005;184:1444-1449.
13. Murgu SD, Colt HG. Description of a multidimensional classification system for patients with expiratory central airway collapse. *Respirology.* 2007;12:543-550.
14. Ernst A, Majid A, Feller-Kopman D, et al. Airway stabilization with silicone stents for treating adult tracheobronchomalacia: a prospective observational study. *Chest.* 2007;132:609-616.
15. Mercer M. Anesthesia for the patient with respiratory disease. *Update in Anaesthesia.* 2000;12:1-3.
16. Ng A, Smith G. Gastroesophageal reflux and aspiration of gastric contents in anesthetic practice. *Anesth Analg.* 2001;93:494-513.
17. Nowbar S, Burkart KM, Gonzales R, et al. Obesity-associated hypoventilation in hospitalized patients: prevalence, effects, and outcome. *Am J Med.* 2004;116:1-7.
18. Scott-Cawiezell J, Vogelsmeier A. Nursing home safety: a review of the literature. *Annu Rev Nurs Res.* 2006;24:179-215.
19. White-Chu EF, Graves WJ, Godfrey SM, et al. Beyond the medical model: the culture change revolution in long-term care. *J Am Med Dir Assoc.* 2009;10:370-378.
20. Baram D, Smaldone G. Tracheal collapse versus tracheobronchomalacia: normal function versus disease. *Am J Respir Crit Care Med.* 2006;174:724.
21. Aquino SL, Shepard JA, Ginns LC, et al. Acquired tracheomalacia: detection by expiratory CT scan. *J Comput Assist Tomogr.* 2001;25:394-399.
22. Stern EJ, Graham CM, Webb WR, et al. Normal trachea during forced expiration: dynamic CT measurements. *Radiology.* 1993;187:27-31.
23. Zhang J, Hasegawa I, Feller-Kopman D, et al. 2003 AUR Memorial Award. Dynamic expiratory volumetric CT imaging of the central airways: comparison of standard-dose and low-dose techniques. *Acad Radiol.* 2003;10:719-724.
24. Gilkeson RC, Ciancibello LM, Hejal RB, et al. Tracheobronchomalacia: dynamic airway evaluation with multidetector CT. *AJR Am J Roentgenol.* 2001;176:205-210.
25. Nuutinen J. Acquired tracheobronchomalacia. *Eur J Respir Dis.* 1982;63:380-387.
26. Boiselle PM, O'Donnell CR, Bankier AA, et al. Tracheal collapsibility in healthy volunteers during forced expiration: assessment with multidetector CT. *Radiology.* 2009;252:255-262.
27. Park JG, Edell ES. Dynamic airway collapse: different from tracheomalacia. *Rev Port Pneumol.* 2005;11:600-602.
28. Park J, Edell E. It's in the definition. *Chest.* 2006;129:497; author reply 497-498.
29. Smaldone GC, Smith PL. Location of flow-limiting segments via airway catheters near residual volume in humans. *J Appl Physiol.* 1985;59:502-508.
30. Hogg JC, Macklem PT, Thurlbeck WM. Site and nature of airway obstruction in chronic obstructive lung disease. *N Engl J Med.* 1968;278:1355-1360.
31. Majid A, Guerrero J, Gangadharan S, et al. Tracheobronchoplasty for severe tracheobronchomalacia: a prospective outcome analysis. *Chest.* 2008;134:801-807.
32. Murgu SD, Pecson J, Colt HG. Bronchoscopy on noninvasive positive pressure ventilation: indications and technique. *Respir Care.* 2010;55:595-600.
33. Ferguson GT, Benoist J. Nasal continuous positive airway pressure in the treatment of tracheobronchomalacia. *Am Rev Respir Dis.* 1993;147:457-461.
34. Adliff M, Ngato D, Keshavjee S, et al. Treatment of diffuse tracheomalacia secondary to relapsing polychondritis with continuous positive airway pressure. *Chest.* 1997;112:1701-1704.
35. FDA Public Health Notification. Complications from metablic tracheal stents in patients with benign airway disorders. 2005; Available at: http://www.fda.gov/MedicalDevices/Safety/Alertsand Notices/PublicHealthNotifications/ucm062115.htm. Accessed February 21, 2011.
36. Wright CD, Grillo HC, Hammoud ZT, et al. Tracheoplasty for expiratory collapse of central airways. *Ann Thorac Surg.* 2005;80:259-267.
37. Gordon RA. Anesthetic management of patients with airway problems. *Int Anesthesiol Clin.* 1972;10:37-59.
38. McMahon CC, Rainey L, Fulton B, et al. Central airway compression: anaesthetic and intensive care consequences. *Anaesthesia.* 1997;52:158-162.
39. Mackie AM, Watson CB. Anesthesia and mediastinal masses. *Anaesthesia.* 1984;39:899-903.
40. Perrin G, Colt HG, Martin C, et al. Safety of interventional rigid bronchoscopy using intravenous anesthesia and spontaneous assisted ventilation: a prospective study. *Chest.* 1992;102:1526-1530.
41. Vaughan RW, Wise L. Intraoperative arterial oxygenation in obese patients. *Ann Surg.* 1976;184:35-42.
42. Watson RA, Pride NB. Postural changes in lung volumes and respiratory resistance in subjects with obesity. *J Appl Physiol.* 2005;98:512-517.
43. Gifford AH, Leiter JC, Manning HL. Respiratory function in an obese patient with sleep-disordered breathing. *Chest.* 2010;138:704-715.
44. Takishima T, Grimby G, Graham W, et al. Flow-volume curves during quiet breathing, maximum voluntary ventilation, and forced vital capacities in patients with obstructive lung disease. *Scand J Respir Dis.* 1967;48:384-393.
45. Bölükbas S, Bergmann T, Fisseler-Eckhoff A, et al. Short- and long-term outcome of sleeve resections in the elderly. *Eur J Cardiothorac Surg.* 2010;37:30-35.
46. Loring SH, O'Donnell CR, Feller-Kopman DJ, et al. Central airway mechanics and flow limitation in acquired tracheobronchomalacia. *Chest.* 2007;131:1118-1124.
47. McMahon CC, Rainey L, Fulton B, et al. Central airway compression: anaesthetic and intensive care consequences. *Anaesthesia.* 1997;52:158-162.
48. Conacher ID. Anaesthesia and tracheobronchial stenting for central airway obstruction in adults. *Br J Anaesth.* 2003;90:367-374.
49. Davoudi M, Shakkottai S, Colt HG. Safety of therapeutic rigid bronchoscopy in people aged 80 and older: a retrospective cohort analysis. *J Am Geriatr Soc.* 2008;56:943-944.
50. Hanowell LH, Martin WR, Savelle JE, et al. Complications of general anesthesia for Nd:YAG laser resection of endobronchial tumors. *Chest.* 1991;99:72-76.
51. Davis S, Jones M, Kisling J, et al. Effect of continuous positive airway pressure on forced expiratory flows in infants with tracheomalacia. *Am J Respir Crit Care Med.* 1998;158:148-152.

Practical Approach to Mediastinal Lymphadenopathy (EBUS and Alternatives)

SECTION 2

Practical Approach to Mediastinal Lymphadenopathy (EBUS and Alternatives)

Chapter 15

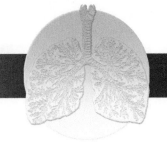

EBUS-TBNA for Right Upper Lobe Mass and Right Lower Paratracheal Lymphadenopathy

> This chapter emphasizes the following elements of the Four Box Approach: techniques and instrumentation.

CASE DESCRIPTION

A 67-year-old male with a 50–pack-year history of smoking presented with fatigue and an unintentional 15-kg weight loss within the last 6 months. His normal weight had been 78 kg. He had a history of oxygen-dependent COPD and hypertension. Blood pressure was 160/80 mm Hg, heart rate 90 bpm, body temperature 37.2° C, and respiratory rate 18 breaths/min. Physical examination showed prolonged expiratory breath sounds and sagging skin over the abdomen. He was a retired mechanical engineer who lived with his wife. He expressed his desire to proceed with available treatment modalities if diagnosed with cancer.

Laboratory data were significant for an albumin level of 2.9 mg/dL. Arterial blood gas analysis showed the following: pH 7.45, $PaCO_2$ 50 mm Hg, and PaO_2 64 mm Hg on 2 L oxygen/min via nasal cannula. Pulmonary function tests revealed FEV_1 of 1.6 L (49% predicted) and DLCO of 50% predicted. A contrast-enhanced chest CT scan (Figure 15-1) followed by whole body integrated PET-CT showed a 3-cm PET-positive right upper lobe mass (SUV max, 7.6) and a 1.7-cm PET-negative right lower paratracheal LN (SUV max, 1.8). CT-guided TTNA of the right upper lobe mass was positive for bronchogenic adenocarcinoma. The patient is referred for mediastinal staging.

DISCUSSION POINTS

1. Describe a step-by-step approach to performing EBUS-TBNA.
2. Describe physics principles of endobronchial ultrasound and their impact on quality image acquisition.
3. Describe the reported relation between PET-negative lymph node size and malignancy.

CASE RESOLUTION

Initial Evaluations

Physical Examination, Complementary Tests, and Functional Status Assessment

This patient presented with significant (>10% from baseline) involuntary weight loss with decreased appetite. These are nearly always signs of a serious medical or psychiatric illness. One study evaluated 154 such patients and found that 36% had cancer, particularly gastrointestinal, lung, lymphoma, renal, and prostate cancers. Twenty-three percent of cases remained unexplained despite extensive evaluation, and remaining patients had primarily other gastrointestinal or psychiatric diseases.[1] Our patient had no evidence of mental illness or another extrathoracic medical disorder to explain weight loss and fatigue. However, he did have moderate chronic obstructive pulmonary disease (COPD), which could be responsible for pulmonary cachexia. The mechanisms that lead to muscle atrophy and weight loss in patients with advanced pulmonary disease are not well understood, but muscle disuse, low-level chronic inflammation, and oxidative stress all appear to contribute to an imbalance between protein degradation and synthesis.[2] Lung cancer could also explain this patient's symptoms. Weight loss and tumor burden, however, may not be closely related, because both increased energy expenditure and reduced energy intake may be present; in lung cancer, these appear to be mediated by enhanced production of cytokines, including tumor necrosis factor (TNF) and interleukin (IL)-6.[3]

Our patient's CT scan showed a 3-cm right upper lobe (RUL) mass and a 1.7-cm right lower paratracheal lymph node (LN). Computed tomography (CT) scanning is usually affordable and is often performed to define the nature of a pulmonary abnormality, to assess potential mediastinal or hilar involvement, and to assist with the clinical diagnosis of suspected lung cancer. Reasons for choosing one sampling approach over another, for example, are governed primarily by anatomic factors (e.g., the location and size of a lung mass or lymph nodes) rather than by metabolic factors (e.g., positron emission tomography [PET] scan uptake). According to intrathoracic radiographic characteristics (including both the primary tumor and the mediastinum), however, patients with known or suspected lung cancer can be separated into four groups to help guide the choice for these subsequent diagnostic studies.[4] These groups include the following:

A. Extensive mediastinal infiltration
B. Enlargement of discrete mediastinal nodes (i.e., measurable size)

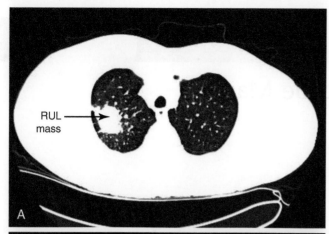

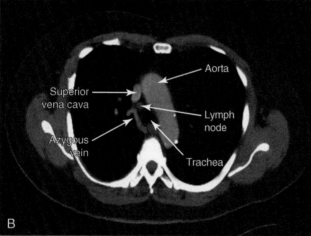

Figure 15-1 **A,** Axial computed tomography (CT) scan view (lung window) shows the 3-cm right upper lobe mass. **B,** Axial view (mediastinal window) shows the 1.7-cm right lower paratracheal lymph node, surrounded by the aorta, the superior vena cava, the azygos vein, and the tracheal lumen.

C. Normal mediastinal nodes identified by CT scan but with a central tumor* or suspected N1 disease
D. Normal mediastinal nodes and a peripheral clinical stage I tumor

Our patient fits into group B because he had a 1.7-cm LN in station 4R. Although contrast CT is very accurate in detecting LN enlargement, the clinical relevance of LN enlargement for staging is poor, because large nodes may be benign and small nodes may contain metastases in up to 20% of cases.[5] A diameter larger than 1 cm in the short axis is generally considered suspicious. In a review article, pooled data on CT performance characteristics for detecting mediastinal involvement showed a sensitivity of 57%, a specificity of 82%, a positive predictive value (PPV) of 56%, and a negative predictive value (NPV) of 83%, with marked heterogeneity across individual studies.[6] This performance is insufficient for

clinical decision making, and in many instances, it is inappropriate to rely solely on CT scan for nodal staging.

Noninvasive staging of lung cancer is further enhanced by the use of positron emission tomography with 18F-fluoro-2-deoxy-D-glucose (FDG-PET). A large number of accuracy studies and meta-analyses have demonstrated that PET is superior to CT for mediastinal LN staging in potentially operable non–small cell lung carcinoma (NSCLC).[7] Sensitivities and NPV were comparable for PET and mediastinoscopy (sensitivity ≈80%, NPV ≈90%). However, the PPV and the specificity of the FDG-PET scan are lower than those of mediastinoscopy owing to the fact that FDG is also taken up by inflammatory processes such as sarcoidosis, fungal disease, or anthracosilicosis. Because of the high NPV of the PET scan, invasive staging procedures generally can be omitted in patients with clinical stage I NSCLC with negative mediastinal PET images. Implementing this strategy warrants caution in patients with central tumors, in those with central hilar N1 disease on CT scan or broncho-alveolar cell carcinoma, in situations with low FDG uptake in the primary tumor, and in cases where mediastinal PET-negative LNs are larger than 16 mm on CT scan, as in our case. For example, in one meta-analysis, a post-test probability for N2 disease of 21% was found in patients with PET-negative nodes larger than 16 mm.[8] In cases of positive mediastinal PET, tissue confirmation is still needed to confirm LN metastasis because the PPV of the PET scan is only 79%. One report that evaluated the role of PET scanning as compared with mediastinoscopy for mediastinal staging in NSCLC found a 26% false positivity rate of PET, a false negativity rate of 25%, sensitivity of 74%, specificity of 73%, and accuracy of only 74%. The NPV of mediastinoscopy was 94%, PPV 100%, sensitivity 84%, specificity 100%, and accuracy 95%. The authors concluded that PET results do not provide acceptable accuracy rates.[9] Therefore, in our patient with an LN larger than 16 mm in the setting of confirmed adenocarcinoma from CT-guided biopsy of the primary lesion, invasive or minimally invasive mediastinal staging procedures are still necessary.

Comorbidities

This patient had COPD with a forced expiratory volume in 1 second (FEV_1) of 49% predicted (moderate, GOLD [Gold Initiative on Obstructive Lung Disease] stage II) but was asymptomatic from a pulmonary standpoint. His hypertension was controlled. No evidence was found of concurrent comorbid conditions such as coronary heart disease, stroke, or obstructive sleep apnea, which could preclude or complicate procedures performed under moderate sedation or general anesthesia.

Support System

Results of studies show that appropriate lung cancer care is affected by sociodemographic factors. In patients with early-stage NSCLC, comorbidities, older age, and low educational level all were found to be associated with a lower probability of receiving surgery. These same factors, as well as being unmarried, were associated with a higher probability of receiving other noncurative care only. Comorbidities and low educational level did not seem to

---

*A tumor is deemed central when its center is located into the inner one third of the lung parenchyma (adjacent to the mediastinum) on transverse CT image. A non–centrally located tumor is a tumor in which the center lies in the outer two thirds of the lung parenchyma on transverse CT image.

affect the more effective patterns of care in the advanced-stage group. When initial patterns of care were controlled for in the early-stage group, age older than 75 years and being unmarried were negative prognostic factors, and survival was completely independent of educational level. Among patients at an advanced stage of disease, only comorbidities had a negative impact on survival.[10] Another study suggested that socioeconomically disadvantaged groups with NSCLC received less-intensive care, but low education remained an independent predictor of poor survival only in women with early-stage disease. The exact underlying mechanisms of these social inequalities are unknown, but differences in access to care, comorbidities, and lifestyle factors all may contribute.[11] Early discussions about quality of life and symptom concerns are justifiable in that patients will commonly develop pain, dyspnea, cough, and fatigue during the course of their illness.[12] These conversations took place repeatedly during initial and subsequent clinical encounters with our patient.

Patient Preferences and Expectations

Evidence indicates that discrepancies exist between preferred and actual roles in decision making for patients suffering from a variety of cancers, including NSCLC.[13] When interviewed, patients wanted a more shared or an active role, across all cancer types, patients wanted more participation than what actually occurred. Role preferences are dynamic, however, and vary greatly during decision making, requiring repeated clinical assessments to help providers meet patients' expectations and improve patient satisfaction with treatment decisions. At the time of our first encounter, this patient had clearly expressed a desire for diagnosis and treatment. He was prepared to consider all available diagnostic options for staging, including conventional TBNA, EBUS-guided TBNA, endoscopic ultrasound (EUS)-guided fine-needle aspiration (FNA), mediastinoscopy, and video-assisted thoracic surgery (VATS).

Procedural Strategies

Indications

For this patient with discrete mediastinal lymph node enlargement and no distant metastases, invasive confirmation of the radiographic stage was recommended, regardless of results of PET scan findings for mediastinal nodes.[4] The status of the mediastinum is, in fact, the most crucial factor in selecting an optimal treatment strategy. It is also fundamental for estimating prognosis. Patients with tumors in clinical stage III are a heterogeneous group, in whom the extent of LN involvement before and after induction therapy determines outcome.[14] If our patient's nodal station 4R is positive for malignancy, his clinical stage is III A-N2. In this subgroup of patients, induction chemotherapy, combined with surgery and/or radiotherapy, has proved effective. If surgical combined-modality treatment is being considered, complete resection is essential in the potential for cure.

If complete resection is unlikely, a nonsurgical multimodality approach is preferred. Therefore, an accurate preoperative and postinduction nodal evaluation is mandatory. For both primary staging and restaging, not every technique is available in every center, and different techniques are advocated in different countries and in different institutions. In many situations, however, an invasive test can provide confirmation of the diagnosis and confirmation of the stage at the same time, thus illustrating the importance of not immediately pursuing a diagnostic test in patients, but rather first thinking through the presumptive diagnosis, the presumptive stage, and the need for additional confirmatory staging tests.

Although the sensitivity of various invasive mediastinal staging tests in clinical N2 and N3 patients appears to be similar, a strict comparison is not justified, because patients undergoing these procedures are not comparable owing to differences in how they are selected for a particular procedure (e.g., the location of the nodes). The primary issue, therefore, is the variability in false-negative rates. If a needle aspiration (NA) technique is chosen, it must be remembered that a negative result is not completely reliable, but at the same time, NA may well be a good first choice because it is less invasive than mediastinoscopy. Sampling station 4R nodes in our patient is essential because the incidence of occult N2* disease in NSCLC patients with negative mediastinal uptake of 18FDG on PET-CT is considered to be approximately 16% (25 of 153 patients). The highest incidence of occult N2 involvement is seen in station 7 (subcarinal) (16 of 25 patients [64%]) followed by station 4 (lower paratracheal) (7 of 25 patients [28%]).[15] Mediastinal LN size is directly related to metastatic involvement. One meta-analysis showed that the prevalence of malignant involvement ranged from 9% to 42% for nodes measuring 10 to 15 mm, from 19% to 75% for nodes measuring 16 to 20 mm, and from 27% to 100% for nodes measuring larger than 20 mm. The probability of nodal metastasis in mediastinal nodes measuring 10 to 15 mm in the short axis on CT is 29% and is consistently twofold higher in larger ones.[8]

Some physicians routinely perform a flexible bronchoscopy before considering curative resection, because evidence indicates that 8% of patients with a small noncalcified pulmonary nodule up to 3 cm in diameter might have an endobronchial lesion that could potentially alter staging and management.[16] Flexible bronchoscopy would allow complete airway inspection to ascertain the absence of endobronchial lesions and to sample the 4R lymph node at the same setting. Although this could be done with the use of conventional TBNA, EBUS-TBNA may increase diagnostic yield at the level 4R compared with conventional sampling techniques (71% to 94% vs. 66%).[17,18]

Contraindications

No absolute contraindications to bronchoscopy with EBUS-TBNA were noted. This procedure, however, is often performed under general anesthesia, which in our patient with COPD and baseline CO_2 retention could

---

*Occult N2 involvement refers to a pathologically positive lymph node in a mediastinal lymph node station that was preoperatively staged as N2/N3 negative by integrated PET-CT.

predispose to bronchospasm, air trapping, and prolonged ventilatory depression, especially if opioids are used.[19] These concerns would have to be addressed with the anesthesiologist before the procedure is undertaken.

Expected Results

We usually perform EBUS-TBNA under general anesthesia with a large endotracheal tube (8.5 or 9 mm) to accommodate the EBUS-TBNA scope (outside scope diameter is 6.2 mm). The EBUS scope would be introduced through the tube once the bite block is secured in place around the tube. Laryngeal mask airway and moderate or deep sedation are feasible alternatives to intubation and general anesthesia. Regardless, in case of general anesthesia, after the airway is secured, complete airway examination would be performed. Station 4R sampling should be accompanied by a complete sonographic mediastinal and hilar nodal assessment because the tumor may be upstaged to N3 (stage IIIB), in case EBUS identifies contralateral lymph nodes from which aspirates are positive for malignancy.[20] The lymph nodes would be systematically visualized by starting with N1 lymph nodes followed by N2 nodes and finally N3 nodes. EBUS-TBNA is then performed first from N3 nodes, followed by N2 nodes, and, if necessary, N1 nodes. If N3 nodes were found to be positive for malignancy on rapid on-site cytologic evaluation, the procedure could be terminated. For this patient, if complete EBUS mediastinal and hilar evaluation reveals no other nodes, then only the CT-documented 4R node should be sampled. In one small study, the diagnostic rate of EBUS-TBNA for station 4R was only slightly better than that of conventional TBNA (71% vs. 66%).[21] However, larger studies have shown high diagnostic yields of 86% to 94% with EBUS for station 4R.[17,22]

Team Experience

A team familiar with the techniques and the equipment is necessary because of the particularities of TBNA, EBUS, and EBUS-TBNA.[23] Because of its availability at our institution, we routinely use on-site cytology to determine the adequacy of specimens obtained and to identify an immediate diagnosis. Experience with sampling this station is high because station 4R and the subcarinal nodes (station 7) are the most commonly biopsied nodes during conventional TBNA and EBUS-TBNA.[17,18]

Risk-Benefit Analysis

Although EBUS-TBNA has a high yield and is a safe procedure,[24] rare clinically significant complications include pericarditis and pneumothorax requiring chest tube drainage.[25] Even when it is performed using moderate sedation, patient satisfaction is high, and no complications occur that might compromise diagnostic yield.[26]

Diagnostic Alternatives

For patients with discrete mediastinal lymph node enlargement and no distant metastases, as in this case, another nonbronchoscopic NA technique (i.e., endoscopic ultrasound-guided needle aspiration [EUS-NA] or transthoracic needle aspiration [TTNA]), mediastinoscopy, or VATS could be performed instead of EBUS or

conventional TBNA. In choosing an invasive staging test, the availability of different procedures has to be considered, because some of these procedures require specialized experience and skill, and those who perform these procedures only occasionally may be unable to achieve performance characteristics comparable with those published in studies performed at high-volume institutions. The location of the suspicious node is important as well, because nodes in one location may be accessible only through a particular approach. Advantages and disadvantages of each of the procedural modalities should be discussed with the patient and his spouse.

1. *TTNA of the mediastinum:* TTNA or biopsy for the diagnosis and staging of the mediastinum is distinct from TTNA of parenchymal masses performed to achieve a diagnosis. The ability to carry out TTNA for this purpose has generally been reported to be high (i.e., >90%), although approximately 10% of patients require the placement of a catheter for evacuation of a pneumothorax. Sensitivity is approximately 90%.[4] Patients selected for this procedure usually have extensive mediastinal involvement (extensive infiltration or LN enlargement), with mediastinal nodes measuring at least 1.5 cm. Extrapolation of these results to patients with lesser amounts of mediastinal involvement, for staging purposes, may be inappropriate. Furthermore, the practical aspects of TTNA make this test unsuited for the biopsy of multiple mediastinal nodes, as would be needed for most patients who require mediastinal staging.

2. *EUS-FNA:* This technique has been used successfully for sampling 4R and reportedly has a diagnostic yield similar to that of EBUS-TBNA.[27] However, this technique is suitable mainly for the assessment of LNs in the posterior part of levels 4L, 5, and 7, and in the inferior mediastinum at levels 8 and 9. Nodes that are anterolateral to the trachea (stations 2R and 4R) are difficult to sample reliably, but these are the nodes more commonly involved in lung cancer. The pretracheal location of 4R in our patient makes it technically inaccessible by EUS-FNA.

3. *Mediastinoscopy:* This method is still considered the gold standard, and it may be recommended for this patient if endoscopic sampling of station 4R is negative for malignancy and is otherwise nondiagnostic.[17] Rates of morbidity and mortality are low (2% and 0.08%, respectively).[4] The average sensitivity of mediastinoscopy for detecting mediastinal node involvement from cancer is approximately 80%, and the average FN rate is approximately 10%.[4] Approximately half (range, 42% to 57%) of FN cases were due to nodes that were not accessible by the mediastinoscope. However, station 4R is usually easily sampled during mediastinoscopy. In our case, the pretracheal location and the 1.7-cm size of the lymph node made it suitable for a less invasive technique such as EBUS-TBNA.

4. *Video-assisted thoracic surgery (VATS):* This approach is usually reserved for subaortic (station 5) and anterior mediastinal (station 6) nodes. It can

also be used for LN levels that are not accessible by routine mediastinoscopy (stations 8 and 9), in case these LN stations cannot be addressed with EUS-FNA, or when EUS-FNA specimens are non-diagnostic. The procedure is limited to assessment of only one side of the mediastinum. Access to nodes on the right side is considered straightforward compared with access to nodes on the left side. Sensitivity varies widely, from 37% to 100%. Even if studies are restricted to patients with enlarged nodes, sensitivity still ranges from 50% to 100%. No mortality has been reported from VATS for mediastinal staging, and complications were noted in only 12 of 669 patients (average, 2%; range, 0% to 9%).[4] VATS was not considered the optimal initial alternative for this patient because less-invasive NA techniques were more feasible and had a high likelihood of diagnostic yield.

Cost-Effectiveness

Based on a review of 12 studies performed between 2004 and 2008, it seems that the sensitivity, specificity, false positivity (FP), and false negativity (FN) of EBUS-TBNA for mediastinal lymph node staging are 93%, 100%, 0%, and 9%, which may be better than findings for cervical mediastinoscopy, for which these values are 78%, 100%, 0%, and 11%, respectively. Sensitivity and false-negative rates for videomediastinoscopy, however, are 90% and 7%, respectively; these rates are similar to those reported for EBUS-TBNA. Three published cost-effectiveness analyses performed in the United States, the United Kingdom, and Singapore, based on mathematical modeling, show that EBUS may be less expensive than mediastinoscopy.[28]

Informed Consent

After they had been advised of all of diagnostic alternatives, the patient and his wife elected to proceed with EBUS-TBNA under general anesthesia. They were informed of the potential for failure to obtain a definitive diagnosis despite successful LN visualization and sampling. Feedback communication techniques were used to confirm patient understanding of the disease. Both the patient and his spouse were able to accurately describe the proposed procedure, alternatives, and potential complications.

Techniques and Results

Anesthesia and Perioperative Care

EBUS-TBNA can be performed under conscious (moderate), deep sedation or under general anesthesia using laryngeal mask airway (LMA) or endotracheal tubes. Moderate sedation offers the advantage of performing the procedure in the bronchoscopy suite and may result in better cost savings/safety ratios when compared with general anesthesia.[29] Because of the relatively small size of the node in this patient with COPD, moderate sedation could have resulted in excessive cough and respiratory movements, significant artifacts, and suboptimal ultrasound image acquisition. The procedure was performed with the patient under general anesthesia in the operating room. LMA No. 4 or 4.5 is preferred by some operators to establish a secure airway,[30] but LMAs may not be appropriate in severely obese patients or in patients with severe untreated gastroesophageal reflux.[31] Endotracheal intubation with a No. 8.5 endotracheal tube (ETT) for female patients and a No. 9 ETT for male patients can be used to secure the airway during bronchoscopy. Because the EBUS scope is directed more centrally in the airway through the ETT, however, coupling of the transducer and the airway wall may be impaired, and biopsies may be more difficult than when the scope is passed directly through an LMA or an oral bite block.[32]

Because we elected to proceed with general anesthesia and endotracheal intubation in this patient with moderate COPD, possible oxygenation, ventilation, and hemodynamic problems were discussed with the anesthesiologist before the procedure was performed. A review of the records revealed no evidence of cor pulmonale or pulmonary hypertension that could result in hypotension during general anesthesia. Preoperative arterial blood gases (ABGs) showed that the patient had baseline hypercapnia; to avoid air trapping, worsening hypoventilation, and hypoxemia, the anesthesia team planned to allow for spontaneous-assisted ventilation with longer expiratory times (normal inspiratory/expiratory [I:E] ratio is 1:2; in COPD, it is 1:3 or 1:4).[33] Peak inspiratory pressures would be closely monitored to avoid intraoperative barotrauma. End-tidal carbon dioxide ($EtCO_2$) should be kept at the patient's baseline because in this patient with baseline CO_2 retention and compensatory metabolic alkalosis, rapid correction could result in post-hypercapnic metabolic alkalosis and its neurologic (seizure) and cardiovascular complications (arrhythmias). To prevent bronchospasm, the anesthesia team planned on using non–histamine-releasing drugs. During the mandatory procedural pause (time-out) process, the need for perioperative antibiotics was readdressed, but in this case they were not necessary because the patient did not have conditions requiring endocarditis prophylaxis, nor did he have an acute upper or lower respiratory tract infection.

Techniques and Instrumentation

EBUS bronchoscopy provides direct real-time ultrasound imaging with a curved array ultrasound transducer incorporated in the distal end of the bronchoscope. As of this writing, various commercially available EBUS bronchoscopes are similar in design but have physical characteristics that are slightly different.[34,34a] We used the Olympus BF-UC160F-OL8 Hybrid scope (Olympus America Inc., Center Valley, PA) with a 2.0-mm working channel, a 6.9-mm outside diameter, and a 7.5-MHz frequency curved linear array transducer. During the procedure, intimate contact between the transducer and the airway wall was required for optimal coupling and image acquisition. Image quality adjustments useful for EBUS-TBNA procedures are usually made by using the gain and Doppler functions on the processor.[35,36] Understanding these functions helps the operator of EBUS to improve image quality to distinguish nodes from vessels and other mediastinal structures, potentially improving the safety of the procedure.

$$\Delta F = Ft - Fr = 2 \times Ft \times (v/c) \times \cos \theta$$

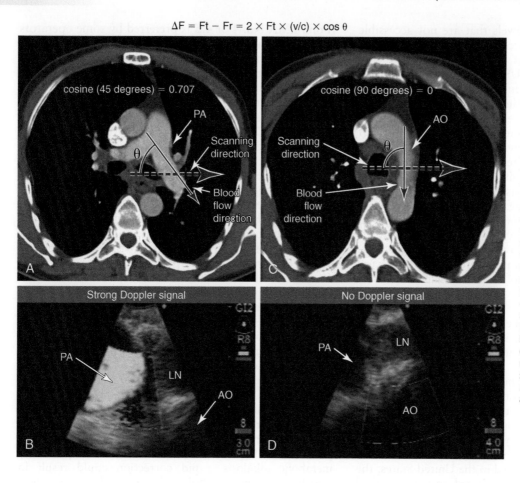

Figure 15-2 This diagram reveals the relationship between scanning plane direction, blood flow direction, and the intensity of the Doppler signal described in the following equation: Doppler frequency shift = $\Delta F = Ft - Fr = 2 \times Ft \times (v/c) \times \cos \theta$, where Ft is transmitted frequency, Fr received frequency, v speed of a moving target, c speed of sound in soft tissue, and θ the angle between the direction of blood flow and the direction of the transmitted sound phase. **A,** In general, the Doppler angle (θ) needs to be 60 degrees or slightly less to the long axis of the vessel (blood flow direction) for the correct velocity to be obtained. **B,** In this example, strong Doppler signal from the pulmonary artery was achieved when the Doppler angle was approximately 45 degrees. **C,** When the aortic arch was scanned, in this case, the Doppler angle was 90 degrees. **D,** Therefore $\Delta F = Ft - Fr = 2 \times Ft \times (v/c) \times \cos 90 = 0$, thus resulting in no frequency shift and no Doppler signal from the aorta. *AO,* Aorta; *LN,* lymph node; *PA,* pulmonary artery.

1. *Gain:* This represents the function for adjusting the brightness of the image in its entirety. The loss in amplitude that occurs as the ultrasound propagates through tissues can be corrected by amplifying the signal in proportion to the depth from which the echo came. The amplifier is controlled by the operator, who sets the gain for various depths of tissue (near or far gain adjustments). Changing the gain makes the whole image brighter (increased gain) or darker (decreased gain), but the difference in brightness between light and dark areas does not change, as can be noted in the video on **ExpertConsult.com** (Video IV.15.1).

2. *Doppler ultrasound:* Doppler effect (shift) represents the phenomenon through which the frequency of the reflected ultrasound wave is changed when it strikes a moving object (e.g., red blood cells within blood vessels). It is described in the following equation: Doppler frequency shift = $\Delta F = Ft - Fr = 2 \times Ft \times (v/c) \times \cos \theta$, where Ft is transmitted frequency, Fr received frequency, v speed of the moving target, c speed of sound in soft tissue, and θ angle between the direction of blood flow and the direction of the transmitted sound phase (Figure 15-2). In general, the Doppler angle (θ) must be 60 degrees or slightly less to the long axis of the vessel for the correct velocity to be obtained. If the angle

is 90 degrees, then $\Delta F = Ft - Fr = 2 \times Ft \times (v/c) \times \cos 90 = 0$, thus resulting in no frequency shift and no "Doppler signal" (see Figure 15-2). Therefore, it is important to understand that if the scanning plane is perpendicular to the direction of blood flow within a vessel, it is possible that no Doppler signal will be noted, and this should not lead to misinterpretation of the vessel as a nonvascular structure (see Figure 15-2). The power Doppler function analyzes returning echoes from blood cells by their power spectrum instead of frequency shift. This method is useful to reliably detect small vessels and is less dependent on speed and direction of flow. Color Doppler (duplex scanning) refers to a color code used for the indications of flow direction and velocity.

Anatomic Dangers and Other Risks

The superior vena cava, the azygos vein, and the lung parenchyma may surround station 4R (see Figures 15-1 and 15-3). The ascending aorta can be visualized distal to the node, especially when 4R is in the pretracheal position. The risk of puncturing these structures may be reduced by using Doppler mode imaging. Minor bleeding at the puncture site was reported, but no instances of major bleeding were described.[37] Pneumothorax after EBUS-TBNA has been very rarely reported in the literature.[24]

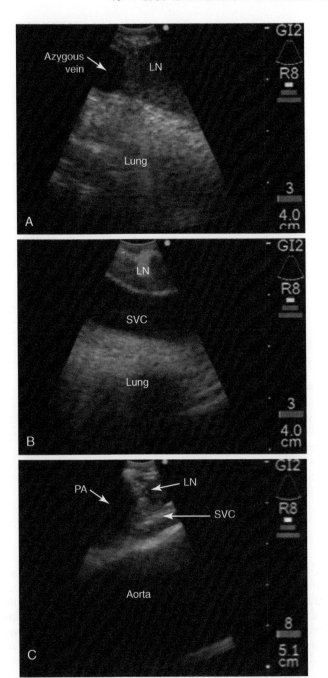

Figure 15-3 Right lower paratracheal lymph node (LN) anatomic relationships as seen on endobronchial ultrasound (EBUS). Different images were obtained from different patients; the distinct anatomic relationships depend on the orientation of the scanning plane and the exact location of the node in relation to the airway, vessels, and lung parenchyma. **A,** The LN is above the azygos vein and is adjacent to lung parenchyma. **B,** The LN is seen in front of the superior vena cava (SVC). **C,** The LN is above the right pulmonary artery (PA) but is in front of the SVC and the aorta.

Results and Procedure-Related Complications

EBUS-TBNA was performed under general anesthesia using a No. 9.0 ETT. Standard white light bronchoscopy was first used to evaluate anatomy, to clear secretions, and to ensure absence of endobronchial disease. Broncho-scopic inspection showed normal airway mucosa without

evidence of endobronchial disease. The EBUS scope was advanced into the trachea (the visualized image is seen at 30 degrees to the long axis of the bronchoscope). Once a complete sonographic evaluation of the mediastinal and hilar structures was performed and showed no other lymph nodes, we positioned the scope just proximal to the main carina and oriented the transducer anterolater-ally toward the 2 o'clock position to visualize the 4R LN station and proceeded with EBUS-TBNA. Once the needle was inside the node, the stylet was advanced and was moved in and out a few times to dislodge any bronchial wall material that could have entered the node; then the stylet was removed, the syringe was attached, suction was applied, and the needle was passed back and forth 10 to 15 times under direct visualization (see video on ExpertConsult.com) (Video IV.15.2). A total of four aspirations were performed. With the use of rapid on-site cytologic examination, no malignant cells were seen, and the specimen was considered representative because of the presence of abundant lymphocytes. The case lasted 30 minutes from induction to extubation. After extu-bation, the patient was monitored for 2 hours and was discharged home the same day. No procedure- or anesthesia-related complications occurred.

Long-Term Management

Outcome Assessment

The final results from EBUS-TBNA showed no malig-nancy. Clinical staging was performed without complica-tions. The patient was discussed in our multidisciplinary chest conference. We noted that the patient's primary tumor was 3 cm in its greatest dimension and was sur-rounded by lung. Because no bronchoscopic evidence of airway involvement was found, this tumor was defined as T1b. In the absence of clinical evidence of mediastinal or hilar LN metastasis after EBUS-TBNA, the N factor was N0; these findings are consistent with clinical stage IA NSCLC.*[38] This stage represents approximately 15% of all patients with NSCLC from the International Asso-ciation for the Study of Lung Cancer (IASLC) database; the estimated 5-year survival for clinical stage IA is 50%, and the median survival time is 60 months. Treatment options were discussed and included right upper lobec-tomy, sublobar resection (wedge or segmentectomy),[39] radiofrequency ablation,[40,41] and stereotactic body radio-therapy.[42] The patient's functional status and pulmonary function tests were reviewed, and he was deemed operable.

Referral

The patient was referred to thoracic surgery. Therapeutic alternatives were discussed, and he underwent right upper lobectomy uneventfully. He was discharged home after 5 days. LN dissection of the hilar and mediastinal nodes showed no malignancy; these findings were consistent

---

*The extent of clinical staging can vary from a clinical evaluation alone (history and physical examination) to extensive imaging (CT/PET scans) or invasive staging techniques; of note, needle aspiration and surgical staging procedures such as mediastinoscopy are still part of clinical staging because surgical resection as a treatment has not taken place.

with pathologic stage IA, for which estimated 5-year survival is 73%, and median survival time is 119 months. A strict focus on prognosis usually leads to an emphasis on pathologic staging because it is most accurate. However, pathologic staging is inherently somewhat academic because it is not available until after major decisions about treatment have been made (i.e., surgical resection in this case).[38]

Follow-up Tests and Procedures

This patient had follow-up within 2 weeks with the thoracic surgeon and had a plan to continue follow-up with the surgical team for at least 3 to 6 months.[43] Post-lobectomy FEV_1 stabilizes (reduced by 10% to 15%) at approximately 6 months post intervention; therefore, at that time, repeat pulmonary function tests (PFTs) are warranted to determine new baseline physiologic parameters. Given that 20% to 40% of confirmed stage I NSCLC recurs during the first 4 years after resection, clinical and imaging surveillance may be warranted. Most recurrences, however, are found outside the thorax, are not amenable to curative resection, and are treated with radiation and chemotherapy. Survival for recurrence is poor, regardless of therapy.[43] Despite these facts, most organizations recommend ongoing surveillance in NSCLC after curative intent therapy. For instance, the American College of Chest Physicians (ACCP) recommends history (Hx), physical examination (PE), chest x-ray (CXR) or chest CT every 6 months for the first 2 years, and then annually. The American Society of Clinical Oncology on the other hand does not recommend imaging but only Hx and PE every 3 months for the first 2 years, every 6 months for years 3 to 5, and then every 12 months after year 5. At this time, none of the national or international societies recommends routine surveillance using PET-CT scanning, tumor markers, or bronchoscopy.[43]

Quality Improvement

In this case, a diagnosis of lung cancer was made quickly, and N2 metastasis was ruled out. Thus the procedure altered management and decision making. At our team meeting, we readdressed whether this patient could have benefited from sublobar (limited) resection. We were aware that sublobar resection is an alternative for patients with limited physiologic reserve and for those with lesions smaller than 2 cm, and that a published randomized controlled study evaluating lobectomy versus sublobar resection established lobectomy with mediastinal nodal staging as the standard of care.[39] In that study, limited resection was associated with a threefold increase in the locoregional recurrence rate compared with lobectomy (6% per person/yr vs. 2% per person/yr; $P = .008$; 4.4% for segmentectomy, 8.6% for wedge resection) and was associated with a 30% non–statistically significant increase in overall death rate (11.7% vs. 8.9%; $P = .088$) and a 50% increase in the death with cancer rate (7.3% vs. 4.9%; $P = .094$). Meta-analysis of mostly retrospective studies and a few nonrandomized prospective trials comparing lobectomy with sublobar resection for stage IA NSCLC showed that combined survival differences at 1, 3, and 5 years after resection were similar.[44] Although pulmonary function is better preserved with the use of sublobar

Table 15-1 Summary of the EBUS-TBNA Technique in a Step-By-Step Approach

Step Number	Description
Step 1	The biopsy needle is passed through the biopsy channel.
Step 2	The housing is secured to the bronchoscope by a flange.
Step 3	The sheath is released by twisting the inferior screw.
Step 4	With the node visualized by ultrasound, the sheath is advanced out of the end of the scope until it slightly touches the airway wall. It is therefore safe to advance the needle.
Step 5	The needle screw, located superiorly, is then released.
Step 6	The needle is advanced into the lymph node using a quick jab. During this process, the needle may push the airway wall away from the balloon. Thus the transducer-wall interface is lost, and the image may show reverberation artifacts. The problem is overcome by gently advancing the scope and/or further inflating the balloon.
Step 7	Visualize the needle entering the target node.
Step 8	Move the stylet in and out a few times to dislodge bronchial wall debris.
Step 9	Remove the stylet.
Step 10	The syringe is applied to the biopsy needle.
Step 11	Suction is applied at usually −20 mL of air.
Step 12	Pass the needle in and out of the node 15 times.
Step 13	Suction is then released.
Step 14	Retract the needle into the sheath.
Step 15	The needle housing is unlocked, and the needle and the sheath are removed together; the aspirated material is smeared onto glass slides.

resection, perioperative mortality is no different than after lobectomy.[45,46] We acknowledged that until prospective randomized controlled studies further clarify the role of sublobar resection, this treatment modality remains indicated in patients with poor cardiopulmonary reserve, cardiac morbidity, old age, or previous surgery, none of which occurred in our patient.

DISCUSSION POINTS

1. Describe a step-by-step approach to performing EBUS-TBNA.

   Once the target node is selected, EBUS-TBNA can be performed in 15 steps, which are summarized in Table 15-1.[47]

2. Describe the physics principles of endobronchial ultrasound and their impact on quality image acquisition.

   Basic ultrasound principles are summarized in Table 15-2 and Figures 15-4 and 15-5. During ultrasound image formation, the transducer sends out a brief pulse of sound that penetrates the tissue. The sound waves are reflected back to the transducer, which serves as the sensor and the source of the signal. Ultrasound is reflected at tissue boundaries and interfaces, similar to the light of a mirror (see Figure 15-4);

Table 15-2   Definitions and Basic Ultrasound Principles

Terminology	Definition	Comments
Ultrasound	Imaging modality based on properties of sound waves; represents the mechanical energy that causes compression and rarefaction of a conducting material or substance known as *medium*.	Refers to sounds with frequencies of 20 kHz or higher, inaudible to humans.
Echogenicity	Represents the extent to which a structure (tissue or substance) gives rise to reflections of ultrasonic waves. When ultrasound (US) images are displayed on a gray scale, the strongest echo signal is white, and when no sound wave is reflected, the image is black or, in ultrasound terms, *anechoic* (see Figure 15-4).	The intensity of the signal, which determines echogenicity, depends on the reflected wave amplitude. The terms used in ultrasonography to describe a certain tissue or structure include the following: *isoechoic*, comparable with surrounding tissue; *hypoechoic*, weaker than surrounding tissue; and *hyperechoic*, stronger than surrounding tissue (see Figure 15-4).
Frequency	Represents a specific number of vibration cycles per second (measured in units of hertz).	Endoscopic US frequencies are in the range of 5 to 30 MHz. Current dedicated endobronchial ultrasound (EBUS)–transbronchial needle aspiration (TBNA) bronchoscopes allow change in frequency from 5 to12 MHz.
Wavelength	Represents the distance between two successive pulses.	The higher the frequency, the shorter the related wavelength.
Propagation	Represents the process through which sound advances through various tissues.	The speed of sound in human tissue is usually 1540 m/sec.
Refraction	Represents a change in direction of the incident ultrasound beam.	Degrades image quality.
Scattering	Represents the spread of the ultrasound beam in different directions.	Degrades image quality.
Attenuation	Represents the loss of energy mainly caused by absorption (when the vibration of the US wave is converted to heat owing to friction).	Attenuation depends on the medium; it is much higher in air than in water and depends on the frequency, increasing with higher frequencies. The bigger the difference in acoustic properties between two media, the larger the proportion of the reflected US and the smaller the transmitted US (see Figure 15-4).
Penetration	Refers to the distance between an imaged area and the transducer. The time delay between the energy going into the body and returning to the US transducer determines the depth from which the signal arises (longer times equal greater depths because Depth = Velocity × Time/2).	Large transducers transmit powerful beams and increase penetration depth (i.e., penetration depth is less in EBUS than in thoracic US) (see Figure 15-4). Depends on the frequency used (indirect relationship): higher frequencies (e.g., 20 MHz) do not penetrate as deeply as lower frequencies (e.g., 7.5 MHz) (see Figure 15-4).
Resolution	Represents the capacity of a system to distinguish small objects from others and is determined by the frequency and duration of the transmitted sound phase.	Depends on the frequency and the size of the transducer. Categorized in two types: axial, representing the ability to resolve objects within the imaging plane at different depths; and lateral, representing the ability to resolve objects in the imaging plane that are located side by side.

it reflects very well wherever a significant change in the propagation medium occurs; the degree of reflection is determined by the acoustic impedance of adjacent tissue, which is largely related to tissue density. When the ultrasound beam strikes an interface, it undergoes refraction, scattering, and attenuation as it passes through tissue, all of which degrade image quality on examination of deeper structures (see Figure 15-4). Ultrasound image distortion is caused by normal phenomena of refraction, scattering, and attenuation and may interfere with the ability to properly identify a target (e.g., lymph node, blood vessel). These artifacts, however, can be useful because they help describe the properties of tissues (e.g., calcification or necrosis within a lymph node). Understanding the different types of artifacts helps us identify and obtain a clear image of a real target and perform safe needle aspiration without puncturing vascular structures or lung parenchyma. Common types of artifacts seen during ultrasound imaging include reverberation and attenuation artifacts.

- Reverberation artifacts occur when a highly reflective tissue is parallel to the transducer, as when the water-filled balloon of the EBUS probe/scope is not in contact with the airway wall, and ultrasound waves are repeatedly reflected between the tissue surface (airway wall) and the transducer.[36] The resulting effect is that strong false echoes appear on the ultrasound image as multiple equally spaced lines (see Figure 15-5).
- Attenuation artifacts include the tadpole tail sign and the acoustic shadow. Tissues with low acoustic impedance (i.e., necrotic lymph nodes, mediastinal cysts) result in lower attenuation than tissues with higher impedance. For the tadpole tail artifact, the echo at the distal border of the low impedance structure will be higher and ultrasound will display the area distal to the low impedance structure more brightly than surrounding tissue (see Figure 15-5). The acoustic shadow artifact is exactly the reverse of the tadpole tail as the area behind a high impedance structure is displayed with lower brightness

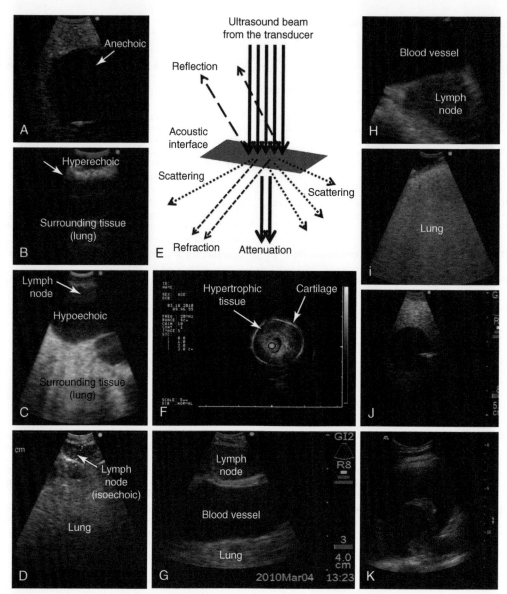

Figure 15-4   Principles and terminology of ultrasound: **A,** A structure (e.g., blood vessel) that does not reflect the sound waves at all is termed *anechoic.* **B,** A hyperechoic pattern (e.g., cartilaginous nodule in tracheopathica osteochondroplastica) occurs when the echoes are stronger than those of surrounding tissues. **C,** A hypoechoic structure (e.g., lymph node) occurs when the echoes are weaker than those from surrounding tissues. **D,** This lymph node is labeled *isoechoic,* because the echoes are of comparable amplitude with surrounding tissue (e.g., lung). **E,** The ultrasound beam undergoes reflection, refraction, scattering, and attenuation as it passes through tissue; all of these degrade image quality upon examination of deeper structures, but the last three processes cause the ultrasound waves reflected back to the transducer to be much weaker. **F,** Increased attenuation and low penetration depth occur when structures are visualized with high-frequency probes: The hypertrophic stenotic tissue and the intact cricoid cartilage are clearly visualized, but the deeper structures are not when a 20-MHz radial probe is used. **G,** When the curved linear endobronchial ultrasound (EBUS) transducer with 7.5-MHz frequency is used, attenuation is decreased, penetration depth is increased, and the EBUS image shows the right lower paratracheal lymph node, the superior vena cava, and the distal normal lung parenchyma, but details of the airway wall structures cannot be assessed. **H,** Attenuation also depends on the medium and is low in fluid (e.g., blood vessels). **I,** Attenuation is high in air (e.g., normal lung tissue). **J,** The depth of penetration is also directly dependent on the size of the transducer. A relatively superficial penetration (e.g., 5 cm) is achieved when the small EBUS curved linear transducer is used. **K,** Deep penetration (e.g., 15 cm) can be obtained by using large thoracic transducers.

than the rest of the surrounding tissue. Because the ultrasound beam is almost completely reflected at the border or attenuated within the high impedance structure, the posterior area does not receive ultrasound waves and appears as a hypoechoic shadow (see Figure 15-5).

3. Describe the reported relation between PET-negative lymph node size and malignancy.

- One report comparing integrated PET-CT scanning with results from surgical resection for mediastinal staging in NSCLC found an incidence of occult N2 disease of 16% (25 of 153), especially at stations 7 and 4[15]; in a different report, the false negativity rate of PET-CT was even higher at 25%.[9]
- Risk factors for occult N2 disease include the following:

Figure 15-5 Image artifacts. **A,** Reverberation artifacts: When the water-filled balloon of the endobronchial ultrasound (EBUS) bronchoscope is not in intimate contact with the airway wall, the ultrasound (US) waves are repeatedly reflected between the highly reflective tissue surface (airway wall) and the transducer; the resulting effect is that strong false echoes appear on the ultrasound image as multiple, equally spaced lines. **B,** In the tadpole tail artifact, the echo at the distal border of the low impedance structure (i.e., the azygos vein) will be higher, and US will display the area distal to the low impedance structure more brightly compared with surrounding tissue (arrows). **C,** The acoustic shadow artifact is the reverse effect of the tadpole tail; the area behind a high impedance structure (i.e., calcification within the lymph node) is displayed with lower brightness than the rest of the surrounding tissue. The US beam is attenuated within the high impedance structure, and the posterior area appears as a hypoechoic shadow (arrows).

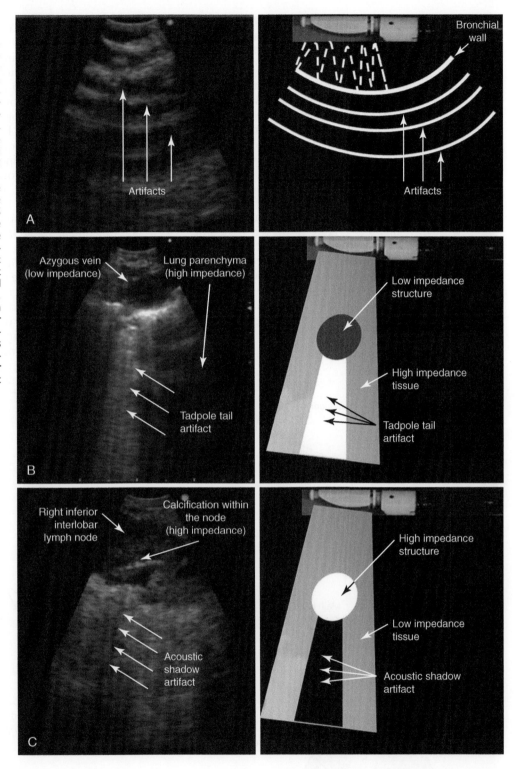

- Central tumors
- Hilar N1 disease on CT scan or PET-CT
- Right upper lobe tumors
- Broncho-alveolar cell carcinoma
- All situations with low FDG uptake in the primary tumor
- Mediastinal PET-negative LNs larger than 16 mm on CT scan: post-test probability for N2 disease is 21% in patients with PET-negative nodes larger

than 16 mm; these patients should be planned for mediastinoscopy or EUS/EBUS before thoracotomy to prevent too many unnecessary surgeries; on the other hand, the post-test probability for N2 disease is 5% for LNs measuring 10 to 15 mm on CT in patients with a negative PET, suggesting that these patients should be planned directly for thoracotomy because the yield of mediastinoscopy will be extremely low.[8]

Expert Commentary

provided by Kenichi Nishina and Kenji Hirooka, Engineers, Olympus Medical Systems Corp., Tokyo, Japan

Understanding the physics principles of ultrasound, their impact on image acquisition, and how they help the physician interpret the ultrasound image is very relevant to clinical care. We agree, therefore, with the authors' perspectives, and we would like to add the following technical and physics-based information with regard to endobronchial ultrasound[36,48]:

1. *Impact of side lobes:* This is the acoustic energy that spreads out from the transducer at angles other than the primary acoustic beam, in other words, "main lobe" (Figure 15-6). When the side lobes are strongly generated, artifacts occur beside highly reflective objects (Figure 15-7). To avoid this artifact, it is useful to change the probe position to a location where there is no image of the highly reflective object, or to adjust the focal point using an ultrasound processor with a variable focus function.

2. *How to distinguish the artifacts:* It is helpful to observe the ultrasound image by maneuvering the ultrasound probe or the endoscope slowly back and forth or left and right to change the angle of observation. Because the position of artifacts is determined by the relative position between the ultrasound source and the object, movements of the artifacts on the ultrasound image are different from the movements of echo images created from the target tissues.

3. *Adjustment of contrast:* Contrast is the image processor function used to adjust brightness between light and dark areas of the image (Figure 15-8). It is desirable to adjust contrast to an even gradation. If the contrast is set too high, the gradation reproduction will be poor, and the middle range of the object will be unrecognizable on the ultrasound image (Figure 15-9).

4. *Adjustment of the monitor:* It is also important to set up the monitor in appropriate conditions to observe distinguishable ultrasound images. The brightness and the contrast of the monitor

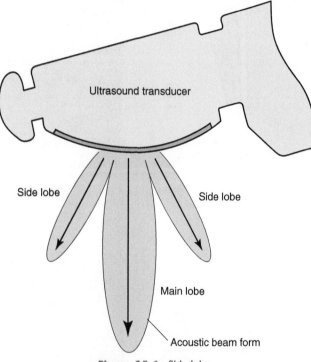

Figure 15-6   Side lobe.

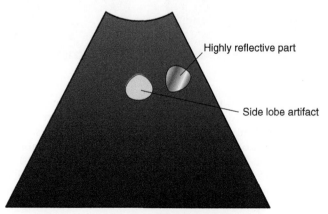

Figure 15-7   Side lobe artifact.

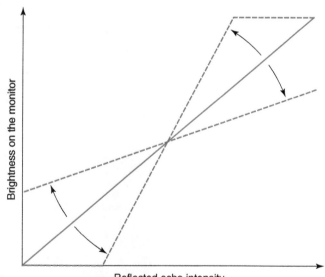

Figure 15-8   Contrast adjustment.

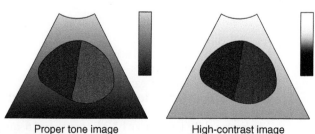

Figure 15-9   Differences in the ultrasound image display due to the contrast setting.

should be adjusted for even distribution of the gray scale (see Figure 15-9). This operation is done separately from any adjustments made on the ultrasound image processor.

5. *Slice resolution:* The ultrasound scanning plane is only as wide as the ultrasound beam. For accurate target sampling (e.g., by TBNA), it is desirable to pierce the target when it appears the largest (in other words, when the largest diameter of the target is visible on the ultrasound image). If a puncture is made toward the periphery of the target, it is possible that the needle will appear as though it is within the target on the ultrasound image, even when the needle is actually located adjacent to the target (Figure 15-10). The authors describe that the ultrasound image may be lost when the needle pierces the target. We believe that this phenomenon is also caused by forward movement of the sheath during EBUS or EBUS-guided TBNA. To remedy this phenomenon, it may be helpful to adjust the sheath once it is completely extended from the distal tip of the endoscope, then to pull the sheath back until it is seen only as a half-moon on the endoscopic view and lock it into position (Figure 15-11). Doing this will reduce the sheath slack in the working channel of the endoscope. Furthermore, creating some distance between the sheath and the bronchial wall will decrease the possibility of losing the ultrasound image, which is caused by pushing against the bronchial wall with the sheath.[36,49]

It is vital to avoid perforation of the working channel of the endoscope during EBUS-guided TBNA. Before the needle is inserted through the working channel of the endoscope, it is necessary to confirm that the needle slider is completely pulled back until it clicks, in such a way that the double-triangle mark appears on the handle section (Figure 15-12). This "step" is readily forgotten after needles have been

removed to extract the specimen from the needle; therefore one should take great care after each extraction to confirm the visibility of the double-triangle mark on the handle section before inserting the needle for an additional pass.

The EBUS-TBNA endoscope is equipped with a curved linear (convex) array scanning ultrasound transducer with a 7.5-MHz center frequency and a scanning direction that is parallel to the insertion axis. This makes it suitable to observe lymph nodes or

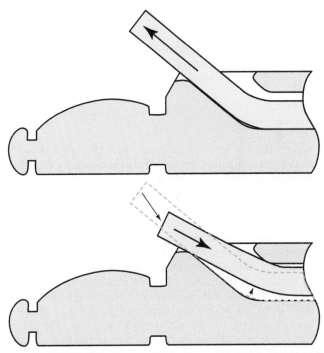

Figure 15-11 The diagram shows how to reduce the sheath advancing phenomenon.

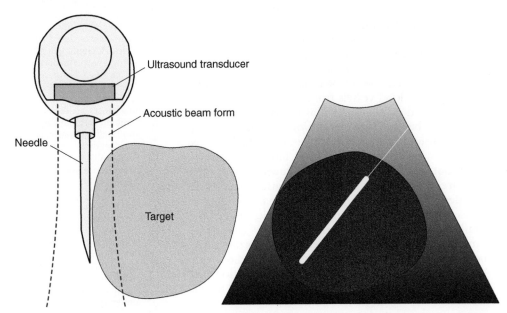

Figure 15-10 The ultrasound image shows the needle as if it is within the target.

Ultrasound transducer

Acoustic beam form

Needle

Target

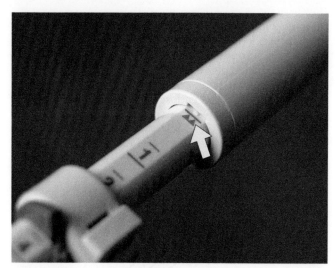

Figure 15-12 Double-triangle mark on the handle of the endobronchial ultrasound (EBUS)–transbronchial needle aspiration (TBNA) needle.

does not exactly correspond. For a more straightforward orientation, it is helpful to rotate the ultrasound image by using the image rotation function on the ultrasound center. It should be rotated to correspond with the movement of the probe on the endoscopic view when the probe is moved by angulating the bronchoscope.[36,50]

In conclusion, endobronchial ultrasound is an exciting and rapidly evolving imaging modality that provides bronchoscopists with several different techniques and technologies with which to care for their patients. Progress to enhance image quality and ease of use is expected. A thorough understanding of physics principles and the effects of image adjustment will help bronchoscopists optimize visualization in both clinical and research environments.

vessels located around the trachea or the bronchi and enables visualization on the ultrasound image of endotherapy accessories inserted through the working channel of the endoscope. When the EBUS-TBNA endoscope is combined with the Olympus endoscopic ultrasound center EU-ME1 (Olympus America Inc.) or designated Aloka diagnostic ultrasound systems (Aloka America, Wallingford, Conn), users can change the frequency of the ultrasound image (this is not the same as the center frequency of the ultrasound transducer, because this is not adjustable). To obtain the best balance of resolution and penetration, the default frequency setting of the ultrasound image is 10 MHz. However, it will be useful to set the frequency to 12 MHz if the region of interest is a small lymph node, or if the target is the detailed structure of tissue in the near field. On the other hand, the frequency should be set at 6 or 7.5 MHz if the region of interest is a large lymph node or a structure located at the farthest end of the depth of penetration. A variable frequency function enables the user to select an appropriate ultrasound image according to the region of interest being scanned. In addition, by using an electronic scanning (array) transducer, one is able to use Doppler function to distinguish blood vessels from tissues.

With regard to endobronchial ultrasound accessories that can be used with conventional bronchoscopes, the ultrasound miniature probe with balloon is equipped with a mechanical radial ultrasound transducer that has a 20-MHz center frequency; its scanning direction is perpendicular to the insertion axis. It provides a high-resolution cross-sectional 360-degree ultrasound image. This makes it suitable to observe detailed structures of the bronchial wall. The ultrasound miniature probe is inserted into the bronchi via the working channel of a conventional bronchoscope. At this point, one will note that the relationship between the endoscopic view and the ultrasound image

REFERENCES

1. Rabinovitz M, Pitlik SD, Leifer M, et al. Unintentional weight loss: a retrospective analysis of 154 cases. *Arch Intern Med.* 1986; 146:186-187.
2. Jackman RW, Kandarian SC. The molecular basis of skeletal muscle atrophy. *Am J Physiol Cell Physiol.* 2004;287:C834-C843.
3. Staal-van den Brekel AJ, Dentener MA, Schols AM, et al. Increased resting energy expenditure and weight loss are related to a systemic inflammatory response in lung cancer patients. *J Clin Oncol.* 1995;13:2600-2605.
4. Detterbeck FC, Jantz MA, Wallace M, et al. American College of Chest Physicians. Invasive mediastinal staging of lung cancer: ACCP evidence-based clinical practice guidelines (2nd ed). *Chest.* 2007;132:202S-220S.
5. De Leyn P, Vansteenkiste J, Cuypers P, et al. Role of cervical mediastinoscopy in staging of non-small cell lung cancer without enlarged mediastinal lymph nodes on CT scan. *Eur J Cardiothorac Surg.* 1997;12:706-712.
6. Toloza EM, Harpole L, McCrory DC. Noninvasive staging of non-small cell lung cancer: a review of the current evidence. *Chest.* 2003;123:137S-146S.
7. Birim O, Kappetein AP, Stijnen T, et al. Meta-analysis of positron emission tomographic and computed tomographic imaging in detecting mediastinal lymph node metastases in nonsmall cell lung cancer. *Ann Thorac Surg.* 2005;79:375-382.
8. de Langen AJ, Raijmakers P, Riphagen I, et al. The size of mediastinal lymph nodes and its relation with metastatic involvement: a meta-analysis. *Eur J Cardiothorac Surg.* 2006;29:26-29.
9. Melek H, Gunluoglu MZ, Demir A, et al. Role of positron emission tomography in mediastinal lymphatic staging of non-small cell lung cancer. *Eur J Cardiothorac Surg.* 2008;33:294-299.
10. Pagano E, Filippini C, Di Cuonzo D, et al. Factors affecting pattern of care and survival in a population-based cohort of non-small-cell lung cancer incident cases. *Cancer Epidemiol.* 2010;34:483-489.
11. Berglund A, Holmberg L, Tishelman C, et al. Social inequalities in non-small cell lung cancer management and survival: a population-based study in central Sweden. *Thorax.* 2010;65:327-333.
12. Podnos YD, Borneman TR, Koczywas M, et al. Symptom concerns and resource utilization in patients with lung cancer. *J Palliat Med.* 2007;10:899-903.
13. Tariman JD, Berry DL, Cochrane B, et al. Preferred and actual participation roles during health care decision making in persons with cancer: a systematic review. *Ann Oncol.* 2010;21:1145-1151.
14. De Leyn P, Lardinois D, Van Schil PE, et al. ESTS guidelines for preoperative lymph node staging for non-small cell lung cancer. *Eur J Cardiothorac Surg.* 2007;32:1-8.
15. Al-Sarraf N, Aziz R, Gately K, et al. Pattern and predictors of occult mediastinal lymph node involvement in non-small cell lung cancer patients with negative mediastinal uptake on positron emission tomography. *Eur J Cardiothorac Surg.* 2008;33:104-109.

16. Chhajed PN, Bernasconi M, Gambazzi F, et al. Combining bronchoscopy and positron emission tomography for the diagnosis of the small pulmonary nodule < or = 3 cm. *Chest*. 2005;128:3558-3564.

17. Herth FJ, Eberhardt R, Vilmann P, et al. Real-time endobronchial ultrasound guided transbronchial needle aspiration for sampling mediastinal lymph nodes. *Thorax*. 2006;61:795-798.

18. Chin R Jr, McCain TW, Lucia MA, et al. Transbronchial needle aspiration in diagnosing and staging lung cancer: how many aspirates are needed? *Am J Respir Crit Care Med*. 2002;166:377-381.

19. Siebeker KL, Curtis JK. Anesthesia for patients with pulmonary emphysema: use of positive-negative pressure respirator during pulmonary surgery. *Anesthesiology*. 1957;18:856-865.

20. Herth FJ, Ernst A, Eberhardt R, et al. Endobronchial ultrasound-guided transbronchial needle aspiration of lymph nodes in the radiologically normal mediastinum. *Eur Respir J*. 2006;28:910-914.

21. Herth F, Becker HD, Ernst A. Conventional vs endobronchial ultrasound-guided transbronchial needle aspiration: a randomized trial. *Chest*. 2004;125:322-325.

22. Herth FJ, Becker HD, Ernst A. Ultrasound-guided transbronchial needle aspiration: an experience in 242 patients. *Chest*. 2003;123:604-607.

23. Colt HG, Murgu S, Davoudi M. EBUS step-by-step. You Tube, posted August 2010. http://www.youtube.com/watch?v=Z9FdgVx_xrM&feature=related. Accessed February 21, 2011.

24. Gu P, Zhao Y, Jiang L, et al. Endobronchial ultrasound–guided transbronchial needle aspiration for staging of lung cancer: a systematic review and meta-analysis. *Eur J Cancer*. 2009;45:1389-1396.

25. Varela-Lema L, Fernandez-Villar A, Ruano-Ravina A. Effectiveness and safety of endobronchial ultrasound–transbronchial needle aspiration: a systematic review. *Eur Respir J*. 2009;33:1156-1164.

26. Steinfort DP, Irving LB. Patient satisfaction during endobronchial ultrasound-guided transbronchial needle aspiration performed under conscious sedation. *Respir Care*. 2010;55:702-706.

27. Herth FJ, Lunn W, Eberhardt R, et al. Transbronchial versus transesophageal ultrasound-guided aspiration of enlarged mediastinal lymph nodes. *Am J Respir Crit Care Med*. 2005;171:1164-1167.

28. Medford AR, Agrawal S, Free CM, et al. A performance and theoretical cost analysis of endobronchial ultrasound-guided transbronchial needle aspiration in a UK tertiary respiratory centre. *Q J Med*. 2009;102:859-864.

29. Kennedy MP, Shweihat Y, Sarkiss M, et al. Complete mediastinal and hilar lymph node staging of primary lung cancer by endobronchial ultrasound: moderate sedation or general anesthesia? *Chest*. 2008;134:1350-1351.

30. Douadi Y, Bentayeb H, Malinowski S, et al. Anaesthesia for bronchial echoendoscopy: experience with the laryngeal mask. *Rev Mal Respir*. 2010;27:37-41.

31. Ng A, Smith G. Gastroesophageal reflux and aspiration of gastric contents in anesthetic practice. *Anesth Analg*. 2001;93:494-513.

32. Sarkiss M, Kennedy M, Riedel B, et al. Anesthesia technique for endobronchial ultrasound-guided fine needle aspiration of mediastinal lymph node. *J Cardiothorac Vasc Anesth*. 2007;21:892-896.

33. Mercer M. Anesthesia for the patient with respiratory disease. *Update in Anaesthesia*. 2000;12:1-3.

34. Pentax. EBUS Pro. Full video endobronchial ultrasound. http://www.pentax.de/en/ebus.php. Accessed February 21, 2011.

34a. Olympus. EBUS bronchoscopes. http://www.olympusamerica.com/msg_section/msg_endoscopy_ebus_bronchoscopes.asp. Accessed February 21, 2011.

35. Kurimoto N. Diagnosis of depth penetration in the tracheobronchial tree. In: Kurimoto N, ed. *Endobronchial Ultrasonography*. Kyoto: Kinpodo; 2001:33-38.

36. Nishina K, Hirooka K, Wiegand J, et al. Principles and practice of endoscopic ultrasound. In: Boliger CT, et al, eds. *Clinical Chest Ultrasound: From the ICU to the Bronchoscopy Suite*. Basel: Karger; 2009:110-127.

37. Yasufuku K, Chiyo M, Sekine Y, et al. Real-time endobronchial ultrasound-guided transbronchial needle aspiration of mediastinal and hilar lymph nodes. *Chest*. 2004;126:122-128.

38. Detterbeck FC, Boffa DJ, Tanoue LT. The new lung cancer staging system. *Chest*. 2009;136:260-271.

39. Ginsberg RJ, Rubinstein LV. Randomized trial of lobectomy versus limited resection for T1 N0 non-small cell lung cancer. Lung Cancer Study Group. *Ann Thorac Surg*. 1995;60:615-622.

40. Chan VO, McDermott S, Malone DE, et al. Percutaneous radiofrequency ablation of lung tumors: evaluation of the literature using evidence-based techniques. *J Thorac Imaging*. 2011;26:18-26.

41. Pennathur A, Abbas G, Schuchert MJ, et al. Image-guided radiofrequency ablation for the treatment of early-stage non-small cell lung neoplasm in high-risk patients. *Semin Thorac Cardiovasc Surg*. 2010;22:53-58.

42. Baba F, Shibamoto Y, Ogino H, et al. Clinical outcomes of stereotactic body radiotherapy for stage I non-small cell lung cancer using different doses depending on tumor size. *Radiat Oncol*. 2010;5:81.

43. Rubins J, Unger M, Colice GL, American College of Chest Physicians. Follow-up and surveillance of the lung cancer patient following curative intent therapy: ACCP evidence-based clinical practice guideline (2nd ed). *Chest*. 2007;132:355S-367S.

44. Nakamura H, Kawasaki N, Taguchi M, et al. Survival following lobectomy vs limited resection for stage I lung cancer: a meta-analysis. *Br J Cancer*. 2005;92:1033-1037.

45. Okada M, Koike T, Higashiyama M, et al. Radical sublobar resection for small-sized non-small cell lung cancer: a multicenter study. *J Thorac Cardiovasc Surg*. 2006;132:769-775.

46. Scott WJ, Howington J, Feigenberg S, et al, American College of Chest Physicians. Treatment of non-small cell lung cancer stage I and stage II: ACCP evidence-based clinical practice guidelines (2nd ed). *Chest*. 2007;132:234S-242S.

47. EBUS Bronchoscopy.wmv. BronchOrg. http://www.youtube.com/watch?v=Z9FdgVx_xrM&feature=related. Accessed October 3, 2010.

48. Nagai H, Itoh K. *Illustrated Textbook of Ultrasound*. 2nd ed. Tokyo: Nankodo; 2000:40-51.

49. Yasufuku K, Nakajima T. *Endobronchial Ultrasound Guided Transbronchial Needle Aspiration Manual*. Tokyo: Kanehara Shuppan; 2009:22-26.

50. Kurimoto N. Diagnosis of depth penetration in the tracheobronchial tree. In: Kurimoto N, ed. *Endobronchial Ultrasonography*. Kyoto: Kinpodo; 2001:7-21.

Chapter 16

EBUS-TBNA of Right Lower Paratracheal Lymph Node (Station 4R)

This chapter emphasizes the following elements of the Four Box Approach: patient's significant comorbidities; patient preferences and expectations (also includes family); risk-benefit analyses and therapeutic alternatives; techniques and instrumentation; and follow-up tests, visits, and procedures.

CASE DESCRIPTION

A 67-year-old Korean man with a 20–pack-year history of smoking was found to have an abnormal chest radiograph showing a right upper lobe pulmonary nodule during a routine preoperative evaluation for hernia repair. The patient had COPD (FEV$_1$ 50% of predicted) and pulmonary hypertension, presumptively related to his COPD (WHO group III*). An echocardiogram performed 3 months earlier showed a normal left ventricular ejection fraction and a pulmonary artery systolic pressure of 59 mm Hg with a tricuspid regurgitant velocity of 3.5 m/sec and an estimated right atrial pressure of 10 mm Hg. Computed tomography of the chest showed a 1.5 × 1-cm right upper lobe nodule and a 1.4-cm right lower paratracheal lymph node. He had no other past medical history and was in excellent health except for mild exertional dyspnea (NYHA class II). The patient was referred for tissue diagnosis (Figure 16-1).

DISCUSSION POINTS

1. Define the borders of station 4R and justify this definition.
2. Describe how the sagittal view of a computed tomography scan is used to plan EBUS-TBNA at station 4R.

CASE RESOLUTION

Initial Evaluations

Physical Examination, Complementary Tests, and Functional Status Assessment

After the pulmonary nodule was discovered on chest radiograph, this patient underwent a chest computed tomography (CT). In addition to the history and physical

examination, CT scan of the chest is recommended in patients suspected of having lung cancer who are eligible for treatment, because its potential benefits for staging and treatment planning outweigh the relatively low risk of radiation-induced damage.[1] CT scan of the chest should be obtained before bronchoscopy because having a more accurate appreciation of the size and location of the tumor increases the diagnostic yield of bronchoscopy, which is low, however, for peripheral pulmonary nodules smaller than 2 cm. Yield is high for diagnosis of larger nodules and for staging of mediastinal lymphadenopathy when sonographic guidance (endobronchial ultrasound–transbronchial needle aspiration [EBUS-TBNA]) is used.

This patient showed evidence of ipsilateral lymph node involvement (right lower paratracheal; 4R), but contralateral lymph node involvement was not suspected on the basis of CT. Positron emission tomography (PET)-CT has greater sensitivity for detecting metastasis in the mediastinum compared with CT, but this procedure had not been performed before the patient was referred to our institution. Nor had other diagnostic studies been performed to search for extrathoracic disease. For example, for patients with clinical stage IB-IIIB being considered for curative treatment, cranial magnetic resonance imaging (MRI) is recommended by some authorities to detect brain metastases, even if clinical examination findings are negative.[1] We elected to perform additional tests on our patient for complete staging after a diagnosis had been made. We chose to recommend bronchoscopy and EBUS-guided TBNA for both diagnosis and mediastinal staging.

Comorbidities

This patient likely had pulmonary hypertension secondary to chronic obstructive pulmonary disease (COPD) based on a Doppler echocardiographic study showing a pulmonary artery systolic pressure (PASP) of 59 mm Hg with a tricuspid regurgitant velocity (TRV) of 3.5 m/sec.[2] In general, pulmonary hypertension is considered likely if the PASP is greater than 50 and the TRV is greater than 3.4; unlikely if the PASP is 36 or less and the TRV is 2.8 or less, and no other suggestive findings are reported; and possible with other combinations of findings. Doppler echocardiography, however, may be misleading in patients with suspected pulmonary hypertension, especially when an inadequate tricuspid regurgitant jet cannot be properly assessed owing to a poor echocardiographic window. This was demonstrated in an observational study† of 65 patients with various types of pulmonary hypertension.[3] The pulmonary arterial pressure estimated by Doppler echocardiography was at least 10 mm Hg higher or lower

---

*This group includes pulmonary hypertension due to COPD, interstitial lung disease, other pulmonary diseases with a mixed restrictive and obstructive pattern, obstructive sleep apnea, alveolar hypoventilation disorders, and other causes of hypoxemia.

†A major limitation of the study was that catheterization and Doppler echocardiography were not performed simultaneously. Doppler echocardiography was performed within 1 hour of a clinically indicated right-heart catheterization.

Figure 16-1 Axial and sagittal chest computed tomography (CT) images showing the 4R lymph node station in its anterior, precarinal position.

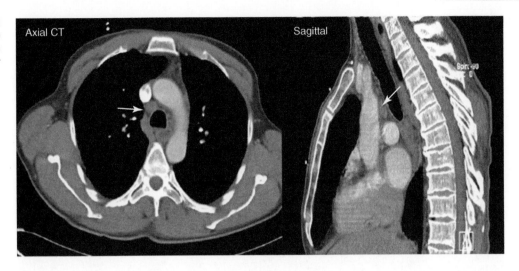

than that obtained by right heart catheterization in 48% of patients.* Therefore, a low threshold for right heart catheterization is warranted when patients with suspected pulmonary hypertension are evaluated. However, perioperative insertion of pulmonary artery catheters is not routinely recommended as a strategy to reduce perioperative mortality or postoperative pulmonary complications, even in high-risk surgical patients.[4]

Support System

The patient lived at home by himself and was independent in his activities of daily living. He had a daughter, who lived far away, and he did not want her involved in decision making about the procedure, but he wanted her to "handle things" once the diagnosis was made.

Patient Preferences and Expectations

The patient expressed his wish to gather information about his disease process so that he could make an informed decision regarding therapies. In general, a decision is seen as autonomous when someone's choice is based on adequate information, taking into account one's values and with appreciation of alternatives and the potential consequences of choosing or refusing a specific procedure or battery of tests. A clear conversation with the patient is warranted to explain the indications and contraindications of diagnostic interventions being proposed and their alternatives.

Procedural Strategies

Indications

This patient likely had primary lung carcinoma. He needed a tissue diagnosis. We proposed bronchoscopy with EBUS-TBNA because the suspected N2 status (right lower paratracheal lymphadenopathy) had to be confirmed to decide on the need for further therapy: If N2 status were negative, therapy would be recommended for

stage I-II non–small cell lung carcinoma (NSCLC) (with likely surgical resection once operability is determined); or for postoperative stage IIIA1* or IIIA2, according to strategies for stage IIIA. If, on the other hand, N2 status is known to be positive preoperatively, the patient would be assigned stage IIIA3 and would be treated according to the algorithm for stage IIIA. Careful white light bronchoscopic examination should be performed at the time of EBUS-TBNA because it may detect mucosal abnormalities, which may be malignant. Such findings would change the stage. For instance, in the setting of mediastinal lymphadenopathy, if the tracheal wall is involved, the tumor would be classified as T4 and therefore stage IIIB, but if no mucosal abnormalities are noted, the patient would have N2 disease, namely, stage IIIA (Figure 16-2); furthermore, if the needle passes through airway wall infiltrated with malignant cells before entering the lymph node target, the lymph node aspirate could become contaminated, and this could represent a false-positive aspirate. Thus we believe that abnormal airway mucosa at the puncture site should be biopsied (see Figure 16-2), and that bronchoscopists should do their best to avoid needle insertion through abnormal appearing tissue, if possible.[†]

EBUS-TBNA can offer diagnosis and staging in one setting. With EBUS, one can potentially sample all stations adjacent to the trachea or bronchi (2, 4, 7, 10, 11) (Figure 16-3), but not level 5, 6, 8, and 9 lymph nodes.[‡]

---

*Stages IIIA1-4 are defined as follows: IIIA1, mediastinal lymph node metastases on postoperative histologic examination at one lymph node level; IIIA2, intraoperative findings of lymph node involvement at one level; IIIA3, involvement of one or more positions identified preoperatively by mediastinoscopy, needle biopsy, or PET. IIIA4, bulky disease (mediastinal lymph nodes >2-3 cm with extracapsular invasion, lymph node involvement of multiple N2 positions, and groups of multiple, positive, 1- to 2-cm lymph nodes).

†The inner stylet does not completely prevent contamination with bronchial wall cells (normal or abnormal).

‡Although sometimes visualized via EBUS but not adjacent to the airway, these stations are not accessible using this technique. Stations 5 and 6 are approached by using anterior mediastinotomy (Chamberlain procedure), and stations 8 and 9 via endoscopic ultrasound-guided fine-needle aspiration (EUS-FNA) or thoracoscopy.

---

*Although overestimations and underestimations occurred with similar frequency, the magnitude of the pressure underestimation was greater than that of overestimation (-30 ± 16 vs. $+19 \pm 11$ mm Hg; $P = .03$).

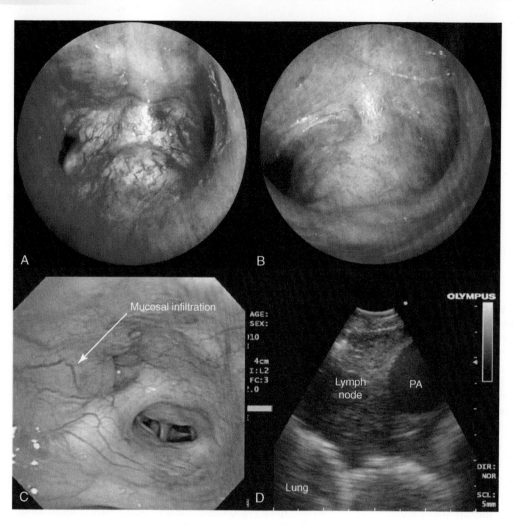

Figure 16-2 **A,** The main carina showing neoplastic mucosal infiltration (carinal invasion, T4 tumor, thus stage IIIB). **B,** Main carinal widening from large subcarinal lymphadenopathy (N2 disease), but no tumor infiltration (possibly stage IIIA). **C,** Left upper lobe lateral wall mucosal infiltration with lymphoma. **D,** Endobronchial ultrasound (EBUS) image of adjacent lymphadenopathy. *PA,* Pulmonary artery.

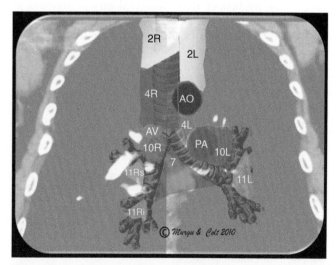

Figure 16-3 Diagram of the lymph node stations usually accessible by endobronchial ultrasound–transbronchial needle aspiration (EBUS-TBNA). Station 4R includes right lower paratracheal nodes and pre-tracheal nodes extending to the left lateral border of the trachea. The upper border is the intersection of the caudal margin of the innominate vein with the trachea; the lower border is the lower border of the azygos vein.

Low-volume cytology specimens such as those obtained via EBUS-TBNA are considered adequate for molecular analysis, as with epidermal growth factor receptor (EGFR) and anaplastic lymphatic kinase (ALK).[5,6] This is increasingly important because whole genome amplification enables multiple molecular analyses and may be used to expand starting deoxyribonucleic acid (i.e., DNA amplification) from low-volume lung biopsies, such as those obtained with EBUS-TBNA, for further analysis of advanced-stage NSCLC.[7] It is noteworthy that even when the primary tumor (the pulmonary nodule) is biopsied and studied for gene alterations, molecular assessment of metastatic sites (e.g., lymph nodes) may change management decisions because of the possibility of genetic differences between primary tumor and metastatic sites caused by tumor heterogeneity.[8,9] Mutations in genes involved in the *EGFR/KRAS/BRAF* pathway, for example, were shown to predict clinical response to EGFR-directed tyrosine kinase inhibitors (TKIs) in NSCLC patients. The presence of activating *EGFR* mutations and the absence of *KRAS* mutations have been shown to be favorable markers for response to EGFR-directed TKI therapy.[9] One study, which compared the mutational status of

EGFR, KRAS, and BRAF in primary tumors* (adenocarcinomas) with that in the corresponding lymph node metastases, found that mutations in primary tumors and lymph node metastases were identical in only 1 of 7 (14%) patients in case of EGFR mutation and in 11of 36 (31%) patients in case of KRAS mutation. Only one patient showed the same EGFR mutation in the primary tumor and corresponding lymph node metastasis. In this study, the remaining 6 patients had EGFR mutations identified in the primary tumor (3 patients) or in the lymph node metastasis (3 patients), but not in both. A different KRAS mutation in the primary tumor and the corresponding metastasis was seen in 1 patient, and 24 patients had KRAS mutations exclusively in primary (16 patients) or metastatic tumor (8 patients).[9] These data suggest that the possibility of differences in the mutational status of EGFR, KRAS,[†] and BRAF[‡] between primary tumors and corresponding lymph node metastases should be considered whenever these mutations are used for the selection of patients for EGFR-directed TKI therapy.[9]

Contraindications

Although no contraindications to bronchoscopy were noted, the patient's COPD and pulmonary hypertension could pose increased risk for hypoventilation, hypoxemia, and hemodynamic instability from worsening pulmonary hypertension during procedures performed under moderate sedation or general anesthesia.

Expected Results

The diagnostic rate of EBUS-TBNA for station 4R is 71% to 94%[10,11] and, as has been mentioned, the likelihood of obtaining sufficient material for use in molecular analysis is high. The prevalence of genetic alterations seems to vary depending on the patient's ethnicity; a meta-analysis of nine published studies showed that among those with adenocarcinoma, EGFR mutations were present in 48% of East Asian patients but in only 12% of those with other ethnicities.[12] Relevant to our patient is that EGFR mutation is frequent among Koreans suffering from lung cancer. In one study, it was seen in 20 of 115 patients (17.4%).[§13] Drugs that target mutant EGFR and ALK are now available, and it is possible that testing for prospective mutations could result in assigning a successful targeted therapy. For instance, erlotinib and gefitinib are already available to target mutant EGFR, and the ALK inhibitor crizotinib has demonstrated remarkable efficacy against ALK fusion–positive lung cancers.[14]

Other lung or nonlung primary tumors could be responsible for this patient's presentation. For neuroendocrine tumors, correct classification of a tumor as small cell lung cancer (SCLC) or as large cell neuroendocrine carcinoma (LCNEC) is a particularly difficult problem because of the many overlapping features of these tumors.[15] In the diagnosis of primary lung lesions, this distinction is important because of different treatment strategies. LCNEC is considered an NSCLC treated by surgical excision, whereas SCLC is usually treated with chemotherapy or chemoradiotherapy. Given the large numbers of background lymphocytes in EBUS-TBNA specimens, the distinction between lymphoid cells and a neuroendocrine tumor can be particularly difficult. If carcinoid is diagnosed, cytology specimens are often inadequate for a definitive diagnosis of typical or atypical morphology[16]—a crucial distinction in determining prognosis.

On a different note, the sensitivity and specificity of EBUS-TBNA for diagnosing mediastinal and hilar lymph node metastasis from nonpulmonary tumors (taken together) have been reported to be as high as 92.0% and 100%, respectively. Tumors encountered included colorectal, head and neck, ovarian, breast, esophageal, hepatocellular, prostate, renal, and germ cell cancers and malignant melanoma.[17] For lymphoma, a small study evaluating patients with high pretest probability for lymphoma in a tertiary cancer center revealed an overall sensitivity of 90.9% and specificity of 100%.[18] Larger, prospective studies showed that the sensitivity and the specificity of EBUS-TBNA for definitive diagnosis of lymphoma were 57% and 100%, respectively. Decreased diagnostic yield may be due in part to problems with the low-volume cytology specimens obtained via EBUS-TBNA. For example, baseline cellularity of the aspirates includes both lymphocytes and bronchial epithelial cells because specimens may be contaminated with bronchial epithelial cells captured when the needle traverses the bronchial wall; in addition, a variety of entities have overlapping cytomorphologic features, and a paucity of published literature pertains to cytomorphology of these tumors.[15] For lymphoma, even though the diagnostic accuracy of EBUS-TBNA is less than that seen for other cancers, the procedure appears justified in patients with isolated mediastinal lymphadenopathy, given the significant proportion (76%) of patients with lymphoma who would thus avoid a surgical biopsy.[19]

Team Experience

Good communication with the cytopathologist is important to increase the yield of the procedure, because sample preparation, triage, and interpretation ultimately depend on the question being asked. The pathologist should be told whether the procedure is performed for suspected primary lung cancer, for staging purposes, or to rule out metastasis or second primaries. In patients with known or suspected lymphoma or infection, additional tests on samples may be warranted.* Failure to begin the

---

*KRAS and BRAF function downstream of EGFR in the signaling pathway, and activating mutations have been described as usually mutually exclusive in EGFR-mutated tumors.

[†]KRAS mutations are detected in 15% to 57% of patients with lung adenocarcinoma from the United States and Europe and are associated with poor response to EGFR-directed TKI therapy.

[‡]BRAF, a serine/threonine kinase, is mutated in only 1% to 2% of lung cancer patients.

[§]EGFR mutations were seen in adenocarcinoma and were more frequent among women and never-smokers. EGFR mutations in adenocarcinomas were not associated with pathologic stage in never-smokers, but were more frequent in pathologic stage II-IV than in stage I disease among current and previous smokers.

---

*For instance, low-grade follicular lymphoma is difficult to distinguish from normal lymph node by morphology alone, so flow cytometry should be performed as well.

procedure with an expected result in mind and failure of the pathologist to understand the question being asked contribute to suboptimal interpretation of cytologic findings.[20]

Diagnostic Alternatives

1. *CT-guided percutaneous needle aspiration of the nodule:* This technique has a high diagnostic rate (91%) but does not provide mediastinal staging and increases the risk for pneumothorax (5% to 60%).[21]
2. *Esophageal ultrasound-guided fine-needle aspiration (EUS-FNA) alone:* EUS alone is suitable for assessing lymph nodes in the posterior aspect of lymph node stations 4L, 5, and 7, and in the inferior mediastinum at stations 8 and 9. EUS alone has limited value for complete staging because right-sided nodes are usually inaccessible.
3. *Mediastinoscopy:* This approach is traditionally considered the gold standard for mediastinal staging. It is more invasive, and bronchoscopic airway inspection might still be required. Mediastinoscopy provides systematic exploration and biopsy under visual guidance of nodal stations 1, 2, 3, 4, and 7.
4. *Combined EUS and EBUS followed by mediastinoscopy:* Because EBUS alone provides no access to lymph node stations 5, 6, 8, and 9, a strategy combining endosonography (EUS and EBUS) and mediastinoscopy (if no nodal metastasis was detected at endosonography) resulted in greater sensitivity for mediastinal nodal metastases and fewer unnecessary thoracotomies (needed in only 1 of 7 patients) in comparison with mediastinoscopy alone.[22] This study used thoracotomy with nodal dissection as the reference standard in both study groups. Although stage IIIA is likely in our patient with ipsilateral mediastinal lymphadenopathy, tissue confirmation was necessary because computed tomography is known to be inaccurate for staging purposes. In one study, up to 28% of patients with high clinical suspicion of nodal disease had mediastinal nodal metastases confirmed by mediastinoscopy despite negative EBUS-TBNA.[23] Therefore, a negative EBUS-TBNA should be followed by mediastinoscopy in patients with suspected mediastinal nodal involvement based on CT or PET.
5. *Thoracotomy with nodal dissection:* In this patient with highly suspected mediastinal nodal disease, this technique is neither cost-effective nor therapeutically advantageous.

Risk-Benefit Analysis

No serious complications are reported in the published literature on EBUS-TBNA, but cough and bleeding at the puncture site are described infrequently, usually when procedures are performed under moderate (conscious) sedation.[24] The benefits of performing this procedure were that diagnosis and staging could be done at the same time, expected yield was excellent, and specimens would be collected for genetic testing that potentially would be useful for selecting targeted therapy based on specific research protocols.

Informed Consent

After the risks, benefits, and alternatives were discussed, our patient chose to proceed with EBUS-TBNA. On further questioning, he stated he had no health care advance directives and had no intention of initiating one at that time. The importance of advance directives may not be equally appreciated by all ethnic groups. In one study, for example, a survey showed that no Korean respondents and few Hispanics had advance directives. Low rates of advance directive completion among nonwhites may reflect health care disparities, distrust of the health care system, different cultural perspectives regarding death and suffering, and differences in family dynamics and parent-child relationships.[25]

Techniques and Results

Anesthesia and Perioperative Care

The patient's pulmonary hypertension could lead to perioperative complications. One study of 28 patients undergoing major or minor surgeries under general and regional anesthesia revealed a perioperative death rate of 7%.* Perioperative complications attributed to pulmonary hypertension occurred in 29% of patients, regardless of the underlying cause of the pulmonary hypertension. Most (92%) of the complications occurred in the first 48 hours following surgery, and risk factors for complications were greater for emergency and major surgery and with a long operative time (193 minutes vs. 112 minutes; $P = .003$).[26] A larger study evaluated 145 surgical patients with pulmonary hypertension, excluding those in whom the condition was due to left heart disease.[27] Complications included respiratory failure (n = 41), cardiac arrhythmia (n = 17), congestive heart failure (n = 16), renal insufficiency (n = 10), and sepsis (n = 10), and risk predictors included a history of pulmonary embolus, NYHA functional class of II or greater, intermediate- or high-risk surgery, and a duration of anesthesia greater than 3 hours.

Our patient underwent the procedure in the operating room, under general anesthesia, and was intubated with a No. 9 endotracheal tube (ETT). With this method, the EBUS scope is directed more centrally in the airway; this could make needle aspirations more difficult, especially if the nodes are laterally located. In such cases, the ETT is moved proximally in the upper trachea—a maneuver that may provide more space for manipulating the scope inside the lower trachea. Laryngeal mask airway (LMA) can also be used instead of ETT for this purpose. In addition, LMA permits evaluation of the upper paratracheal nodes, which may not be accessible if an ETT is used.[†28] EBUS can also be performed under moderate sedation in the bronchoscopy suite. This may result in safety and cost savings compared with general anesthesia, but aspiration of smaller nodes is technically more difficult.[29]

---

*At the time of surgery, 75% of patients were in NYHA functional class I-II.

†This is because the EBUS scope is directed more centrally in the airway through the ETT, and coupling of the transducer and the airway wall may be impaired and biopsies may be more difficult than when the scope is passed directly through an LMA.

Furthermore, at the time of this writing, most published studies of EBUS-TBNA showing high diagnostic rates were done with the patient under general anesthesia.

Technique and Instrumentation

We used a dedicated EBUS bronchoscope (BF-UC180 F, Olympus, Tokyo, Japan) with an integrated convex transducer at the tip of the scope, which scans parallel to the insertion direction of the bronchoscope, and a 22-gauge needle to perform TBNA (NA-201SX-4022, Olympus). After the lymph node had been penetrated, the internal stylet was used to push out the bronchial wall debris, which may clog the internal lumen, and then the stylet was removed. Negative pressure can be applied with a syringe and the needle moved back and forth inside the target 10 to 15 times over 30 to 60 seconds.[30] In some instances, the bronchoscopist may choose to avoid suction, having obtained the specimen simply through needle insertion into the node.

Many times, the bronchoscopist notices the needle in the lesion, but aspirates are acellular, or only blood or bronchial cells are seen. From a "targeting" perspective, the node is properly accessed, but acquisition of lymph node material is suboptimal. The question that may have to be asked is not whether the needle is in the lesion, but whether the lesion is in the node.[31] This means that penetration of the needle into the node does not guarantee the presence of lymph node tissue inside the needle. In this regard, the principles of any fine-needle aspiration technique include the following: (1) Ensure the cutting action of the needle by performing a fast, downstroke movement (see video on ExpertConsult.com) (Video IV.16.1); and (2) minimize the amount of blood in the sample by following a straight needle trajectory, for instance, if the node is sampled from different entry locations, the needle should be repositioned outside the target first, thus avoiding tissue tearing and minimizing suction within the target, especially for vascular nodes (i.e., renal cell carcinoma, melanoma). High negative pressure may rupture nodal capillaries (see video on ExpertConsult. com) (Video IV.16.2). Minimizing or eliminating suction altogether, while moving the needle fewer than a dozen times inside the node, reduces transit time and potentially decreases the chance for retrieving blood clot rather than a tissue sample.[31] With a cytologist available for rapid on-site examination (ROSE) of the aspirates, TBNA is continued until adequate sampling is confirmed. Without ROSE, three aspirates per lymph node station or two aspirations with one core tissue specimen is recommended.[32] Feedback from the cytopathologist, whether obtained at the time of ROSE or later after final results are available, is important to improve one's technique. Operators can examine the quality of their stained smears to judge adequacy and quality of the aspirates.* In

addition to technique, other reasons for false-negative aspirates have been identified, including partial tumor invasion within the lymph node. Complementary optical technologies such as spectroscopy or optical coherence tomography may have a role in the future by directly guiding needle aspiration toward abnormal zones within lymph nodes.[33,34]

After we retrieved our specimen, the aspirated material was pushed onto a glass slide. We did not retrieve a core of tissue,* but if this had been obtained, it could have been placed on filter paper to absorb excess blood and then fixed with 10% neutral buffered formalin, so that a formalin-fixed paraffin-embedded sample would have been made and further stained with hematoxylin and eosin for histologic diagnosis.[†30] The rest of the material was smeared onto glass slides for both air-dried smears and was immediately fixed with 95% ethanol smears. The air-dried smears were stained by Diff-Quick staining for ROSE or Giemsa stain solution. The ethanol-fixed smears were sent for Papanicolau staining. The contents of the EBUS-TBNA needle were washed into a tube containing saline and were used for molecular testing if warranted.

Anatomic Dangers and Other Risks

At station 4R, the major blood vessels include pulmonary artery, azygos vein, superior vena cava, and ascending aorta. The lung is also visualized (Figure 16-4). The risk of penetrating a major vessel may be reduced with Doppler mode imaging (see Figure 16-4). To date, no cases of major bleeding have been reported.[35] It has been shown that dedicated EBUS-TBNA needles can release metal particles consisting of iron, titanium, nickel, and chromium, probably resulting from friction between the stylet and the needle. A potential risk is involved in injecting particles into nodes. The long-term consequences of lymph node contamination are currently unknown.[36]

Results and Procedure-Related Complications

Bronchoscopy inspection showed normal airway mucosa. EBUS mediastinal exploration showed no lymphadenopathy other than in station 4R. ROSE showed NSCLC (likely adenocarcinoma) after the second aspirate. Two more aspirates were obtained and were sent for genetic analysis. The procedure lasted 30 minutes. The patient was extubated, recovered in the postanesthesia care unit (PACU) for 2 hours, and was discharged home the same day. No perioperative complications occurred.

Long-Term Management

Outcome Assessment

At the time of final interpretation, Papanicolaou- and Diff-Quick–stained smears, as well as hematoxylin and eosin (H&E)-stained sections of the formalin-fixed cell block, showed adenocarcinoma. The procedure was

---

*EBUS-guided FNAs or a nondiagnostic or negative specimen can be very cellular with numerous reactive bronchial cells (if nondiagnostic) and numerous lymphocytes (if diagnostic). This high cellularity creates a large number of diagnostic difficulties and makes these cases difficult to screen at the time of ROSE. Thus, the focus is not so much on the quantitative features, but is more on the qualitative features and the need to determine whether a sufficient number of the correct cells are present to indicate sampling of the target.

---

*Part of the core tissue can be stored with the use of stabilizing solutions for extraction of RNA.

†This specimen can be used for in situ hybridization, and DNA/RNA can be extracted for genetic analysis.

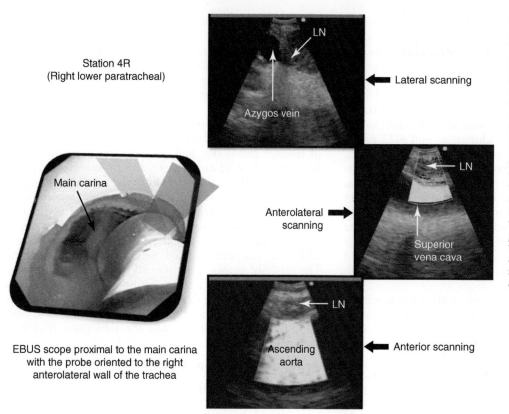

Station 4R
(Right lower paratracheal)

LN

Azygos vein

◄— Lateral scanning

LN

Superior vena cava

Anterolateral scanning ■►

Main carina

LN

Ascending aorta

◄— Anterior scanning

EBUS scope proximal to the main carina
with the probe oriented to the right
anterolateral wall of the trachea

Figure 16-4 Three different sonographic patterns of station 4R, depending on the scanning plane. To visualize this station, the endobronchial ultrasound (EBUS) scope is placed just proximal to the main carina and is turned toward the 3 o'clock position (lateral scanning) when the azygos vein is identified *(top panel)*. Very often 4R is pretracheal, in a more anterior position, so the scope has to be turned counterclockwise toward the 12 o'clock position. During this process, the transducer is oriented anterolaterally and the lymph node can be seen in front of the superior vena cava *(middle panel)*. In the bottom panel, the transducer is oriented anteriorly, and the station 4R lymph node is seen in front of the ascending aorta.

considered successful because a diagnosis was obtained by using a minimally invasive technique. Findings were shared with the patient's daughter, who asked us to refrain from informing the patient of his diagnosis. She believed that learning he had cancer would cause him unnecessary anxiety and depression. Being asked to avoid truthfulness regarding diagnosis or prognosis often poses a significant ethical dilemma for health care providers, who must juggle with the principles of autonomy, beneficence, nonmaleficence, and justice in their daily practices.[37] Truth telling respects the rights of patients and their families to receive accurate information about their illness. In fact, several studies demonstrate that most patients expect and desire truthfulness about their health. Nondisclosure can be viewed as a betrayal of trust, a rupture of the tacit agreement between patient and physician that both shall be forthright in their dialogue.

On the other hand, we were aware that certain ethnic groups prefer not to be directly informed of a life-threatening diagnosis, and that on many occasions, families might make medical decisions without disclosing the whole truth when one of its family members is ill. A long tradition of family-centered health care decisions[38] has been noted, for example, in South America, where more than 60% of physicians reported informing families only in cases of a patient's fatal prognosis.[39] In Japan, Taiwan, and China, however, most patients with cancer were more likely than their families to believe that they should be informed of their diagnosis.[40,41] In the culturally diverse United States, investigators compared persons of black and European descent versus those of Korean and Mexican American descent and found that Koreans and Mexican Americans were more likely to consider family members, rather than the patient alone, as holding decision-making power regarding life support.[42] Even with acculturation, minorities may still view the decision-making process as a family-centered process.[43] Among Asian cultures, family-based medical decisions are viewed as a function of filial devoutness, with an orientation toward the extended family as opposed to individual patient self-interest.[43] Hence, illness is often considered a family affair rather than an individual event, and a sense of obligation can make it difficult for relatives to accept anything other than extraordinary measures of care.[44]

When treating patients from cultures with norms of nondisclosure, physicians might offer to provide diagnostic and treatment information to the patients themselves. Physicians can ask patients how they would like treatment decisions to be made, to help them determine the extent to which patients and family members wish to be involved in the decision-making process. By offering autonomy to patients,* cultural customs are respected, while rights to independent decision making are simultaneously acknowledged. A patient who refuses diagnostic information and prefers family- or physician-centered decision making has made a clear, voluntary choice. If a patient prefers that family members receive information,

---

*This can be done by asking the following question: "Some patients want to know everything about their medical condition, but others do not. What is your preference?"

the physician should find out which family member(s) will be responsible for decision making. In our case, based on his request, the patient's daughter was clearly identified as the primary decision maker.

Follow-up Tests and Procedures

We discussed with our pathologist and oncologist the rationale for sending specimens for genetic analysis. Advances in targeted therapies may lead to an era of personalized medicine. This is particularly important because lung cancer is proving to be a heterogeneous collection of diseases with highly diverse pathogeneses and molecular characteristics, even within a single histologic type such as adenocarcinoma.[45] As of this writing, several biomarkers are thought to predict the likelihood of a patient's response to a specific chemotherapeutic drug for NSCLC. Some oncologists apply testing and treatment algorithms when they encounter any new patient with advanced NSCLC,[45] first, *EGFR* mutation analysis: If a mutation is present, the patient is a candidate for EGFR-TKI.[46] If no response is noted, or if the mutation is not present, the tumor is assessed for EML4/ALK rearrangements and, if present, is treated with crizotinib.[14] If no response or evidence of EML4/ALK fusion is noted, the tumor is assessed for ERCC1 and RRM1.* Patients with low levels are treated with a platinum plus gemcitabine combination.[47] If no response is seen, levels of ERCC1† and TS‡ are assessed. Patients with low ERCC1 and TS levels are treated with a platinum plus pemetrexed combination. For those in whom these treatments are ineffective and for those who have high levels of ERCC1, default treatment with a taxane plus a nonplatinum drug is provided. For practical purposes, bronchoscopists may need to perform additional aspirates, ideally obtaining core biopsies so that specimens can be preserved for further molecular analysis if necessary. This is especially important today because almost 70% of patients with lung cancer are diagnosed on the basis of small biopsy or cytology specimens.[48] In our patient, *EGFR* and *EML/ALK4* mutations were negative. Testing for other biomarkers was deferred until a formal oncology consultation could be obtained.

Referrals

Targeted therapy is highly dependent on which pathway is activated for a particular tumor. In this regard, erlotinib targets EGFR signaling, sorafenib, ras/raf signaling, vandetanib, vascular endothelial growth factor (VEGF) and EGFR signaling, and bexarotene, the retinoid X receptor for signaling.[49] The patient was referred to an oncologist, who actively practiced targeted therapy. This appointment was arranged to occur within 10 days after the procedure.

---

*Regulatory subunit of ribonucleotide reductase.

†Excision repair cross-complementation group 1; high levels of this protein in NSCLC tumors predict longer survival in patients randomized to treatment without chemotherapy and a lower likelihood of response to platinum-based chemotherapy.

‡Thymidylate synthase: Low expression of this protein in NSCLC predicts better outcome regardless of treatment and potentially better response to neoadjuvant chemotherapy with pemetrexed.

Quality Improvement

In this case, the EBUS-TBNA aspirate showed adenocarcinoma, confirming the diagnosis and staging the tumor as stage IIIA. The specimen was adequate for interpretation. Lymph node sampling is represented by abundant dispersed lymphocytes, lymphoid aggregates, anthracotic histiocytes, granulomatous aggregates, or tumor. The "adequate sampling" definition is controversial, prompting some experts to recommend using the term *nondiagnostic* only for those cases that truly have no evidence of lymph node sampling. Cases with sparse evidence of lymph node sampling should be reported as such, with the understanding that the chance of false-negative results may be increased.[20]

DISCUSSION POINTS

1. Define the borders of station 4R and justify this definition.

   Station 4R includes right lower paratracheal nodes and pretracheal nodes extending to the left lateral border of the trachea. Lymphatic drainage in the superior mediastinum predominantly occurs to the right paratracheal area and extends past the midline of the trachea; therefore the boundary between lymph nodes of the right- and left-sided levels 2 and 4 has been reset to the left lateral wall of the trachea.[50] When the scope is oriented anteriorly in the lower trachea or in the right mainstem bronchus at the level of the main carina, the node seen is still the right lower paratracheal node (station 4R). The Doppler-positive vessel behind it could represent the superior vena cava or the ascending aorta, depending on the actual orientation of the scope (Figure 16-5). Based on IASLC definitions, the upper border of station 4R is the intersection of the caudal margin of the innominate vein with the trachea, and the lower border is represented by the lower border of the azygos vein (see Figure 16-3).[50]

2. Describe how the sagittal view of a computed tomography scan is used to plan EBUS-TBNA at station 4R.

   A sagittal (aka median) plane is perpendicular to the ground; this separates left from right. The midsagittal plane is the specific sagittal plane that is exactly in the middle of the body. To visualize station 4R in its anterior carinal position, the scope is positioned just proximal to the main carina and is oriented anteriorly toward the 12 o'clock position; therefore when 4R has a pretracheal component, the sagittal view is useful and the ascending aorta will be visualized just distal to the node; the superior vena cava (SVC) can be seen most times when the transducer is oriented slightly toward the right anterolateral wall (1 o'clock position), and the azygos vein, when oriented toward the right lateral wall (3 o'clock position) (see Figures 16-4 and 16-5). In this patient, the EBUS image at station 4R shows the pattern in Figure 16-6, when the scanning plane is anterior toward the ascending aorta (Doppler mode on). The scanning plane for the EBUS scope is the same as in the sagittal CT view (see Figure 16-6). However, although the sagittal CT view is projected as if the scope is vertical, the EBUS image is

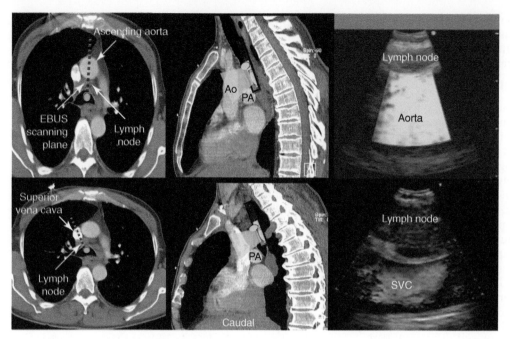

Figure 16-5 Two different sonographic images at station 4R, depending on the scanning plane orientation. In the upper panel, the scanning plane is anterior and the ascending aorta is seen just distal to the lymph node on both axial *(left)* and sagittal *(center)* computed tomography (CT) views. The Doppler-positive vascular structure seen on the corresponding endobronchial ultrasound (EBUS) image *(right)* therefore represents the ascending aorta. In the lower panel, the scanning plane is right anterolateral and the superior vena cava (SVC) is visualized on axial *(left)* and sagittal *(center)* CT views. The Doppler-positive vascular structure seen on the corresponding EBUS image *(right)* therefore represents the SVC. *Ao,* Aorta; *PA,* pulmonary artery.

projected as if the scope is horizontal. Thus, to understand the reasons for use of the sagittal CT view, one must understand the reference points on the EBUS image (see Figure 16-6). The green dot on the monitor represents the point where the needle exits the scope and corresponds to the superior (cephalad) aspect of the body. This dot is by default toward the 1 o'clock position on the screen (see Figure 16-6). Reorientation of the sagittal CT image is necessary to bring the scope to a horizontal position and to bring the green dot cephalad (toward the 1 o'clock position on the screen) to match the EBUS image. For practical purposes, one can print out or save the sagittal CT image showing station 4R as a separate picture. This picture is flipped over like a page, then is rotated clockwise to "horizontalize" the scope and bring the green dot cephalad toward the 1 o'clock position (see Figure 16-6), so that the two images (EBUS and CT) now correlate and show the lymph node and the aorta in similar positions.

Expert Commentary

provided by Ibrahim Ramzy, MD, FRCPC

This case provides an opportunity to discuss sampling adequacy and diagnostic difficulties related to the interpretation of cytologic material obtained by needle aspiration in patients with known or suspected central airway disorders involving the lung or mediastinum. In the following paragraphs, I will focus on adequacy of sampling and issues pertaining to interpretation.

Malignant tumors often produce cellular aspirates, a manifestation of decreased cell cohesion. Establishing adequacy of the sample is not a problem when malignant cells are identified, because the specificity is close to 100%. However, in cases in which no

malignant cells are readily identified (i.e., negative cases), classifying the sample as adequate is more challenging. The presence of abundant lymphocytes in an aspirate is a good indication that the needle was in a lymph node, and multiple passes usually ensure that the nodes were thoroughly sampled. However, the presence of a few lymphocytes, particularly in a background of mucus and bronchial epithelial cells, calls into question the adequacy of the sample and probably should not be classified as an indication of absence of malignancy.[51]

One of the main factors contributing to the diagnostic success of needle aspiration is on-site assessment of the aspirate by an expert cytopathologist. This close, real-time coordination between the physician performing the procedure and the cytopathologist ensures that an adequate sample is procured with a minimal number of passes, thus reducing morbidity and discomfort to the patient, lessening the duration of the procedure, diminishing the potential risk of needle-induced damage to the bronchoscope, and, depending on the medical fiscal environment, limiting health care expenditures, particularly in countries where cytopathologists bill per sample examined, rather than per procedure performed.

The multidisciplinary approach also allows for optimal triaging of sampled material, and conversations with the cytopathologist can help identify and prioritize those tests that will prove most useful for diagnosis or treatment planning. Rinsing the needle to obtain material for cell block and histologic processing is extremely valuable, because such processing is optimal for immunocytochemistry; several molecular tests for diagnostic and prognostic markers such as gene rearrangements, overexpressions, and deletions can have an impact on making the diagnosis, refining

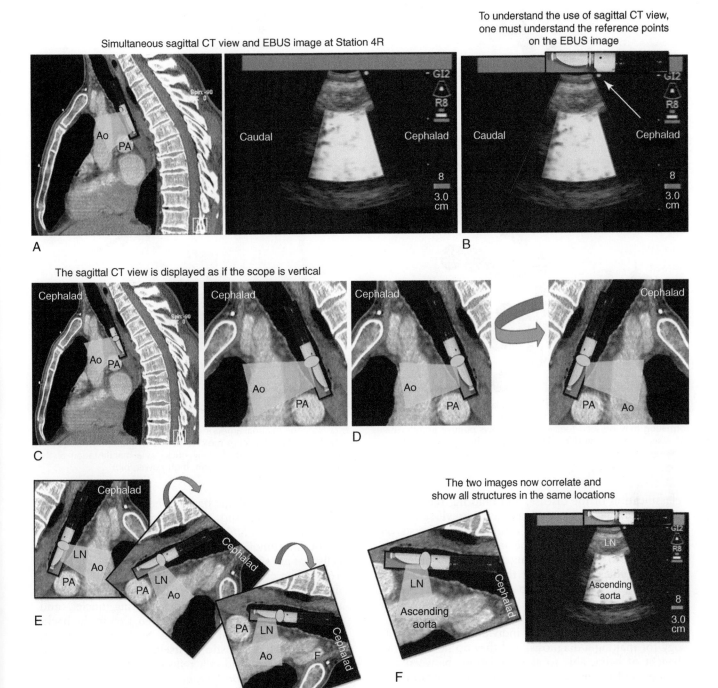

Figure 16-6 Computed tomography–endobronchial ultrasound (CT-EBUS) correlations for station 4R. **A,** The sagittal CT view and the EBUS image of station 4R when the EBUS scope is oriented anteriorly toward the ascending aorta. **B,** To understand the correlation between the two images (CT and EBUS), the reference points on the EBUS image must be identified. The EBUS image is projected on the monitor as if the scope is horizontal; the green dot on the monitor represents the point where the needle exits the scope and corresponds to the superior (cephalad) aspect of the body; this dot is by default toward the 1 o'clock position of the screen. **C,** Because the sagittal CT view is displayed as if the scope is vertical, several adjustments can be made to the sagittal CT image to bring the scope to a horizontal position: the green dot turned cephalad (toward the 1 o'clock position on the screen) to match the EBUS image. **D,** To do this, the image is flipped over like a page, then it is rotated clockwise to horizontalize the scope and bring the green dot cephalad toward the 1 o'clock position. **E,** Now, the scope is horizontalized, the green dot is toward the 1 o'clock position, and the cephalad section of the image is toward the right side, as it is displayed by default on the EBUS screen. **F,** The two images now correlate and show the lymph node and the aorta in the same location.

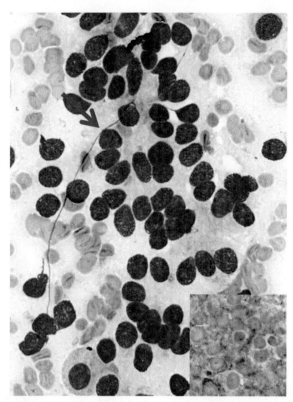

Figure 16-7 Carcinoid tumor. The neoplastic cells are fairly uniform, with moderate amounts of granular cytoplasm. Attempts at rosette formation may be seen *(arrow)*. Insert shows positive immunostains for synaptophysin. (Air-dried, Diff-Quik stain, high power, oil.)

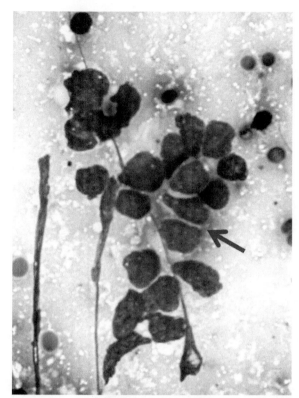

Figure 16-8 Small cell carcinoma. The nuclei of the neoplastic cells are larger than the few round lymphocytes in the background *(upper left)*. Note the minimal amount of cytoplasm, the tendency of irregularly shaped bare nuclei to mold to fit into neighboring cells *(arrow)*, and the linear smearing of some nuclei as a manifestation of their fragility (Air-dried, Diff-Quik stain, high power, oil.)

classification of the disease, and tailoring therapy for certain tumors, as was outlined in the previous discussion of this case. Obtaining a full battery of tests on all samples may not always be necessary, but it is most important to note that failing to obtain samples for specific studies may decrease the chance of diagnosis. For example, an additional pass may be warranted to specifically procure material for flow cytometry when aspirates are lymphocyte rich.

Cytopathologists rely on individual cell morphology for making a diagnosis, and they do not have the benefit of being able to assess relations between cell groups and tissues, as do their colleagues examining histopathologic material. Differentiation between some neoplasms based solely on isolated cytologic criteria can be difficult. The use of immunocytochemical ancillary techniques, however, greatly enhances the ability of cytopathology to close this gap.[16]

Differentiation between carcinoid tumor, small cell carcinoma, and lymphoma can be challenging cytologically. *Carcinoid tumors* produce cellular specimens with fairly uniform round to oval nuclei that have a characteristic "salt and pepper" chromatin clumping and occasionally an attempt at rosette formation (Figure 16-7). The granular cytoplasm stains positively for neuroendocrine markers such as chromogranin and synaptophysin. Differentiation between typical and atypical carcinoid tumors, however, is not always

feasible on a cytologic basis alone, and requires additional sampling and correlation with clinical and imaging studies. *Small cell carcinoma*, another neuroendocrine tumor, is characterized by undifferentiated cells that are small, yet larger than lymphocytes (Figure 16-8). The cytoplasm is scant at best, unlike that of neuroendocrine large cell carcinoma. The nuclei show molding to accommodate neighboring nuclei, and streaks of nuclear material are often seen in the background as a result of smearing. Such crush artifact, although not diagnostic by itself, raises a red flag to the microscopist and is a reflection of the fragility of the nuclei. *Malignant lymphoma* is another tumor that enters into the differential diagnosis of small cell tumors. It can involve the lung as a primary lesion, or more often as part of systemic disease. The cytomorphology depends on the type of neoplasm. When an abundant infiltrate by lymphocytes is encountered in the aspirate, particularly if lymphocytes show atypia or the presence of nucleoli, a second aspirate dedicated to flow cytometric evaluation is recommended. If not, a cell block may be prepared and stained for various lymphocyte markers to establish monoclonality, and thus neoplasia (Figure 16-9). The sensitivity and specificity of cytologic diagnosis of non-Hodgkin lymphoma show variability among different studies; they are dependent on the availability of an adequate number of lymphocytes for flow cytometry analysis and

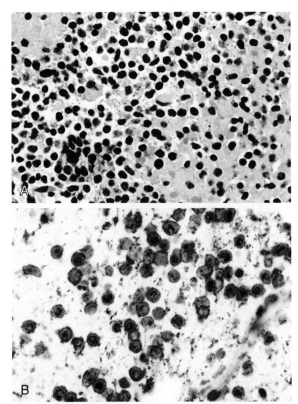

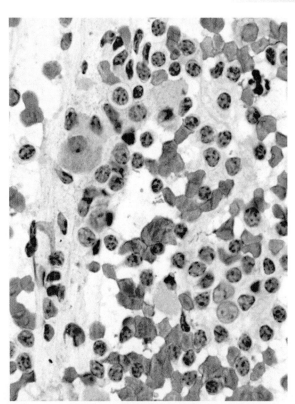

Figure 16-9 Non-Hodgkin malignant lymphoma, small lymphocytic. **A,** The atypical small lymphocytic population in this cell block preparation is monomorphous. **B,** The neoplastic lymphocytes stained positively (brown) with CD20. Staining for CD3 was negative in this case. (**A,** Hematoxylin and eosin; **B,** CD20 immunoperoxidase stain, both at high power, oil.)

Figure 16-10 Sarcoidosis. The aspirate shows an abundance of macrophages among a mixture of inflammatory cells. No evidence of caseous necrosis is seen, and microbiologic studies failed to reveal any organisms. (Papanicolaou stain, medium power.)

dilution of the sample by a significant component of bronchial columnar cells and blood. Hodgkin lymphoma can be diagnosed if the clinical and cytologic characteristics are taken in consideration, but greater sampling is often necessary to subclassify the disease. *Reactive lymph node aspirates* demonstrate a polymorphous population of lymphocytes at various stages of maturation, unlike the monomorphous population encountered in aspirates from lymphomas that can be easily established by flow cytometric immunophenotyping. Identification of histiocytic cells with phagocytized material in their cytoplasm (tingible body macrophages) is also helpful in supporting a benign diagnosis. In cases where abundant histiocytes are encountered, a granulomatous reaction should be considered, and material should be reserved for microbiologic studies (Figure 16-10).

Neoplasms with large cells form a heterogeneous group that includes squamous cell carcinomas, adenocarcinomas, large cell carcinomas, metastatic carcinomas, and melanomas, among others. The cytologic characteristics of these tumors can establish the diagnosis in many cases, or at least can narrow the differential diagnosis. Immunohistochemical stains can further refine or confirm the diagnosis in cases where cytomorphologic features overlap. A detailed discussion of the specific morphologic characteristics of this

heterogeneous group of tumors is beyond the scope of this commentary,* but a description of a few basic principles and problem areas is appropriate. *Adenocarcinomas*, for example, can present particular challenges in terms of their classification. The cytologic patterns of a tumor can be variable and often overlap with those of other tumor types. Decisions as to whether the tumor is primary or metastatic, the type of primary lesion, and the source of metastasis can be difficult to ascertain, particularly in the absence of a known primary. In general, malignant glandular cells tend to have abundant cytoplasm with evidence of polarization of their nuclei to one end. *Bronchioloalveolar carcinomas (BACs)*, on histologic examination, have a characteristic pattern of spread along alveolar septa. Such a pattern, however, can be encountered with other adenocarcinomas, including metastasis.

Cytologic samples can be difficult to interpret because cells may be quite bland with minimal evidence of malignancy. Other BACs show abundant mucinous

---

*Detailed discussions of specific morphologic characteristics of these is tumors is available in *A Colour Atlas of Endoscopic Diagnosis in Early Stage Lung Cancer* by Kato H, Horai T (Mosby 1991); in *Pulmonary Cytopathology* by Erozan Y, Ramzy I (Springer 2009); and in online cytopathology and pathology resources (http://137.189.150.85/cytopathology/link.html).

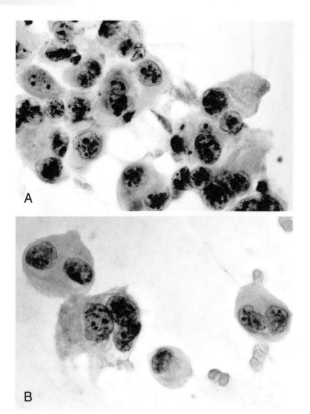

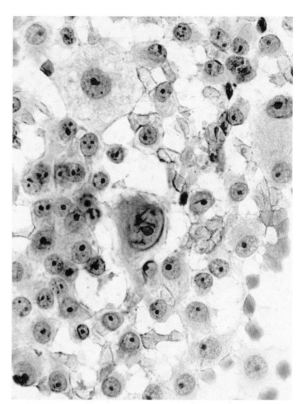

Figure 16-11   Giant cell carcinoma. **A,** A poorly differentiated epithelial malignancy, with pleomorphic cells that vary in shape and size. The abundant cytoplasm surrounds large, irregularly shaped nuclei. **B,** Multinucleation and prominent nucleoli are evident in several cells. Immunocytochemistry is critical in an attempt to further classify poorly differentiated tumors. (Papanicolaou stain, high power, oil.)

Figure 16-12   Malignant melanoma. The cells have abundant cytoplasm, large nuclei with prominent nucleoli, and multinucleation. Despite lack of melanin pigment, the nature of the lesion can be confirmed using immunocytochemical markers such as Melan-A. (Papanicolaou stain, high power, oil.)

cells. Cytologic parameters for adenocarcinomas will have to be adapted to the classification of non–small cell carcinoma (NSCC) recently developed by the International Association for the Study of Lung Cancer and other American and European organizations. Data on patient survival support the validity of this new classification. In situ, minimally invasive and lepidic-predominant adenocarcinomas have excellent 5-year survival rates, and micropapillary-predominant and solid with mucin-predominant tumors are associated with poor survival. Papillary and acinar-predominant tumors have an intermediate survival rate.[52] *Giant cell tumors,* as illustrated in Figure 16-11, are poorly differentiated neoplasms associated with aggressive behavior. Careful examination of the material in some of these tumors may reveal subtle clues of differentiation into a glandular or squamous cell line. By using immunocytochemical and molecular marker studies, as discussed later, our ability to further characterize these tumors may be enhanced, decreasing the number of tumors that cannot be further categorized. One has also to recognize that some neoplasms can show differentiation along two or more cell lines, such as squamous cell and/or small cell and/or adenocarcinoma.

Last, metastatic neoplasms may present with poorly differentiated highly atypical cells, and some aspirates fail to elucidate the source of the primary tumor, unless

a history of another primary has been reported. In some cases, cytologic criteria point to a specific tumor type. The presence of elongated cigar-shaped nuclei and a necrotic background often points to metastasis from the colon, rather than a primary lung adenocarcinoma. Prominent nucleoli, intranuclear cytoplasmic inclusions, and multinucleation point to a malignant melanoma, even in the absence of melanin pigment (Figure 16-12). In many cases, confirmation rests on positive staining with immunocytochemical markers, such as Melan-A and chromogranin.

The role of immunocytochemistry warrants a final comment. Some of the immunohistochemical stains used most frequently to diagnose lung tumors are epithelial cell markers such as TTF-1, various cytokeratin markers, EMA, and lymphocytic cell markers. Immunohistochemistry should be used judiciously in view of the scant material procured and the cost involved. Most of the techniques commonly used, such as keratin markers, are reimbursed by insurers and Medicare. Others are still considered experimental, are not Food and Drug Administration (FDA) approved, and should be used only with this stipulation. The selection of a specific battery of stains depends on the question confronting the pathologist. If the cytomorphology, for example, is that of a small basophilic cell with minimal amounts of cytoplasm, the so called small blue cell tumor, the differential will encompass small cell carcinoma, lymphoma, and Merkel cell carcinoma. In such cases, a likely panel would include CK20, TTF-1, and Ker 903. When a patient with a past history of breast cancer develops a pulmonary tumor, a panel of TTF-1, GCDFP-15, and ER would be an appropriate selection, and if the history was that of a melanoma, Melan-A or HMB-45 should be included. Cytokeratins such as CK7, CK20, and pancytokeratin are helpful in sorting out the source of a lung metastasis from different gastrointestinal organs. Little doubt remains that among the many new diagnostic and prognostic markers being introduced, some will prove to be of little value because of low specificity, low sensitivity, or high cost. Others, such as PSA, EGFR, p53, p63, and ER/PR steroid receptors, will stand the test of time and the rigor of critical evaluation in large controlled studies. It is the responsibility of both the pathologist and the treating physician to select what is optimal for their patient.

REFERENCES

1. Goeckenjan G, Sitter H, Thomas M, et al. Prevention, diagnosis, therapy, and follow-up of lung cancer: interdisciplinary guideline of the German Respiratory Society and the German Cancer Society. *Pneumologie*. 2011;65:39-59.
2. Task Force for Diagnosis and Treatment of Pulmonary Hypertension of European Society of Cardiology (ESC), European Respiratory Society (ERS), International Society of Heart and Lung Transplantation (ISHLT), et al. Guidelines for the diagnosis and treatment of pulmonary hypertension. *Eur Respir J*. 2009;34: 12-19.
3. Fisher MR, Forfia PR, Chamera E, et al. Accuracy of Doppler echocardiography in the hemodynamic assessment of pulmonary hypertension. *Am J Respir Crit Care Med*. 2009;179:615-621.
4. Sandham JD, Hull RD, Brant RF, et al. A randomized, controlled trial of the use of pulmonary-artery catheters in high-risk surgical patients. *N Engl J Med*. 2003;348:5.
5. Garcia-Olivé I, Monsó E, Andreo F, et al. Endobronchial ultrasound-guided transbronchial needle aspiration for identifying EGFR mutations. *Eur Respir J*. 2010;35:391-395.
6. Sakairi Y, Nakajima T, Yasufuku K, et al. EML4-ALK fusion gene assessment using metastatic lymph node samples obtained by endobronchial ultrasound-guided transbronchial needle aspiration. *Clin Cancer Res*. 2010;16:4938-4945.
7. Lim EH, Zhang SL, Li JL, et al. Using whole genome amplification (WGA) of low-volume biopsies to assess the prognostic role of EGFR, KRAS, p53, and CMET mutations in advanced-stage non-small cell lung cancer (NSCLC). *J Thorac Oncol*. 2009;4:12-21.
8. Park S, Holmes-Tisch AJ, Cho EY, et al. Discordance of molecular biomarkers associated with epidermal growth factor receptor pathway between primary tumors and lymph node metastasis in non-small cell lung cancer. *J Thorac Oncol*. 2009;4:809-815.
9. Schmid K, Oehl N, Wrba F, et al. EGFR/KRAS/BRAF mutations in primary lung adenocarcinomas and corresponding locoregional lymph node metastases. *Clin Cancer Res*. 2009;15:4554-4560.
10. Herth F, Becker HD, Ernst A. Conventional vs endobronchial ultrasound-guided transbronchial needle aspiration: a randomized trial. *Chest*. 2004;125:322-325.
11. Herth FJ, Eberhardt R, Vilmann P, et al. Real-time endobronchial ultrasound guided transbronchial needle aspiration for sampling mediastinal lymph nodes. *Thorax*. 2006;61;795-798.
12. Shigematsu H, Gazdar AF. Somatic mutations of epidermal growth factor receptor signaling pathway in lung cancers. *Int J Cancer*. 2006;118:257-262.
13. Bae NC, Chae MH, Lee MH, et al. EGFR, ERBB2, and KRAS mutations in Korean non-small cell lung cancer patients. *Cancer Genet Cytogenet*. 2007;173:107-113.
14. Kwak EL, Bang YJ, Camidge DR, et al. Anaplastic lymphoma kinase inhibition in non-small-cell lung cancer. *N Engl J Med*. 2010;363:1693-1703.
15. Monaco SE, Schuchert MJ, Khalbuss WE. Diagnostic difficulties and pitfalls in rapid on-site evaluation of endobronchial ultrasound guided fine needle aspiration. *Cyto J*. 2010;7:9.
16. Erozan YS, Ramzy I. Primary epithelial malignancies. In: Rosenthal DL, ed. *Pulmonary Cytopathology: Essential in Cytopathology Series*. New York: Springer; 2008:146-153.
17. Nakajima T, Yasufuku K, Iyoda A, et al. The evaluation of lymph node metastasis by endobronchial ultrasound-guided transbronchial needle aspiration: crucial for selection of surgical candidates with metastatic lung tumors. *J Thorac Cardiovasc Surg*. 2007;134: 1485-1490.
18. Kennedy MP, Jimenez CA, Bruzzi JF, et al. Endobronchial ultrasound-guided transbronchial needle aspiration in the diagnosis of lymphoma. *Thorax*. 2008;63:360-365.
19. Steinfort DP, Conron M, Tsui A, et al. Endobronchial ultrasound-guided transbronchial needle aspiration for the evaluation of suspected lymphoma. *J Thorac Oncol*. 2010;5:804-809.
20. Stewart J. EBUS: a cytopathologist's perspective. In: *Interventional Pulmonology in Cancer Patients*. Conference syllabus 2011; 175-183. MD Anderson Cancer Center, Houston Texas, February 10-12, 2011.
21. Toloza EM, Harpole L, Detterbeck F, et al. Invasive staging of non-small cell lung cancer: a review of the current evidence. *Chest*. 2003;123:157S-166S.
22. Annema JT, van Meerbeeck JP, Rintoul RC, et al. Mediastinoscopy versus endosonography for mediastinal nodal staging of lung cancer: a randomized trial. *JAMA*. 2010;304:2245-2252.
23. Defranchi SA, Edell ES, Daniels CE, et al. Mediastinoscopy in patients with lung cancer and negative endobronchial ultrasound guided needle aspiration. *Ann Thorac Surg*. 2010;90:1753-1758.
24. Varela-Lema L, Fernandez-Villar A, Ruano-Ravina A. Effectiveness and safety of endobronchial ultrasound–transbronchial needle aspiration: a systematic review. *Eur Respir J*. 2009;33:1156-1164.
25. Blackhall LJ, Murphy ST, Frank G, et al. Ethnicity and attitudes toward patient autonomy. *JAMA*. 1995;274:820-825.
26. Price LC, Montani D, Jaïs X, et al. Noncardiothoracic nonobstetric surgery in mild-to-moderate pulmonary hypertension. *Eur Respir J*. 2010;35:1294-1302.
27. Ramakrishna G, Sprung J, Ravi BS, et al. Impact of pulmonary hypertension on the outcomes of noncardiac surgery: predictors of perioperative morbidity and mortality. *J Am Coll Cardiol*. 2005; 45:1691-1699.
28. Douadi Y, Bentayeb H, Malinowski S et al. Anaesthesia for bronchial echoendoscopy: experience with the laryngeal mask. *Rev Mal Respir*. 2010;27:37-41.
29. Sarkiss M, Kennedy M, Riedel B, et al. Anesthesia technique for endobronchial ultrasound-guided fine needle aspiration of mediastinal lymph node. *J Cardiothorac Vasc Anesth*. 2007;21:892-896.
30. Nakajima T, Yasufuku K. How I do it—optimal methodology for multidirectional analysis of endobronchial ultrasound-guided transbronchial needle aspiration samples. *J Thorac Oncol*. 2011; 6:203-206.
31. Papanicolau Society of Cytopathology. Optimal FNA techniques. www.papsociety.org/fna.html. Accessed April 23, 2011.
32. Lee HS, Lee GK, Lee HS, et al. Real-time endobronchial ultrasound-guided transbronchial needle aspiration in mediastinal staging of non-small cell lung cancer: how many aspirations per target lymph node station? *Chest*. 2008;134:368-374.
33. Kanick SC, van der Leest C, Aerts JG, et al. Integration of single-fiber reflectance spectroscopy into ultrasound-guided endoscopic lung cancer staging of mediastinal lymph nodes. *J Biomed Opt*. 2010;15:017004.
34. McLaughlin RA, Scolaro L, Robbins P, et al. Imaging of human lymph nodes using optical coherence tomography: potential for staging cancer. *Cancer Res*. 2010;70:2579-2584.
35. Yasufuku K, Chiyo M, Sekine Y, et al. Real-time endobronchial ultrasound-guided transbronchial needle aspiration of mediastinal and hilar lymph nodes. *Chest*. 2004;126:122-128.
36. Gounant V, Ninane V, Janson X, et al. Release of metal particles from needles used for transbronchial needle aspiration. *Chest*. 2011;139:138-143.

37. Brody H, Tomlinson T. Commentary. *J Fam Pract*. 1988;26: 404-406.
38. Searight HR, Gafford J. Cultural diversity at the end of life: issues and guidelines for family physicians. *Am Fam Physician*. 2005;71: 515-522.
39. de Souza Trindade E, de Azambuja LE, Andrade JP, et al. O médico frente ao diagnóstico e prognóstico do câncer avançado. *Rev Assoc Med Bras*. 2007;53:68-74.
40. Fujimori M, Parker PA, Akechi T, et al. Japanese cancer patients' communication style preferences when receiving bad news. *Psychooncology*. 2007;16:617-625.
41. Jiang Y, Liu C, Li JY, et al. Different attitudes of Chinese patients and their families toward truth telling of different stages of cancer. *Psychooncology*. 2007;16:928-936.
42. Blackhall L, Murphy S, Frank G, et al. Ethnicity and attitudes toward patient autonomy. *JAMA*. 1995;274:820-825.
43. Kagawa-Singer M, Blackhall LJ. Negotiating cross-cultural issues at the end of life: "you got to go where he lives." *JAMA*. 2001;286:2993-3001.
44. Frank G, Blackhall LJ, Michel V, et al. A discourse of relationships in bioethics: patient autonomy and end-of-life decision making among elderly Korean Americans. *Med Anthropol Q*. 1998;12: 403-423.
45. Gadgeel SM, Cote ML, Schwartz AG, et al. Parameters for individualizing systemic therapy in non-small cell lung cancer. *Drug Resist Update*. 2010;13:196-204.
46. Mok TS, Wu YL, Thongprasert S, et al. Gefitinib or carboplatin-paclitaxel in pulmonary adenocarcinoma. *N Engl J Med*. 2009;361: 947-957.
47. Reynolds C, Obasaju C, Schell MJ, et al. Randomized phase III trial of gemcitabine-based chemotherapy with in situ RRM1 and ERCC1 protein levels for response prediction in non-small-cell lung cancer. *J Clin Oncol*. 2009;27:5808-5815.
48. Travis WD, Brambilla E, Noguchi M, et al. International Association for the Study of Lung Cancer/American Thoracic Society/European Respiratory Society international multidisciplinary classification of lung adenocarcinoma. *J Thorac Oncol*. 2011;6: 244-285.
49. Printz C. BATTLE to personalize lung cancer treatment: novel clinical trial design and tissue gathering procedures drive biomarker discovery. *Cancer*. 2010;116:3307-3308.
50. Rusch VW, Asamura H, Watanabe H, et al, Members of IASLC Staging Committee. The IASLC lung cancer staging project: a proposal for a new international lymph node map in the forthcoming seventh edition of the TNM classification for lung cancer. *J Thorac Oncol*. 2009;4:568-577.
51. Baker JJ, Solanki PH, Schenk DA, et al. Transbronchial needle aspiration of the mediastinum: importance of lymphocytes as an indicator of specimen adequacy. *Acta Cytol*. 1990;34:517-523.
52. Russell PA, Wainer Z, Wright GM, et al. Does lung adenocarcinoma subtype predict patient survival? A clinicopathologic study based on the New International Association for the Study of Lung Cancer/American Thoracic Society/European Respiratory Society International Multidisciplinary Lung Adenocarcinoma Classification. *J Thorac Oncol*. 2011 Jun 2 [Epub ahead of print].

Chapter 17

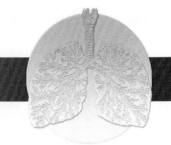
EBUS-TBNA of a Left Lower Paratracheal Node (Level 4 L) in a Patient with a Left Upper Lobe Lung Mass and Suspected Lung Cancer

This chapter emphasizes the following elements of the Four Box Approach: operator and team experience and expertise, and techniques and instrumentation.

CASE DESCRIPTION

A 72-year-old man with 40–pack-year history of smoking presented with chronic cough. Computed tomography of the chest showed a 2.8 × 1.7 cm left upper lobe mass and a 1.57 cm short diameter left lower paratracheal lymph node (Figure 17-1). The patient was referred for diagnosis and staging. He had a history of COPD (post bronchodilator FEV_1 was 58% predicted) and stable angina pectoris treated medically by his cardiologist. On chest auscultation, decreased air entry bilaterally and prolonged exhalation were noted. He was independent in his daily activities but performed them with effort. Karnofsky performance status was 80. Resting and two-dimensional dobutamine stress echocardiography was normal. He lived with his wife at home, desired a prompt diagnosis, and was willing to consider all available treatment options.

DISCUSSION POINTS

1. Describe the diagnostic yield of EBUS-TBNA versus conventional TBNA and EUS-FNA at station 4 L.
2. Describe how the coronal view of a computed tomography scan can be used to help plan EBUS-TBNA.
3. Describe endobronchial sonographic findings, including adjacent vascular structures at and around lymph node station 4 L.

CASE RESOLUTION

Initial Evaluations

Physical Examination, Complementary Tests, and Functional Status Assessment

This patient had decreased air entry bilaterally and prolonged exhalation, consistent with his obstructive ventilatory impairment detected on spirometry. He had grade II functional status based on the World Health Organization scale, specifically, mild limitation of physical activity was noted; no discomfort was reported at rest, but normal physical activity caused increased symptoms.[1]

Other measurement instruments that can be used to accurately assess impaired health, perceived well-being, dyspnea, and quality of life in patients with chronic obstructive pulmonary disease (COPD) are St. George's Respiratory Questionnaire, the Borg Baseline Dyspnea Index (BDI), and the modified Medical Research Council (MRC) Dyspnea Scales.[2]

Results from prospective studies of COPD patients with a mean age of 65 years and a mean value of post bronchodilator forced expiratory volume in 1 second (FEV_1) of 44% of the predicted value show that the all-cause mortality rate is 12% to 16% at 3 years.[3] Our patient, however, additionally had a lung nodule, ipsilateral mediastinal lymphadenopathy, and a positive smoking history. These findings are highly suspicious for primary lung carcinoma. If non–small cell lung cancer (NSCLC) were diagnosed, the primary tumor size would be staged as T1; in conjunction with positive N2 nodal staging (ipsilateral mediastinal lymphadenopathy), this patient would be staged clinically as having IIIA disease with an estimated 5 year survival of 19% and a median survival of 14 months despite treatment.[4] Because his risk of dying from cancer far outweighs that of dying from COPD, prompt diagnosis, staging, and treatment of his lung cancer are warranted.

Survival estimates are critical factors in patient and physician decision making in all phases of cancer diagnosis and treatment. These estimates are not perfect and of course may not apply to the particular "individual" faced with a cancer diagnosis. One measure that has been used to predict survival and consequently has been used as an entry criterion for oncology clinical trials is performance status. The Karnofsky Performance Scale, for example, is a commonly used general measure of functional impairment that allows comparison of the effectiveness of various therapies and prognosis considerations in individual patients: The lower the score, the worse the chance of survival.[5]

Comorbidities

This patient had COPD with FEV_1 of 58% predicted (moderate; Gold Initiative on Obstructive Lung Disease [GOLD] stage II). He was taking tiotropium 18 mcg/day and albuterol by metered dose inhaler (MDI) as needed. He had stable angina pectoris managed medically with nitrates and calcium channel blockers. The patient had

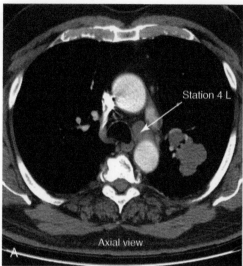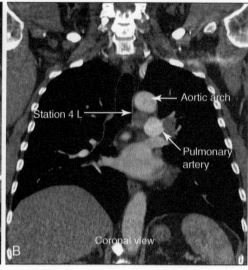

Figure 17-1 **A,** Axial computed tomography (CT) view reveals the left upper lobe mass and the 1.7 cm left paratracheal lymph node (station 4 L) to the left of the left lateral border of the trachea. **B,** Coronal CT view reveals the relationship between the left paratracheal node, the pulmonary artery, and the aortic arch.

no signs or symptoms of other illnesses. Careful examination and review of systems are warranted because COPD is linked to many comorbid conditions such as hypertension, coronary heart disease, stroke, obstructive sleep apnea, psychiatric illness (e.g., depression, anxiety), and cognitive decline, which could preclude or complicate interventions provided under general anesthesia.[6,7]

Support System

Our patient was married and lived with his wife, who was very supportive. Cancer, as suspected in this patient, is often considered a "family matter" with significant psychological and emotional impact on family members.[8] Because significant others are often involved in caregiving to a considerable extent during a patient's illness, involvement of family members in discussions about diagnosis and prognosis is warranted. Additionally, health care providers should be concerned about the caregiver's health because several investigators have found that caregiving, although it is not always judged to be a negative experience, can contribute to mental and physical ill health and can have a negative impact on social functioning.[9]

Patient Preferences and Expectations

This patient had clearly expressed a desire for treatment. He was prepared to consider all available diagnostic options, including conventional transbronchial needle aspiration (TBNA), endobronchial ultrasound (EBUS)-guided TBNA, endoscopic ultrasound (EUS)-guided fine-needle aspiration (FNA), computed tomography (CT)-guided biopsy, mediastinoscopy, or video-assisted thoracic surgery (VATS).

Although increasing emphasis is now placed on patient empowerment, results of studies show that many patients do not wish to be involved in decisions about their own care. Patient preferences regarding involvement in decision making vary with age, socioeconomic status, and illness experience, as well as the gravity of the decision. Evidence suggests that even if patients wish to be informed about their illness and treatment alternatives, they might not wish to be actively involved in making the treatment

decision.[10] Therefore the distinction between providing information, evaluating the information given, and taking responsibility for deciding on treatment may be important. In our case, the patient explicitly asked that all information and alternatives be discussed with both him and his wife, so they could make medical decisions together.

Procedural Strategies

Indications

Tissue diagnosis and sampling of station 4 L (left lower paratracheal node) for staging purposes were warranted because mediastinal lymph node involvement is found in approximately 26% of patients with newly diagnosed lung cancer.[11] Sampling of the 4 L lymph node station is important because the presence of mediastinal lymph node metastasis remains one of the most adverse prognostic factors in NSCLC. This tumor can be subclassified as IIIA3 with significant implications for additional management decisions. This is the largest subgroup of IIIA NSCLC patients and consists of patients with clinical ipsilateral lymph node invasion demonstrated by minimally invasive techniques or noninvasive imaging. Patients are often considered resectable or marginally resectable, depending on the number and the location of the lymph nodes involved.[12] However, the American College of Chest Physicians (ACCP) states that in NSCLC patients with stage IIIA-N2 disease identified preoperatively, induction therapy followed by surgery is not recommended, except as part of a clinical trial. Furthermore, although the use of any induction chemotherapy followed by surgery in stage IIIA lung cancer appears feasible, published data do not support this treatment as the standard of care in the community.[13] In fact, concomitant chemoradiation is increasingly becoming the standard of care in selected patients in clinical stage IIIA3 with a good risk profile, that is, low comorbidity, good performance and pulmonary function, and adequately staged disease.[12]

Although imaging studies are helpful for identifying lung parenchyma and mediastinal abnormalities, they do not provide a tissue diagnosis. Flexible bronchoscopy would allow complete airway inspection to ascertain the absence of endobronchial lesions, to potentially obtain samples from the lung mass itself, and to sample the mediastinal lymph node at the same setting. This could be done with the use of conventional transbronchial needle aspiration; however, the use of EBUS-TBNA significantly increases diagnostic yield (96% vs. 41%) at the level 4 L region compared with conventional sampling techniques.[14,15] By sampling station 4 L, both diagnosis and staging can be accomplished during a single procedure. Complete sonographic mediastinal lymph node assessment is warranted, however, because the tumor may be upstaged to N3 (stage IIIB), in case EBUS identifies contralateral lymph nodes and aspirates are positive for malignancy.[16] One study showed that compared with radiologic staging, EBUS-TBNA downstaged 18 of 113 (15.9%) and upstaged 11 of 113 (9.7%) patients.[17] Therefore ultrasound examination is done in a stepwise fashion, usually beginning at the highest-level node in relation to the lung mass in staging procedures: Contralateral lymph nodes, when identified, are sampled first and are immediately stained and read by an on-site pathologist. If no malignant cells are seen, subcarinal or ipsilateral lymph nodes are sampled. All aspirates are stained immediately for rapid on-site interpretation; aspirates are obtained until a preliminary cytologic diagnosis of malignancy is given, or until the cytologist determines that an adequate quantity of representative tissue has been obtained (usually four aspirates per lesion).[18] For this patient, if complete EBUS mediastinal and hilar evaluation reveals no contralateral nodes, the CT-documented 4 L node should be sampled.

Contraindications

No absolute contraindications to EBUS-TBNA were noted. This procedure is often performed under general anesthesia, which in our patient could predispose to myocardial ischemia as the result of volume shifts and increased myocardial oxygen demand from elevations in heart rate and blood pressure. Patients with major cardiac predictors for anesthesia risk such as unstable coronary syndrome, decompensated heart failure, significant arrhythmia, and severe valvular disease warrant intensive management, which may lead to delay in cancellation of an operative procedure. Other clinical predictors that require careful assessment include a history of ischemic heart disease (as seen in our patient), diabetes mellitus, compensated heart failure, and renal insufficiency. It is noteworthy that diagnostic endoscopic procedures such as bronchoscopy are considered low risk with a reported rate of cardiac death or nonfatal myocardial infarction of less than 1%; therefore preoperative cardiac testing usually is not necessary.[19] The negative stress test performed several weeks earlier was reassuring because of its high negative predictive value (90% to 100%) for postoperative cardiac complications.[20]

Expected Results

We usually perform EBUS-TBNA with a large endotracheal tube (8.5 or 9 mm) with the patient under general anesthesia. The EBUS scope would be introduced through the tube once the bite block is secured in place around the tube. Some practitioners prefer using a laryngeal mask airway or inserting the EBUS bronchoscope through the mouth with the use of a bite block under moderate or deep sedation. Complete airway examination would be performed and attention would be paid to both contralateral and ipsilateral mediastinal lymph node stations with EBUS.

In one small study, the diagnostic rate of EBUS-TBNA for station 4 L was equal to that of conventional TBNA (72% vs. 71%), but lymphocytes (indicative of an adequate sample) were more often present on EBUS-TBNA specimens (82% vs. 71%).[21] Several larger studies, however, have shown high diagnostic yields of 88% to 96% with EBUS for station 4 L.[14,22,23]

Team Experience

Although the yield of EBUS-TBNA has generally been reported to be as low as 70% for all lymph node stations,[24] it has become standard practice in most institutions that can offer it. An experienced team of doctors and nurses familiar with the techniques and the equipment is necessary. On-site cytology is preferred to provide immediate diagnosis, or at the least to know whether representative samples are being obtained. However, many bronchoscopists do not use rapid on-site cytologic examination because of cost, logistics, and organizational issues, stating instead that because the operator visualizes nodal sampling, immediate cytology is not necessary. On the other hand, having an immediate result of malignancy might increase the yield of the procedure and prevent the need for additional specimens from other nodal sites, thus potentially decreasing the time required for the procedure and potentially the associated complications. This issue continues to be debated within professional circles. A systematic review and meta-analysis showed that on-site evaluation of cytologic specimens had the highest pooled sensitivity at 0.97 (95% confidence interval [CI], 0.94 to 0.99); however, because of potential heterogeneity, when pooled sensitivity was compared with that of other subgroups, no statistical significance was found ($P > .05$).[25] In addition, for pathologists, this is a relatively time-consuming procedure, with a mean of 22 minutes spent on an average of three passes performed, with six slides prepared per lymph node site.[26]

Risk-Benefit Analysis

EBUS-TBNA has a high yield and is a safe same-day procedure.[25] One serious complication (pneumothorax requiring chest tube drainage) was reported in a meta-analysis of 1299 patients. Cough and the presence of blood at the needle puncture site are infrequent.[27] Even when performed by a single individual using moderate sedation in a single center, patient satisfaction was high, and no complications occurred that might have compromised diagnostic yield.[28]

Anecdotal reports show evidence of clinically significant bacteremia and polymicrobial pericarditis with tamponade physiology after EBUS-TBNA; these complications were considered to be caused by direct inoculation of oropharyngeal flora into mediastinal tissue during full EBUS-TBNA with needle extension to 3.6 cm.[29] Some investigators have suggested that contamination of the TBNA needle by oropharyngeal flora is common and may predispose patients to clinically significant infection, although this occurs rarely.[30] Results from a prospective study document the presence of bacteremia, confirmed by blood culture within 60 seconds of EBUS-TBNA, in 7% (3/43) of patients, compared with 0% to 6% rates following routine bronchoscopy, but no clinically significant infections have been described (none of the three bacteremic patients had clinical features suggestive of infection within 1 week of EBUS-TBNA). Bacteremia, universally caused by oropharyngeal commensal organisms, is considered by some investigators to be the likely result of insertion of the bronchoscope itself. Investigators postulate that as the bronchoscope traverses the naso-oropharyngeal region, the working channel becomes contaminated. As a result, when the transbronchial needle passes through the working channel, it becomes contaminated and can potentially inoculate the sampled tissue. Although the needle designed for the EBUS scope has an outer sheath, which could minimize sample contamination, this sheath is still passed through the working channel. When the needle is advanced at the site of interest, it is passed through the distal end of this sheath and could become contaminated. In addition, needle penetration depth may contribute to contamination and infection, especially if the tip of the fully extended needle is out of the scanning plane, and the pericardium or vessels can be violated but not visualized.[29]

Diagnostic Alternatives

Various alternatives are available, each with its advantages and disadvantages. It is ethical to share a description of these alternatives with the patient and his spouse:

1. *CT-guided percutaneous needle aspiration of the left upper lobe nodule* could be performed because the diagnostic rate (91%) is high. This would not provide information on staging, is associated with increased risk for pneumothorax (5% to 60%),[31] and provides no information regarding airway lesions and potential resectability. If cancer were diagnosed, mediastinal sampling would still be warranted for staging purposes.
2. *EUS-FNA (endoscopic ultrasound-guided fine-needle aspiration)* could be performed because the 4 L lymph node station is accessible via the esophagus. Overall reported sensitivity is 81% to 97%, and specificity is 83% to 100%.[32] For station 4 L in particular, EUS-FNA has a diagnostic yield similar to EBUS-TBNA.[23] Some might argue that bronchoscopy would still need to be performed to identify possible airway abnormalities. Rates of bacteremia following upper EUS are similar whether or not FNA is performed and are equal to those seen in routine gastroscopy (6%).[33]
3. *Mediastinoscopy* is still considered the gold standard and may be recommended if endoscopic sampling of station 4 L is negative for malignancy and is otherwise nondiagnostic.[14] This invasive procedure is performed in the operating room with the patient under general anesthesia. It has associated morbidity and mortality of 2% and 0.08%,

respectively.[34] Mediastinoscopy has a specificity of 100% and offers good access to lymph node stations 2, 4, and 7, but access to posterior and inferior mediastinal nodes is limited, which explains its overall sensitivity of 80% to 90%.[31]
4. *Video-assisted thoracic surgery (VATS)* is another invasive alternative but provides access to ipsilateral nodes only and has 75% sensitivity overall.[35] Its benefits include access to inferior mediastinal nodes and definitive lobar resection at the same time if nodes are negative.

Cost-Effectiveness

In two separate decision-analysis models, EUS-FNA + EBUS-TBNA and conventional TBNA + EBUS-FNA were more cost-effective approaches than mediastinoscopy for staging patients with NSCLC and abnormal mediastinal lymph nodes on noninvasive imaging.[36,37] The strategy of adding EUS-FNA to a conventional lung cancer staging approach (mediastinoscopy and thoracotomy) reduced costs by 40% per patient.[38] The two procedures (EUS-FNA and EBUS-TBNA) can be performed with the use of a dedicated linear EBUS bronchoscope in one setting and by one operator. Procedures are complementary and their combined use provides better diagnostic accuracy than is attained with either procedure alone.[39] This approach may reduce costs and enhance efficiency if one person can perform the combined procedure; simultaneously scheduling two skilled endoscopists with different subspecialties is often difficult.

EBUS-TBNA may actually increase health care costs if done in low-volume centers by inexperienced operators.[40] In fact, start-up costs are significant because of the need for training (participation in national and international hands-on workshops), equipment costs, and the risk that costly repairs will be needed in cases of instrument damage.[41]

Informed Consent

After they had been advised of all of the diagnostic alternatives, the patient and his wife elected to proceed with EBUS-TBNA under general anesthesia. No barriers to learning were identified. They were informed of potential failure to obtain a definitive diagnosis despite successful lymph node visualization and sampling. Feedback communication techniques were used to confirm patient understanding of his disease. Both the patient and his spouse were able to accurately describe the proposed procedure, alternatives, and potential complications.

Techniques and Results

Anesthesia and Perioperative Care

EBUS-TBNA can be performed with the patient under conscious (moderate) sedation or under general anesthesia with the use of a laryngeal mask airway or endotracheal tubes:

1. *Conscious (moderate) sedation:* In a single center, it was shown that despite frequent cough (70% of patients), patient satisfaction was high and diagnostic yield remained 90%.[28] Moderate sedation offers the advantage of performing the procedure in the

bronchoscopy suite and results in better cost savings/safety ratios when compared with general anesthesia.[42] Cough and respiratory movements, however, may impair coupling of the transducer with the airway wall and may result in significant artifacts and suboptimal ultrasound imaging. Sampling of smaller nodes may be technically more difficult than that done with the patient under general anesthesia.

2. *General anesthesia with laryngeal mask airway (LMA)* is preferred in many institutions. It is possible to establish a secure airway and maintain oxygenation using the LMA during bronchoscopy without diminishing the chances for a successful procedure.[24] At least a No. 4 or a No. 4.5 LMA should be used to allow straightforward manipulation of the scope inside the airway.[43] LMAs of this size allow passage of endotracheal tubes (ETTs) if necessary. Anesthesia given by LMA allows visualization of higher mediastinal structures and lymph nodes at stations 1 and 2 compared with ETTs for obvious reasons: After intubation, the distal extremity of the ETT is at least 3 cm below the vocal cords because the distance between the tip of the tube and the cuff of the tube is usually 1 cm, and the cuff length is approximately 2 cm. Were the tube higher within the trachea, the cuff would abut or sit within the larynx. If an ETT is used, it will have to be mobilized proximally to allow examination of stations 1 and 2. General anesthesia and the LMA are used in the bronchoscopy suite in some centers and in the operating room in others, depending on logistics, personnel, and institutional policies. Patients should be selected carefully because use of an LMA may not be appropriate in severely obese patients or in patients with severe untreated gastroesophageal reflux (GERD) because of the known reduction in barrier pressure at the lower esophageal sphincter and increased risk for aspiration of gastric contents.[44]

3. *General anesthesia with endotracheal tube (ETT):* A No. 8.5 ETT for female patients and a No. 9 ETT for male patients should be used to allow for proper ventilation and to potentially prevent elevated peak airway pressures and development of auto–positive end-expiratory pressure (PEEP) during the procedure. These tubes provide at least a 2 mm difference between the scope diameter and that of the ETT because the outer diameter of the EBUS-TBNA scope is 6.2 mm. This bronchoscope/ETT ratio may prevent critical alterations in ventilatory parameters.[45] The procedure is usually performed in the operating room. Because the EBUS scope is directed more centrally in the airway through the ETT, coupling of the transducer and the wall may be impaired, and biopsy may be more difficult to perform than with LMA or moderate sedation techniques.[43]

During the time-out process, the need for perioperative antibiotics is readdressed by the anesthesia team. Current evidence suggests that given a bacteremia rate comparable with that of routine flexible bronchoscopy, recommendations for the use of prophylactic antibiotics for the prevention of infective endocarditis in patients undergoing EBUS-TBNA should not differ from those for routine bronchoscopy. The latest guidelines recommend antibiotic prophylaxis for bronchoscopic procedures only in patients with cardiac conditions such as congenital heart disease, prosthetic heart valves, or previous history of infectious endocarditis.[46] Our patient had no such conditions.

Instrumentation

The EBUS bronchoscopes used for diagnosing and staging mediastinal lymph nodes in lung cancer are dedicated real-time EBUS-TBNA scopes.[47,48] These scopes are similar in design, but their physical characteristics may be slightly different (Table 17-1).

The bronchoscope used in our case had a curved array 7.5 MHz ultrasound transducer incorporated into its distal end (BF-UC 160F, Olympus Optical Co., Ltd., Tokyo, Japan) (Figure 17-2, *A*). Resolution is low, but optimal depth of penetration is approximately 5 cm, which allows clear visualization of mediastinal structures surrounding the airways. The ultrasound processor (Figure 17-2, *B*) (Olympus Endo Echo EU C2000) allows for adjustable gain and depth to improve image quality and has Doppler capabilities that help to distinguish lymph nodes from mediastinal vascular structures (see video on ExpertConsult.com) (Video IV.17.1). The dedicated 22 gauge acrogenic needle has a stylet and a lockable sheath. Precise needle projection is up to 4 cm (Figure 17-2, *C* and *D*). The stylet allows the operator to expel bronchial cells inside the node that might otherwise contaminate the specimen during the aspiration process (see video on ExpertConsult.com) (Video IV.17.2).

Anatomic Dangers and Other Risks

The pulmonary artery and the aortic arch surround station 4 L (see Figure 17-1). The risk of puncturing these and other major vessels may be reduced by using real-time B-mode and Doppler mode imaging. Minor bleeding at the puncture site has been reported but no cases of major bleeding have been described.[49] Pneumothorax and pericarditis have occurred after conventional TBNA but are very rarely reported in the EBUS-TBNA literature.[25,29]

Results and Procedure-Related Complications

EBUS-TBNA was performed with the patient under general anesthesia using a 9.0 ETT. Bronchoscopic inspection showed normal airway mucosa without evidence of endobronchial disease. A total of three aspirates were performed from station 4 L. With the use of rapid on-site cytology examination, a diagnosis of non–small cell carcinoma (likely adenocarcinoma) was made. No procedure-related complications were reported.

When EBUS-TBNA is performed, a cytology specimen can be considered adequate or representative if frankly malignant cells are present, as in our case. Lymphocytes, lymphoid tissue, and clusters of anthracotic pigment-laden macrophages are also signs of a representative (being within the lymph node) sample.[50] The specimen is considered inadequate or nonrepresentative if no cellular

Table 17-1 Specifications for Commercially Available Endobronchial Ultrasound Bronchoscopes

Bronchoscope Type	BF-UC160F-OL8 (Olympus)	BF-UC180F (Olympus)	EB-1970UK (Pentax)
Field of view	80 degrees	80 degrees	100 degrees
Direction of view	35 degrees forward oblique	35 degrees forward oblique	45 degrees forward oblique
Depth of field	2-50 mm	2-50 mm	3-100 mm
Distal end outer diameter	6.9 mm	6.9 mm	7.45 mm
Insertion tube outer diameter	6.2 mm	6.2 mm	6.3 mm
Working length	600 mm	600 mm	600 mm
Channel inner diameter	2.0 mm	2.2 mm	2.0 mm
Angulation range	Up 120 degrees Down 90 degrees	Up 120 degrees Down 90 degrees	Up 120 degrees Down 90 degrees
Display mode	B mode CPD mode	B mode, M mode, D mode, Flow mode Power flow mode*	B mode, color Doppler, pulse Doppler
Scanning method	Electrical curved linear array	Electrical curved linear array	Electrical curved linear array
Scanning direction	Parallel to the insertion direction (longitudinal)	Parallel to the insertion direction (longitudinal)	Parallel to the insertion direction (longitudinal)
Frequency	7.5 MHz	5/7.5/10/12 MHz	5/6.6/7.5/9/10 MHz
Tissue harmonic echo	N/A	5OP/6OS/6OR/7.5 H	N/A
Focusing point	Fixed	Maximum of 4 focusing points*	N/A
Scanning range	50 degrees	60 degrees	75 degrees
Contacting mode	Balloon method Direct contact mode	Balloon method Direct contact mode	Balloon method Direct contact mode

CPD, Color power Doppler; *N/A*, not applicable or reported.
*With Aloka Prosound α5 (Aloka America, Wallingford, Conn).

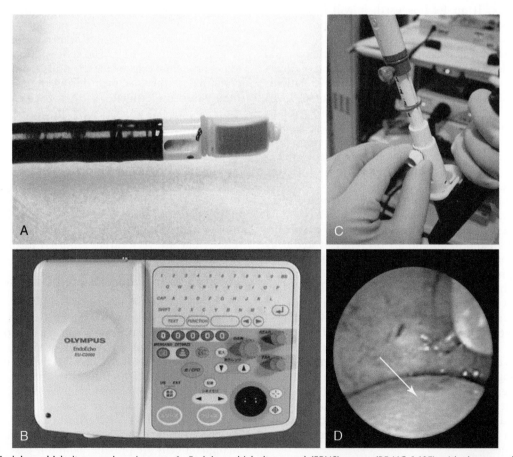

Figure 17-2 Endobronchial ultrasound equipment. **A,** Endobronchial ultrasound (EBUS) scope (BF-UC 160F) with the curved array 7.5 MHz ultrasound transducer incorporated into the distal end of the bronchoscope. **B,** The ultrasound processor unit (EU C 2000) allows for adjustable gain and depth to improve image quality and has Doppler capabilities. **C,** The 22 gauge needle system is being locked to the bronchoscope. **D,** Endoscopic view showing the water-inflated balloon *(arrow)* against the airway wall and the needle extended out of its sheath, penetrating the airway wall.

components are present, and if the specimen contains scant lymphocytes (defined as <40 per high-power field [HPF]) and blood only, cartilage, or bronchial epithelial cells only.[51] A quantitative cutoff value of at least 30% cellularity composed of lymphocytes has been arbitrarily proposed by some experts.[52] Higher yields may be obtained by taking aspirates from the periphery of the node. The case lasted 30 minutes from induction to extubation. Extubation was uneventful, and the patient was transferred to the postanesthesia care unit for 2 hour observation, during which no complications were noted. He was discharged home the same day.

We chose to use rapid on-site examination (ROSE) because of its availability at our institution. The procedure was stopped once the pathologist determined specimen adequacy. A firm and unquestionable diagnosis at the time of EBUS-TBNA was not required. Literature shows that if ROSE is not utilized, the greatest diagnostic yield is obtained by performing three aspirates per lymph node station (reported sensitivity of 95% and specificity of 100%).[51] Two aspirations per lymph node station seem to be acceptable if at least one tissue core specimen is obtained. If the operator believes that targeting is inadequate or insufficient, additional aspirates should probably be obtained, regardless of the number of passes.

Long-Term Management

Outcome Assessment

The patient was discussed in a multidisciplinary chest conference attended by chest radiologists, along with representatives from cardiothoracic surgery, oncology, and radiation oncology. He was potentially eligible to be enrolled in a clinical trial of neoadjuvant treatment of stage IIIA adenocarcinoma of the lung.[13] Five-year survival for all treated patients with clinical stage IIIA non–small cell lung cancer is 19%.[4] Patients with stage IIIA disease usually are stratified radiographically into those with nonbulky (stage IIIA3) or bulky (stage IIIA4) mediastinal lymph node disease.[12] The definition of bulky mediastinal lymphadenopathy varies in the literature, but it is reasonably defined as lymph nodes larger than 2 cm in short-axis diameter, as measured by CT, groupings of multiple smaller lymph nodes, or involvement of more than two lymph node stations.[13] The distinction between nonbulky and bulky stage IIIA and IIIB disease is useful primarily in selecting patients for surgical resection after neoadjuvant therapy. Our patient's mediastinal lymphadenopathy included only one station, and the node was smaller than 2 cm; the disease was therefore determined to be stage IIIA3 (see Figure 17-1).

Referral

The patient was referred to oncology and radiation oncology for further discussion of treatment options. Therapeutic alternatives included definitive combined chemotherapy and radiotherapy or consideration for surgical resection following neoadjuvant chemotherapy alone, radiation therapy alone, or combined modality treatment. Enrollment in clinical research trials was also discussed.

Follow-up Tests and Procedures

The final diagnosis 2 days after the procedure confirmed primary lung adenocarcinoma. Complete staging included whole body positron emission tomography (PET)-CT scanning and brain magnetic resonance imaging (MRI). These tests showed no extrathoracic disease. A follow-up appointment was arranged 2 weeks after EBUS-TBNA to ensure involvement of subspecialty physicians as part of a multidisciplinary approach to lung cancer management.

Discussion with the oncologist and the pathologist was necessary to determine whether the EBUS-TBNA specimen should be sent for genetic testing. Evidence suggests that patient outcomes are optimized by testing for specific mutated pathways against which treatment may be directed.[53-55]

Quality Improvement

In this case, a diagnosis of lung cancer was made quickly, and N2 metastasis was identified using a single outpatient procedure, resulting in cost-effective, quality care. At our team meeting, we discussed whether general anesthesia had been necessary for this procedure. We concluded that although some evidence indicates that moderate sedation is sufficient and safe for performing EBUS-TBNA, our physicians and nurses preferred general anesthesia if patients had no contraindications. Reasons for this preference include having a secure airway in case of problems (e.g., hypoxemia, aspiration, bleeding), perceived patient comfort in case the bronchoscope needs to be removed and introduced several times, virtual absence of patient agitation and cough during general anesthesia, and an ability to routinely obtain high-quality images and representative specimens in a timely manner.

DISCUSSION POINTS

1. Describe the diagnostic yield of EBUS-TBNA versus conventional TBNA and EUS-FNA at station 4 L.

   According to a study that directly evaluated the yield of EBUS-TBNA versus conventional TBNA for separate lymph node stations, the diagnostic yield of EBUS-TBNA was similar to that of conventional TBNA (72% vs. 71%) at station 4 L, but lymphocyte-positive aspirates were retrieved more commonly with EBUS-TBNA (82% vs. 71%). In a more recent paper with a large number of patients, the yield of EBUS-TBNA for diagnosing station 4 L was as high as 96% in expert hands[14] and was much higher than the yield of 41% reported with conventional TBNA for this lymph node station.[15] For station 4 L, EUS-FNA has a diagnostic yield similar to that of EBUS-TBNA.[23]

2. Describe how the coronal view of a computed tomography scan can be used to help plan EBUS-TBNA.

   According to the International Association for the Study of Lung Cancer (IASLC) lymph node map,[56] station 4 L includes nodes to the left of the left lateral border of the trachea, medial to the ligamentum arteriosum. The upper border is the upper margin of the aortic arch, and the lower border is the upper rim of the left main pulmonary artery (see Figure 17-1). Both axial and coronal CT views are useful to define station

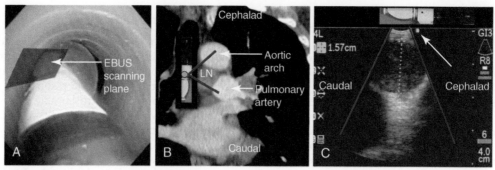

Figure 17-3 **A,** Bronchoscopic view shows the endobronchial ultrasound (EBUS) scope with the transducer oriented toward the left lateral wall of the trachea at the 9 o'clock position when the patient is bronchoscoped from the head; the scanning plane is parallel to the insertion direction and is oriented toward the left side of the trachea. **B,** Close view coronal computed tomography (CT) image reveals station 4 L (lymph node [LN]), the aortic arch (cephalad), and the pulmonary artery (caudal). Schematic representation of the EBUS scope inside the trachea and the scanning range of 50 degrees. **C,** Bronchoscopic ultrasound image is projected as if the EBUS scope were horizontal. The green dot *(arrow)* is oriented toward the cephalad portion of the body.

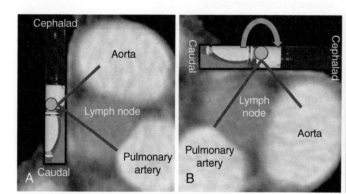

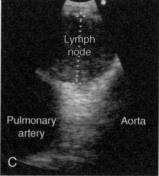

Figure 17-4 **A,** Coronal computed tomography (CT) image adjustments are made to bring the green dot cephalad, as in the endobronchial ultrasound (EBUS) image. **B,** Coronal CT image is projected as if the EBUS scope were horizontal. The aortic arch is cephalad, and the pulmonary artery is caudal. **C,** The EBUS image, projected by default as if the scope were horizontal, shows the same structures that are seen on the adjusted coronal CT image.

4 L and identify adjacent vascular structures. The coronal CT view, however, is more useful for correlation with the EBUS image, as is explained later.[57]

To visualize the left paratracheal node (4 L), the operator turns the bronchoscope laterally to the 9 o'clock position and scans the area of lymph node station 4 L (Figure 17-3, *A*). Therefore the scanning plane for the EBUS scope is the same as that for the coronal CT view (Figure 17-3, *B*). However, although the coronal CT view is projected as if the scope is vertical, the EBUS image is projected as if the scope is horizontal (Figure 17-3, *C*). Thus to understand the use of the coronal CT view, one must understand the reference points on the EBUS image (see Figure 17-3, *C*). The green dot on the monitor represents the point where the needle exits the scope and corresponds to the superior (cephalad) aspect of the body. This dot is by default toward the 1 o'clock position on the screen (see Figure 17-3, *C*). Reorientation of the coronal CT image is necessary to bring the scope to a horizontal position and to bring the green dot cephalad (toward the 1 o'clock position on the screen) to match the EBUS image. For practical purposes, one can print out or save the coronal CT image showing station 4 L as a separate picture. This picture is then rotated clockwise to "horizontalize" the scope and bring the green dot cephalad toward the 1 o'clock position (Figure 17-4).

3. Describe endobronchial sonographic findings, including adjacent vascular structures at and around lymph node station 4 L.

The coronal CT image and the EBUS image correlate and show the same structures in the same locations, as well as the characteristic EBUS image at station 4 L (see Figure 17-4).

Expert Commentary

provided by Kenneth Chang, MD

The authors have presented a thorough and comprehensive review of the diagnosis, staging, and therapeutic strategies for this illustrative case. An alternative approach would have been to perform EUS-FNA at the same time (or before) EBUS. The instrumentation, technique, and expected results of EUS-FNA at station 4 L will be discussed.

Instrumentation

With EUS, two different scopes can be used alone or in combination. Radial instruments utilize a mechanical or an electronic rotating transducer that creates a 360 degree ultrasonographic image that is perpendicular to the axis plane of the echoendoscope. In the esophagus, this gives a spatial orientation of the image similar to that obtained with CT of the chest. Current radial echoendoscopes have the ability to switch frequencies from 5 MHz up to 10 MHz to optimize imaging. The main limitation of the radial echoendoscope is its inability to safely perform FNA, because the needle path cannot be tracked accurately.

On the other hand, linear-array echoendoscopes permit the performance of FNA. The ultrasound transducer generates a 100 to 180 degree image that is parallel to the shaft of the echoendoscope, allowing full visualization of a needle that is passed through the working channel of the device. The anatomic orientation is at an angle of 90 degrees to the radial anatomy. Linear echoendoscopes also have a frequency range of 5 to 10 MHz. The needle for FNA can be tracked in its entirety from exiting the biopsy channel to entering and aspirating the target lesion. Linear echoendoscopes also provide the ability for color flow and Doppler imaging to choose an FNA needle path that avoids vascular structures by combining simultaneous real-time ultrasonography with Doppler ability. For mediastinal nodal staging, we prefer to start with the radial echoendoscope, which provides 360 degree imaging, followed by the linear echoendoscope for performing FNA.

Technique

A vast majority of cases are performed with the patient under moderate sedation, usually with a combination of meperidine and midazolam. General anesthesia is reserved for those patients with sleep apnea, previously failed moderate sedation, severe comorbidities, or age over 80. The echoendoscope is advanced by direct visualization through the mouth into the proximal esophagus. For acoustic coupling, the water balloon surrounding the transducer can be inflated. Water balloon imaging is always used to couple the entire esophageal lumen when performing radial EUS. Unlike EBUS, the esophageal lumen can be completely occluded during sustained imaging. For linear EUS, minimal balloon coupling may be used to improve surface contact. Staging of lung cancer usually begins by imaging the liver for possible metastasis. The right lobe is imaged through the duodenum, and the left lobe is imaged through the gastric fundus. In addition, the left adrenal gland is imaged, because lung cancer not infrequently can metastasize to the adrenal gland.[58] The right adrenal is more difficult to image through the duodenum, in which case the scope is positioned in the gastric cardia, where the aorta is positioned at 6 o'clock (similar to CT of chest) and is followed proximally from the level of the celiac artery. The hepatic veins merging into the inferior vena cava can be imaged at this level as well. The next structure that is visualized during scope withdrawal is the base of the heart, including the right atrium. Next, the left atrium is most prominent when a four-chambered view of the heart and the descending aorta is obtained. Slightly more proximal, the pulmonary veins coming into the left atrium can be seen, along with the aortic outflow tract, the azygos vein, and the superior vena cava (SVC). Further withdrawal brings to view the subcarinal region, with visualization of the right and left

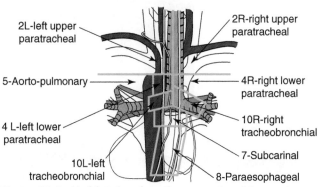

Anatomy of the mediastinum
Mediastinal lymph node stations

2L-left upper paratracheal
2R-right upper paratracheal
5-Aorto-pulmonary
4R-right lower paratracheal
4 L-left lower paratracheal
10R-right tracheobronchial
10L-left tracheobronchial
7-Subcarinal
8-Paraesophageal

Figure 17-5 Nodal stations from the perspective of the esophagus.

mainstem bronchi. Next is the region of the descending aorta and pulmonary arteries (the right pulmonary artery is prominently visualized as it comes under the ascending aorta and SVC). More proximally, the aortic arch comes into view, followed by the right and left carotid arteries and internal jugular veins. Thus all lymph node stations can be assessed with the exception of 10 L and 10R (Figure 17-5).

Performing FNA

The most commonly used FNA needle size has changed in many institutions, including ours, from the 22 gauge to the 25 gauge needle. The technique involves having the lesion to be biopsied placed in the center or just to the left of center in the imaging field.[59] If concern arises regarding surrounding vascular structures, Doppler imaging can be used to better define potential vessels. The needle is then advanced through the biopsy channel and can be seen exiting the biopsy channel into the lymph node under real-time ultrasonography. Although suction with a 10 mL syringe has been used for two decades, advancements have led to the use of no suction or the "stylet pull-back" technique while quick to-and-fro movements of the needle are made within the node. Studies have shown that suction creates a bloody specimen, especially when FNA is performed in lymph nodes. The needle is removed and is immediately placed onto a glass slide and is processed by a cytopathology technician within the unit. We now place the first and last drops on the slide and the remainder of the material into the formalin bottle for cell block. While the first slide is being processed and reviewed, we may take a second pass while waiting for the preliminary cytologic interpretation from the preceding pass. This continues until cytologic adequacy for interpretation is attained. Typically, only one or two passes are required to yield an adequate specimen.

The specific technique for assessing and performing FNA of station 4 L lymph nodes is as follows. The linear echoendoscope is advanced into the distal esophagus. With the descending aorta in the longitudinal position, the scope is withdrawn while the aorta

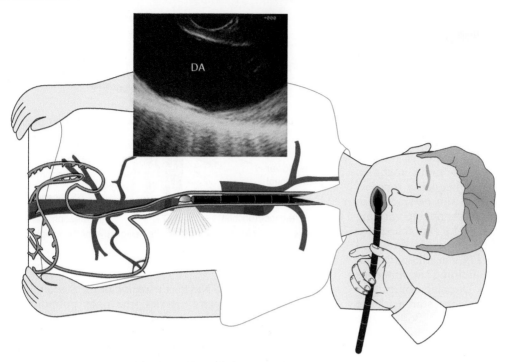

Figure 17-6 Linear endoscopic ultrasound (EUS) position in the distal esophagus following the descending aorta.

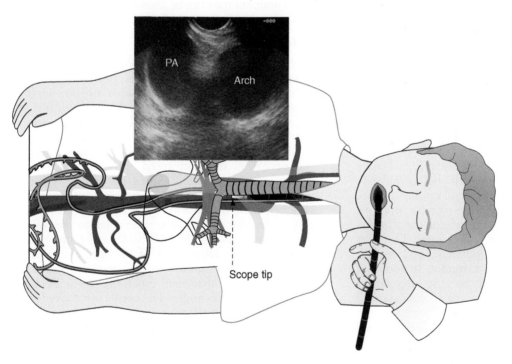

Figure 17-7 Linear endoscopic ultrasound (EUS) scope in the area of the aortopulmonary window and the left lower paratracheal node station (4 L).

is kept in view at the 6 o'clock position (Figure 17-6) until the aortic arch is identified. At this point, rotation of the scope will allow visualization of the aortopulmonary window and left lower paratracheal (4 L) nodes (Figure 17-7).

Concluding Comments

With the advent of endobronchial and esophageal endoscopic ultrasound (EUS), current data suggest that most mediastinal stations can be reached with minimally invasive staging, with the exception of stations 5 and 6. EUS fine-needle aspiration (FNA) is a minimally invasive technique that allows sampling of mediastinal lymph nodes relevant to lung cancer staging, particularly in the subcarinal area (station 7), the lower paraesophageal lymph nodes (station 8), the inferior pulmonary ligament lymph nodes (station 9), and the celiac lymph nodes. In addition, EUS-FNA is capable of sampling metastatic sarcoidosis and lymphoma-harboring lymph nodes. The left adrenal gland is easily sampled by EUS-FNA through the transgastric approach. EUS-FNA can also be used to sample central primary lung masses abutting the esophagus, particularly when other techniques fail.

The accuracy of single-modality EUS-guided FNA of lymph nodes in the setting of lung cancer is approximately 85%. When combined with EBUS-TBNA, accuracy approaches 100%. We would prefer to start with EUS because it can be used to assess the liver and left adrenal glands, and if found positive would preclude the need for further local staging. If EUS is negative, then EBUS could be performed, preferably during the same sedation.

REFERENCES

1. World Health Organization. The WHO family of international classifications. Available at: http://www.who.int/classifications/en/ Accessed August 22, 2010.
2. Hajiro T, Nishimura K, Tsukino M, et al. Analysis of clinical methods used to evaluate dyspnea in patients with chronic obstructive pulmonary disease. *Am J Respir Crit Care Med.* 1998;158:1185-1189.
3. Calverley PM, Anderson JA, Celli B, et al, TORCH Investigators. Salmeterol and fluticasone propionate and survival in chronic obstructive pulmonary disease. *N Engl J Med.* 2007;356: 775-789.
4. Goldstraw P, Crowley J, Chanksy K, et al. The IASLC Lung Cancer Staging Project: proposals for the revision of the TNM stage groupings in the forthcoming (seventh) edition of the TNM classification of malignant tumours. *J Thorac Oncol.* 2007;2:706-714.
5. Schag CC, Heinrich RL, Ganz PA. Karnofsky performance status revisited: reliability, validity, and guidelines. *J Clin Oncol.* 1984;2:187-193.
6. Sin DD, Man SF. Chronic obstructive pulmonary disease as a risk factor for cardiovascular morbidity and mortality. *Proc Am Thorac Soc.* 2005;2:8-11.
7. Omachi TA, Katz PP, Yelin EH, et al. Depression and health-related quality of life in chronic obstructive pulmonary disease. *Am J Med.* 2009;122:778.e9-e15.
8. Duhamel F, Dupuis F. Guaranteed returns: investing in conversations with families of patients with cancer. *Clin J Oncol Nurs.* 2004;8:68-71.
9. Persson C, Ostlund U, Wennman-Larsen A, et al. Health-related quality of life in significant others of patients dying from lung cancer. *Palliat Med.* 2008;22:239-247.
10. Robinson A, Thomson R. Variability in patient preferences for participating in medical decision making: implication for the use of decision support tools. *Qual Health Care.* 2001;10(suppl 1):134-138.
11. Spira A, Ettinger DS. Multidisciplinary management of lung cancer. *N Engl J Med.* 2004;350:379-392.
12. van Meerbeeck JP, Surmont VF. Stage IIIA-N2 NSCLC: a review of its treatment approaches and future developments. *Lung Cancer.* 2009;65:257-267.
13. Robinson LA, Ruckdeschel JC, Wagner H, et al. Treatment of nonsmall cell lung cancer-stage IIIA: ACCP evidence-based clinical practice guidelines (2nd edition). *Chest.* 2007;132:243-265.
14. Herth FJ, Eberhardt R, Vilmann P, et al. Real-time endobronchial ultrasound guided transbronchial needle aspiration for sampling mediastinal lymph nodes. *Thorax.* 2006;61:795-798.
15. Chin R Jr, McCain TW, Lucia MA, et al. Transbronchial needle aspiration in diagnosing and staging lung cancer: how many aspirates are needed? *Am J Respir Crit Care Med.* 2002;166: 377-381.
16. Herth FJ, Ernst A, Eberhardt R, et al. Endobronchial ultrasound-guided transbronchial needle aspiration of lymph nodes in the radiologically normal mediastinum. *Eur Respir J.* 2006;28:910-914.
17. Vincent BD, El-Bayoumi E, Hoffman B, et al. Real-time endobronchial ultrasound-guided transbronchial lymph node aspiration. *Ann Thorac Surg.* 2008;85:224-230.
18. Wallace MB, Ravenel J, Block MI, et al. Endoscopic ultrasound in lung cancer patients with a normal mediastinum on computed tomography. *Ann Thorac Surg.* 2004;77:1763-1768.
19. Fleisher LA, Beckman JA, Brown KA, et al. ACC/AHA 2007 guidelines on perioperative cardiovascular evaluation and care for noncardiac surgery: a report of the American College of Cardiology/ American Heart Association Task Force on Practice Guidelines. *J Am Coll Cardiol.* 2007;50:e159-e241.
20. Auerbach A, Goldman L. Assessing and reducing the cardiac risk of non-cardiac surgery. *Circulation.* 2006;113:1361.
21. Herth F, Becker HD, Ernst A. Conventional vs endobronchial ultrasound-guided transbronchial needle aspiration: a randomized trial. *Chest.* 2004;125:322-325.
22. Herth FJ, Becker HD, Ernst A. Ultrasound-guided transbronchial needle aspiration: an experience in 242 patients. *Chest.* 2003; 123:604-607.
23. Herth FJ, Lunn W, Eberhardt R, et al. Transbronchial versus transesophageal ultrasound-guided aspiration of enlarged mediastinal lymph nodes. *Am J Respir Crit Care Med.* 2005;171:1164-1167.
24. Fournier C, Boutemy M, Ramon PP, et al. Developing real time lymph node aspiration under endobronchial ultrasound control: one year's French experience in two different pulmonary departments. *Rev Mal Respir.* 2008;25:847-852.
25. Gu P, Zhao Y, Jiang L, et al. Endobronchial ultrasound-guided transbronchial needle aspiration for staging of lung cancer: a systematic review and meta-analysis. *Eur J Cancer.* 2009;45: 1389-1396.
26. Alsharif M, Andrade RS, Groth SS, et al. Endobronchial ultrasound-guided transbronchial fine-needle aspiration: the University of Minnesota experience, with emphasis on usefulness, adequacy assessment, and diagnostic difficulties. *Am J Clin Pathol.* 2008; 130:434-443.
27. Varela-Lema L, Fernandez-Villar A, Ruano-Ravina A. Effectiveness and safety of endobronchial ultrasound-transbronchial needle aspiration: a systematic review. *Eur Respir J.* 2009; 33:1156-1164.
28. Steinfort DP, Irving LB. Patient satisfaction during endobronchial ultrasound-guided transbronchial needle aspiration performed under conscious sedation. *Respir Care.* 2010;55:702-706.
29. Haas AR. Infectious complications from full extension endobronchial ultrasound transbronchial needle aspiration. *Eur Respir J.* 2009;33:935-938.
30. Steinfort DP, Johnson DF, Irving LB. Incidence of bacteraemia following endobronchial ultrasound-guided transbronchial needle aspiration. *Eur Respir J.* 2010;36:28-32.
31. Toloza EM, Harpole L, Detterbeck F, et al. Invasive staging of nonsmall cell lung cancer: a review of the current evidence. *Chest.* 2003;123:157S-166S.
32. Fritscher-Ravens A. Endoscopic ultrasound evaluation in the diagnosis and staging of lung cancer. *Lung Cancer.* 2003;41:259-267.
33. Janssen J, König K, Knop-Hammad V, et al. Frequency of bacteremia after linear EUS of the upper GI tract with and without FNA. *Gastrointest Endosc.* 2004;59:339-344.
34. Detterbeck FC, DeCamp MM Jr, Kohman LJ, et al, American College of Chest Physicians. Lung cancer: invasive staging: the guidelines. *Chest.* 2003;123:167S-175S.
35. Detterbeck FC, Jantz MA, Wallace M, et al, American College of Chest Physicians. Invasive mediastinal staging of lung cancer: ACCP evidence-based clinical practice guidelines (2nd edition). *Chest.* 2007;132:202S-220S.
36. Savides TJ. EUS for mediastinal disease. *Gastrointest Endosc.* 2009;69:S97-S99.
37. Kunst P, Eberhardt R, Herth F. Combined EBUS real time TBNA and conventional TBNA are the most cost-effective means of lymph node staging. *J Bronchol.* 2008;15:17-20.
38. Kramer H, van Putten JW, Post WJ, et al. Oesophageal endoscopic ultrasound with fine needle aspiration improves and simplifies the staging of lung cancer. *Thorax.* 2004;59:596-601.
39. Hwangbo B, Lee GK, Lee HS, et al. Transbronchial and transesophageal fine-needle aspiration using an ultrasound bronchoscope in mediastinal staging of potentially operable lung cancer. *Chest.* 2010;138:795-802.
40. de Romijn BJ, van den Berg JM, Uiterwijk H, et al. Necessity of centralization of EBUS. *Lung Cancer.* 2009;64:127-128.

41. Bowling MR, Perry CD, Chin R Jr, et al. Endobronchial ultrasound in the evaluation of lung cancer: a practical review and cost analysis for the practicing pulmonologist. *South Med J.* 2008;101:534-538.

42. Kennedy MP, Shweihat Y, Sarkiss M, et al. Complete mediastinal and hilar lymph node staging of primary lung cancer by endobronchial ultrasound: moderate sedation or general anesthesia? *Chest.* 2008;134:1350-1351.

43. Sarkiss M, Kennedy M, Riedel B, et al. Anesthesia technique for endobronchial ultrasound-guided fine needle aspiration of mediastinal lymph node. *J Cardiothorac Vasc Anesth.* 2007;21:892-896.

44. Ng A, Smith G. Gastroesophageal reflux and aspiration of gastric contents in anesthetic practice. *Anesth Analg.* 2001;93:494-513.

45. Lawson RW, Peters JI, Shelledy DC. Effects of fiberoptic bronchoscopy during mechanical ventilation in a lung model. *Chest.* 2000; 118:824-831.

46. Wilson W, Taubert KA, Gewitz M, et al, American Heart Association Rheumatic Fever, Endocarditis, and Kawasaki Disease Committee; American Heart Association Council on Cardiovascular Disease in the Young; American Heart Association Council on Clinical Cardiology; American Heart Association Council on Cardiovascular Surgery and Anesthesia; Quality of Care and Outcomes Research Interdisciplinary Working Group. Prevention of infective endocarditis: guidelines from the American Heart Association: a guideline from the American Heart Association Rheumatic Fever, Endocarditis, and Kawasaki Disease Committee, Council on Cardiovascular Disease in the Young, and the Council on Clinical Cardiology, Council on Cardiovascular Surgery and Anesthesia, and the Quality of Care and Outcomes Research Interdisciplinary Working Group. *Circulation.* 2007;116:1736-1754.

47. Pentax EBUS Pro. Full video endobronchial ultrasound. Available at: http://www.pentax.de/en/ebus.php. Accessed March 20, 2011.

48. Olympus EBUS bronchoscopes overview. Available at: http://www.olympusamerica.com/msg_section/msg_endoscopy_ebus_bronchoscopes.asp. Accessed March 20, 2011.

49. Yasufuku K, Chiyo M, Sekine Y, et al. Real-time endobronchial ultrasound-guided transbronchial needle aspiration of mediastinal and hilar lymph nodes. *Chest.* 2004;126:122-128.

50. Alsharif M, Andrade RS, Groth SS, et al. Endobronchial ultrasound-guided transbronchial fine-needle aspiration: the University of Minnesota experience, with emphasis on usefulness, adequacy assessment, and diagnostic difficulties. *Am J Clin Pathol.* 2008; 130:434-443.

51. Lee HS, Lee GK, Lee HS, et al. Real-time endobronchial ultrasound-guided transbronchial needle aspiration in mediastinal staging of non-small cell lung cancer: how many aspirations per target lymph node station? *Chest.* 2008;134:368-374.

52. Trisolini R, Lazzari Agli L, Patelli M. Conventional vs endobronchial ultrasound-guided transbronchial needle aspiration of the mediastinum. *Chest.* 2004;126:1005-1006.

53. Lynch TJ, Bell DW, Sordella R, et al. Activating mutations in the epidermal growth factor receptor underlying responsiveness of non-small-cell lung cancer to gefitinib. *N Engl J Med.* 2004;350: 2129-2139.

54. Paez JG, Jänne PA, Lee JC, et al. EGFR mutations in lung cancer: correlation with clinical response to gefitinib therapy. *Science.* 2004;304:1497-1500.

55. Pao W, Miller V, Zakowski M, et al. EGF receptor gene mutations are common in lung cancers from "never smokers" and are associated with sensitivity of tumors to gefitinib and erlotinib. *Proc Natl Acad Sci U S A.* 2004;101:13306-13311.

56. Rusch VW, Asamura H, Watanabe H, et al, Members of IASLC Staging Committee. The IASLC Lung Cancer Staging Project: a proposal for a new international lymph node map in the forthcoming seventh edition of the TNM classification for lung cancer. *J Thorac Oncol.* 2009;4:568-577.

57. Bronchoscopy International. Available at: http://www.bronchoscopy.org/downloads/BiDown_asp. Accessed March 20, 2011.

58. Chang KJ, Erickson RA, Nguyen P. Endoscopic ultrasound (EUS) and EUS-guided fine-needle aspiration of the left adrenal gland. *Gastrointest Endosc.* 1996;44:568-572.

59. Chang KJ. Maximizing the yield of EUS-guided fine-needle aspiration. *Gastrointest Endosc.* 2002;56:S28-S34.

Chapter 18

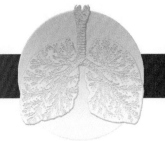

EBUS-TBNA for Subcentimeter PET-Negative Subcarinal LAD (Station 7) and a Right Lower Lobe Pulmonary Nodule

> This chapter emphasizes the following elements of the Four Box Approach: risk-benefit analysis and therapeutic alternatives, anatomic dangers and other risks, and results and procedure-related complications.

CASE DESCRIPTION

An 81-year-old man was referred for a 1.5 cm solitary pulmonary nodule in the medio-basal segment of the RLL, incidentally noted while he was undergoing CT of the abdomen for nephrolithiasis. An integrated emission tomography with CT/18F-fluoro-2-deoxy-D-glucose PET scan confirmed the nodule, showing a 5.5 SUV max on PET, and revealed a PET-negative 7 mm subcarinal lymph node (Figure 18-1). Vital signs and physical examination were unremarkable. Complete blood count, coagulation, chemistry panel, and spirometry and DLCO were normal. A treadmill stress test performed 6 months earlier was normal. PPD was negative, and the patient had no known exposure to tuberculosis. He smoked 1 pack/day for 25 years but quit 20 years before the time of his presentation. He was still working and active, playing golf 3 times a week. He lived with his wife, who was very involved in his care. He desired all available treatment options in case this was lung cancer.

DISCUSSION POINTS

1. Describe the major elements of informed consent.
2. Describe pros and cons pertaining to staging the PET-CT–negative mediastinum in patients with known or suspected lung cancer.
3. List five reasons for a poor sample on a nodal aspiration smear.

CASE RESOLUTION

Initial Evaluations

Physical Examination, Complementary Tests, and Functional Status Assessment

Assessment of this patient's functional status at the initial visit could guide additional diagnostic and therapeutic interventions. His age, smoking history, and imaging studies increased the likelihood that he had primary lung carcinoma. Treatment of lung cancer, whether with surgery, chemotherapy, radiation therapy, or a combination of these, can be associated with substantial toxicity. Patients with significant functional impairment due to their lung cancer or to comorbid conditions may not be able to withstand resection or, alternatively, aggressive chemoradiotherapy. The Karnofsky Performance Status (KPS) is a general measure of functional impairment that is used to compare the effectiveness of various therapies and to assess prognosis in individual patients: The lower the score, the worse the survival for most serious illnesses.[1] The Eastern Cooperative Oncology Group (ECOG) Performance Scale uses a five-point scale and has been shown to be a better predictor of prognosis than KPS.[2,3] Relevant to this case suspicious of smoking-related malignancy is that if diagnosis performed is locally advanced cancer (stage IIIA) based on his pulmonary nodule and the subcentimeter subcarinal lymph node (LN), this patient's operability or eligibility for chemoradiotherapy could be precluded by poor performance status. However, his performance status was excellent, with KPS of 100 and ECOG score of 0.

Computed tomography (CT) scan showed a 1.5 cm right lower lobe (RLL) nodule and a 0.7 cm subcarinal LN. Although CT is accurate in detecting LN enlargement, the clinical relevance of LN enlargement for staging is poor, because large nodes may be benign and small nodes contain metastases in approximately 20% of cases.[4] Of importance to this patient, 5.6% of patients with radiographic stage I disease in one study were eventually found to have N2 disease.[5] Multiple studies and meta-analyses have demonstrated that noninvasive staging of lung cancer is improved by the use of positron emission tomography (PET) scanning.[6] Owing to a high negative predictive value (NPV) of PET scanning of approximately 90%, invasive staging procedures are generally omitted in patients with clinical stage I non–small cell lung cancer (NSCLC) and negative mediastinal PET images. This strategy warrants caution, however, in the following situations, which increase the risk for occult N2 disease: larger tumor size (≥6.0 cm)—57% prevalence; central location—21.6% prevalence; high standardized uptake value (SUV) in the primary tumor (≥4.0)—10.5% prevalence; and adenocarcinoma cell type—9.0% prevalence.[7] In these instances, PET results do not provide acceptable accuracy rates for mediastinal staging. Therefore invasive staging is usually advocated for patients with one or more risk factors for occult N2 disease.[5,7,8] Routine use of invasive lymph node staging for patients with clinical stage I NSCLC and no risk factors for occult N2 disease, however, is neither

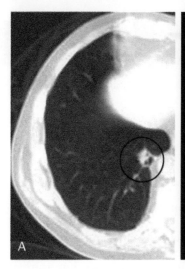 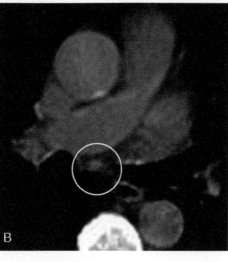

Figure 18-1 A, Chest computed tomography (CT) scan (lung window) shows the 1.5 cm right lower lobe pulmonary nodule. **B,** Chest CT scan (mediastinal window) reveals a 7 mm subcarinal lymph node.

necessary nor considered to be cost-effective.[5] In our patient with a maximal standardized uptake value (SUV max) greater than 4.0 in the nodule, small but measurable LN (<10 mm), and suspected NSCLC, mediastinal staging was considered necessary.

Comorbidities

The patient had normal lung function and was asymptomatic from a pulmonary standpoint. Despite an extensive smoking history, he did not meet clinical or spirometry criteria for chronic obstructive pulmonary disease (COPD). Nor was evidence of other smoking-related comorbid conditions found, such as coronary heart disease, stroke, or obstructive sleep apnea, which could preclude or complicate procedures performed under moderate sedation or general anesthesia.

Support System

His wife and son accompanied him at the time of our clinical encounter and were very supportive. He lived with his wife. Both were independent in their activities of daily living.

Patient Preferences and Expectations

The patient clearly expressed a desire to consider all available options for diagnosis and staging, including CT-guided biopsy of the pulmonary nodule, conventional transbronchial needle aspiration (TBNA) of the subcarinal LN, endobronchial ultrasound (EBUS)-guided TBNA, endoscopic ultrasound (EUS)-guided FNA, mediastinoscopy, and video-assisted thoracic surgery (VATS).

Procedural Strategies

Indications

The status of the mediastinum is a most crucial factor in selection of an optimal treatment strategy for NSCLC; invasive confirmation of the radiographic stage is recommended, regardless of results of PET scan findings for mediastinal nodes.[9] If our patient's nodal station 7 is positive for malignancy, his clinical stage is IIIA-N2. Sampling station 7 in our patient is essential because the

incidence of occult N2* disease in NSCLC patients with negative mediastinal uptake of 18F-fluoro-2-deoxy-D-glucose (18FDG) on PET-CT is reportedly around 16% (25 of 153 patients). The highest incidence of occult N2 involvement is seen in fact in station 7 (subcarinal) (16 of 25 patients; 64%) followed by station 4 (lower paratracheal) (7 of 25 patients; 28%).[10] Flexible bronchoscopy in this patient would allow complete airway inspection to ascertain the absence of endobronchial lesions that could potentially alter staging and management,[11] and to sample LN 7 at the same setting. Although nodal sampling could be done with the use of conventional TBNA, EBUS-TBNA might increase diagnostic yield, even at level 7, because of small lymph node size.[12,13]

Contraindications

No absolute contraindications to bronchoscopy with EBUS-TBNA were identified. We usually perform this procedure with the patient under general anesthesia; however, in our elderly patient, this approach could result in a number of physiologic changes that affect respiratory and cardiovascular function and may complicate the procedure.[14] These age-related changes include lung parenchymal changes resulting in impaired gas exchange and reduced partial pressure of oxygen in arterial blood (PaO_2); decreased lung elasticity and increased ventilation-perfusion mismatch; decreased chest wall compliance and respiratory muscle strength, leading to increased work of breathing and higher risk of respiratory failure; reduced cough and mucociliary clearance, and possibly neuromuscular deconditioning, increasing the risk for aspiration; and reduced responsiveness of brain respiratory centers to hypoxemia and hypercarbia and diminished overall cardiopulmonary reserve, resulting in heightened sensitivity to the negative inotropy and vasodilatory effects of induction agents and other vasoactive drugs. These concerns must be addressed with the anesthesiologist before the procedure is begun.

---

*Occult N2 involvement refers to a pathologically positive lymph node in a mediastinal lymph node station that was preoperatively staged by integrated PET-CT as N2/N3 negative.

Expected Results

After complete airway examination has been performed with white light bronchoscopy, a complete sonographic mediastinal and hilar nodal assessment would be completed because of potential upstaging to N3 disease (stage IIIB),[15] in case EBUS identified contralateral LNs positive for malignancy (microscopic N3 disease, which could render the patient unresectable). If complete EBUS mediastinal and hilar evaluation reveals no other nodes, then CT documenting LN 7 only would be sampled. EBUS-TBNA can reliably sample enlarged mediastinal LNs in patients with NSCLC, but most studies have addressed nodes visible on CT (>1 cm) or PET (SUV max >2.5). However, in one study, 100 patients highly suspicious for NSCLC on CT scans showing no enlarged lymph nodes (no node >1 cm) and a negative PET of the mediastinum underwent EBUS-TBNA. Identifiable LNs at locations 2R, 2 L, 4R, 4 L, 7, 10R, 10 L, 11R, and 11 L were aspirated, and all patients underwent subsequent surgical staging; diagnoses based on aspiration results were compared with those based on surgical results. The sensitivity of EBUS-TBNA for detecting malignancy was 89%, the specificity was 100%, and the NPV was 98.9%. Overall, 17 of 97 patients had stage N2 or N3 disease, of whom 16 were identified from EBUS-TBNA, and 4 had stage N1 disease, of whom 3 were identified by EBUS-TBNA. Investigators concluded that EBUS-TBNA could accurately sample and stage patients with clinical stage I lung cancer without evidence of mediastinal involvement on CT and PET. Based on these data, open surgical exploration could be avoided in 1 of 6 patients without CT evidence of mediastinal disease. If nonmalignant results are obtained from EBUS-TBNA, however, this should be followed by mediastinoscopy. Because potentially operable patients with no signs of mediastinal involvement may benefit from presurgical staging by EBUS-TBNA, even when LNs are small,[16] we decided to proceed with EBUS-TBNA under general anesthesia.*

Team Experience

The team should be familiar with techniques and equipment because of the particularities of TBNA, EBUS, and EBUS-TBNA.[17] Experience with sampling this station is high because LN 7 and right lower paratracheal nodes (station 4R) are the most commonly sampled nodes during conventional TBNA and EBUS-TBNA.[12,13] At the time of this writing, American College of Chest Physicians (ACCP) guidelines for interventional pulmonary procedures state that trainees should be supervised for 50 EBUS procedures, and that a chest physician should perform 5 to 10 procedures per year to maintain competency.[18] The European Respiratory Society/American Thoracic Society joint statement on interventional pulmonology recommends that initial training should consist of 40 supervised procedures, and 25 procedures should be done per year to maintain competency.[19] The chest physician learning EBUS probably should be well acquainted with needle aspiration principles and should be trained to interpret endobronchial ultrasound images.[20]

Risk-Benefit Analysis

Although EBUS-TBNA has a high diagnostic yield and is safe, clinically significant and rare complications include pericarditis and pneumothorax requiring chest tube drainage.[21] The risk of pericarditis is particular to this station because the subcarinal node could be adjacent to the pericardium (Figure 18-2); with the needle at its full extension (i.e., 4 cm), the operator may inadvertently penetrate the pericardium during EBUS-TBNA at this station. A false-negative result may be considered a "complication" because it could lead to death if inappropriate decisions are made (e.g., pulmonary resection in case of unrecognized N3, absence of indicated induction therapy in case of missed N2 disease).[22] Thus the complication rate of EBUS-TBNA is higher than that of mediastinoscopy (24% false-negative rate for EBUS as compared with 10% for mediastinoscopy).[9] We considered that the benefits of making a diagnosis and

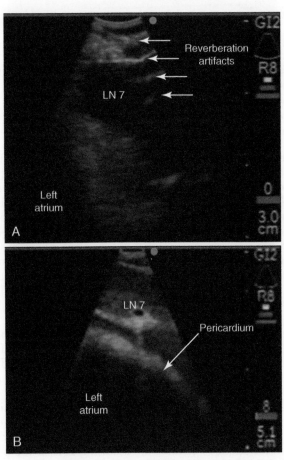

Figure 18-2 A, The small subcarinal lymph node (LN 7) is seen despite reverberation artifacts caused by lack of intimate contact between the endobronchial ultrasound (EBUS) scope balloon and the airway wall when the image was captured. **B,** The subcarinal lymph node from a different patient shows its proximity to the pericardium and only 2 cm distant from the exit point of the needle (*green dot*).

---

*It is noteworthy that in the published articles previously mentioned, most EBUS examinations were done immediately before the scheduled surgical procedure and were therefore performed with the patient under general anesthesia; this may explain in part the high yield of this procedure for such small lymph nodes.

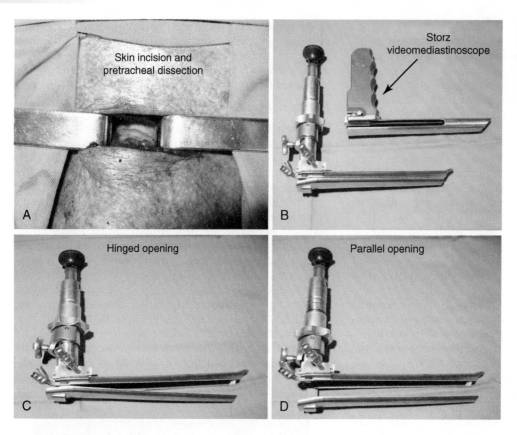

Figure 18-3 **A,** Transverse skin incision and pretracheal dissection for mediastinoscopy. **B,** Different brands of mediastinoscopes and (**C** and **D**) different opening systems. *(Courtesy Ramon Rami-Porta, MD, Barcelona, Spain.)*

staging this patient outweighed the minimal associated risks.

Diagnostic Alternatives

For Diagnosis and Staging of the Mediastinum

For patients with discrete (measurable) mediastinal LN enlargement on CT scan and no obvious distant metastases, another nonbronchoscopic needle aspiration (NA) technique (i.e., EUS-NA or transthoracic needle aspiration [TTNA]), mediastinoscopy, or VATS could be performed instead of conventional or EBUS-guided TBNA. When a procedure is selected, the location of the suspicious LN is important because nodes in one location may be accessible only through a particular approach. Advantages and disadvantages of each alternative modality should be discussed with the patient and his spouse.

1. *Conventional TBNA:* In one study, the yield of conventional TBNA for station 7 was 74% compared with 86% in the EBUS-guided group (difference not statistically significant).[23] Other studies have shown higher diagnostic yields of 96% with EBUS for station 7.[12]
2. *EUS-FNA* has been used successfully for sampling station 7 and reportedly has a diagnostic yield similar to that of EBUS-TBNA.[24] Although this technique is suitable for assessing LNs in the posterior part of levels 4 L, 5, and 7, and in the inferior mediastinum at levels 8 and 9, EUS alone has limited value for complete staging because right-sided LNs usually are inaccessible. Therefore EUS was not offered in this case.

3. *Mediastinoscopy:* This open surgical biopsy technique is performed with the patient under general anesthesia. It could be recommended in this patient if endoscopic sampling of station 7 is negative for malignancy or is otherwise nondiagnostic.[12] Rates of morbidity and mortality are low (2% and 0.08%, respectively).[9] The average sensitivity of mediastinoscopy in detecting mediastinal node involvement from cancer is approximately 80%, and the average false-negative (FN) rate is approximately 10%[9]; half (range, 42% to 57%) of FN cases were due to nodes that were not accessible by the mediastinoscope. Sampling of station 7 is usually straightforward. The procedure involves an incision just above the suprasternal notch (Figure 18-3), insertion of a mediastinoscope alongside the trachea (Figure 18-4) and, ideally, systematic exploration and biopsy under visual guidance of at least one node from up to five nodal stations (2R, 4R, 7, 4 L, and 2 L), unless none are present after dissection in the nodal region. It is recommended to always biopsy the right and left lower paratracheal and subcarinal nodes. In this case, after risks and benefits were discussed, our patient preferred that we proceed with an endoscopic needle aspiration technique.
4. *Video-assisted thoracic surgery (VATS):* This procedure is usually reserved for subaortic (station 5) and anterior mediastinal (station 6) nodes. It can also be used for LN levels that are not accessible by routine mediastinoscopy (stations 8 and 9), in case these LN stations cannot be accessed by EUS-FNA, or when EUS-FNA specimens are nondiagnostic.

Figure 18-4 Mediastinoscopy step by step. **A,** Palpation. **B,** Dissection. **C,** Test puncture. **D,** Biopsy. (*Courtesy Ramon Rami-Porta, MD, Barcelona, Spain.*)

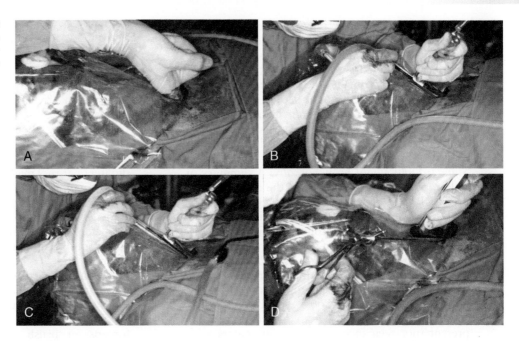

The procedure is limited to assessment of only one side of the mediastinum (i.e., the side of the thoracoscopy). Sensitivity varies from 37% to 100%. Even in studies restricted to patients with enlarged nodes, sensitivity ranges from 50% to 100%. No mortality is reported from VATS for mediastinal staging, and complications are few, occurring in only 12 of 669 patients (average, 2%; range, 0 to 9%).[9] VATS can also be used to further evaluate T stage, especially for detecting or excluding T4 lesions that preclude resection. True disease has been shown to be absent in 38% of patients (range, 29% to 50%) with radiographically suspected T4 involvement. Our patient did not have a separate tumor nodule in an ipsilateral lobe, and the primary tumor was not adjacent to the heart, trachea, carina, recurrent laryngeal nerve, or esophagus; however, it was relatively close to the aorta and the vertebral body (see Figure 18-1).

5. *Combined EUS and EBUS:* This should enable a complete evaluation of the mediastinum because of the complementary reach of each technique. Hwangbo et al.[25] and Herth et al.[26] reported on complete endosonographic staging of NSCLC using just a single EBUS scope to perform both EBUS and EUS. EUS-FNA using the same EBUS scope could be used as an add-on to EBUS only for those patients in whom nodes were inaccessible or difficult to reach by EBUS. As expected, this approach proved useful for sampling left lower paratracheal nodes (4 L), the aortopulmonary window (station 5), and the lower mediastinum (stations 8 and 9) but not for sampling station 7.

For Diagnosing the Pulmonary Nodule

An alternative approach in this case is to proceed directly with diagnosing the pulmonary nodule rather than sampling the PET-negative subcentimeter LN 7. In fact, a bayesian model suggests that the post-test probability of malignant involvement is very low (6%) if the mediastinum is normal on both CT and PET.[27] One meta-analysis found a similar post-test probability for N2 disease of 5% for LNs smaller than 15 mm in the short axis on CT in patients with a negative PET result. Some experts suggest that patients in this group should be referred for thoracotomy and complete lymph node dissection, without prior mediastinoscopy.[28] This approach could be justifiable in our patient with a high pretest probability for malignancy, and one could argue that even biopsying the pulmonary nodule may not be necessary before surgery because the risk for malignancy is high, given the patient's history. Moreover, diagnostic bronchoscopic modalities have poor NPV for pulmonary nodules, prompting some authorities to advise against their routine use in patients with a high clinical likelihood of early-stage and surgically resectable lung cancer. In such cases, a negative result would still require surgical resection. Surgical removal of ultimately benign nodules has been reported in 20% and 49% of cases, meaning that many patients with benign nodules have been unnecessarily subjected to surgical resection.[29]

Bronchoscopic procedures might be best applied to confirm a cancer diagnosis in patients when an extensive resection is planned, in high-risk patients before surgery, in medically inoperable patients with early-stage disease who are candidates for high-dose radiation treatments, and in patients with advanced disease but without alternatives for safer, less-invasive biopsy (e.g., solitary lung mass with brain metastasis). In such cases, a CT-guided approach may be reasonable, especially if the lesion is accessible (pleural based) and the risk of pneumothorax is not consequential. The patient and his spouse were provided with descriptions of the following modalities:

1. *CT-guided transthoracic needle aspiration (TTNA):* This technique has a high yield and low cost for pulmonary nodule diagnosis but is associated with

frequent occurrence of pneumothorax (20% to 50%), with approximately 7% of patients requiring chest tube drainage.[30] Certain lesions, such as the one seen in our patient, are difficult to access or increase risk for pneumothorax because of their small size or their location, or because of surrounding emphysematous lung parenchyma.[31] Distance from the pleura affects diagnostic accuracy, which drops to 60% or less when the needle path length exceeds 40 mm.[32]

2. *Standard white light bronchoscopy:* A summary of publications prepared as part of the dissemination of ACCP lung cancer guidelines suggests that for lesions smaller than 2 cm, the sensitivity of bronchoscopy is only 34%.[33] Bronchoscopic lung biopsy is unreliable for biopsies of small peripheral lesions, and diagnostic yields as low as 14% have been reported for peripheral lesions smaller than 2 cm.[34] This has led to recommendations for CT-guided approaches and suggestions that bronchoscopy should be performed only if an air bronchogram is present (not seen in our case) or in centers with expertise in using newer techniques.[35]

3. *Ultrathin bronchoscopy:* Bronchoscopes with working channels of 1.2 to 1.7 mm allow insertion of small biopsy forceps. One study targeted peripheral lesions with a mean diameter of 21.7 mm (range, 10 to 40 mm).[36] The overall diagnostic yield was 60%, which was incrementally only 8.6% greater than that attained after the use of standard bronchoscopy. In a second phase of this study, 40.6% of patients with lesions measuring 12 to 55 mm (mean, 24.4 mm) and with negative on-site rapid cytology after standard bronchoscopy had a diagnosis confirmed by ultrathin bronchoscopy. In the largest case series published to date, 102 patients with peripheral lung lesions underwent bronchoscopy with a 3.5 mm thin bronchoscope with a 1.7 mm working channel.[37] Transbronchial biopsies (1.5 mm forceps) and bronchial washings with 10 to 20 mL of saline were performed under fluoroscopic guidance. An overall diagnostic yield of 69% was attained in lesions measuring between 1.1 and 7.6 cm (mean, 3.4 cm).

4. *Electromagnetic navigational bronchoscopy (ENB):* This technique uses an electromagnetic field to track a locatable guide in real time, correlating its position in the airways with a patient's CT scan. A path to a peripheral lung lesion can be planned and the locatable guide advanced toward it with the use of a steerable probe through the working channel of a standard bronchoscope. Once the guide has reached the lesion, it is removed, leaving a guide sheath (GS) in place through which forceps, brushes, or needles can be advanced. Data from a total of 285 patients showed diagnostic yields between 59% and 77% overall, and between 54% and 75% in nodules measuring 3 cm or less.[30] Actual yields may be lower given concerns with study design; inclusion of nonspecific benign features is confirmed only by clinical follow-up, but they are included in the definition of positive results. Another

concern pertains to the high cost of disposables. At the time of this writing, the list price of an ENB system is $150,000 or more with various other charges.[38] The ENB system has been found to be safe, however, with an average pneumothorax rate of less than 3%. It appears particularly effective in patients whose lesion size and location are beyond those ensuring effectiveness of conventional white light bronchoscopy, who have a history of nondiagnostic procedures, and who are not surgical candidates or are not medically suitable for transthoracic needle aspiration or surgery.

5. *High-frequency endobronchial ultrasonography:* Radial-type 20 MHz ultrasound probes with outer diameters of 1.4 mm and 1.8 mm coupled with corresponding guiding sheaths, which can fit into 2.0 mm and 2.8 mm working channels, respectively, can be used to visualize pulmonary nodules (current cost in the United States ranges from $3000 to $6000, but probes can potentially last for 50 to 75 examinations).[39] These guide a needle, forceps, or brush placed through the sheath to perform the biopsy. EBUS-guided biopsies of peripheral pulmonary lesions improve accuracy and sensitivity compared with conventional transbronchial biopsies; improved sensitivity is most apparent in smaller peripheral lesions, and when the EBUS probe is seen within rather than adjacent to the lesion.[30] Investigators have compared 140 prospective EBUS-GS bronchoscopies versus a retrospective analysis of 121 CT-TTNA procedures performed in the same institution during the same time period. Although lesion size was slightly smaller in the EBUS group (2.9 cm vs. 3.7 cm), the overall diagnostic sensitivity was similar (EBUS 66% and CT-TTNA 64%).[40] EBUS-GS had higher sensitivity for lesions not touching the visceral pleura compared with lesions touching the visceral pleura (74% vs. 35%). Rates of pneumothorax and tube thoracostomy were significantly greater in the CT-TTNA group compared with the EBUS-GS group (28% vs. 1% for pneumothorax; 6% vs. 0% for tube thoracostomy; $P < .001$), and fewer pneumothoraces were observed in the CT-TTNA group when lesions were pleural based (2.6% vs. 31.7%). These results suggest that pleural-based lesions are preferably accessed using CT-TTNA, given the low risk of pneumothorax and the poor yield of EBUS in this setting.

6. *Multimodal bronchoscopic approach:* Some systems provide bronchoscopists with information on the best path to take, offer the ability to take that path, and confirm that the destination has been reached.[30] The combination of ENB, which offers maneuverability and the path to the nodule, and EBUS, which confirms that the destination has been reached, has been the subject of a randomized trial. Once the GS position is confirmed via EBUS to be in the lesion of interest, the ultrasound probe is removed and a biopsy forceps advanced to the correct location. In a three-way study design, 118 patients with peripheral lung lesions (mean size, 2.6 cm) underwent

ENB, EBUS, or a combination of techniques using diagnostic yield as the primary outcome measure.[41] Diagnostic yields for ENB (59%), EBUS (69%), and the combination (88%) were statistically significant. The NPV for combined ENB and EBUS was 75%, which is similar to that for CT-TTNA.[33]

Cost-Effectiveness

Our patient's nodule was too peripheral and too small to be visualized or sampled by standard bronchoscopy. After discussion of the case with our interventional radiology colleagues, its size and location were deemed not suitable for CT-TTNA (it was small, far from the pleura, and close to the descending aorta). The patient could possibly have benefited from one of the newer bronchoscopic modalities but also had evidence of a small subcarinal LN, sampling of which offered diagnosis and staging simultaneously. He could have been offered mediastinoscopy, but according to some data, sensitivity and FN rates appear similar for videomediastinoscopy and EBUS-TBNA, especially for the subcarinal node, a very easily sampled node, during EBUS-TBNA. In general, however, EBUS-TBNA studies have tended to include patients with discreet LN enlargement, in whom TBNA was done more for confirmation of suspected mediastinal LN disease than for ruling out LN disease that was believed was unlikely to be present, given findings on imaging. This would clearly tend to inflate the sensitivity of EBUS-TBNA and to reduce the false-negative rate.[22]

Published cost-effectiveness analyses based on mathematical modeling in the United States, the United Kingdom, and Singapore show that EBUS may be less expensive than mediastinoscopy.[42-44] If one considers the need for general anesthesia, as is seen in most studies showing high yields, then EBUS-TBNA may not be a cheaper alternative to mediastinoscopy, especially when the latter is performed as part of thoracotomy, as is standard in many centers.[22]

Informed Consent

The concept of informed consent protects patients by providing them with complete information on which to base an informed decision. This is of particular importance when choices among interventions are complex. Informed consent also helps to protect health care providers from liability, provided that procedures are properly executed according to prevailing community standards of care and without negligence. From a legal standpoint, consent for a medical procedure must be both informed and effective: (1) To be informed, patients must be given information about the procedure relevant to their individual situation; (2) for consent to be effective, persons undergoing the procedure should be able to demonstrate, in their own words, their understanding of the procedure or treatment.

Most important, the informed consent process gives health care providers and patients an opportunity to consider and reconsider diagnostic and therapeutic strategies that have been proposed, while respecting the patient's wishes and values; it allows for discussion of possible risks and benefits and preparation for procedure-related events. After they had been advised of all diagnostic

alternatives, the patient and his wife agreed to proceed with EBUS-TBNA under general anesthesia. They were informed of potential failure to obtain a definite diagnosis despite successful LN visualization and sampling. Feedback communication techniques were used to confirm patient understanding of his disease process and the procedure being proposed. Both the patient and his spouse were able to accurately describe the procedure, its alternatives, and potential adverse events.

Techniques and Results

Anesthesia and Perioperative Care

EBUS-TBNA is performed with the patient under moderate or deep sedation or under general anesthesia using laryngeal mask airway (LMA) or endotracheal tubes. Moderate sedation may result in better cost savings/safety ratios when compared with general anesthesia.[45] One study evaluated two different techniques for topically anesthetizing the airway with lidocaine during EBUS-TBNA under moderate sedation: standard injection through the working channel, and the spray catheter application. All patients received nebulized lidocaine followed by posterior oropharyngeal lidocaine via atomizer and a cotton ball swab using McGill forceps. Lidocaine delivery via the spray catheter reduced the number of significant coughing episodes compared with standard working channel injection, but no statistical differences between groups in terms of dosage of lidocaine or intravenous sedation medications used were noted.[46] Because of the subcentimeter size of the node in this elderly patient, moderate sedation could have resulted in excessive cough and respiratory movements, significant artifacts, suboptimal ultrasound image acquisition, and potentially nondiagnostic intervention. General anesthesia and endotracheal intubation with a No. 9 ETT were planned to secure the airway during EBUS bronchoscopy.

For this elderly patient, possible difficult airway, oxygenation, ventilation, and hemodynamic problems need to be discussed with the anesthesiologist before the procedure is begun. Attention should be paid to edentulous elderly patients, who are harder to ventilate with a bag-valve mask. Loss of upper airway muscle tone and loose lips unsupported by teeth make mask seal and maintenance of a patent airway more difficult.[47] However, this patient had normal teeth. Because baseline oxygen saturation is often low in the elderly, adequate preoxygenation may be difficult or impossible. In addition, elders desaturate more rapidly than healthy, younger patients. The safe apnea period before the airway is secured therefore is decreased despite best attempts at preoxygenation compared with routine intubation in younger, healthy adults.[48] Oxyhemoglobin saturation should be maintained above 90% whenever possible, because elderly patients are more susceptible to hypoxic insult with even brief periods of oxygen desaturation, resulting in permanent cardiac and neurologic damage. Because the medications used for intubation cause more pronounced hypopnea and hypotension in the elderly than in younger, healthy patients, it is generally best to reduce the doses of short-acting opioids used for pretreatment and of induction agents by approximately 30% to 50%.[49] These issues were readdressed during the mandatory procedural pause (time-out) process before induction and intubation.

Technique and Instrumentation

We used the Olympus BF-UC 160F-OL8 Hybrid scope with a 2.0 mm working channel, a 6.9 mm outside diameter, and a 7.5 MHz frequency curved linear array transducer (Olympus Optical Co., Ltd., Tokyo, Japan).

Anatomic Dangers and Other Risks

The subcarinal node is usually safe to sample because of the lack of major blood vessels or lung parenchyma adjacent to the node. However, the left atrium is inferior to the node (see Figure 18-2), and a potential risk for penetrating the pericardium, especially with the needle at its full extension, is present.[21] The risk of puncturing this structure may be reduced by using Doppler mode imaging, locking the needle at the desired length, and maintaining visual control of the tip of the needle at all times (see video on ExpertConsult.com) (Video IV.18.1). Although sterile, the needles used for EBUS-TBNA may become contaminated by oropharyngeal secretions, resulting in bacteremia.[50] This risk may be higher and clinically significant when multiple passes are performed, and when immunosuppressive therapies are initiated shortly after the procedure.[51] During the time-out process, we addressed the need for antibiotics. Although no evidence for routine use of antibiotic prophylaxis with EBUS has been found, some EUS researchers report use of a 3 day course for patients with necrotic lymph nodes.[52]

Results and Procedure-Related Complications

After intubation with a No. 9.0 ETT, we performed standard white light bronchoscopy to clear secretions and ensure absence of endobronchial disease. Then a complete sonographic evaluation of the mediastinal and hilar structures performed using the EBUS scope showed no other LNs; we positioned the scope in the right mainstem bronchus at the level of the main carina and oriented the transducer medially toward the 9 o'clock position to visualize the subcarinal node and proceeded with EBUS-TBNA in a step-by-step fashion.[53] A total of four aspirates were performed. No core tissue was obtained. With the use of rapid on-site cytology examination (ROSE), malignant cells were seen, suggesting adenocarcinoma. If ROSE is not utilized, the best yield seems to occur with three aspirates per station (sensitivity 91.7%, NPV 96.0%, and accuracy 97.2%). Two aspirates per LN station can be acceptable when at least one tissue core specimen is obtained.[54] However, if the operator believes that targeting is inadequate or insufficient, another aspirate should be performed. In our case, the diagnosis was made after the second aspirate; two additional aspirates were performed to prepare a cell block for staining and potential assessment of epidermal growth factor receptor mutation if considered appropriate by the oncology team.[55] The case lasted 35 minutes from induction to extubation. After extubation, the patient was monitored for 2 hours and was discharged home the same day.

No procedure- or anesthesia-related complications were reported.

Long-Term Management

Outcome Assessment

Final results from EBUS-TBNA showed primary lung adenocarcinoma (Figure 18-5). Further clinical staging was performed, and the patient was discussed in our multidisciplinary chest conference, noting that the primary tumor was 1.5 cm in its greatest dimension and without bronchoscopic evidence of airway involvement could be classified as T1a. He underwent brain magnetic resonance imaging (MRI), which showed no metastases. Results of EBUS-TBNA sampling of the subcarinal node prompted N factor designation as stage N2, prompting disease classification as clinical stage IIIA NSCLC.[56*] Nodal metastases (single or multiple station) recognized by prethoracotomy staging (mediastinoscopy, other nodal biopsy such as EBUS, or PET scan) prompted subclassification as IIIA3.[57] Stage IIIA represents approximately 20% of all patients with NSCLC from the International Association for the Study of Lung Cancer (IASLC) database; this information is useful for assessing prognosis but not necessarily for dictating treatment, especially in cases of stage III lung cancer; the estimated 5 year survival for clinical stage IIIA is 19%, and the median survival time is 14 months (cases treated by all modalities of care, including multimodality treatment). Treatment options were discussed, and given the patient's normal lung function and excellent performance status, he was deemed both resectable and operable.

Referral

The patient was referred for thoracic surgery. Therapeutic alternatives were discussed, and right lower lobectomy with complete lymph node dissection was performed. His hospital course was complicated by aspiration pneumonia in the remaining right lung, but he was discharged home on oral antibiotics after 7 days; a surgical specimen revealed a 1.8 × 1.3 × 1.3 cm adenocarcinoma without visceral pleural invasion but with lymphatic invasion and two mediastinal stations positive for metastatic disease (station 4R and station 7); these findings were consistent with pathologic stage IIIA, for which estimated 5 year survival is 24% and median survival time is 22 months.[56] The patient was referred to oncology for adjuvant treatment.

Follow-up Tests and Procedures

Post discharge, the patient had a follow-up visit within 2 weeks with the thoracic surgeon and a plan to continue follow-up with the surgical team for at least 3 to 6 months.[58] Surveillance chest radiographs showed resolution of the pneumonic infiltrate. The medical oncologist recommended initiation of carboplatin/pemetrexed for

---

*The extent of clinical staging can vary from a clinical evaluation alone (history and physical examination) to extensive imaging (CT-PET scans) or invasive staging techniques; of note, needle aspiration and surgical staging procedures such as mediastinoscopy are still part of clinical staging because surgical resection as a treatment has not taken place.

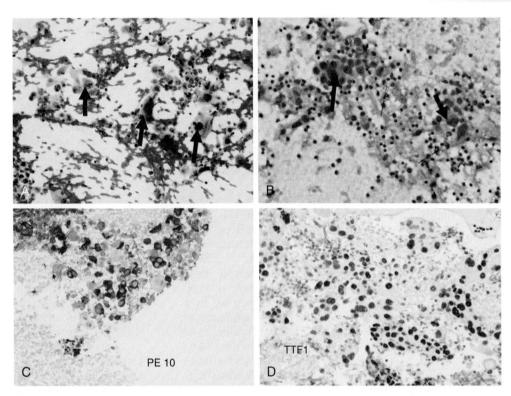

Figure 18-5 Subcarinal fine-needle aspiration with the 22 gauge endobronchial ultrasound (EBUS) needle shows poorly differentiated adenocarcinoma. Immunohistochemistry shows the malignant cells to be positive for CK7, PE10, and TTF1—an immunoprofile that supports the diagnosis of lung primary. **A,** PAP and **(B)** Diff-Quick stains show lymphocytes and macrophages with anthracotic pigment *(thin arrow)*. Also, malignant cells are noted in groups and singly with a high nuclear/cytoplasmic ratio and large nuclei and a vacuolated cytoplasm consistent with adenocarcinoma *(thick arrows)*. **C,** Cytoplasmic stain: PE10 is a monoclonal antibody that recognizes the surfactant apoprotein A in type II pneumocytes and is very specific for adenocarcinoma of the lung. **D,** Nuclear stain: TTF1 is the thyroid transcription factor-1; it is sensitive but not specific for neoplasms of primary lung and is most common in adenocarcinoma of the lung.

four cycles every 3 weeks, followed by daily radiotherapy (RT), in view of this patient's multinodal N2 disease. Analysis of 7465 patients with stage II or III NSCLC found that patients with N2 involvement had a statistically significant improved 5 year survival rate with adjuvant RT (27% vs. 20%; $P = .0077$).[59] However, the outcome of postoperative RT could be affected both by the extent of nodal involvement and by the use of adjuvant chemotherapy. For example, survival is reportedly longer among patients with N2 disease who receive postoperative RT, with a trend toward longer median survival rates noted in the chemotherapy than in the observation group.[60] Our patient completed adjuvant therapy without significant toxicity and was alive and functional 6 months later. Clinical and imaging surveillance to detect recurrence, although controversial, is being continued by the treating team in accordance with ACCP recommendations.[58]

Quality Improvement

In this case, a diagnosis of lung cancer and N2 metastasis was made using minimally invasive technology. The procedure altered management and decision making by avoiding riskier interventions. At our team meeting, we discussed the results of surgery as compared with EBUS-TBNA with regard to mediastinal staging. We questioned whether visualizing and sampling station 4R (although not identified on CT or integrated PET-CT) during EBUS would have changed management. In this case, the patient would have had multistation, microscopic N2 disease diagnosed preoperatively. Indeed, EBUS missed microscopic N2 disease in the 4R station, which could make a stronger argument for neoadjuvant chemotherapy.

We also readdressed whether we could have prevented the episode of aspiration and subsequent pneumonia that prolonged the length of stay after lung resection. Aspiration is known to be more common among the elderly with comorbid conditions and may lead to alterations in mental status. This group includes patients with swallowing dysfunction, disruption of the gastroesophageal junction, or anatomic abnormalities of the upper airway or digestive tract. Our patient had no such comorbidities, but any situation in which altered mental status and loss of airway protection mechanisms occurs creates a risk for aspiration.[61] During the perioperative period, these factors include depressed consciousness related to general anesthesia, supine position, and drugs such as propofol and opioids that reduce lower esophageal sphincter pressure and promote gastroesophageal reflux. Aspiration of gastric contents during anesthesia can be prevented by adhering to National Anesthesiology Society guidelines.[62] Water and other clear liquids (e.g., tea, coffee, soda water, apple and pulp-free orange juice) are allowed up to 2 hours before anesthesia in otherwise healthy adults scheduled for elective surgery. The fasting period after intake of solids should not be shorter than 6 hours. Careful review of the medical record revealed that all of these recommendations had been followed in this patient.

DISCUSSION POINTS

1. Describe major elements of informed consent.

   The American Medical Association states that informed consent is a process that should disclose and discuss the following:

- Patient diagnosis and related clinical issues
- Nature and purpose of the proposed procedure
- Risks and benefits of the proposed procedure
- Alternatives, regardless of cost or coverage by health insurance
- Potential risks and benefits associated with choosing the alternatives
- Risks and benefits of not receiving or undergoing treatments or procedures

2. Describe pros and cons pertaining to staging the PET-CT–negative mediastinum in patients with known or suspected lung cancer.

   2.1. *Pro:* Several studies have evaluated patients highly suspicious for NSCLC with CT scans showing no enlarged LNs (no node >1 cm) and a negative PET finding of the mediastinum in those who underwent EBUS-TBNA.[15,16] EBUS-TBNA was found to accurately sample even small mediastinal nodes (5 to 10 mm), thereby avoiding unnecessary surgical exploration in 1 out of 6 patients who had no CT evidence of mediastinal disease. The 17% prevalence of mediastinal LN metastases detected with EBUS-TBNA was similar to that of surgical studies evaluating patients with negative mediastinal CT. Thus some authorities suggest that EBUS-TBNA should be used to accurately sample and stage patients with clinical stage I lung cancer with no evidence of mediastinal involvement on CT and PET, and that potentially operable patients with no signs of mediastinal involvement may benefit from presurgical staging with EBUS-TBNA.

   2.2. *Con:* Surgical resection is the treatment of choice for patients who appear to have clinical stage I or II disease when pathologic involvement of mediastinal LNs is not detected preoperatively or by frozen section before definitive tumor resection.

      2.2.1. According to some data, the post-test probability for N2 disease is 5% for LNs measuring less than 15 mm on CT in patients with a negative PET, suggesting that these patients should be referred directly for thoracotomy, because the yield of mediastinoscopy will be extremely low.[63] Despite careful preoperative staging, mediastinal nodal involvement is identified in the final pathologic specimen in up to 20% of these patients. For patients found to have such microscopic nodal disease, studies have demonstrated that adjuvant chemotherapy can result in a significant survival benefit. Treatment guidelines for NSCLC recommend cisplatin-based regimens in patients with resected stage III disease if the patient's overall medical condition permits.[64]

      2.2.2. In patients with NSCLC who have incidental (occult/microscopic) N2 disease (IIIA2) found at surgical resection, and in whom complete resection of the LN and primary tumor is technically possible, completion of the planned lung resection and mediastinal lymphadenectomy is recommended.[57]

      2.2.3. Results from studies show that patients with nonbulky (i.e., <2 cm) and non-multistation N2 LN involvement have acceptable cure rates after primary surgical resection. In fact, induction therapy was never compared with postoperative chemotherapy for patients with stage IIIA (N2) disease. The only studies that showed a benefit of preoperative chemotherapy for patients with stage IIIA (N2) disease included many patients who had more than what would be considered microscopically involved N2 disease.[22]

      2.2.4. In view of these data, it may not be particularly important to identify preoperatively patients with microscopic N2 disease; thus preoperative invasive or minimally invasive staging (needle aspiration techniques) of CT-PET–negative mediastinum may not be justified.

3. List five reasons for a poor sample on a nodal aspiration smear.

   3.1. *Sample coagulation:* Any delay in processing the sample may result in coagulation in the needle lumen or on the slide surface and may completely hinder the process of smearing on the slide.

   3.2. *Air drying artifacts:* If a Papanicolaou stain is required (Figure 18-6), the smear must be wet when fixative is applied. Otherwise, staining artifacts are the rule. Conversely, with Diff-Quick stain, the quantity of sample fluid must be just enough to smear, enabling the sample to dry as soon as possible.

   3.3. *Air bubbles:* Their presence in the material smeared on the slide causes uneven distribution.

   3.4. *Thick smear:* The correct smear technique results in a monolayer of cell distribution on the slide surface. Overlapping cells, which can be avoided by placing only a small drop of sample on the slide surface, hinder precise evaluation of cellular details, making diagnosis difficult or impossible.

   3.5. *Crushed smear:* This results from excessive pressure applied while the sample is smeared. This can completely destroy diagnostic material.

Expert Commentary

provided by Kemp H. Kernstine Sr., MD, PhD

This interesting case illustrates several important features pertaining to evaluation and treatment of solitary pulmonary nodules and early non–small cell lung cancer (NSCLC). This patient is elderly—over 80 years of age; the average age of the lung cancer patient is approximately 70 to 72 years.[65] The patient is asymptomatic with an Eastern Cooperative Oncology Group (ECOG) or a Zubrod Performance status score of 0.

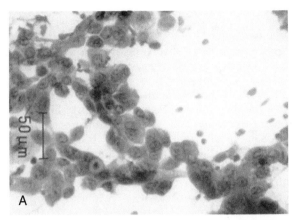

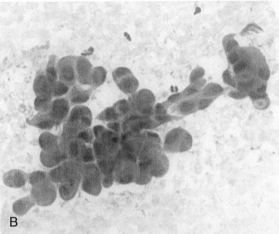

Figure 18-6 Needle biopsy of peripheral lung nodule from a different patient shows adenocarcinoma. Figure parts **A** and **B** are from the same sampling and staining process. **A,** The slide was correctly smeared and fixed while wet, giving a precise color profile (pale blue). **B,** The slide was correctly smeared but fixed when completely dried, giving a wrong color profile (pinkish): same neoplastic cells, same staining procedure, but different color profile. *(Courtesy G. Marciano, with permission.)*

Zubrod Performance status seems to be less subjective than Karnofsky Performance status.[3] To stage the mediastinum and evaluate for potential metastatic disease, positron emission tomography (PET)-computed tomography (CT) was performed (superior to CT or PET alone[66]). The right lower lobe lesion is small, close to the mediastinum and diaphragm, where diaphragmatic motion and high fluorodeoxyglucose (FDG) uptake of the heart can make it difficult to assess FDG uptake, also referred to as the standard uptake value (SUV), in a solitary pulmonary nodule.[67] The patient also has an FDG-PET–negative and subcentimeter subcarinal lymph node, along with the non-hilar solitary pulmonary nodule, which has a low probability of possessing metastatic disease; yet endobronchial ultrasound (EBUS) was performed and demonstrated metastatic mediastinal involvement.[68]

Rather than attempting to diagnose the solitary pulmonary nodule, clinicians first performed mediastinal evaluation using EBUS. By identifying subcarinal metastatic disease, they were able to achieve a diagnosis and stage the patient with this low-risk technique. The specificity of this test is 100%.[69] The discovery of malignant disease speaks to the inaccuracy of CT, PET, and PET-CT in staging mediastinal lymph nodes. For CT, the pooled sensitivity is 51% and the specificity is 86%, whereas the pooled sensitivity of PET is 74% and the specificity is 85%.[70] PET-CT is the better test, given the coincident anatomic and metabolic assessment. Its sensitivity ranges from 40% to 84%, and its specificity ranges from 80% to 98%.[66,68] However, for specifically addressing the prediction of N2 disease, the negative predictive value is 12% to 81%, and the positive predictive value is 41% to 83%.[71] This case also illustrates the inaccuracy of EBUS, a procedure that not only is dependent on the experience and skill of the professionals performing it, but also is associated with a certain false negativity rate of up to 28%.[72] The 4R nodal station was staged as negative for metastatic disease, whereas the thoracotomy demonstrated malignant disease. Had this information been available, this patient might have been encouraged to pursue nonsurgical treatment options.

In spite of the discovery that the patient had mediastinal metastatic disease, with a clinical stage of T1aN2M0, stage IIIA (UICC 7), surgical resection was chosen as the primary method of treatment, rather than definitive chemoradiotherapy or possibly treatment with induction/neoadjuvant therapy. Guidelines of the American College of Chest Physicians (ACCP) and the European Society of Medical Oncology (ESMO) advocate that stage IIIA patients treated surgically should be in clinical trials, representing a distinct divergence from what had been recommended in the past, and that chemoradiotherapy should be considered the standard of care.[57] Surgical resection in elderly patients is associated with significant morbidity and mortality, as is illustrated in this case.[73] Also, it is unclear whether the surgical resection offered a survival benefit for this patient.

Concerning the choice of a neoadjuvant chemotherapy treatment plan versus surgical resection, one of several strategies recommended in the National Comprehensive Cancer Network (NCCN) guidelines is that once the patient has completed two cycles of therapy, he should be reassessed with PET-CT, and the size and SUV of the primary lesion calculated to assess response, looking again for metastatic disease.[74] EBUS and endoscopic ultrasound (EUS) could be repeated to determine whether the mediastinum responded to therapy and to ascertain the absence of subdiaphragmatic disease. If the primary lesion does not respond and/or newly discovered metastatic disease is present, and/or if the patient's clinical status deteriorates, the patient could be treated with definitive chemoradiotherapy or with alternative neoadjuvant chemotherapy, or radiotherapy (or both radiation and chemotherapy) could be added, followed by surgical resection. This last approach is most certainly very aggressive in this elderly patient. If repeat EBUS/EUS is negative for metastatic disease, then cervical mediastinoscopy could be recommended.[72] If results show no metastatic disease, the patient would be an appropriate candidate for lobectomy. If EBUS/EUS or mediastinoscopy demonstrates continued mediastinal metastatic disease, on the other hand, then surgical resection provides no survival advantage,[75] especially given the surgical risks in an 80+-year-old patient.

The performance of a thorough inspection bronchoscopy should be highlighted. Performed during the EBUS/EUS procedure, it provides critical information before surgical resection is undertaken. The surgeon needs to know of any anatomic airway variation, especially in cases for which a minimally invasive approach is planned. Synchronous lung cancers or premalignant lesions that may change the surgical approach may be found. These are more common in patients with squamous cell lung cancers. The presence of airway edema, erythema, excessive or turbid secretions, or foreign bodies may alter the surgical timing and approach.

Ruckdeschel grading of nodal involvement provides this patient with a IIIA3 designation.[57] We know that the CT finding of grossly enlarged, multidensity mediastinal lymph nodes—Ruckdeschel nodal grading IIIA4—portends a poor prognosis, and that these patients are much less likely to benefit from surgical resection. Other features of lymph node pathology that are important to assess include the presence or absence of (1) contralateral involvement, (2) multinodal station involvement, (3) transcapsular involvement, (4) complete replacement of the lymph node architecture with tumor, (5) matted nodes and the total number of involved nodes, and (6) the percentage of lymph nodes that are involved. The discovery of gross nodal involvement on CT has a high degree of specificity and, if necessary, is easily confirmed with EBUS/EUS or other minimally invasive techniques, such as mediastinoscopy.

Given the plan for surgical resection, and given the patient's age, cervical mediastinoscopy might have been helpful. A frequent misunderstanding among lung cancer specialists is that mediastinoscopy is the same across all institutions. It is not. Results are dependent on the training and experience of the surgeon, available technology in the institution, and the technique used by the surgeon, that is, fine-needle aspiration cytology, whole node biopsy, or complete nodal resection through a mediastinoscope,[76] a video-assisted mediastinoscope,[77] or a transcervical extended mediastinal lymphadenectomy (TEMLA).[78,79] To illustrate the status of mediastinoscopy in the United States, Little et al. reviewed the American College of Surgeons Commission on Cancer database and found that 53% of mediastinoscopies involved no nodal tissue.[80] In an additional 25%, only one node was biopsied, totaling nearly 75% of all mediastinoscopies in which insufficient tissue was obtained to adequately stage the mediastinum. It is this author's opinion that it is likely that most patients undergoing mediastinoscopy do not meet the ACCP recommendation of resecting at least five lymph node station biopsies/resections, that is, stations 2R, 4R, 7, 2 L, and 4 L.[70] Resection of nodes

and perinodal tissue appears to improve the sensitivity of the technique.[78]

Had the patient's suspicious nodule been found in the left upper lobe, left video-assisted thoracic surgery (VATS) biopsy or resection of the aorto-pulmonary (AP) window node might have been performed to assess the AP window. As an alternative, historically, a mediastinotomy (aka Chamberlain procedure) can approach the AP window directly.[81] Today, many clinicians use instead a mediastinoscope through a second intercostal space incision to accomplish the same goal, with less postoperative pain. A transcervical approach (i.e., extended transcervical mediastinoscopy or Ginsberg procedure[82]) may also be used. Each of these procedures requires experience and knowledge of indications and limitations, but all provide a sufficient sampling of AP window tissue.

Another interesting feature of this patient's case is the surgical approach selected. It is likely that the patient would have benefited from a minimally invasive resection performed by VATS[83] or by a robotic technique.[84] The likelihood of sufficient surgical resection is equally as good as with a conventional open technique, but reduced pain, an earlier return to preoperative functional status, and a shorter hospital stay are likely.[83] In patients who have not undergone induction therapy, we attempt to resect at least 15 or 16 lymph nodes from three or four nodal stations.[85]

This patient aspirated and developed pneumonia during the postoperative period—not an uncommon finding. The surgical team must be acutely aware of this complication. These patients are intubated, often with large double-lumen endotracheal tubes that stretch the posterior pharynx. This potentially affects swallowing coordination. In addition, sedatives and narcotics used postoperatively have varying degrees of effects on normal swallowing. Many of these patients, especially the elderly, have dysphagia before undergoing surgery. As a result, 20% to 30% of post lung resection patients aspirate—a rate that increases with age.[86,87] Having a high index of suspicion, delaying oral intake until the patient is fully awake, and consulting with the speech therapist should help to minimize this complication. The patient was discharged in 7 days, however, which is within the average amount of time that the typical patient remains hospitalized, in spite of the pneumonia.

The estimate of this patient facing a 5 year survival of 24% is fairly generous. In my opinion, survival is likely to be less than 10% because the patient has disease in two different mediastinal nodal stations and is older than 80 years of age. His comorbidities are low and he has an excellent performance status, but the overwhelming issue is the extent of his metastatic disease and his capability for tolerating adjuvant therapy. Typically, 60% of postsurgical NSCLC patients will tolerate such treatment, a therapy that for this patient is absolutely essential for long-term survival. In my opinion, given this patient's age, postoperative status, and course, he is much less likely to tolerate therapy. The most likely sites for recurrence are local and systemic and are fairly equally distributed. Concurrent or sequential radiation therapy might be of benefit for reducing the likelihood of local recurrence, although concurrent therapy is aggressive and may reduce his ability to tolerate the four to six cycles of intended treatment. With excellent care and preemptive support, this patient might have 1 to 2 years of good quality of life.

REFERENCES

1. Schag CC, Heinrich RL, Ganz PA. Karnofsky performance status revisited: reliability, validity, and guidelines. *J Clin Oncol.* 1984; 2:187-193.
2. Oken MM, Creech RH, Tormey DC, et al. Toxicity and response criteria of the Eastern Cooperative Oncology Group. *Am J Clin Oncol.* 1982;5:649-655.
3. Buccheri G, Ferrigno D, Tamburini M. Karnofsky and ECOG performance status scoring in lung cancer: a prospective, longitudinal study of 536 patients from a single institution. *Eur J Cancer.* 1996;32:1135-1141.
4. De Leyn P, Vansteenkiste J, Cuypers P, et al. Role of cervical mediastinoscopy in staging of non-small cell lung cancer without enlarged mediastinal lymph nodes on CT scan. *Eur J Cardiothorac Surg.* 1997;12:706-712.
5. Meyers BF, Haddad F, Siegel BA, et al. Cost-effectiveness of routine mediastinoscopy in computed tomography- and positron emission tomography-screened patients with stage I lung cancer. *J Thorac Cardiovasc Surg.* 2006;131:822-829.
6. Birim O, Kappetein AP, Stijnen T, et al. Meta-analysis of positron tomographic and computed tomographic imaging in detecting mediastinal lymph node metastases in nonsmall cell lung cancer. *Ann Thorac Surg.* 2005;79:375-382.
7. Lee PC, Port JL, Korst RJ, et al. Risk factors for occult mediastinal metastases in clinical stage I non-small cell lung cancer. *Ann Thorac Surg.* 2007;84:177-181.
8. De Leyn P, Lardinois D, Van Schil PE, et al. ESTS guidelines for preoperative lymph node staging for non-small cell lung cancer. *Eur J Cardiothorac Surg.* 2007;32:1-8.
9. Detterbeck FC, Jantz MA, Wallace M, et al, American College of Chest Physicians. Invasive mediastinal staging of lung cancer: ACCP evidence-based clinical practice guidelines (2nd edition). *Chest.* 2007;132(3 suppl):202S-220S.
10. Al-Sarraf N, Aziz R, Gately K, et al. Pattern and predictors of occult mediastinal lymph node involvement in non-small cell lung cancer patients with negative mediastinal uptake on positron emission tomography. *Eur J Cardiothorac Surg.* 2008;33:104-109.
11. Chhajed PN, Bernasconi M, Gambazzi F, et al. Combining bronchoscopy and positron emission tomography for the diagnosis of the small pulmonary nodule < or = 3 cm. *Chest.* 2005;128: 3558-3564.
12. Herth FJ, Eberhardt R, Vilmann P, et al. Real-time endobronchial ultrasound guided transbronchial needle aspiration for sampling mediastinal lymph nodes. *Thorax.* 2006;61:795-798.
13. Chin R Jr, McCain TW, Lucia MA, et al. Transbronchial needle aspiration in diagnosing and staging lung cancer: how many aspirates are needed? *Am J Respir Crit Care Med.* 2002;166: 377-381.
14. Sevransky JE, Haponik EF. Respiratory failure in elderly patients. *Clin Geriatr Med.* 2003;19:205-224.
15. Herth FJ, Ernst A, Eberhardt R, et al. Endobronchial ultrasound-guided transbronchial needle aspiration of lymph nodes in the radiologically normal mediastinum. *Eur Respir J.* 2006;28: 910-914.
16. Herth FJ, Eberhardt R, Krasnik M, et al. Endobronchial ultrasound-guided transbronchial needle aspiration of lymph nodes in the radiologically and positron emission tomography-normal mediastinum in patients with lung cancer. *Chest.* 2008;133:887-891.
17. Colt HG, Murgu S, Davoudi M. EBUS step-by-step, You Tube, posted August 2010. Available at: http://www.youtube.com/watch?v=Z9FdgVx_xrM&feature=related. Accessed February 20, 2011.
18. Ernst A, Silvestri GA, Johnstone D, American College of Chest Physicians. Interventional pulmonary procedures: guidelines from the American College of Chest Physicians. *Chest.* 2003;123: 1693-1717.
19. Bolliger CT, Mathur PN, Beamis JF, et al. European Respiratory Society/American Thoracic Society. ERS/ATS statement on interventional pulmonology. *Eur Respir J.* 2002;19:356-373.
20. Murgu S, Saffari A, Davoudi M, et al. Physics of endobronchial ultrasound, You Tube, posted October 2010. Available at: http://www.youtube.com/watch?v=5cxwBjOlF-M&feature= related.Accessed February 20, 2011.
21. Varela-Lema L, Fernandez-Villar A, Ruano-Ravina A. Effectiveness and safety of endobronchial ultrasound-transbronchial needle aspiration: a systematic review. *Eur Respir J.* 2009;33:1156-1164.
22. Shrager JB. Mediastinoscopy: still the gold standard. *Ann Thorac Surg.* 2010;89:S2084-S2089.
23. Herth F, Becker HD, Ernst A. Conventional vs endobronchial ultrasound-guided transbronchial needle aspiration: a randomized trial. *Chest.* 2004;125:322-325.
24. Herth FJ, Lunn W, Eberhardt R, et al. Transbronchial versus transesophageal ultrasound-guided aspiration of enlarged mediastinal lymph nodes. *Am J Respir Crit Care Med.* 2005;171:1164-1167.
25. Hwangbo B, Lee GK, Lee HS, et al. Transbronchial and transesophageal fine-needle aspiration using an ultrasound bronchoscope in mediastinal staging of potentially operable lung cancer. *Chest.* 2010;138:795-802.
26. Herth FJ, Krasnik M, Kahn N, et al. Combined endoscopic-endobronchial ultrasound-guided fine-needle aspiration of mediastinal lymph nodes through a single bronchoscope in 150 patients with suspected lung cancer. *Chest.* 2010;138:790-794.
27. Gould MK, Kuschner WG, Rydzak CE, et al. Test performance of positron emission tomography and computed tomography for mediastinal staging in patients with non-small-cell lung cancer: a meta-analysis. *Ann Intern Med.* 2003;139:879-892.
28. de Langen AJ, Raijmakers P, Riphagen I, et al. The size of mediastinal lymph nodes and its relation with metastatic involvement: a meta-analysis. *Eur J Cardiothorac Surg.* 2006;29:26-29.
29. Bernard A, The Thorax Group. Resection of pulmonary nodules using video-assisted thoracic surgery. *Ann Thorac Surg.* 1996; 61:202-204.
30. Hergott CA, Tremblay A. Role of bronchoscopy in the evaluation of solitary pulmonary nodules. *Clin Chest Med.* 2010;31:49-63.
31. Heyer CM, Reichelt S, Peters SA, et al. Computed tomography-navigated transthoracic core biopsy of pulmonary lesions: which factors affect diagnostic yield and complication rates? *Acad Radiol.* 2008;15:1017-1026.
32. Ohno Y, Hatabu H, Takenaka D, et al. CT-guided transthoracic needle aspiration biopsy of small (< or = 20 mm) solitary pulmonary nodules. *AJR Am J Roentgenol.* 2003;180:1665-1669.
33. Rivera MP, Mehta AC, American College of Chest Physicians. Initial diagnosis of lung cancer: ACCP evidence-based clinical practice guidelines (2nd edition). *Chest.* 2007;132(3 suppl): 131S-148S.
34. Gildea TR, Mazzone PJ, Karnak D, et al. Electromagnetic navigation diagnostic bronchoscopy: a prospective study. *Am J Respir Crit Care Med.* 2006;174:982-989.
35. Gould MK, Fletcher J, Iannettoni MD, et al, American College of Chest Physicians. Evaluation of patients with pulmonary nodules: when is it lung cancer? ACCP evidence-based clinical practice guidelines (2nd edition). *Chest.* 2007;132(3 suppl):108S-130S.
36. Yamamoto S, Ueno K, Imamura F, et al. Usefulness of ultrathin bronchoscopy in diagnosis of lung cancer. *Lung Cancer.* 2004; 46:43-48.
37. Oki M, Saka H, Kitagawa C, et al. Novel thin bronchoscope with a 1.7-mm working channel for peripheral pulmonary lesions. *Eur Respir J.* 2008;32:465-471.
38. Edell E, Krier-Morrow D. Navigational bronchoscopy: overview of technology and practical considerations—new Current Procedural Terminology codes effective 2010. *Chest.* 2010;137:450-454.
39. Sheski FD, Mathur PN. Endobronchial ultrasound. *Chest.* 2008;133:264-270.
40. Fielding DI, Robinson PJ, Kurimoto N. Biopsy site selection for endobronchial ultrasound guide-sheath transbronchial biopsy of peripheral lung lesions. *Intern Med J.* 2008;38:77-84.
41. Eberhardt R, Anantham D, Ernst A, et al. Multimodality bronchoscopic diagnosis of peripheral lung lesions: a randomized controlled trial. *Am J Respir Crit Care Med.* 2007;176:36-41.
42. Medford AR, Agrawal S, Free CM, et al. A performance and theoretical cost analysis of endobronchial ultrasound-guided

transbronchial needle aspiration in a UK tertiary respiratory centre. *Q J Med.* 2009;102:859-864.

43. Harewood GC, Pascual J, Raimondo M, et al. Economic analysis of combined endoscopic and endobronchial ultrasound in the evaluation of patients with suspected non-small cell lung cancer. *Lung Cancer.* 2010;67:366-371.

44. Ang SY, Tan RW, Koh MS, et al. Economic analysis of endobronchial ultrasound (EBUS) as a tool in the diagnosis and staging of lung cancer in Singapore. *Int J Technol Assess Health Care.* 2010;26:170-174.

45. Kennedy MP, Shweihat Y, Sarkiss M, et al. Complete mediastinal and hilar lymph node staging of primary lung cancer by endobronchial ultrasound: moderate sedation or general anesthesia? *Chest.* 2008;134:1350-1351.

46. Lee HJ, Haas AR, Sterman DH, et al. Pilot randomized study comparing two techniques of airway anesthesia during curvilinear probe endobronchial ultrasound bronchoscopy (CP-EBUS). *Respirology.* 16:102-106, 2011.

47. Langeron O, Masso E, Huraux C, et al. Prediction of difficult mask ventilation. *Anesthesiology.* 2000;92:1229-1236.

48. Benumof JL, Dagg R, Benumof R. Critical hemoglobin desaturation will occur before return to an unparalyzed state following 1 mg/kg intravenous succinylcholine. *Anesthesiology.* 1997;87:979.

49. Vuyk J. Pharmacodynamics in the elderly. *Best Pract Res Clin Anaesthesiol.* 2003;17:207-218.

50. Steinfort DP, Johnson DF, Irving LB. Incidence of bacteraemia following endobronchial ultrasound-guided transbronchial needle aspiration. *Eur Respir J.* 2010;36:28-32.

51. Kouskov OS, Almeida FA, Eapen G, et al. Mediastinal infection after ultrasound-guided needle aspiration. *J Broncol Intervent Pulmonol.* 2010;17:338-341.

52. Aerts JG, Kloover J, Los J, et al. EUS-FNA of enlarged necrotic lymph nodes may cause infectious mediastinitis. *J Thorac Oncol.* 2008;3:1191-1193.

53. Colt HG, Murgu S, Davoudi M. EBUS step-by-step, You Tube, posted August 2010. Available at: http://www.youtube.com/watch?v=Z9FdgVx_xrM&feature=related. Accessed February 20, 2011.

54. Lee HS, Lee GK, Lee HS, et al. Real-time endobronchial ultrasound-guided transbronchial needle aspiration in mediastinal staging of non-small cell lung cancer: how many aspirations per target lymph node station? *Chest.* 2008;134:368-374.

55. Nakajima T, Yasufuku K, Suzuki M, et al. Assessment of epidermal growth factor receptor mutation by endobronchial ultrasound-guided transbronchial needle aspiration. *Chest.* 2007;132:597-602.

56. Detterbeck FC, Boffa DJ, Tanoue LT. The new lung cancer staging system. *Chest.* 2009;136:260-271.

57. Robinson LA, Ruckdeschel JC, Wagner H Jr, Stevens CW. Treatment of non-small cell lung cancer-stage IIIA: ACCP evidence-based clinical practice guidelines (2nd edition). *Chest.* 2007;132:243S-265S.

58. Rubins J, Unger M, Colice GL, American College of Chest Physicians. Follow-up and surveillance of the lung cancer patient following curative intent therapy: ACCP evidence-based clinical practice guideline (2nd edition). *Chest.* 2007;132:355S-367S.

59. Lally BE, Zelterman D, Colasanto JM, et al. Postoperative radiotherapy for stage II or III non-small-cell lung cancer using the surveillance, epidemiology, and end results database. *J Clin Oncol.* 2006;24:2998-2306.

60. Douillard JY, Rosell R, De Lena M, et al, Adjuvant Navelbine International Trialist Association. Impact of postoperative radiation therapy on survival in patients with complete resection and stage I, II, or IIIA non-small-cell lung cancer treated with adjuvant chemotherapy: the adjuvant Navelbine International Trialist Association (ANITA) Randomized Trial. *Int J Radiat Oncol Biol Phys.* 2008;72:695-701.

61. Ng A, Smith G. Gastroesophageal reflux and aspiration of gastric contents in anesthetic practice. *Anesth Analg.* 2001;93:494-513.

62. Søreide E, Eriksson LI, Hirlekar G, et al. Pre-operative fasting guidelines: an update. *Acta Anaesthesiol Scand.* 2005;49:1041-1047.

63. de Langen AJ, Raijmakers P, Riphagen I, et al. The size of mediastinal lymph nodes and its relation with metastatic involvement: a meta-analysis. *Eur J Cardiothorac Surg.* 2006;29:26-29.

64. Pisters KM, Evans WK, Azzoli CG, et al, Cancer Care Ontario, American Society of Clinical Oncology. Cancer Care Ontario and American Society of Clinical Oncology adjuvant chemotherapy and adjuvant radiation therapy for stages I-IIIA resectable non small-cell lung cancer guideline. *J Clin Oncol.* 2007;25:5506-5518.

65. SEER Cancer Statistics Review 1975-2007, updated October 8, 2010. Available at: http://seer.cancer.gov/csr/1975_2007/. Accessed February 20, 2011.

66. Fischer B, Lassen U, Mortensen J, et al. Preoperative staging of lung cancer with combined PET-CT. *N Engl J Med.* 2009;361: 32-39.

67. Erasmus JJ, Macapinlac HA, Swisher SG. Positron emission tomography imaging in nonsmall-cell lung cancer. *Cancer.* 2007; 110:2155-2168.

68. Al-Sarraf N, Gately K, Lucey J, et al. Lymph node staging by means of positron emission tomography is less accurate in non-small cell lung cancer patients with enlarged lymph nodes: analysis of 1,145 lymph nodes. *Lung Cancer.* 2008;60:62-68.

69. Wallace MB, Pascual JM, Raimondo M, et al. Minimally invasive endoscopic staging of suspected lung cancer. *JAMA.* 2008; 299:540-546.

70. Silvestri GA, Gould MK, Margolis ML, et al. Noninvasive staging of non-small cell lung cancer: ACCP evidenced-based clinical practice guidelines (2nd edition). *Chest.* 2007;132:178S-201S.

71. Lee HJ, Kim YT, Kang WJ, et al. Integrated positron-emission tomography for nodal staging in lung cancer. *Asian Cardiovasc Thorac Ann.* 2009;17:622-626.

72. Defranchi SA, Edell ES, Daniels CE, et al. Mediastinoscopy in patients with lung cancer and negative endobronchial ultrasound guided needle aspiration. *Ann Thorac Surg.* 2010;90:1753-1758.

73. Kates M, Perez X, Gribetz J, et al. Validation of a model to predict perioperative mortality from lung cancer resection in the elderly. *Am J Respir Crit Care Med.* 2009;179:390-395.

74. Non-small cell lung cancer guidelines, 2009. Available at: www.nccn.org. Accessed February 20, 2011.

75. Jaklitsch MT, Herndon JE 2nd, DeCamp MM Jr, et al. Nodal downstaging predicts survival following induction chemotherapy for stage IIIA (N2) non-small cell lung cancer in CALGB protocol #8935. *J Surg Oncol.* 2006;94:599-606.

76. Whitson BA, Groth SS, Maddaus MA. Surgical assessment and intraoperative management of mediastinal lymph nodes in non-small cell lung cancer. *Ann Thorac Surg.* 2007;84:1059-1065.

77. Witte B. New developments in videomediastinoscopy: video-assisted mediastinoscopic lymphadenectomy and mediastinoscopic ultrasound. *Front Radiat Ther Oncol.* 2010;42:63-70.

78. Kuzdzal J, Zielinski M, Papla B, et al. The transcervical extended mediastinal lymphadenectomy versus cervical mediastinoscopy in non-small cell lung cancer staging. *Eur J Cardiothorac Surg.* 2007; 31:88-94.

79. Zielinski M, Hauer L, Hauer J, et al. Non-small-cell lung cancer restaging with transcervical extended mediastinal lymphadenectomy. *Eur J Cardiothorac Surg.* 2010;37:776-780.

80. Little AG, Rusch VW, Bonner JA, et al. Patterns of surgical care of lung cancer patients. *Ann Thorac Surg.* 2005;80:2051-2056.

81. Olak J. Parasternal mediastinotomy (Chamberlain procedure). *Chest Surg Clin N Am.* 1996;6:31-40.

82. Call S, Rami-Porta R, Serra-Mitjans M, et al. Extended cervical mediastinoscopy in the staging of bronchogenic carcinoma of the left lung. *Eur J Cardiothorac Surg.* 2008;34:1081-1084.

83. Cheng D, Downey RJ, Kernstine K, et al. Video-assisted thoracic surgery in lung cancer resection: a meta-analysis and systematic teview of controlled trials. *Innovations.* 2007;2:261-292.

84. Anderson CA, Falabella A, Lau CS, et al. Robotic-assisted lung resection for malignant disease. *Innovations.* 2007;2:254-258.

85. Ou SH, Zell JA. Prognostic significance of the number of lymph nodes removed at lobectomy in stage IA non-small cell lung cancer. *J Thorac Oncol.* 2008;3:880-886.

86. Keeling WB, Lewis V, Blazick E, et al. Routine evaluation for aspiration after thoracotomy for pulmonary resection. *Ann Thorac Surg.* 2007;83:193-196.

87. Keeling WB, Hernandez JM, Lewis V, et al. Increased age is an independent risk factor for radiographic aspiration and laryngeal penetration after thoracotomy for pulmonary resection. *J Thorac Cardiovasc Surg.* 2010;140:573-577.

Chapter 19

EBUS-Guided TBNA for Isolated Subcarinal Lymphadenopathy (Station 7)

> This chapter emphasizes the following elements of the Four Box Approach: techniques and instrumentation; results and procedure-related complications; and follow-up tests, visits, and procedures.

CASE DESCRIPTION

The patient is a 51-year-old male with a 10–pack-year history of smoking. His past medical history includes COPD (FEV$_1$ 60% predicted) controlled on tiotropium and albuterol inhalers and right toe amputation for melanoma 3 years earlier. A surveillance chest CT ordered by his oncologist showed a 2.5 × 2.7 cm subcarinal lymph node and no other abnormalities (Figure 19-1). The PET scan showed increased activity (SUV max 6) in the subcarinal node but no evidence of other thoracic or extrathoracic abnormalities. His physical examination was normal. He lives alone and is extremely concerned about a possible recurrence of melanoma. He has been referred for convex probe EBUS-guided TBNA.

DISCUSSION POINTS

1. Describe how the coronal view of a computed tomography scan can be used to help plan the procedure in this patient.
2. Describe the yield of EBUS-guided TBNA versus conventional TBNA for sarcoidosis.
3. Describe the clinical implications of granulomatous inflammation detected on an EBUS-guided TBNA specimen.
4. List six sonographic criteria of morphology that can be used to describe mediastinal and hilar lymph nodes.

CASE RESOLUTION

Initial Evaluations

Physical Examination, Complementary Tests, and Functional Status Assessment

Chest computed tomography (CT) showed a large* 2.5 cm subcarinal lymph node with no associated pulmonary

---

*The short axis or least diameter in cross-section should be used in measuring lymph node size; this value more closely reflects the actual node diameter when nodes are obliquely oriented relative to the scan plane and shows less variation among normal subjects than the long axis.

†Metastases to mediastinal or hilar lymph nodes from extrathoracic tumors usually occur from carcinomas of the head and neck, genitourinary tract, and breast, as well as melanoma.

‡Round, smooth, sharply defined; 50% are subcarinal.

nodules, masses, or infiltrates. Although variations in normal node size are significant, depending on the location of the node, by convention, the upper limit of normal for mediastinal lymph nodes is considered to be 1 cm in the short axis, except in the subcarinal region, where an upper limit of 1.5 cm is generally used.[1] Micrometastasis can be present, however, in the absence of lymph node enlargement in patients with known or suspected lung cancer or other malignancy. Conversely, enlarged lymph nodes may just be post inflammatory or hyperplastic, especially in a patient without cancer risk factors. Very large lymph nodes (short axis >2 cm) in the middle mediastinum, including the subcarinal region, often reflect metastatic primary lung carcinoma, metastatic extrapulmonary carcinoma,† lymphoma, tuberculosis, fungal disease (e.g., histoplasmosis, coccidioidomycosis), or sarcoidosis. A careful review of the chest CT is always warranted to avoid confusion with a bronchogenic cyst,‡ a dilated azygos vein, esophageal varices, or a hiatal hernia.

This patient does not have a high pretest probability for sarcoidosis or another granulomatous disorder. In sarcoidosis, lymph node enlargement is seen in more than 80% to 95% of cases but predominates in the right paratracheal, aorto-pulmonary window, and hilar regions. CT scans show enlarged subcarinal lymph nodes in approximately 65% of patients.[2]

Although enlargement of lymph nodes in a single station can be seen in patients with Hodgkin's disease, this most often occurs in the anterior mediastinum. Non-Hodgkin's lymphoma, on the other hand, may show involvement of only one node group in 40% of cases, most commonly involving the superior mediastinum. Another lymphoproliferative disorder, the hyaline vascular type of Castleman's disease, is often asymptomatic, presents as a hilar or localized mediastinal mass in any mediastinal compartment, and could be responsible for this patient's large subcarinal lymph node.[2] The lack of multiple enlarged lymph nodes, constitutional symptoms, and normal laboratory markers makes rare lymphoproliferative disorders or leukemia less likely to explain this patient's isolated subcarinal lymphadenopathy.

In active tuberculosis, right-side lymphadenopathy predominates (i.e., right paratracheal), but subcarinal nodes are abnormal in 50% of patients. Histoplasmosis and coccidioidomycosis are well-known causes of hilar and mediastinal lymphadenopathy. In view of the lack of pulmonary or systemic symptoms; chest radiograph or CT parenchymal abnormalities such as infiltrates, masses, or nodules; immunosuppression; or travel history to endemic regions, infectious causes are unlikely. This

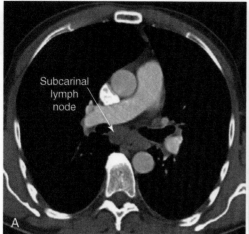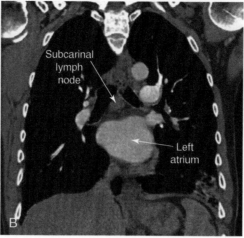

Figure 19-1 Axial **(A)** and coronal **(B)** computed tomography images show the large subcarinal lymph node located cephalad from the left atrium.

could, of course, represent primary lung carcinoma or metastatic adenocarcinoma, given the patient's age, medical history, and smoking history. This could also be recurrent melanoma with mediastinal metastasis. Indeed, settings in which biopsy remains mandatory, even if imaging findings may suggest an alternative diagnosis (e.g., sarcoidosis), are represented by human immunodeficiency virus (HIV)-positive patients or patients presenting with lung infiltrates and/or enlarged hilar mediastinal positron emission tomography (PET)-positive lymph nodes with a clinical history of neoplasm. From this patient's history and physical examination, review of imaging studies, and laboratory workup, no diagnosis could be made, thus warranting tissue diagnosis.

Comorbidities

Chronic obstructive pulmonary disease (COPD) is reportedly associated with an increased complication rate after bronchoscopy compared with that seen in patients with normal lung function. Concern for bronchospasm is increased, but premedication with inhaled short-acting agonists is not routinely recommended.[3]

Support System

This patient lived alone and had very few acquaintances. Given that our main differential diagnoses were cancer and sarcoidosis, we wondered whether he might eventually benefit from participation in support groups. For people with sarcoidosis, many of these groups are available online, and they may become necessary when physical and emotional problems associated with this disease arise. In self-help groups, patients might better cope with problems and concerns related to their disease and feelings of isolation.[4] Similarly, for cancer, support groups focus on behavioral issues and symptoms, or on the expression of emotions. Most of these support programs are structured to ensure delivery of information and to provide emotional and social support, stress management strategies based on cognitive-behavioral approaches, and relaxation techniques. Group therapy helps patients gain emotional support from others with similar experiences and learn to use these experiences to reduce their fear of dying and uncertainty.[5]

Patient Preferences and Expectations

Our patient was anxious about his potential diagnosis and had many questions regarding his health. In such circumstances, effective communication skills improve a patient's understanding of the condition and promote adherence to potential treatment regimens. Having good communication skills helps health care providers use time efficiently, avoid burnout, and enhance feelings of professional fulfillment. Blocking,* lecturing, depending on a routine, collusion,† coercion, and premature reassurance are usually ill advised. One well-recognized and effective communication skill is the "ask-tell-ask technique," which is based on the notion that providing patient education requires knowing what the patient already knows and building on that knowledge. Of course, building a relationship with a patient requires that the physician listen to the patient, understand and empathize with his perspectives, show compassion, and respect the patient's agenda, even if it is not quite in line at all times with the way the physician might want to do things.[6]

Procedural Strategies

Indications

In general, proposed indications for endobronchial ultrasound (EBUS)-guided transbronchial needle aspiration (TBNA) include nondiagnostic conventional TBNA, staging of the radiologically normal mediastinum in case of suspected or confirmed lung cancer, mediastinal restaging after induction chemotherapy, and, more commonly, diagnosis of mediastinal or hilar lymphadenopathy.[7] In patients with a history of cancer, such as ours, the diagnosis of new mediastinal adenopathy suggests recurrence of malignancy; therefore this diagnosis needs to be excluded or confirmed. Because not all cases of PET-positive mediastinal adenopathy are due to cancer recurrence, lymph node sampling is usually warranted. In this patient with a

---

*Blocking occurs when a patient raises a concern, but the physician either fails to respond or redirects the conversation.

†Collusion occurs when patients hesitate to bring up difficult topics and their physicians do not ask them specifically about them.

newly discovered large subcarinal lymph node, a tissue diagnosis was going to be obtained using EBUS-guided TBNA with the patient under general anesthesia.

Contraindications

No contraindications to bronchoscopy under general anesthesia were noted.

Expected Results

The yield of EBUS-guided TBNA varies depending on the ultimate diagnosis and usually is higher for malignant than for benign disorders.

1. *In patients with previous malignancy* and PET-positive lymph nodes, EBUS-TBNA has a yield greater than 90%. In one study, 73 lymph nodes from 48 patients were sampled, with each patient undergoing mediastinoscopy or thoracoscopy immediately after needle aspiration for histologic confirmation. The sensitivity, specificity, positive predictive value (PPV), negative predictive value (NPV), and accuracy of EBUS-TBNA were 97.4%, 100%, 100%, 87.5%, and 97.7%, respectively.[8] In another study, similarly high sensitivity, specificity, diagnostic accuracy, and NPV of EBUS-TBNA for the diagnosis of mediastinal and hilar lymph node metastasis were found (92.0%, 100%, 95.3%, and 90%, respectively). Tumors encountered included colorectal, head and neck, ovarian, breast, esophageal, hepatocellular, prostate, renal, and germ cell cancers and melanoma.[9]

2. *For primary lung carcinoma*, a meta-analysis of 11 studies with 1299 patients found that overall, EBUS-guided TBNA (using both radial and convex probes) had a pooled sensitivity of 93% and a pooled specificity of 100%. The subgroup of patients selected on the basis of CT- or PET-positive results had higher pooled sensitivity (94%) than the subgroup of patients not selected on the basis of CT or PET findings (76%).[10]

3. *The diagnosis of lymphoma* may be controversial, although the use of flow cytometry, molecular biology techniques, and immunohistochemistry on cell block preparations may provide enough information for definitive diagnosis. Results from EBUS-TBNA were compared with a reference standard of pathologic tissue diagnosis of lymphoma or a composite of greater than 6 months of clinical follow-up with radiographic imaging. Nodes studied were larger than 5 mm and had a standardized uptake value (SUV) max higher than 4. Sensitivity was 90.9%, specificity 100%, PPV 100%, and NPV 92.9%.[11] In another study, EBUS-TBNA had a sensitivity of 76%, but 20% of patients required surgical biopsy to completely characterize lymphoma subtypes, resulting in overall sensitivity of 57% and specificity of 100%.[12]

4. *For fungal or mycobacterial infection*, no studies have specifically addressed the yield of EBUS-TBNA. For patients with tuberculosis, however, in endemic areas, conventional TBNA has sensitivity of 83%, specificity of 100%, PPV of 100%, NPV of 38%, and accuracy of 85%.[13] Future studies are

necessary to determine whether EBUS-TBNA offers similar or better results.

5. *For sarcoidosis*, several studies have reported yields ranging from 82% to 95% for EBUS-TBNA.[14-17]

Team Experience

A single-institution study suggested that the learning curve for EBUS-TBNA for thoracic surgeons requires 10 procedures to reach the high yields reported in controlled clinical trials.[18] In reality, however, the actual number of any given procedure performed does not account for the different rates at which people learn. With regard to EBUS-TBNA, one study assessed the learning curves of five independent operators by retrospectively applying cusum analysis* to the first 100 cases of each[19]; over a wide range of time, EBUS-TBNA competence was attained and the pooled sensitivity of EBUS-TBNA under conscious (moderate) sedation was 67.4%—lower than the high (>90%) rates reported in clinical trials.[19]

The usefulness of EBUS-TBNA resides in its clinical significance, accuracy, and reproducibility, which are usually shown to be excellent among pathologists experienced with these types of samples. Pathologists with little experience must climb what appears to be a steep learning curve.[20]

Diagnostic Alternatives

1. *Conventional TBNA:* For cancer, the yield of conventional TBNA for large subcarinal lymph nodes is similar to that of EBUS-TBNA, but EBUS guidance increases the yield of TBNA in all other stations.[21] In the diagnosis of sarcoidosis, the overall diagnostic accuracy of TBNA cytology is as high as 86.2%.[22]

2. *Endoscopic ultrasound (EUS)-FNA:* EUS alone is suitable for assessing lymph nodes in the posterior aspect of lymph node stations 4L, 5 (when significantly enlarged), and 7, and in the inferior mediastinum at stations 8 and 9 (Figure 19-2); data from lung cancer studies show that EUS-FNA and EBUS-TBNA have similarly high yields for diagnosing cancer involving lymph node station 7 (subcarinal).[23] The overall diagnostic accuracy and sensitivity of EUS-FNA in the diagnosis of sarcoidosis were found to be 94% and 100%, respectively.[24] A disadvantage of EUS-FNA is its lesser ability to access different hilar lymph nodes and nodes situated anterior and to the right of the trachea. These nodes are in fact those most commonly involved in sarcoidosis.

3. *Mediastinoscopy:* Mediastinoscopy provides systematic exploration and biopsy under visual guidance of stations 1, 2, 3, 4, and 7 (see Figure 19-2); mediastinoscopy is more invasive and has higher complication rates than are seen with needle aspiration techniques. With regard to suspected lung cancer, it was shown that up to 28% of patients with a high clinical suspicion of nodal disease had mediastinal nodal metastases confirmed by mediastinoscopy despite negative EBUS-TBNA[25]; therefore a negative EBUS-TBNA

---

*Cusum analysis is a method of continuously assessing the performance of an individual or process against a predetermined standard to detect adverse trends and to allow for early intervention (e.g., retraining).

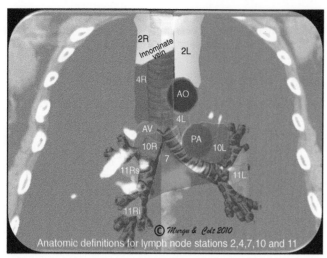

Figure 19-2 Schematic map of commonly sampled hilar and mediastinal lymph node stations. Anatomic borders are based on the International Association for the Study of Lung Cancer (IASLC) lymph node staging system.

should be followed by mediastinoscopy when cancer is suspected. For sarcoidosis, mediastinoscopy is used as the gold standard for histologic confirmation.[26] For patients with isolated mediastinal lymphadenopathy, the sensitivity of mediastinoscopy is 96%, and before the introduction of dedicated EBUS-TBNA, some experts recommended it as a procedure of choice to diagnose lesions in the axial (middle) mediastinum.[27]

Cost-Effectiveness

It is debatable whether EBUS-TBNA is more cost-effective than mediastinoscopy for evaluation of mediastinal lymphadenopathy in non–small cell lung cancer.[28] In patients with a benign disease such as sarcoidosis, this issue has not been studied in a systematic fashion. Mediastinoscopy is usually considered the gold standard approach for undiagnosed mediastinal adenopathy, including sarcoidosis,[29] and before the introduction of EBUS in clinical practice, one cost-benefit analysis of mediastinoscopy for patients with suspected stage I sarcoidosis (asymptomatic bilateral hilar adenopathy) showed that benefits of mediastinoscopy would be minimal and likely would be offset by the procedure's morbidity and mortality.[30]

Informed Consent

The patient showed understanding of the indications, expected results, and potential complications, as well as alternative procedures, including observation, conventional TBNA, EUS-FNA, and mediastinoscopy. He preferred to proceed with EBUS-guided TBNA under general anesthesia.

Techniques and Results

Anesthesia and Perioperative Care

We performed the procedure with the patient under general anesthesia, but many operators perform it with the patient under moderate (conscious) sedation. Many studies reporting a high yield for the procedure were conducted with patients under general anesthesia.[28]

Instrumentation

A dedicated EBUS bronchoscope, which offers direct real-time ultrasound imaging with a curved linear array transducer, was used. The frequency was set to 10 MHz. The associated ultrasound processor has adjustable gain and depth to optimize image quality, along with Doppler capabilities to distinguish vascular structures such as the heart and the inferior pulmonary veins; this is useful in sampling the subcarinal node. The 22 gauge acrogenic needle with an inner stylet allows for dislodgment of bronchial wall debris from the needle. This theoretically enhances the adequacy of the specimen (Figure 19-3). The needle guide system locks to the scope, and precise needle projection up to 4 cm is possible.

Anatomic Dangers and Other Risks

Concern has arisen regarding mediastinal abscess after EBUS-TBNA.[31] In addition, pericarditis may occur in cases of inadvertent contamination of the pericardial space.[32] With full-needle extension, the needle tip can be difficult to visualize, because small changes in the ultrasound angle can cause the needle tip to be out of plane with the ultrasound wave (see video on ExpertConsult. com) (Video IV.19.1). As a result, the pericardium (or vascular structures) may be violated but not visualized.[32]

Results and Procedure-Related Complications

Under general anesthesia, the patient was intubated without difficulty using a 9.0 endotracheal tube. Bronchoscopic inspection showed normal airway mucosa and no endobronchial lesions. EBUS showed a subcarinal node greater than 1 cm in the short axis, of oval shape, homogeneous echogenicity, and indistinct margins; the node did not have a central necrosis sign (CNS),* nor did it have a central hilar structure (CHS)† (Figure 19-4). Studies show that sonographic features can be useful in evaluating lymph node metastasis in head and neck cancers, breast cancers, and thoracic malignancies.[33,34] For example, operators may wish to avoid necrotic regions and obtain aspirates from the periphery of the node.[35]

In one study of 1061 lymph node stations from 487 patients with confirmed or suspected lung cancer, morphologic sonographic features of mediastinal and hilar lymph nodes reportedly helped predict the presence or absence of metastasis.[36] The presence of CNS had the highest specificity (92.6%) and the highest hazard ratio (5.6) for prediction of metastatic lymph nodes. This evidence does not obviate the need for sampling the node, but the high negative predictive values could be useful in certain clinical scenarios. For instance, if EBUS-TBNA of a lymph node in a patient with suspected lung cancer provides an adequate cytologic specimen revealing only

---

*CNS is a hypoechoic area within the lymph node without blood flow.
†CHS is defined as a linear, flat, hyperechoic area in the center of the lymph node.

Figure 19-3 Images **A, B, C,** and **D** are consecutive still images captured from a video showing endobronchial ultrasound–transbronchial needle aspiration (EBUS-TBNA) during needle aspiration. **A,** The stylet pushed the bronchial wall debris inside the node. **B,** The needle is retracted, and the debris becomes evidently dislodged from the needle. **C,** The needle is advanced while aspiration is in process. **D,** The debris has completely disappeared, having been aspirated into the syringe. This probably explains how bronchial cells were present in the cytology specimen.

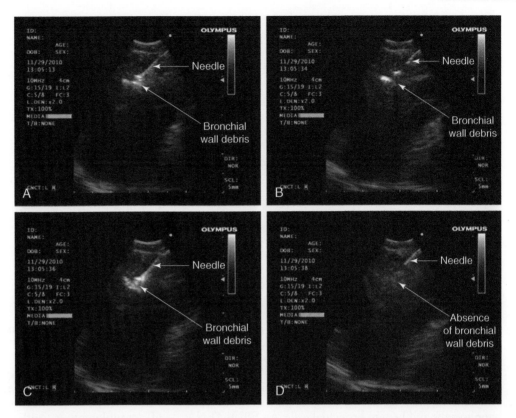

Figure 19-4 **A,** This patient's homogeneous subcarinal lymph node is adjacent to the pericardium and left atrium. **B,** Right paratracheal lymph node (from a different patient) showing hypoechoic areas without blood flow, consistent with coagulation necrosis sign (CNS). **C,** Right paratracheal lymph node (from a different patient) showing a flat hyperechoic area in the center of the node, consistent with central hilar structure (CHS) sign. **D,** Doppler-positive anechoic linear structure within the lymph node is consistent with a blood vessel.

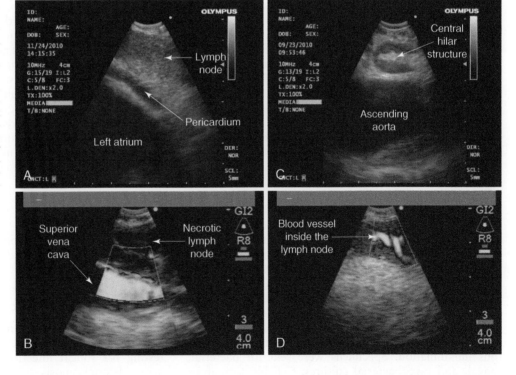

benign lymphocytes, then the lack of EBUS-related malignant lymph node characteristics could reinforce suspicions of true negativity.

Immediately after completing the first aspiration, while watching the needle deep within a lymph node (Figure 19-5, *A*), the operating room nurse interrupted the operator to ask whether she should record a video. After the operator answered her, a different image was apparent on the display monitor (Figure 19-5, *B*). It is likely that the operator rotated his wrist in such a way that the scanning plane of the ultrasound was changed while the needle remained in the same position (see video on

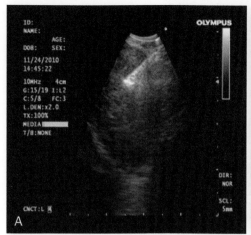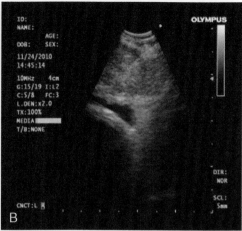

Figure 19-5 A, The needle is visualized inside the lymph node during the aspiration process. **B,** The needle tip is difficult to visualize because a small change in the ultrasound angle (scanning plane) caused the needle tip to be out of plane with the ultrasound. It is likely that in turning the head to speak with the nurse, the operator rotated his wrist in such a way that he changed the scanning plane of the ultrasound while the needle remained in the same position.

ExpertConsult.com) (Video IV.19.1). This may not affect diagnostic yield but could result in accidental puncture of adjacent structures, because the tip of the needle is not seen.[32]

The first aspirate was prepared using a Diff-Quik stain, was read by the on-site cytologist, and showed scant lymphocytes and benign bronchial cells. An EBUS-TBNA cytology specimen is considered adequate or representative if frankly malignant cells, granulomas or lymphocytes, lymphoid tissue, or clusters of anthracotic pigment-laden macrophages are present.[37] An EBUS-TBNA specimen is considered inadequate or nonrepresentative if no cellular components, scant lymphocytes (defined as <40 per high-power field [HPF]), and blood only, cartilage, or bronchial epithelial cells are noted.[38] A quantitative cutoff value of at least 30% cellularity composed of lymphocytes has been arbitrarily proposed.[39] In our case, aborting the procedure because lymphocytes were seen or assuming that the specimen was representative would have been premature.

The second aspirate was bloody but had been obtained from a different part of the subcarinal lymph node. The inferior pulmonary vein or left atrium could have been inadvertently penetrated. This was not the case, however, because the needle was seen in its entirety throughout the procedure. Blood vessels inside a lymph node are not uncommon and often appear as hypoechoic linear or circular structures that are Doppler positive. Their presence could explain bloody aspirates, even when the needle is well visualized inside the node (see Figure 19-4). The third and fourth aspirates were adequate and showed abundant lymphocytes and a suggestion of granulomatous inflammation. Specimens were sent for bacterial, fungal, and mycobacterial cultures. Cell block analysis was added to conventional cytologic evaluation because, in addition to increasing the yield for malignancy, it may result in a higher yield for granulomas in patients with suspected sarcoidosis.[40] After the fourth aspirate, the procedure was terminated. No complications occurred, and the patient was discharged home after having been monitored in the postanesthesia care unit for 2 hours.

Long-Term Management

Outcome Assessment

Adequate specimens were obtained, but no specific diagnosis was made. However, the differential diagnosis was narrowed to infectious and noninfectious causes of granulomatous inflammation. If granulomatous inflammation is identified by EBUS-TBNA in a patient with suspected cancer recurrence, a reasonable clinical approach is to follow the patient radiographically without performing additional invasive testing, unless radiographic progression is noted.[41] This is recommended because at least 5% of patients undergoing EBUS-TBNA in a tertiary cancer center were found to have a sarcoid-like lymphadenopathy mimicking cancer recurrence. Long-term follow-up imaging studies did not confirm tumor recurrence. The precise origin, natural history, and prognosis of this phenomenon are not yet known, but proposed mechanisms include immunologic dysfunction and a reaction due to previously administered chemotherapy.[41]

Referrals

The patient was referred back to his oncologist to continue follow-up clinical and imaging studies for possible melanoma recurrence.

Follow-up Tests and Procedures

Final culture results were negative for bacterial, fungal, tuberculous, and nontuberculous mycobacteria. Serologic testing for fungal infection was negative. In endemic areas, histoplasmosis or coccidioidomycosis must be excluded, especially before immunosuppressive medications are administered to patients with presumed sarcoidosis. Negative results do not entirely exclude infectious causes and, in such patients, the response to immunosuppressive agents must be carefully monitored.

In view of the lack of evidence for infectious causes, the diagnosis of sarcoidosis or sarcoid-like reaction was made. No evidence of granulomatous inflammation was found at other sites to suggest sarcoidosis, nor were biochemical abnormalities such as hypercalcemia, hypercalciuria, hyperuricemia, elevated serum aminotransferase, alanine aminotransferase, or alkaline phosphatase present. The serum angiotensin-converting enzyme (SACE)* level was normal. Demonstration of granulomas remains an essential criterion for sarcoidosis, but because granulomatous inflammation can be seen in several conditions, it is necessary to exclude all possible causes and to correlate histology with other findings.[42] To establish a diagnosis of sarcoidosis, for example, granulomas must be present in two or more organs and no agent known to cause a granulomatous response must be identified.[43] This was not the case in our patient; therefore a diagnosis of sarcoid-like reaction was ultimately made. Because mediastinoscopy had been deferred, CT was scheduled 3 months later to re-evaluate the mediastinum; no change was noted. Continued surveillance scans during the next 12 months remained unchanged. We planned to monitor for stability for a total of 2 years.

Quality Improvement

No diagnosis was made on EBUS-TBNA, but we did not find evidence of primary lung tumor or recurrent melanoma. Attributing mediastinal lymphadenopathy to cancer recurrence without tissue confirmation can lead to unnecessary and toxic therapy[44]; therefore we certainly believed the procedure was warranted. We wondered, however, whether more aspirates should have been performed. For sarcoidosis, the yield of EBUS-TBNA exceeds 80% with five passes in one study and no further increase in yield, even after seven passes.[15] For malignancy, however, the yield plateaus after a mean of only three aspirates.[45] Therefore continuing the procedure "indefinitely" in the belief that eventually a diagnosis will be made is not warranted and probably increases the costs and risks for procedure-related complications or scope damage.

DISCUSSION POINTS

1. Describe how the coronal view of a computed tomography scan can be used to help plan the procedure in this patient.

    Based on the International Association for the Study of Lung Cancer (IASLC) lymph node map, the upper border of the subcarinal lymph node station is the carina of the trachea; the lower border is the upper border of the lower lobe bronchus on the left and the lower border of the bronchus intermedius on the right.[46] This lymph node is located medial to the left or right mainstem bronchi, below the level of the main carina (see Figure 19-2). The EBUS scope should be placed in the right or left mainstem bronchus and the transducer turned medially to allow visualization of the subcarinal region. A coronal (aka frontal) plane is

perpendicular to the ground and in humans separates the anterior from the posterior regions of the body (see Figure 19-1). The coronal CT view identifies the EBUS scanning plane and reveals the same structures but in different positions (Figure 19-6). To understand the EBUS image based on the coronal CT scan, however, several reference points should be recognized:
- The EBUS image is displayed as if the scope is horizontal (Figure 19-6, D).
- The green dot on the monitor represents the point where the needle exits the scope and corresponds to the superior (cephalad) aspect of the body (see Figure 19-6, D).
- The position of this dot, although adjustable, is located by default toward the 1 o'clock position of the screen (see Figure 19-6, D).

    The coronal CT view is displayed as if the scope is nearly vertical (Figure 19-6, A). If one rotates the CT coronal image clockwise to horizontalize the scope and bring the green dot cephalad toward the 1 o'clock position, the two images (CT and EBUS) correlate and show all structures in the same locations (Figure 19-7). Because the green dot corresponds to the more cephalad, and therefore proximal, aspect of the body, the structure adjacent to the airway at approximately 1 o'clock is the subcarinal lymph node, and the anechoic structure at 7 o'clock is the left atrium (distal) (see Figure 19-7).

2. Describe the yield of EBUS-guided TBNA versus conventional TBNA for sarcoidosis.

    Several studies have shown that conventional TBNA (61% to 72%) with 19 gauge needles has an incremental diagnostic yield over other bronchoscopic techniques, including endobronchial biopsy (EBB) (45%) and transbronchial lung biopsy (TBLB) (40% to 52%), for stage I sarcoidosis. TBNA may actually have a higher yield than bronchioloalveolar lavage (BAL), EBB, or even TBLB alone.[47,48] EBUS-TBNA was shown to significantly add to the yield of combined BAL and TBLB or EBB and TBLB for patients with suspicious stage I sarcoidosis.[49,50] Both conventional and EBUS-TBNA procedures have a high yield.
- Nonrandomized studies showed the sensitivity of conventional TBNA cytology specimens for sarcoidosis to be as high as 86% to 92%.[22,51]
- Nonrandomized studies have showed the diagnostic yield of real-time EBUS-TBNA to be 85% to 95%.[14-17]
- As of this writing, one study has prospectively compared the diagnostic yield of EBUS-TBNA versus that of conventional TBNA performed with a standard 19 gauge needle in 50 patients (24 EBUS, 26 conventional) with mediastinal adenopathy and clinical suspicion of stage I sarcoidosis. The diagnostic yield was 53.8% versus 83.3% in favor of the EBUS-TBNA group.[52]

3. Describe the clinical implications of granulomatous inflammation detected on EBUS-guided TBNA specimen.
- Granulomatous inflammation can coexist with malignancy and may be an epiphenomenon. Lymph nodes that harbor both necrotizing and

---

*Elevated serum angiotensin-converting enzyme levels are seen in fact in only 50% to 60% of patients with sarcoidosis. Although these levels may reflect the total granuloma burden, they do not reliably correlate with disease activity nor with its prognosis.

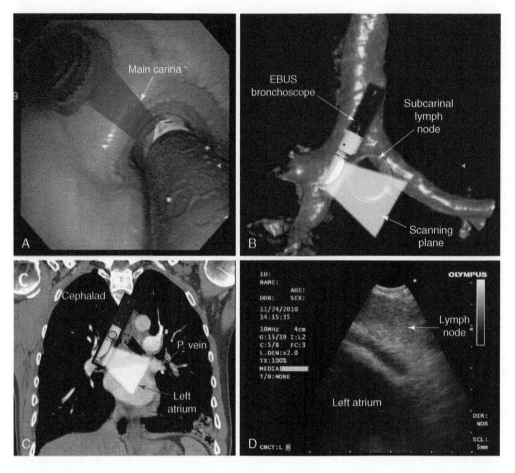

Figure 19-6 **A,** Picture taken inside an airway model shows the endobronchial ultrasound (EBUS) scope placed in the right main bronchus with the transducer turned medially to scan the subcarinal region. **B,** Three-dimensional computed tomography (CT)-based diagram shows the EBUS scope and its scanning plane for visualizing the subcarinal region. **C,** The coronal CT view identifies the EBUS scanning plane. **D,** The EBUS image is projected on the monitor as if the scope were horizontal. The same structures are visualized but in different positions.

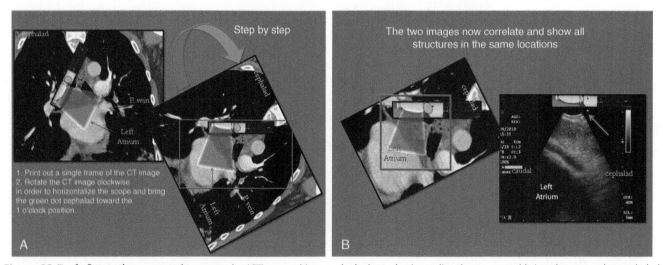

Figure 19-7 **A,** Rotate the computed tomography (CT) coronal image clockwise to horizontalize the scope and bring the green dot cephalad toward the 1 o'clock position. **B,** CT and endobronchial ultrasound (EBUS) images correlate, showing all structures in the same locations.

non-necrotizing granulomas and metastatic malignancies have been reported.[53]

- In a study of 153 patients with mediastinal lymphadenopathy on CT imaging at a cancer institution, however, noncaseating granulomas were detected by EBUS-TBNA in 17 of 153 (11%) patients with no concurrent evidence of cancer; 8 of 153 patients (5.2%) had sarcoid-like lymphadenopathy

mimicking cancer recurrence (5/5 PET positive), but 8 of 153 (5.2%) patients had new mediastinal lymphadenopathy and no prior history of cancer and had a clinical syndrome consistent with sarcoidosis.[41]

- Sarcoid-like reactions have been reported in patients with various lymphomas, non–small cell carcinoma of the lung (NSCLC), and germ cell neoplasms in lymph nodes draining the malignancy or in remote lymph node stations.[54] The overall incidence of sarcoidal reactions occurring in regional lymph nodes of NSCLC patients was 4.3%. Findings were confined to patients with stage I disease, with an incidence of 7.7%. The mechanism of granuloma formation in such patients is an important area of future research that may allow improved understanding of effective antitumor responses.

4. List six sonographic criteria of morphology that can be used to describe mediastinal and hilar lymph nodes[36]:
   - *Size (in short axis):* smaller or larger than 1 cm
   - *Shape:* oval or round; when the ratio of the short versus the long axis of lymph nodes is smaller than 1.5, the lymph node is defined as round; when the ratio is larger than 1.5, it is oval
   - *Margin:* indistinct or distinct; if most of the margin (>50%) is clearly visualized with a high echoic border, lymph nodes are declared distinct. If the margin is unclear, they are declared indistinct.
   - *Echogenicity:* homogeneous or heterogeneous
   - *Presence or absence of central hilar structure (CHS),* defined as a linear, flat, hyperechoic area in the center of the lymph node
   - *Presence or absence of coagulation necrosis sign (CNS),* defined as a hypoechoic area* within the lymph node without blood flow

Expert Commentary

provided by Carlos A. Jimenez, MD

Linear or convex probe endobronchial ultrasound-guided transbronchial needle aspiration (CP EBUS-TBNA) has revolutionized the evaluation of mediastinal lymph nodes since its introduction to clinical practice in 2004. Many studies have been published, but almost all of them have failed to meet rigorous proposed guidelines for the study of new diagnostic tests[55]—a problem also encountered when the published literature on cervical mediastinoscopy is reviewed. For example, to date, only two studies have directly compared cervical mediastinoscopy versus CP EBUS-TBNA alone[56] or combined with transesophageal ultrasound.[57]

Despite the lack of rigorous clinical studies evaluating the diagnostic accuracy of both cervical mediastinoscopy and CP EBUS-TBNA, the use of endobronchial ultrasound has spread rapidly. Because of its straightforwardness when performed by trained bronchoscopists, consistent published results, low rate of complications, and high levels of physician and patient satisfaction, it has clearly replaced mediastinoscopy as the first choice for sampling mediastinal lymph nodes.

This case of isolated, enlarged fluoro-2-deoxy-D-glucose (FDG)–avid subcarinal (station 7) lymphadenopathy allows discussion of two important issues:

The first is whether conventional TBNA could be as helpful in this situation as CP EBUS-TBNA or cervical mediastinoscopy; the second addresses the clinical significance of granulomatous inflammation detected on an EBUS-TBNA specimen.

The mobility of mediastinal lymph nodes during the respiratory cycle has been blamed for the poor yield of conventional TBNA.[58] The results of the only study that directly compared CP EBUS-TBNA versus cervical mediastinoscopy (diagnostic yield 98% vs. 78%; P = .007) suggest that CP EBUS-TBNA is superior when station 7 lymph nodes are evaluated.[56] Conventional TBNA has not been compared directly with CP EBUS-TBNA but rather with radial probe EBUS,[21] which does not allow real-time visualization of the needle as it enters the lymph node. In this study, conventional TBNA performed as well as radial probe EBUS-guided TBNA (diagnostic yields 72% vs. 80%; P = .3) in lymph nodes that measured 0.8 to 4.3 cm. CP EBUS-TBNA studies have consistently reported diagnostic yields above 90% in subcarinal lymph nodes. Therefore CP EBUS-TBNA could be recommended as the first diagnostic technique with which an isolated subcarinal lymphadenopathy can be evaluated, but if not readily available, conventional TBNA should be attempted.

Regarding the second point for discussion, I would like to use a simplified Bayesian approach. Given the clinical and radiographic information provided, I assume that our patient's pretest probability of having a malignant condition (primary lung cancer or metastatic melanoma) is 70% (I am being pessimistic), and therefore, the pretest probability of having a benign condition is 30%. Based on all the published data, I also assume that the sensitivity and specificity of EBUS-TBNA in diagnosing a malignant condition is at least 90%, and that the positive likelihood ratio (sensitivity/[1-specificity]) and the negative likelihood ratio ([1-sensitivity]/specificity) are 9 and 0.11, respectively. Once we have a negative result for malignancy, the post-test probability of having primary lung cancer or metastatic melanoma decreases significantly, to approximately 20%, and the probability of a benign condition increases to roughly 80%.

With regard to excluding other benign diagnoses, if final cultures and serologic testing were negative, infectious causes would be less likely, although they could not be completely excluded. A single mediastinal lymph node with granulomatous inflammation without additional manifestations, however, should hardly prompt one to give a patient the diagnosis of sarcoidosis, let alone begin inmunosuppressive therapy to treat it.

In fact, the association between granulomatous inflammation and cancer has been recognized for over a century. Although this phenomenon has been reported more frequently in patients with testicular germ cell tumor, it presents with other cancer types as well, as described by our group,[41] affecting patients treated with chemotherapy or surgical resection only. No clarity on the cause of the association has been

---

*Typical CNS is described as one low echoic area within the lymph node, but sometimes it may occupy most of the lymph node.

obtained, but proposed explanations include an immunologic dysfunction shared by cancer and sarcoidosis, side effects of cancer therapy, and "antigenic shedding" from the malignant tumor, leading to granuloma formation. In our report, this phenomenon occurred in only 5.2% of patients studied, but we could expect a higher prevalence because before EBUS-TBNA became available in our institution, patients with a history of cancer and new onset of hilar or mediastinal lymphadenopathy might have often been treated for cancer recurrence without histologic confirmation. We recommend that with radiographic findings suggestive of cancer recurrence, such as enlarged or FDG-avid mediastinal lymph nodes, patients should undergo histologic confirmation of the recurrence to avoid unnecessary and toxic therapies.

Cervical mediastinoscopy might be difficult to perform when prior instrumentation or radiation therapy to the mediastinum has been provided. On the other hand, EBUS-TBNA allows for safe, repeated hilar and mediastinal lymph node sampling. I concur with the proposed diagnosis of sarcoid-like reaction and the established follow-up battery of tests and procedures. The patient will require continued surveillance using CT of the chest for a total of 2 years to demonstrate stability of the lymphadenopathy. CT might then be repeated at intervals that vary from 3 to 12 months, becoming less frequent as repeated surveillance images demonstrate no changes. If at some point during the surveillance the lymph node clearly decreases in size, no additional CT images are needed. On the other hand, if the lymph node increases in size or in FDG activity, a repeated EBUS-TBNA would be warranted.

Finally, interventional pulmonology physicians and thoracic surgeons should be encouraged to join efforts to properly conduct a few well-designed studies. Although these may be difficult to organize, they are likely to provide more accurate, more readily generalizable, and more reliable information than has been obtained from results of a myriad of poorly designed studies. Six years has passed since the introduction of CP EBUS-TBNA into clinical practice, yet complete agreement has not been reached regarding the roles for this and other new endosonography technologies alongside or instead of mediastinoscopy in evaluating mediastinal lymph nodes.

REFERENCES

1. Glazer GM, Gross BH, Quint LE, et al. Normal mediastinal lymph nodes: number and size according to American Thoracic Society mapping. *AJR Am J Roentgenol.* 1985;144:261-265.
2. Webb R. The mediastinum: mediastinal masses. In: Richard Webb, Charles Higgins, eds. *Thoracic Imaging.* Philadelphia: Lippincott Williams & Wilkins; 2005:212-270.
3. Stolz D, Pollak V, Chhajed PN, et al. A randomized, placebo-controlled trial of bronchodilators for bronchoscopy in patients with COPD. *Chest.* 2007;131:765-772.
4. Swayze S. Helping them cope. *J Psychosoc Nurs Ment Health Serv.* 1991;29:35-37.
5. Weis J. Support groups for cancer patients. *Support Care Cancer.* 2003;11:763-768.
6. Back AL, Arnold RM, Baile WF, et al. Approaching difficult communication tasks in oncology. *CA Cancer J Clin.* 2005;55:164-177.
7. Yasufuku K, Nakajima T, Chiyo M, et al. Endobronchial ultrasonography: current status and future directions. *J Thorac Oncol.* 2007;2:970-979.
8. Nosotti M, Tosi D, Palleschi A, et al. Transbronchial needle aspiration under direct endobronchial ultrasound guidance of PET-positive isolated mediastinal adenopathy in patients with previous malignancy. *Surg Endosc.* 2009;23:1356-1359.
9. Nakajima T, Yasufuku K, Iyoda A, et al. The evaluation of lymph node metastasis by endobronchial ultrasound-guided transbronchial needle aspiration: crucial for selection of surgical candidates with metastatic lung tumors. *J Thorac Cardiovasc Surg.* 2007; 134:1485-1490.
10. Gu P, Zhao Y, Jiang L, et al. Endobronchial ultrasound-guided transbronchial needle aspiration for staging of lung cancer: a systematic review and meta-analysis. *Eur J Cancer.* 2009;45: 1389-1396.
11. Kennedy MP, Jimenez CA, Bruzzi JF, et al. Endobronchial ultrasound-guided transbronchial needle aspiration in the diagnosis of lymphoma. *Thorax.* 2008;63:360-365.
12. Steinfort DP, Conron M, Tsui A, et al. Endobronchial ultrasound-guided transbronchial needle aspiration for the evaluation of suspected lymphoma. *J Thorac Oncol.* 2010;5:804-809.
13. Bilaçeroğlu S, Günel O, Eris N, et al. Transbronchial needle aspiration in diagnosing intrathoracic tuberculous lymphadenitis. *Chest.* 2004;126:259-267.
14. Oki M, Saka H, Kitagawa C, et al. Real-time endobronchial ultrasound-guided transbronchial needle aspiration is useful for diagnosing sarcoidosis. *Respirology.* 2007;12:863-868.
15. Garwood S, Judson MA, Silvestri G, et al. Endobronchial ultrasound for the diagnosis of pulmonary sarcoidosis. *Chest.* 2007; 132:1298-1304.
16. Wong M, Yasufuku K, Nakajima T, et al. Endobronchial ultrasound: new insight for the diagnosis of sarcoidosis. *Eur Respir J.* 2007;29:1182-1186.
17. Yasufuku K, Chiyo M, Sekine Y, et al. Real-time endobronchial ultrasound-guided transbronchial needle aspiration of mediastinal and hilar lymph nodes. *Chest.* 2004;126:122-128.
18. Groth SS, Whitson BA, D'Cunha J, et al. Endobronchial ultrasound-guided fine-needle aspiration of mediastinal lymph nodes: a single institution's early learning curve. *Ann Thorac Surg.* 2008;86:1104-1109; discussion 1109-1110.
19. Kemp SV, El Batrawy SH, Harrison RN, et al. Learning curves for endobronchial ultrasound using Cusum analysis. *Thorax.* 2010; 65:534-538.
20. Skov BG, Baandrup U, Jakobsen GK, et al. Cytopathologic diagnoses of fine-needle aspirations from endoscopic ultrasound of the mediastinum: reproducibility of the diagnoses and representativeness of aspirates from lymph nodes. *Cancer.* 2007;111:234-241.
21. Herth F, Becker H, Ernst A. Conventional versus ultrasound-guided transbronchial needle aspiration: a randomized trial. *Chest.* 2004; 125:322-325.
22. Smojver-Jezek S, Peros-Golubicic T, Tekavec-Trkanjec T, et al. Transbronchial fine needle aspiration cytology in the diagnosis of mediastinal/hilar sarcoidosis. *Cytopathology.* 2007;18:3-7.
23. Herth FJ, Lunn W, Eberhardt R, et al. Transbronchial versus transesophageal ultrasound-guided aspiration of enlarged mediastinal lymph nodes. *Am J Respir Crit Care Med.* 2005;171:1164-1167.
24. Fritscher-Ravens A, Sriram PV, Topalidis T, et al. Diagnosing sarcoidosis using endosonography-guided fine-needle aspiration. *Chest.* 2000;118:928-935.
25. Defranchi SA, Edell ES, Daniels CE, et al. Mediastinoscopy in patients with lung cancer and negative endobronchial ultrasound guided needle aspiration. *Ann Thorac Surg.* 2010;90:1753-1758.
26. Pakhale SS, Unruh H, Tan L, Sharma S. Has mediastinoscopy still a role in suspected stage I sarcoidosis? *Sarcoidosis Vasc Diffuse Lung Dis.* 2006;23:66-69.
27. Porte H, Roumilhac D, Eraldi L, et al. The role of mediastinoscopy in the diagnosis of mediastinal lymphadenopathy. *Eur J Cardiothorac Surg.* 1998;13:196-199.
28. Shrager JB. Mediastinoscopy: still the gold standard. *Ann Thorac Surg.* 2010;89:S2084-S2089.
29. Hunninghake GW, Costabel U, Ando M, et al. ATS/ERS/WASOG statement on sarcoidosis: American Thoracic Society/European

Respiratory Society/World Association of Sarcoidosis and other Granulomatous Disorders. *Sarcoidosis Vasc Diffuse Lung Dis.* 1999;16:149-173.

30. Reich JM, Brouns MC, O'Connor EA, et al. Mediastinoscopy in patients with presumptive stage I sarcoidosis: a risk/benefit, cost/benefit analysis. *Chest.* 1998;113:147-153.
31. Moffatt-Bruce SD, Ross P Jr. Mediastinal abscess after endobronchial ultrasound with transbronchial needle aspiration: a case report. *J Cardiothorac Surg.* 2010;5:33.
32. Haas AR. Infectious complications from full extension endobronchial ultrasound transbronchial needle aspiration. *Eur Respir J.* 2009;33:935-938.
33. Lee N, Inoue K, Yamamoto R, et al. Patterns of internal echoes in lymph nodes in the diagnosis of lung cancer metastasis. *World J Surg.* 1992;16:986-994.
34. Bhutani MS, Hawes RH, Hoffman BJ. A comparison of the accuracy of echo features during endoscopic ultrasound (EUS) and EUS-guided fine-needle aspiration for diagnosis of malignant lymph node invasion. *Gastrointest Endosc.* 1997;45:474-479.
35. Fujiwara T, Yasufuku K, Nakajima T, et al. The utility of sonographic features during endobronchial ultrasound-guided transbronchial needle aspiration for lymph node staging in patients with lung cancer: a standard endobronchial ultrasound image classification system. *Chest.* 2010;138:641-647.
36. Wallace M, Hoffman B. Needle device systems for interventional endoscopic ultrasound and general technique of endoscopic ultrasound-guided fine-needle aspiration. *Tech Gastrointest Endosc.* 2000;2:136-141.
37. Alsharif M, Andrade RS, Groth SS, et al. Endobronchial ultrasound-guided transbronchial fine-needle aspiration: the University of Minnesota experience, with emphasis on usefulness, adequacy assessment, and diagnostic difficulties. *Am J Clin Pathol.* 2008;130:434-443.
38. Lee HS, Lee GK, Lee HS, et al. Real-time endobronchial ultrasound-guided transbronchial needle aspiration in mediastinal staging of non-small cell lung cancer: how many aspirations per target lymph node station? *Chest.* 2008;134:368-374.
39. Trisolini R, Lazzari Agli L, Patelli M. Conventional vs endobronchial ultrasound-guided transbronchial needle aspiration of the mediastinum. *Chest.* 2004;126:1005-1006.
40. von Bartheld MB, Veselic Charvat M, Rabe KF, et al. Endoscopic ultrasound-guided fine-needle aspiration for the diagnosis of sarcoidosis. *Endoscopy.* 2010;42:213-217.
41. Kennedy MP, Jimenez CA, Mhatre AD, et al. Clinical implications of granulomatous inflammation detected by endobronchial ultrasound transbronchial needle aspiration in patients with suspected cancer recurrence in the mediastinum. *J Cardiothorac Surg.* 2008;3:8.
42. Mehrotra R, Dhingra V. Cytological diagnosis of sarcoidosis revisited: a state of the art review. *Diagn Cytopathol.* 2010;39:541-548.
43. Barnett BP, Sheth S, Ali SZ. Cytopathologic analysis of paratracheal masses: a study of 737 cases with clinicoradiologic correlation. *Acta Cytol.* 2009;5:672-678.
44. Kok TC, Haasjes JG, Splinter TA, et al. Sarcoid-like lymphadenopathy mimicking metastatic testicular cancer. *Cancer.* 1991;68:1845-1847.
45. Lee HS, Lee GK, Lee HS, et al. Real-time endobronchial ultrasound-guided transbronchial needle aspiration in mediastinal staging of non-small cell lung cancer: how many aspirations per target lymph node station? *Chest.* 2008;134:368-374.
46. Rusch VW, Asamura H, Watanabe H, et al; Members of IASLC Staging Committee. The IASLC lung cancer staging project: a proposal for a new international lymph node map in the forthcoming seventh edition of the TNM classification for lung cancer. *J Thorac Oncol.* 2009;4:568-577.
47. Bilaceroglu S, Perim K, Gunel O, et al. Combining transbronchial aspiration with endobronchial and transbronchial biopsy in sarcoidosis. *Monaldi Arch Chest Dis.* 1999;54:217-223.
48. Trisolini R, Agli LL, Cancellieri A, et al. The value of flexible transbronchial needle aspiration in the diagnosis of stage I sarcoidosis. *Chest.* 2003;124:2126-2130.
49. Nakajima T, Yasufuku K, Kurosu K, et al. The role of EBUS-TBNA for the diagnosis of sarcoidosis—comparisons with other bronchoscopic diagnostic modalities. *Respir Med.* 2009;103:1796-1800.
50. Navani N, Booth HL, Kocjan G, et al. Combination of endobronchial ultrasound-guided transbronchial needle aspiration with standard bronchoscopic techniques for the diagnosis of stage I and stage II pulmonary sarcoidosis. *Respirology.* 2011;16:467-472.
51. Pisircriler R, Atay Z, Lang W. Cytological diagnosis of intrathoracic epithelioid cellular inflammatory process. *Pneumologie.* 1990;44:767-770.
52. Tremblay A, Stather DR, Maceachern P, et al. A randomized controlled trial of standard vs endobronchial ultrasonography-guided transbronchial needle aspiration in patients with suspected sarcoidosis. *Chest.* 2009;136:340-346.
53. Laurberg P. Sarcoid reactions in pulmonary neoplasms. *Scand J Respir Dis.* 1975;56:20-27.
54. Steinfort DP, Irving LB. Sarcoidal reactions in regional lymph nodes of patients with non-small cell lung cancer: incidence and implications for minimally invasive staging with endobronchial ultrasound. *Lung Cancer.* 2009;66:305-308.
55. Schunemann HJ, Oxman AD, Brozek J, et al. Grading quality of evidence and strength of recommendations for diagnostic tests and strategies. *BMJ.* 2008;336:1106-1110.
56. Ernst A, Anantham D, Eberhardt R, et al. Diagnosis of mediastinal adenopathy-real-time endobronchial ultrasound guided needle aspiration versus mediastinoscopy. *J Thorac Oncol.* 2008;3:577-582.
57. Annema JT, van Meerbeeck JP, Rintoul RC, et al. Mediastinoscopy vs endosonography for mediastinal nodal staging of lung cancer: a randomized trial. *JAMA.* 2010;304:2245-2252.
58. Piet AH, Lagerwaard FJ, Kunst PW, et al. Can mediastinal nodal mobility explain the low yield rates for transbronchial needle aspiration without real-time imaging? *Chest.* 2007;131:1783-1787.

SECTION 5

Practical Approach to Malignant Central Airway Obstruction

Chapter 20

Stent Insertion for Extrinsic Tracheal Obstruction Caused by Thyroid Carcinoma

This chapter emphasizes the following elements of the Four Box Approach: indications, contraindications, and expected results; anesthesia and other perioperative care; techniques and instrumentation; and follow-up tests, visits, and procedures.

CASE DESCRIPTION

This patient was a 67-year-old obese (BMI, 37 kg/m²) African American female with a 25–pack-year history of smoking who developed progressive dyspnea on exertion, cough, and hoarseness. She had a history of COPD (FEV₁ 45% predicted) and obstructive sleep apnea (OSA) treated with CPAP of 10 cm H₂O. Physical examination was remarkable for biphasic stridor, heard best during forced inspiratory and expiratory maneuvers. Computed tomography scanning showed the intrathoracic extension of a thyroid mass, narrowing the trachea (Figure 20-1). Ultrasound-guided fine-needle aspiration of the thyroid mass revealed papillary thyroid carcinoma. The patient was referred for evaluation and management of her tracheal obstruction before performance of a complete thyroidectomy. Flexible bronchoscopy performed under moderate sedation with the patient in a semi-upright position showed redundant pharyngeal and laryngeal tissues; the arytenoid cartilages were edematous and were collapsing over the vocal folds during inspiration (see video on ExpertConsult.com) (Video V.20.1). Tracheal narrowing was due to pure extrinsic compression without mucosal infiltration or exophytic endoluminal abnormalities. The stenotic segment was located 3.5 cm below the cords and extended for 3 cm. The degree of narrowing was 60% during inspiration and 70% during tidal expiration as compared with the normal airway lumen (see Figure 20-1).

DISCUSSION POINTS

1. List four indications for airway stent insertion in this patient.
2. List and justify four anesthesia considerations of rigid bronchoscopy in view of this patient's medical history, physical examination, and tracheal obstruction.
3. Describe and justify one indication for prolonged indwelling airway stent placement if this patient undergoes successful thyroidectomy.

CASE RESOLUTION

Initial Evaluations

Physical Examination, Complementary Tests, and Functional Status Assessment

Thyroid disease with airway obstruction has been described in patients with thyroid carcinoma and in those with benign goiters.[1,2] Mechanisms of airway obstruction include extrinsic compression (e.g., benign intrathoracic or substernal goiter), airway invasion by tumor (e.g., thyroid cancer), tracheomalacia (e.g., after thyroidectomy or long-term compression from goiter), vocal cord paralysis (e.g., recurrent nerve paralysis due to tumor or after thyroidectomy), and a combination of these.[3] The most frequent cause of airway obstruction in the presence of thyroid disease is substernal (benign or malignant) goiter compressing the trachea with or without associated tracheomalacia.[4] In the setting of thyroid carcinoma, symptoms associated with mucosal invasion such as hemoptysis (seen in 11% to 39% of patients) and airway obstruction causing dyspnea (seen in 5% to 89% of patients) underestimate the depth of airway invasion because they are usually present in patients with a most advanced degree of invasion (i.e., when the tumor is already intraluminal). Even deep tumor invasion into the tracheal wall often is not identified before surgery unless fixation of the gland is obvious on physical examination.[5] In this regard, physical examination during initial evaluation of patients with thyroid carcinoma may not suffice to identify a thyroid mass as a cause of respiratory problems. In fact, in one small series of five patients with acute airway obstruction, goiters were palpable in three patients, whereas the other two goiters were diagnosed by emergency computed tomography (CT) of the thorax.[6]

Malignant airway obstruction caused by a primary tumor or by recurrent disease is the cause of death in one half of all patients with thyroid carcinoma.[7] In general, well-differentiated thyroid carcinoma is considered an indolent disease with an 80% to 95% 10 year survival rate.[8] In about 5.7% to 7% of cases of well-differentiated thyroid carcinoma, the tumor invades adjacent laryngotracheal structures,[9] and changes in clinical status may occur only when it reaches the mucosa. It is important that patients with malignant thyroid disease be evaluated by CT imaging of the neck and chest and by flexible bronchoscopy to assess the extent and the severity of the narrowing, and to determine whether intraluminal tumor

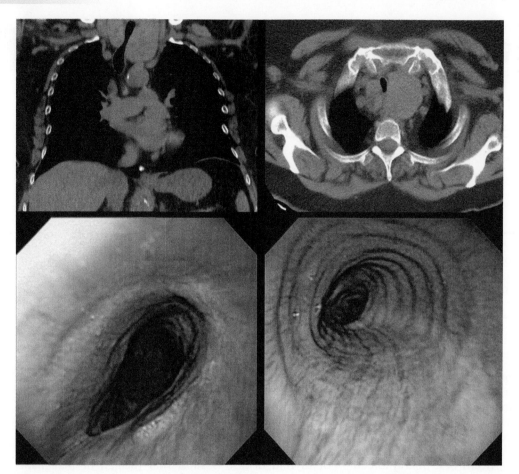

Figure 20-1 Coronal *(top left)* and axial *(top right)* computed tomography (CT) images show tracheal narrowing from a large thyroid mass. The tracheal lumen is seen at the level of the stenosis *(bottom left)* and distal to it *(bottom right)*.

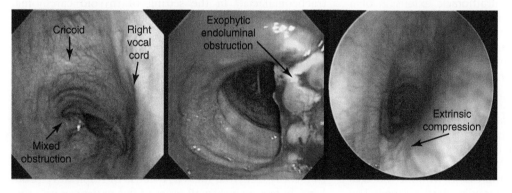

Figure 20-2 Three types of tracheal obstruction caused by thyroid cancer. Mixed endoluminal and extrinsic compression type *(left)*, pure exophytic endoluminal *(center)*, and pure extrinsic compression *(right)*.

or extrinsic compression is the main cause of obstruction, especially if patients are being considered for complete thyroidectomy. Some patients, such as those for whom radical surgery for laryngotracheal invasion is not feasible owing to poor physical condition or those who are symptomatic from airway narrowing, may not be candidates for curative surgery but may be suitable for palliative bronchoscopic interventions.

In our patient, bronchoscopic inspection was conducted to evaluate for possible vocal cord paralysis, airway tumor invasion, and the mechanism of obstruction: exophytic endoluminal versus pure extrinsic versus mixed extrinsic and intraluminal (Figure 20-2).[10] In fact, one study found unilateral vocal cord paralysis in 83% of patients with thyroid carcinoma.[11] During

bronchoscopy, if the airway mucosa is abnormal, biopsy of the intraluminal tumor can and should be performed because positive results predict a worse prognosis.[12] Indeed, the depth of airway invasion appears to predict outcome, with shorter survival reported in patients with endoluminal tumor.[13] Other bronchoscopic findings in patients with thyroid disease–induced airway involvement include erythema and edema, neovascular formation, and frank mucosal invasion.[12] Tracheal invasion should be clearly documented by the bronchoscopist; this is of particular interest to surgeons because it is a marker for more aggressive tumors and defines a patient population at greater risk for death.[5,7] Results from one study of 18 cases of thyroid cancer infiltrating the trachea showed poor tumor differentiation in 50% of papillary and follicular carcinomas compared with 11.4% when airways were not invaded.[14] Among 292 patients with well-differentiated papillary carcinoma, the most commonly encountered histology, authors identified laryngotracheal invasion in 124 patients (41%) as a significant independent predictor of death.[15] An additional study found that laryngotracheal or esophageal invasion was an important negative prognostic factor, indicating that tracheal invasion lowers long-term survival.[16]

Usually identified at the time of operation, extraluminal airway invasion demands a decision regarding the extent of resection. The proportion of patients with thyroid cancer involving the larynx and the trachea depends not only on histology but also on the definition of invasion. Invasion into the tracheal wall or the larynx in the form of external adherence was noted in surgical studies to vary from 3.6% to 22.9% of all patients undergoing thyroidectomy.*[5] The most advanced stage of invasion constitutes intraluminal tumor, which is more rare and is detected on bronchoscopy in only 0.5% to 1.5% of patients presenting for resection. Radiologic criteria such as compression or displacement by tumor, which occurred in up to 35%, may overestimate invasion. Thus bronchoscopy remains essential in determining endoluminal involvement, surgical strategy, and outcome.[5] In our patient, who had no evidence of endoluminal invasion, bronchoscopy was necessary to determine the site, severity, and length of the tracheal obstruction to allow selection of a tracheal stent of appropriate length and size to relieve her symptoms.

Comorbidities

Obesity, chronic obstructive pulmonary disease (COPD), and obstructive sleep apnea (OSA) could increase the risk for complications during or after procedures performed with the patient under general anesthesia.

Support System

The patient had one daughter who was very involved in her care and accompanied her to all of her clinic appointments. Her daughter was present in the room during our diagnostic flexible bronchoscopy.

Patient Preferences and Expectations

The patient understood her diagnosis. She and her daughter had already talked about it in detail with the treating surgeon. At the time of our encounter, the patient did not have an advance directive and was reluctant to initiate one. In this regard, it is possible that among African Americans, nonacceptance of advance directives may be part of a different set of values regarding quality of life and trust in health care professionals.[†] Do not resuscitate (DNR) orders may be viewed as a way of limiting health care expenditures or cutting costs by stopping care

prematurely.[17] Furthermore, the reluctance of African Americans to address end-of-life care in a formal fashion may originate from a history of health care discrimination. Evidence indicates that nonwhites, even after controls for income, insurance status, and age are applied, are less likely to receive a range of common medical interventions such as analgesics for acute pain, cardiac catheterization, and even immunizations.[17] Overall, African American patients are about one half as likely to accept DNR status and are more likely than whites to later change DNR orders to more aggressive levels of care.[18]

Procedural Strategies

Indications

Clinically manifest airway obstruction due to thyroid enlargement is considered to be an absolute indication for surgical intervention. In general, treatment of differentiated primary thyroid cancer consists of total thyroidectomy followed by adjuvant radioiodine treatment and suppressive thyroxine therapy. Indications for bronchoscopic treatment in benign and malignant thyroid disorders causing airway obstruction include refusal of surgery, medical or surgical inoperability, tracheomalacia, and acute severe respiratory insufficiency with imminent respiratory failure. An indication specific to malignant disease is recurrence after previous surgery.[3] In one series, among patients requiring bronchoscopic treatment for malignant disease, 10 patients (77%) had purely extrinsic compression of the trachea requiring stent insertion, 1 with associated bilateral vocal cord paralysis, and 3 patients (23%) showed mixed obstruction with extrinsic tracheal compression associated with exophytic endoluminal disease (see Figure 20-2).[3] Indications for interventional bronchoscopy in our patient included stridor, dyspnea, and potential avoidance of tracheomalacia post thyroidectomy. Tracheal stent insertion could provide our patient with symptomatic relief of her respiratory difficulties while subsequently allowing the surgical team to perform a potentially curative resection. In one study, for example, airway patency was maintained with covered retrievable self-expandable nitinol stents until surgery was performed. Stents were successfully removed within 3 weeks after surgery.[19]

In patients who are not operable, however, stent insertion, by improving functional status, allows the medical team to proceed with palliative chemotherapy or radiotherapy. Tracheal stents should not be placed prophylactically in these patients just because the airway is extrinsically compressed or invaded by tumor. Airway involvement should cause symptoms that warrant stent insertion. This is especially true in patients with thyroid cancer because most tumors (≈80%) are located in the larynx and at the level of the cricoid cartilage—a region where stents are at high risk for migration and may not be well tolerated owing to their close proximity to the vocal cords.[12] Even in mixed forms of obstruction, ablation of the intraluminal lesion is the first-line procedure (see video on ExpertConsult.com) (Video V.20.2), but stent insertion becomes necessary when symptomatic airway stenosis results from increased

---

*The surgeon's definition of invasion, ranging from any attachment of the gland to gross tumor transgression, further influences this proportion.

†This perspective may originate from a long history of distrust of the white-dominated health care system. One example is the Tuskegee syphilis study, in which infected African American men were followed for 40 years and were not informed of the availability of penicillin treatment.

extrinsic compression, or when repeated removal of an intraluminal lesion at short intervals is due to a fast-growing tumor. In one study, this approach was shown to succeed in maintaining airway patency, and the cause of death in two thirds of patients was not airway obstruction but progression of preexisting lung metastases or carcinomatous pleuritis.[12]

Contraindications

No contraindication to general anesthesia or stent placement was noted.

Expected Results

In multiple reports, researchers have revealed their experience with tracheal stent placement for palliation in patients with thyroid disease such as benign intrathoracic or substernal goiter, thyroid cancer, thyroid lymphoma, and tracheomalacia after thyroidectomy. For this purpose, they have used silicone stents, covered or uncovered metallic stents, T-tubes, or tracheostomy tubes.[3,11] In one series of 16 patients with malignant thyroid disease, neodymium-doped yttrium aluminum garnet (Nd:YAG) laser treatment (n = 3) and stent insertion* (n = 13) resulted in restoration of airway patency and symptomatic improvement in 92% of patients (see video on ExpertConsult.com) (Video V.20.3). Data revealed 15% short-term[†] and 8% long-term complications[‡] and a median survival time (MST) of 17 months.[3] Shorter survival times of only 4 months were reported, however, by other investigators.[20] In a large retrospective study of 35 patients with advanced thyroid cancer requiring stent insertion for managing airway obstruction, the authors compared studded silicone stents (Novatech, Aubagne, France) and T-tubes (Koken, Tokyo, Japan) versus self-expandable metallic stents—covered and uncovered Ultraflex (Boston Scientific, Natick, Mass) and Spiral Z (Medico's Hirata, Tokyo, Japan).[11] All patients reported immediate symptomatic relief objectively documented by improvements in both Eastern Cooperative Oncology Group (ECOG) performance status and the Hugh-Jones dyspnea scale. MST was 8 months. One-year survival was 40%, but death was due to progression of disease at sites other than the airway.[11] In this series, almost all stent-related complications requiring further intervention occurred in patients who had a studded silicone stent or a T-tube inserted. These included stent migration, retained secretions, granulation tissue formation, and tumor overgrowth. Critical complications of stent insertion included supraglottic stenosis (5 cases, 14% of stent implantations) and migration within 1 week of insertion (4 cases, 11% of stent implantations). These were associated with studded silicone stents in the proximity of the cricoid cartilage, indicating that migration occurred in as many as 40% of all studded silicone stent placements.[11]

Team Experience

For inoperable patients requiring bronchoscopic treatments, procedures are usually performed with the patient under general anesthesia and using rigid bronchoscopy.[3,11] Therefore referral to a center experienced in this procedure is warranted. For operable patients, the surgeon who is unfamiliar with techniques of open tracheal resection has several options when encountering tracheal invasion, including operative exploration without thyroidectomy, or leaving complete, combined resection to the surgeon trained in thyroid and airway procedures. Alternatively, combined resection may be performed by a multidisciplinary team of thyroid and tracheal surgeons. If thyroidectomy has been completed with a shave resection, tracheal or laryngotracheal resection may then be performed after referral to a surgeon experienced in airway surgery.[5]

Therapeutic Alternatives

Endoscopic tumor ablation by debulking with an Nd:YAG laser has been performed for patients with endoluminal tumor involvement in whom radical operations are contraindicated. In one study, 22 consecutive patients underwent endoscopic tumor ablation* for well-differentiated thyroid carcinoma. During a follow-up period of up to 125 months, 6 of 22 patients died (median survival, 50 months), mainly of lung metastases, but all had a patent airway at the time of death. The authors noted that post intervention extraluminal lesion growth is indolent, and because relapse of the intraluminal lesion is the main cause of symptoms, local control could be obtained by repeat ablation of the mucosal lesion.[12]

Tracheostomy is the traditional method used for primary treatment of acute airway obstruction due to malignant invasion and compression of the trachea from thyroid carcinoma. However, insertion of tracheal stents may obviate the need for tracheostomy.[11] Indeed, emergent stent insertion in 10 patients with a severe, mixed type of airway obstruction caused by various malignancies, including papillary thyroid carcinoma, resulted in a median survival time of 8 months.[21] Patients with repeated local recurrence over a long period from the time of initial treatment often are unable to undergo radical surgery, in which case tracheotomy could be performed to establish a patent airway. Tracheostomy may be technically difficult, however, in the case of a large, bulky thyroid mass,[22] in which case a tracheal stent is often a feasible alternative.

Surgical airway resection when performed immediately after detection of airway invasion at the time of thyroidectomy is associated with longer disease-free survival compared with later resection (after a mean period of 67 months, at recurrence).[23] In our patient, no airway mucosal invasion was evident on bronchoscopy; however, if detected at the time of surgery, airway resection could become necessary. In general, strategies for surgical

---

*Stents used included 10 Dumon (Bryan Corp., Woburn, Mass), 3 Noppen-Tygon (Reynders Medical Supply, Lennik, Belgium), and 1 Ultraflex.

[†]One patient had tumor recurrence requiring laser resection at 9 days and 20 days after the initial treatment. One patient had stent migration at 1 week, requiring stent replacement.

[‡]One patient had tumor recurrence at 18 months, requiring laser resection and stent repositioning.

---

*In this particular study, debulking by Nd:YAG laser was followed by electrocoagulation and microwave coagulation for the residual tumor base.

resection of the airway for laryngotracheal invasion are considered in five different clinical settings[5]: (1) when the thyroid gland adheres to the airway at the time of initial thyroidectomy; (2) in cases referred after incomplete tangential excision* of tumor; (3) when invasion with airway obstruction is detected before the time of surgical therapy; (4) in cases of local recurrence with airway obstruction late after thyroidectomy; and (5) in some cases of airway obstruction in the presence of distant metastatic disease.[†] Several surgical alternatives have been described and include tangential excision of tumor, tracheal or laryngotracheal sleeve resection,[‡] and laryngectomy with cervical exenteration,[§] all of which usually are considered salvage resections for patients with extensive invasive disease or locoregional recurrent disease following previous resection or radiation.[5,24]

Self-expandable metallic stents are a reasonable alternative to silicone stent insertion in inoperable patients with malignant thyroid tumor and airway obstruction.[11] Placement of covered retrievable self-expandable nitinol stents was safe and effective in patients with airway obstruction caused by benign or malignant thyroid disease, and in some patients served as an effective bridge to surgery.[19] For patients with thyroid carcinoma, one study showed that the uncovered Ultraflex stent was associated with fewer complications (supraglottic obstruction and migration) than were observed with silicone stents.[11]

Radioactive iodine (RAI) therapy: This is usually indicated alone for metastatic or locally advanced disease when surgical options are exhausted. Postoperatively, this adjuvant therapy for residual disease in the tracheal wall may have limited effectiveness because tumors invading the airway are often less differentiated, may have less RAI uptake, and may be resistant to therapy. However, postoperative adjuvant RAI is commonly administered after surgical resection.[5]

External beam radiation therapy (EBRT): Adjuvant or palliative radiation is proposed to improve local control for patients with advanced cancer after incomplete resection. EBRT may potentially improve recurrence rates[25] in patients with resected locally advanced disease.

Cost-Effectiveness

It is difficult to draw conclusions about the most cost-effective stent insertion strategy in this patient. One study showed that self-expanding metallic stents (SEMS) may represent a better choice than silicone stents in terms of complications[11]; other studies, using predominantly silicone stents, showed symptomatic benefit without significant complications.[3] We chose to proceed with an easily retrievable stent because we considered that stent

insertion was a temporary measure that would allow our patient to undergo surgical resection.

Informed Consent

The patient showed understanding of the indications, benefits, and potential complications of silicone stent insertion. The informed consent form was signed by the patient.

Techniques and Results

Anesthesia and Perioperative Care

In obese patients, similar to our patient, the pharmacokinetics of anesthetic drugs is different from that in individuals of normal weight. This should be carefully considered to reduce any risks for intraoperative or postoperative complications. For instance, in one study that evaluated the pharmacokinetics of remifentanil in 12 obese patients compared with 12 control subjects of normal weight, obese subjects had significantly higher plasma concentrations compared with normal subjects after a loading dose, suggesting that to avoid an overdose, remifentanil should be administered on the basis of ideal body weight (IBW) or lean body mass (LBM), rather than on the basis of total body weight (TBW).[26] Another study compared the plasma concentrations of fentanyl measured in normal (body mass index [BMI] <30) and obese (BMI >30) subjects undergoing major surgery with a fentanyl infusion based on TBW, finding that this led to an overestimation of fentanyl dose requirements in obese patients.[*27]

We do not use neuromuscular blockers in our patients who undergo rigid bronchoscopy, but these drugs may be employed in cases of rigid bronchoscopy and high-frequency jet ventilation. The polar, hydrophilic nature of nondepolarizing neuromuscular blockers tends to limit their volume of distribution. Vecuronium has a prolonged duration of action if it is administered on the basis of TBW. If it is administered on the basis of IBW, the volume of distribution, total clearance, and elimination half-life have been shown to be equivalent between obese and normal subjects.[28] The same principles apply to rocuronium and cisatracurium, with dosage guided by TBW leading to a prolonged duration of action.[29]

With regard to the commonly used drug propofol, a comparison study with controls of normal weight showed that administering doses of propofol on the basis of TBW resulted in an unchanged initial volume of distribution; clearance was related to body weight, and the volume of distribution at steady state correlated with body weight. No evidence suggested propofol accumulation when dosing was based on TBW.[30]

Induction of anesthesia must be performed cautiously in patients with obesity. For endotracheal intubation using an endotracheal tube (ETT), an awake intubation

---

*Tangential excision of tumor (aka "shaving") consists of sharp separation of the gland from the wall of the airway with a knife; the surface of the trachea is scraped or is tangentially cut to remove a further layer of airway tissue for microscopic analysis.

†Categories 4 and 5 are performed mainly for palliative reasons.

‡Consists of en bloc resection of the thyroid gland and attached trachea when the discovered invasion is limited to two or three tracheal rings, allowing a short tracheal resection.

§Exenteration refers to the combined removal of larynx, pharynx, cervical esophagus, thyroid, and lymph nodes with intestinal reconstruction using stomach (gastric pull-up), jejunum, or colon.

---

*The authors derived a parameter that they refer to as *pharmacokinetic mass*, which could be used to linearly predict fentanyl clearance and thus accurately guide fentanyl infusions. For patients weighing 140 to 200 kg, the pharmacokinetic mass was 100 to 108 kg, which illustrates the magnitude of dosing errors that can result from using TBW with fentanyl.

technique should be considered if the adequacy of the mask ventilation is questionable. In cases of rigid bronchoscopy, the operator has to be positioned at the head of the table, ready to intervene and secure the airway in case of loss of airway patency or inability to mask ventilate patients after induction. Proper positioning for direct laryngoscopy will maximize the likelihood of success on the first attempt. This may require significant elevation of the upper body and head. Positioning obese patients in a "ramped" position (with blankets used to elevate both the upper body and the head of the patient or by raising the head of the table) has been shown to result in improved laryngeal exposure with direct laryngoscopy, which could result in fewer failed intubations.[31] In addition, because hypoxemia may occur post induction, improvements in oxygenation can be achieved with the preinduction use of positive end-expiratory pressure (PEEP), which will increase the time before desaturation begins.*[32] It is unclear whether obese patients have more frequent complications resulting from positioning during anesthesia than patients of normal weight. The standard supine position traditionally used creates some difficulties because some patients have such a large body habitus that standard operating room tables are too small or are unable to handle the patient's weight. In addition, prolonged surgery (3 to 5 hours) in the supine position has been anecdotally associated with rhabdomyolysis of the gluteal muscles, leading to renal failure.[33] Health care organizations should plan appropriately for the care of morbidly obese patients and should consider the safety of health care workers involved in caring for these patients.†[34]

Obese patients are more likely to become hypoxic during anesthesia and surgery than patients of normal weight.[34] Morbid obesity (BMI >40 kg/m^2) is associated with reductions in expiratory reserve volume (ERV), forced vital capacity (FVC), forced expiratory volume in 1 second (FEV$_1$), maximum voluntary ventilation (MVV), and functional residual capacity (FRC).[35] Subjects often have FRC reduced to near residual volume (RV); the reduction in FRC is even greater in the supine position.[36] Marked changes in lung and chest wall mechanics, including reduced respiratory system compliance, increased respiratory system resistance, severely reduced FRC, and impaired arterial oxygenation, have been described in mechanically ventilated and paralyzed morbidly obese patients.[37] One of the mechanisms of hypoxemia during mechanical ventilation in obese patients is increased intra-abdominal pressure that reduces lung volumes, resulting in ventilation-perfusion mismatch.[38] Results from a physiologic study showed that severely obese supine subjects at relaxation volume have positive pleural pressure (Ppl) throughout the chest, as suggested by high esophageal pressure (PEs) measurements or inferred from airway pressure and flow measurements.* Both lung and respiratory system compliances were found to be low because of breathing at abnormally low lung volumes. High pleural pressure causes tidal breathing to be initiated from low end-expiratory volumes, where the lungs are less compliant and airways are prone to close on exhalation.[39] The positive pleural pressure and the early small airway closure could result in worsening of the expiratory central airway collapse, as was seen in our patient (see video on ExpertConsult.com) (Video V.20.4).

Regarding postanesthesia care, sedation and narcotic-based analgesia may exacerbate symptoms of sleep apnea. Therefore, if the patient has a difficult airway, extubation should be accomplished in a conservative fashion with careful assessment of the patient's level of consciousness. It is noteworthy that the pharyngeal cross-sectional area is larger in the lateral position than in the supine position, and this may limit airway obstruction in patients with OSA.[40] In addition, given that the rigid bronchoscope is positioned in the larynx, close postsurgical observation for laryngeal edema is mandatory.

Instrumentation

Stent selection traditionally has been based on an operator's previous experience with a particular stent and the local availability of various stents. Stent retrievability is important in patients with benign disease and in those with malignancy for which a temporary stent placement is expected; these include patients with malignant central airway obstruction who will undergo further surgical or systemic chemotherapy and/or radiation therapy. In patients with thyroid disease and airway obstruction, it was possible to safely remove polymer stents 6 months after surgery in all patients.[3]

In addition to the morphology and consistency of the tumor, mechanical properties of the stent should be considered in selecting the appropriate stent.[41] Expansile force (strength) and ability to withhold angulation (buckling) vary among different types of stents. For our patient with extrinsic compression, we believe that the most important attribute of a stent would be its expansile force, because this determines whether the stent is likely to expand fully. In this regard, the studded-silicone–type stent has high expansile force and was thus selected for our patient.[42] However, for a distorted, curved airway, angulation properties become important because they determine whether the stent can conform to an acutely angulated airway and still remain patent. This was not the case in our patient with tracheal obstruction but should be considered in patients with curved, distorted

---

*Preoxygenation with 100% fraction of inspired oxygen (FiO$_2$) and PEEP of 10 cm H$_2$O for 5 minutes before the induction of general anesthesia, followed by PEEP of 10 during mask ventilation and after intubation, reduces immediate post intubation atelectasis as assessed by CT scan and improves immediate post intubation arterial oxygenation on 100% FiO$_2$ (partial pressure of oxygen in arterial blood [PaO$_2$] of 457 ± 130 mm Hg vs. 315 ± 100 mm Hg in the control group); this strategy has to be carefully considered in obese patients with gastroesophageal reflux, who are at higher risk for aspiration during noninvasive application of PEEP.

†If it is necessary to move an anesthetized morbidly obese patient, a roller may be used under the patient, or a sufficient number of personnel may be required to minimize the risk of injury for those moving the patient.

*Respiratory system compliance (C[RS]) was lower in obese than in control subjects (0.032 ± 0.008 vs. 0.053 ± 0.007 L/cm H$_2$O), principally as the result of lower lung compliance (0.043 ± 0.016 vs. 0.084 ± 0.029 L/cm H$_2$O) rather than chest wall compliance (obese 0.195 ± 0.109, control 0.223 ± 0.132 L/cm H$_2$O).

Figure 20-3 Rigid bronchoscopy picture after stent placement *(left)*: Airway patency is restored and the stent is in intimate contact with the airway wall. Flexible bronchoscopy after thyroidectomy shows the loose stent and no evidence of extrinsic compression *(right)*.

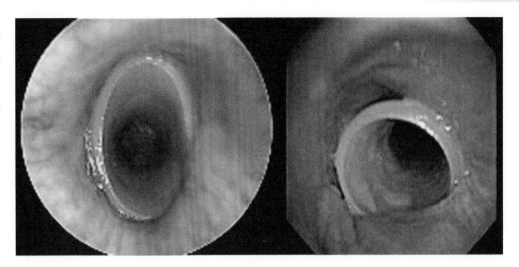

airways such as those with left main bronchial obstruction. In these cases, the Ultraflex stent may be a better choice than a straight silicone stent because of the Ultraflex stent's known resistance to angulation.[43]

Anatomic Dangers and Other Risks

One critical complication of interventional bronchoscopy for advanced thyroid cancer is temporary bilateral vocal cord paralysis or supraglottic stenosis caused by laryngeal edema.*[20] During treatment of laryngeal lesions, the tip of the rigid bronchoscope is positioned adjacent to the vocal cords; furthermore, because most patients have pre-existing unilateral vocal cord paralysis (up to 80%), the risk for airway obstruction is high if bronchoscopy results in temporary paralysis of the unaffected vocal cord.

Results and Procedure-Related Complications

After induction with propofol and remifentanil, the patient was intubated with a 12 mm rigid bronchoscope (EFER-Dumon bronchoscope, Bryan Corporation, Boston, Mass) through an open-tube technique, which allows insertion of the flexible bronchoscope. Redundant pharyngeal tissues and arytenoid cartilage edema were again noticed. The site of tracheal obstruction was carefully inspected, and no evidence of endoluminal disease or mucosal infiltration was found. The proximal aspect of the stricture was 3.5 cm below the vocal cords. The distal and proximal margins of the stenotic segment were visualized, and the total length of the stenosis was 3 cm. Distal to the obstruction, we noted excessive dynamic airway collapse of moderate severity, likely worsened by the supine position and general anesthesia **(see video on ExpertConsult.com)** (Video V.20.4) when compared with images obtained during flexible bronchoscopy with the patient in a semi-upright position and use of moderate sedation. The distal aspect of the scope was positioned just distal to the stenotic segment, and a 16 × 40 mm

studded Dumon-type silicone stent was inserted and positioned with its proximal aspect seated 3 cm below the cords, and its distal aspect seated 5 cm above the main carina (Figure 20-3). Anesthetic drug infusion was then stopped, and once the patient showed signs of awakening (she began bucking and coughing), the head of the operating room table was raised so that the patient could lie in the ramp position, the rigid scope was removed, and an oral airway was inserted. She was placed on oxygen via mask and was transferred to the postanesthesia care unit (PACU) in stable condition. The patient was discharged home the next day.

Long-Term Management

Outcome Assessment

Airway patency was restored satisfactorily and without complications. We contacted the referring physician and recommended that in case of thyroidectomy, she should be intubated using a flexible bronchoscope to avoid dislodgment and migration of the stent.

Follow-up Tests and Procedures

Once surgery was completed, 2 months after stent placement, the patient returned for follow-up bronchoscopy, which showed that the stent was now loose in her upper trachea (see Figure 20-3). Rigid bronchoscopy was performed, and the stent was safely removed. No evidence of residual extrinsic compression or of malacia was found. Occasionally, however, post thyroidectomy, these patients may have persistent airway compromise, primarily caused by tracheomalacia. In such cases, several techniques of tracheal support have been advocated, including endotracheal stent placement, tracheoplasty, tracheal suspension, and insertion of prosthetic rings. In our case, had malacia occurred, we would have left the stent in place and proceeded with routine follow-up bronchoscopy every 1 to 4 months, depending on our patient's clinical status.[11] The literature suggests that most cases of tracheomalacia post thyroidectomy will resolve if patients are left intubated for a few days. Some authors choose this technique, reserving endotracheal stent placement for patients with persistent airway compromise who fail

---

*Supraglottic stenosis from laryngeal edema is a life-threatening condition that requires emergency airway control and reinsertion of a rigid bronchoscope, or endotracheal intubation could be problematic in severe cases.

extubation.[44] In patients with thyroid carcinoma, follow-up bronchoscopy post thyroidectomy is probably warranted, even if patients do not have indwelling airway stents. Evidence suggests that in postoperative patients, cancer recurrence and progression may occur predominantly inside the lumen rather than extraluminally. A pathologic study of 22 cases of papillary carcinoma with tracheal invasion indicated that tracheal invasion occurs directly from the primary thyroid cancer extending between the cartilaginous rings and the ligaments of the trachea, where the vessels penetrate perpendicular to the lumen, allowing an invasion pathway. Scar tissue formation and adhesion following effective surgical resection of the extraluminal lesion may prevent extraluminal proliferation of the existing differentiated thyroid carcinoma of the tracheal wall. The tumor may slowly penetrate into the airway lumen through the laryngotracheal wall, and once it reaches the mucosa, it may grow to involve portions of the airway where tissue resistance is weak. More aggressive tumors may grow extraluminally, resulting in recurrent extrinsic compression.[13]

Referrals

Our patient underwent adjuvant RAI and continued her care with the referring pulmonologist for her OSA and COPD and for follow-up bronchoscopies.

Quality Improvement

One could argue that our patient had alternative explanations for her dyspnea (i.e., COPD) and even for her stridor (i.e., bronchoscopic finding of floppy and edematous arytenoids), and that insertion of the stent therefore was not warranted. In addition, prophylactic stent insertion is not routinely recommended to prevent malacia post thyroidectomy.[11] However, in symptomatic extrinsic compression from thyroid carcinoma, stent insertion is an accepted practice.[12] In our patient, extrinsic compression in the intrathoracic airway and stridor on exhalation were clear, suggesting that the intrathoracic obstruction was contributory to the patient's symptoms. In addition, in one case series of five patients (four patients with benign substernal goiter and one patient with follicular carcinoma of the thyroid), airway stents prevented airway collapse due to tracheomalacia after thyroidectomy.[44] However, although postoperative tracheomalacia has been well described, its incidence is low (1 case in 116 thyroidectomies in one study)[45]; therefore the indication for preventive stent placement can be questioned, even in patients with long-standing thyroid masses. Perhaps a more conservative strategy such as awaiting results of extubation after thyroidectomy is justified, and stent insertion should be performed only after the diagnosis of postsurgical tracheomalacia has been confirmed.[3]

DISCUSSION POINTS

1. List four indications for airway stent insertion in this patient.
   - Avoid respiratory failure[44,46]
   - Maintain airway patency during anesthesia[47]
   - Improve airflow and symptoms[3]
   - Maintain airway patency post thyroidectomy[48]

2. List and justify four anesthesia considerations of rigid bronchoscopy in view of this patient's medical history, physical examination, and tracheal obstruction.
   - Loss of airway due to severe tracheal obstruction[47]
   - Auto-PEEP during positive-pressure ventilation in the setting of COPD[49]
   - Decreased FRC, ventilation-perfusion mismatch, and hypoxemia due to severe obesity[34]
   - Potentially difficult intubation and postoperative respiratory failure, given the patient's OSA[34]

3. Describe and justify one indication for prolonged indwelling airway stent placement if this patient undergoes successful thyroidectomy.

Tracheomalacia: This results from long-standing compression by a large thyroid mass wherein rings of the trachea may be completely destroyed or considerably weakened. The airway is prone to collapse after thyroidectomy, resulting in postoperative stridor and potentially in respiratory failure.* The incidence of tracheomalacia has been reported between 0.001% and 1.5%[50-52] with the highest incidence (1.5%) reported in substernal goiter.[53] Clinical findings thought to be associated with tracheomalacia include a preoperative history of stridor, radiologic evidence of tracheal deviation or compression, retrosternal goiter, cancer, post thyroidectomy status, long-term compression, and difficulty in intubation.†[54,55]

Expert Commentary

provided by Chris T. Bolliger, MD, PhD

As I read this detailed approach to a 67-year-old female patient with thyroid carcinoma and symptomatic tracheal stenosis, I asked myself whether I too would have inserted a stent, or perhaps would have chosen a different approach?

Well, let's look at this patient's detailed description again. She reported exertional dyspnea, but she did not report dyspnea at rest. Apart from her tracheal obstruction, she had been diagnosed with chronic obstructive pulmonary disease (COPD) (her forced expiratory volume in 1 second [FEV_1] was only 45% of predicted) and with obstructive sleep apnea (OSA), which was being treated by continuous positive airway pressure (CPAP). Although the patient had clearly audible stridor, it is possible that the cause of her exertional dyspnea might have been multifactorial. On bronchoscopy, a clearly relevant obstruction was noted at the level of the upper trachea. This obstruction was

---

*If patients develop stridor along with desaturation despite the administration of increasing FiO_2, it is also important to rule out bilateral vocal cord paralysis and glottic/subglottic edema, which are more common causes of stridor than tracheomalacia.

†The intraoperative diagnosis of tracheomalacia during thyroid surgery is reportedly made possible by identifying one or more of the following criteria: (1) soft and floppy trachea on palpation by the surgeon at the end of thyroidectomy; because of the splinting effect of the indwelling endotracheal tube, however, it may be difficult to appreciate a soft trachea; (2) obstruction to spontaneous respiration during gradual withdrawal of the ETT after thyroidectomy; (3) difficulty in advancing the suction catheter beyond the ETT after gradual withdrawal; and (4) absence of peritubal leak on deflation of the ETT cuff.

estimated to decrease the airway lumen by 70% during tidal breathing expiration but decreased it to only 60% of normal on inspiration. From an airway dynamics point of view, this means that the obstruction was not completely fixed.

The extent of the stenotic segment was 3 cm, beginning 3.5 cm below the vocal cords. It is important to note that the stenosis was entirely extrinsic: It was caused by outside compression, and the tracheal mucosa looked normal. As far as I can make out on the available computed tomography (CT) scan images provided, no evidence of any tumor infiltration of the tracheal wall was found. In this scenario, a multidisciplinary team had decided to perform a thyroidectomy but wanted an opinion as to the potential danger of post resectional tracheal collapse due to tracheomalacia. The recommendation to insert a tracheal stent perioperatively resulted in subsequent placement of a silicone stent via rigid bronchoscopy, which relieved the stridor. The patient underwent thyroidectomy uneventfully, and the tracheal stent could be successfully removed 2 months later, because repeat bronchoscopy showed it to be loose in the upper trachea.

From my perspective, the management of this patient was appropriate, accompanied by sound medical reasoning resulting in an uneventful outcome. If one chooses to insert a stent in this situation, one should primarily opt for a silicone stent, which can always be removed with ease, even years after placement, whereas self-expanding metal stents (SEMS), which are very popular because of their ease of insertion, can become impossible to remove after some weeks or months. Because of many problems associated with SEMS, the U.S. Food and Drug Administration (FDA) issued an official warning against their use in patients with benign disease.[56] For purposes of choosing a stent, the patient described in this scenario should be considered to have a "benign" trachea, because a thyroidectomy will most likely cure the patient. The inserted stent had adequate dimensions—slightly longer and slightly larger than the obstructed airway. This is of paramount importance to avoid migration of the stent within a smooth airway, where the actions of anchoring studs located on the external surface of silicone stents are suboptimal.

So the question is, would I have done the same thing? My answer is No. In fact, I would have done nothing! Let me defend this approach. A 70% stenosis of the trachea is a matter of concern, but the fact that it decreased from 70% to 60% on inspiration showed that it was fairly stable. Total obstruction within days before surgery, therefore, was highly unlikely. According to the literature (extensively discussed in the text), the incidence of post thyroidectomy tracheomalacia varies from 0.001% to a maximum of 1.5% and is highest in patients with substernal goiter. Let us assume that the risk for obstructive malacia in this patient might have been 1%. This is a very low risk by surgical standards, and from my point of view is perfectly acceptable, because the occurrence of this complication could have been

treated successfully by reintubation and mechanical ventilation for some days, as supported by the literature. In the worst case scenario, stent insertion would have become necessary after prolonged intubation, but with a stenotic portion of the trachea not longer than 3 cm, an anterior surgical stabilization procedure of the malacic segment or even a sleeve resection of the stenosis could have been planned.

Another aspect of care that I should mention is the need for numerous procedures, especially if they necessitate a general anesthetic. This is particularly important in this patient because of her significant comorbidities. With temporary stent placement, she needed three procedures under general anesthesia for stent, thyroidectomy, and stent removal. In addition to increased risk to the patient, one must consider the increased costs of such a strategy.

So in conclusion, I would have favored an expectant approach, similar to the one described by the authors at the end of their report. In my opinion, the chances of this patient having post thyroidectomy obstructive malacia requiring bronchoscopic intervention were low; an expectant approach would have resulted in considerable cost-savings, and, very likely, this patient would have been immediately extubated uneventfully in the operating theater after her thyroidectomy.

REFERENCES

1. Cady B. Management of tracheal obstruction from thyroid diseases. *World J Surg.* 1982;6:696-701.
2. Raftos JR, Ethell AT. Goitre causing acute respiratory arrest. *Aust N Z J Surg.* 1996;66:331-332.
3. Noppen M, Poppe KD, Haese J, et al. Interventional bronchoscopy for treatment of tracheal obstruction secondary to benign or malignant thyroid disease. *Chest.* 2004;125:723-730.
4. Anders HJ. Compression syndromes caused by substernal goiters. *Postgrad Med J.* 1998;74:327-329.
5. Honings J, Stephen AE, Marres HA, Gaissert HA. The management of thyroid carcinoma invading the larynx or trachea. *Laryngoscope.* 2010;120:682-689.
6. Geelhoed GW. Tracheomalacia from compressing goitre: management after thyroidectomy. *Surgery.* 1988;104:1100-1108.
7. Ishihara T, Yamazaki S, Kobayashi K, et al. Resection of the trachea infiltrated by thyroid carcinoma. *Ann Surg.* 1982;195:496-500.
8. Hay ID, Thompson GB, Grant CS, et al. Papillary thyroid carcinoma managed at the Mayo Clinic during six decades (1940-1999): temporal trends in initial therapy and long-term outcome in 2444 consecutively treated patients. *World J Surg.* 2002;26:879-885.
9. Batsakis JG. Laryngeal involvement by thyroid disease. *Ann Otol Rhinol Laryngol.* 1987;96:718-719.
10. Randolph GW, Kamani D. The importance of preoperative laryngoscopy in patients undergoing thyroidectomy: voice, vocal cord function, and the preoperative detection of invasive thyroid malignancy. *Surgery.* 2006;139:357-362.
11. Tsutsui H, Kubota M, Yamada M, et al. Airway stenting for the treatment of laryngotracheal stenosis secondary to thyroid cancer. *Respirology.* 2008;13:632-638.
12. Tsutsui H, Usuda J, Kubota M, et al. Endoscopic tumor ablation for laryngotracheal intraluminal invasion secondary to advanced thyroid cancer. *Acta Otolaryngol.* 2008;128:799-807.
13. Shin DH, Mark EJ, Suen HC, et al. Pathologic staging of papillary carcinoma of the thyroid with airway invasion based on the anatomic manner of extension to the trachea: a clinicopathologic study based on 22 patients who underwent thyroidectomy and airway resection. *Hum Pathol.* 1993;24:866-870.

14. Tsumori T, Nakao K, Miyata M, et al. Clinicopathologic study of thyroid carcinoma infiltrating the trachea. *Cancer*. 1985;56: 2843-2848.
15. Czaja JM, McCaffrey TV. The surgical management of laryngotracheal invasion by well-differentiated papillary thyroid carcinoma. *Arch Otolaryngol Head Neck Surg*. 1997;123:484-490.
16. McCaffrey JC. Aerodigestive tract invasion by well-differentiated thyroid carcinoma: diagnosis, management, prognosis, and biology. *Laryngoscope*. 2006;116:1-11.
17. Candib LM. Truth telling and advance planning at the end of life: problems with autonomy in a multicultural world. *Fam Syst Health*. 2002;20:213-228.
18. Steinbrook R. Disparities in health care—from politics to policy. *N Engl J Med*. 2004;350:1486-1488.
19. Kim WK, Shin JH, Kim JH, et al. Management of tracheal obstruction caused by benign or malignant thyroid disease using covered retrievable self-expandable nitinol stents. *Acta Radiol*. 2010;51: 768-774.
20. Ribechini A, Bottici V, Chella A, et al. Interventional bronchoscopy in the treatment of tracheal obstruction secondary to advanced thyroid cancer. *J Endocrinol Invest*. 2006;29:131-135.
21. Wassermann K, Eckel HE, Michel O, et al. Emergency stenting of malignant obstruction of the upper airways: long-term follow-up with two types of silicone prostheses. *J Thorac Cardiovasc Surg*. 1996;112:859-866.
22. Gunasekaran S, Osborn JR, Morgan A, et al. Tracheal stenting: a better method of dealing with airway obstruction due to thyroid malignancies than tracheostomy. *J Laryngol Otol*. 2004;118: 462-464.
23. Gaissert HA, Honings J, Grillo HC, et al. Segmental laryngotracheal and tracheal resection for invasive thyroid carcinoma. *Ann Thorac Surg*. 2007;83:1952-1959.
24. Kim KH, Sung MW, Chang KH, et al. Therapeutic dilemmas in the management of thyroid cancer with laryngotracheal involvement. *Otolaryngol Head Neck Surg*. 2000;122:763-767.
25. Farahati J, Reiners C, Stuschke M, et al. Differentiated thyroid cancer: impact of adjuvant external radiotherapy in patients with perithyroidal tumor infiltration (stage pT4). *Cancer*. 1996;77: 172-180.
26. Egan TD, Hulzinga B, Gupta SK, et al. Remifentanil pharmacokinetics in obese versus lean patients. *Anesthesiology*. 1998;89: 562-573.
27. Shibutani K, Inchiosa MA, Sawada K, et al. Accuracy of pharmacokinetic models for predicting plasma fentanyl concentrations in lean and obese surgical patients: derivation of dosing weight ("pharmacokinetic mass"). *Anesthesiology*. 2004;101: 603-613.
28. Schwartz AE, Matteo RS, Ornstein E, et al. Pharmacokinetics and pharmacodynamics of vecuronium in the obese surgical patient. *Anesth Analg*. 1992;74:515-518.
29. Leykin Y, Pellis T, Lucca M, et al. The effects of cisatracurium on morbidly obese women. *Anesth Analg*. 2004;99:1090-1094.
30. Servin F, Farinotti R, Haberer JP, et al. Propofol infusion for maintenance of anesthesia in morbidly obese patients receiving nitrous oxide: a clinical and pharmacokinetic study. *Anesthesiology*. 1993; 78:657-665.
31. Collins JS, Lemmens HJ, Brodsky JB, et al. Laryngoscopy and morbid obesity: a comparison of the "sniff" and "ramped" positions. *Obes Surg*. 2004;14:1171-1175.
32. Coussa M, Proietti S, Schnyder P, et al. Prevention of atelectasis formation during the induction of general anesthesia in morbidly obese patients. *Anesth Analg*. 2004;98:1491-1495.
33. Bostanjian D, Anthone GJ, Hamouti N, et al. Rhabdomyolysis of gluteal muscles leading to renal failure: a potentially fatal complication of surgery in the morbidly obese. *Obes Surg*. 2003;13:302-305.
34. Passannante AN, Rock P. Anesthetic management of patients with obesity and sleep apnea. *Anesthesiol Clin North Am*. 2005;23: 479-491.
35. Biring MS, Lewis MI, Liu JT, et al. Pulmonary physiologic changes of morbid obesity. *Am J Med Sci*. 1999;318:293-297.
36. Yap JC, Watson RA, Gilbey S, et al. Effects of posture on respiratory mechanics in obesity. *J Appl Physiol*. 1995;79:1199-1205.
37. Pelosi P, Croci M, Ravagnan I, et al. Total respiratory system, lung, and chest wall mechanics in sedated-paralyzed postoperative morbidly obese patients. *Chest*. 1996;109:144-151.
38. Pelosi P, Croci M, Ravagnan I, et al. Respiratory system mechanics in sedated, paralyzed, morbidly obese patients. *J Appl Physiol*. 1997;82:811-818.
39. Behazin N, Jones SB, Cohen RI, et al. Respiratory restriction and elevated pleural and esophageal pressures in morbid obesity. *J Appl Physiol*. 2010;108:212-218.
40. Isono S, Tanaka A, Nishino T. Lateral position decreases collapsibility of the passive pharynx in patients with obstructive sleep apnea. *Anesthesiology*. 2002;97:780-785.
41. Chan AC, Shin FG, Lam YH, et al. A comparison study on physical properties of self-expandable esophageal metal stents. *Gastrointest Endosc*. 1999;49:462-465.
42. Freitag L, Eicker K, Donovan TJ, et al. Mechanical properties of airway stents. *J Bronchol*. 1995;2:270-278.
43. Chhajed PN, Somandin S, Baty F, et al. Therapeutic bronchoscopy for malignant airway stenoses: choice of modality and survival. *J Cancer Res Ther*. 2010;6:204-209.
44. Kadhim AL, Sheahan P, Timon C. Management of life-threatening airway obstruction caused by benign thyroid disease. *J Laryngol Otol*. 2006;120:1038-1041.
45. Ratnarathorn B. Tracheal collapse after thyroidectomy: case report. *J Med Assoc Thai*. 1995;78:55-56.
46. Shaha AR, Burnett C, Alfonso A, et al. Goiters and airway problems. *Am J Surg*. 1989;158:378-380.
47. McMahon CC, Rainey L, Fulton B, et al: Central airway compression: anaesthetic and intensive care consequences. *Anaesthesia*. 1997;52:158-162.
48. De Leo S, Giustozzi GM, Boselli C, et al. Complications after total thyroidectomy in thyroid carcinoma. *Minerva Chir*. 1991;46: 1251-1254.
49. Grichnik KP, Hill SE. The perioperative management of patients with severe emphysema. *J Cardiothorac Vasc Anesth*. 2003;17: 364-387.
50. Sitges-Serra A, Sancho J. Surgical management of recurrent and intrathoracic goiter. In: Clark O, Duh Q-Y, Kebebew E, eds. *Textbook of Endocrine Surgery*. Philadelphia: WB Saunders; 1997.
51. Green WE, Shepperd HW, Stevenson HM, et al. Tracheal collapse after thyroidectomy. *Br J Surg*. 1979;66:554.
52. Peterson JL, Rovenstine EA. Tracheal collapse complicating thyroidectomy: a case report. *Curr Res Anesth Analg*. 1936;15:300.
53. Singh B, Lucente FE, Shaha AR. Substernal goiter: a clinical review. *Am J Otolaryngol*. 1994;15:409-416.
54. Chen WJ, Deng Y, Liang ZY. Acute respiratory tract obstruction during thyroid operation: analysis of 10 cases. *Di Yi Jun Yi Da Xue Xue Bao*. 2003;23:507-509.
55. Agarwal A, Mishra AK, Gupta SK, et al. High incidence of tracheomalacia in longstanding goiters: experience from an endemic goiter region. *World J Surg*. 2007;31:832-837.
56. Food and Drug Administration. Metallic tracheal stents in patients with benign airway disorders, 2005. Available at: www.fda.gov/Safety/MedWatch/SafetyInformation/SafetyAlertsforHuman MedicalProducts/ucm153009.htm. Accessed June 1, 2011.

Chapter 21

Rigid Bronchoscopic Tumor Debulking and Silicone Stent Insertion for Mixed Malignant Tracheal Obstruction Caused by Esophageal Carcinoma

This chapter emphasizes the following elements of the Four Box Approach: physical examination; complementary tests and functional status assessment; risk-benefit analyses and therapeutic alternatives; and techniques and instrumentation.

CASE DESCRIPTION

The patient is a 67-year-old male who presents with several weeks of progressive dysphagia, 25 lb weight loss, and dyspnea with activities of daily living. He recently developed intractable nausea and vomiting and was admitted to the hospital because of difficulty swallowing and choking. His medical history was unremarkable. He had a 40–pack-year history of tobacco smoking and a significant history of alcohol use. Head and neck examination revealed limited cervical range of motion and a two-fingerbreadth mouth opening. Lung examination showed a prolonged expiratory phase and bilateral rhonchi. Esophagogastroduodenoscopy (EGD) showed a mass protruding from the posterior mid-esophagus. After the EGD, his breathing became labored, prompting intubation with a No. 8 endotracheal tube and placement on mechanical ventilation. Bronchoscopy performed on mechanical ventilation revealed a 2 cm obstructing mass in the mid-trachea. Broad-spectrum antibiotics (levofloxacin and piperacillin/tazobactam) were initiated for presumed aspiration pneumonia, after which the patient was transferred to our tertiary care center.

Chest radiograph showed a soft tissue mass density projecting to the right of the trachea. Lung volumes appeared to be enlarged bilaterally (Figure 21-1). Laboratory markers revealed WBC 21.3, Hb 12, and Plt 164. Results from the esophageal mass biopsy showed squamous cell carcinoma. Ventilator settings included assist-control volume-control ventilation with a tidal volume of 500 mL, rate 16, PEEP 5, and FiO_2 0.5. At these settings, peak airway pressure was 60 cm H_2O and plateau pressure 28 cm H_2O. Weaning was attempted but failed. Rigid bronchoscopy was performed, revealing extrinsic compression and an exophytic endoluminal mass protruding from the posterior wall, completely occluding the mid-trachea (see

Figure 21-1). The mass was 2 cm in length and was located 5 cm above the carina and 5 cm below the vocal cords. The endoluminal tumor was cored out using Nd:YAG laser for hemostasis. Airway patency was improved, but tracheal obstruction from extrinsic compression (>70%) remained significant. A 16 × 50 mm straight studded silicone stent was therefore placed in the mid-trachea, restoring airway patency satisfactorily. The patient was successfully extubated the next day (see Figure 21-1).

DISCUSSION POINTS

1. Describe three patient-related factors associated with difficult rigid bronchoscopic intubation.
2. Explain the rationale for stent insertion after tumor debulking in this patient.
3. List at least three strategies to prevent airway perforation and hemorrhage during rigid bronchoscopy.
4. Describe five ways to avoid complications of rigid bronchoscopy.

CASE RESOLUTION

Initial Evaluations

Physical Examination, Complementary Tests, and Functional Status Assessment

Advanced, unresectable esophageal cancer with airway invasion has a very poor prognosis (5 year survival rate <10%).[1] Patients with this disease have not only a limited life expectancy but also many potentially debilitating complications from the local effects of their tumors. These include dysphagia, dysphonia, dyspnea from airway involvement, chest pain, and, rarely, massive fatal hemorrhage from aortic erosion.[2,3] Airway involvement in the setting of esophageal carcinoma includes tissue invasion, infiltration, or the presence of an esophago-respiratory fistula (ERF).* Airway complications may be caused (1) by extrinsic compression on the airways by the tumor or by an esophageal stent and (2) by direct invasion by the tumor into the airways. These processes can result in severe airway narrowing or ERF. Among a large series of 372 patients seen over the 14 year study period, 74 (20%) were found to have airway involvement: 35 (47%) of these patients had an ERF; in the absence of ERF, airway involvement identified as invasion or

---

Juxtaposition, abutment, bulge, and deviation are terms used to describe extrinsic compression, which is not considered adequate evidence of true airway involvement.

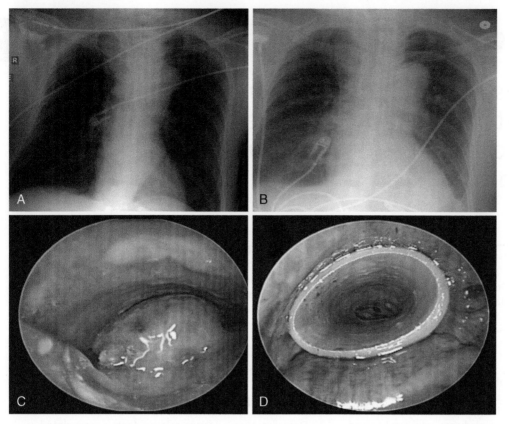

Figure 21-1 A, Chest x-ray (CXR) before the bronchoscopy showed a soft tissue mass density projecting to the right of the trachea, enlarged lung volumes bilaterally, and the endotracheal tube (ETT). **B,** The day after the rigid bronchoscopy, the ETT was removed, and air trapping had resolved. **C,** Rigid bronchoscopic view of the mixed airway obstruction, which consisted of exophytic endoluminal mass and extrinsic compression. **D,** Indwelling silicone stent after rigid bronchoscopy restored airway patency but is still partially compressed in the anteroposterior diameter.

infiltration was biopsy proven in 29 of 39 patients (74%).[4] Other investigators report airway involvement in 10.9% to 62% of cases.[4,5] Because of the proximity of the major airways to the upper two thirds of the esophagus in the thorax, major airway obstruction is also common. In fact, patients with esophageal tumors above the level of the main carina have a worse prognosis than those with lower tumors because of this anatomic relationship with the large airways.[6] Hence, up to 25% of patients with advanced esophageal cancer may require airway stent insertion to alleviate airway obstruction.[7-10] The mean duration of survival for patients requiring airway stent insertion for obstruction due to esophageal cancer reportedly ranges from only 35 to 121 days, with many patients dying at home or in hospice.[9]

Severe respiratory symptoms in these patients may occur because of ERF or severe airway narrowing. For tumors extending into the airway lumen, as is seen in our patient, primary goals of therapy include palliative relief of the malignant obstruction of the esophageal lumen and central airway. If present, attempts can be made to close fistulas between the esophagus and the central airway or, at the least, to alleviate or diminish risks of aspiration and inability to swallow. Recurrent aspiration pneumonia may be caused by dysphagia due to esophageal obstruction or by ERF and can lead to respiratory failure. Initial chest radiographs are often normal; in these cases, they are useful for excluding other causes of respiratory symptoms such as pneumonia, pneumothorax, and pleural effusion.[11] In our patient, for example, pneumonia was not evident on chest x-ray (CXR) nor was ERF on bronchoscopy. The critical airway obstruction was therefore

the likely culprit for respiratory failure in view of notably high peak airway pressures and normal plateau pressures, which point to an airway resistance process. In the absence of evidence for bronchospasm, mucus plugging, or kinking of the endotracheal tube, the most plausible explanation for high peak airway pressures and respiratory failure in this patient was tracheal obstruction by the esophageal mass. This was probably worsened by the moderate sedation used for EGD.

On bronchoscopy, this patient's central airway obstruction was classified as mixed because it comprised an endoluminal component and extrinsic compression (Figure 21-2).[12] In addition to bronchoscopy, computed tomography (CT) provides a noninvasive means of confirming the presence and severity of suspected airway involvement and is valuable in assessing the length of a stenosis, especially when a bronchoscope may not be passable beyond the stenosis. Before bronchoscopy, CT may help to determine whether double stent insertion is necessary (Figure 21-3). In cases of suspected ERF, a barium swallow is usually performed.

Comorbidities

It is possible that our patient had hypoventilation post EGD, caused by sedation-induced reduction in minute ventilation in the setting of critical tracheal obstruction, or possibly by upper airway obstruction unmasked by sedatives. The redundant pharyngeal and laryngeal tissues, as seen in patients with obstructive sleep apnea (OSA), may further lose tonicity, contributing to the hypoventilation and hypoxemia induced by moderate sedation, which potentially leads to respiratory failure and endotracheal

Figure 21-2 Central airway obstruction classification on the basis of mechanism. The bottom photos represent endoluminal papillomas *(left)*, extrinsic compression from the sarcoma *(center)*, and mixed extrinsic compression and endoluminal obstruction from the thyroid carcinoma *(right)*.

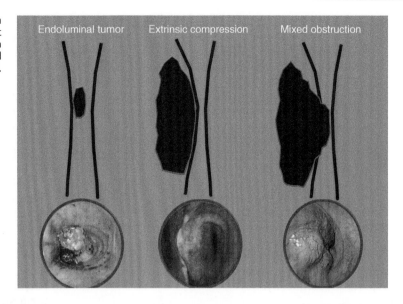

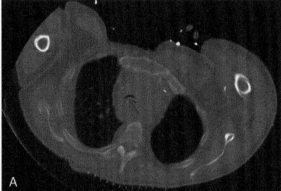

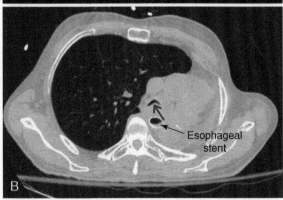

Figure 21-3 **A,** Computed tomography shows severe tracheal obstruction in a patient with esophageal cancer scheduled for esophageal stent placement. **B,** In a different patient with left pneumonectomy, the lower trachea and the right mainstem bronchus were severely narrowed post esophageal stent placement, resulting in respiratory failure.

arrhythmias, and myocardial infarction.[13] Results of observational studies show that most patients with OSA who are undergoing surgery have not been diagnosed before surgery. In a study of 2877 elective surgery patients, 24% were found to be at risk for having OSA, and 81% of these had not been diagnosed previously.[14] These data raise the question whether all patients undergoing surgery should be screened for OSA.

Support System

The patient had been married for 47 years and had no children. He had no living will and no advance health care directives. His wishes were not known.

Patient Preferences and Expectations

The prognosis was discussed with the patient's wife. By investing in patient-centered conversations with family members, health care providers can better meet the needs of families and patients during a medical crisis such as respiratory failure or admission to the intensive care unit.[15] His wife hoped he could be weaned from the ventilator, so she could speak with him about his wishes.

Procedural Strategies

Indications

The primary goal was to restore airway patency to facilitate extubation and change the level of care. Interventional bronchoscopic procedures have been reported to facilitate weaning from mechanical ventilation.[16] Relevant to this patient's condition, in a study of 11 inoperable patients with esophageal carcinoma and airway involvement treated with a combination of rigid bronchoscopy, neodymium-doped yttrium aluminum garnet (Nd:YAG) laser resection, and silicone stent placement, authors noted that 4 patients who required mechanical ventilation for respiratory failure were successfully weaned from mechanical ventilation after the procedure.[9] Overall, airway stent insertion is considered a palliative intervention for airway complications in patients with unresectable esophageal cancer.[9] Airway stents are effective for

intubation (see video on ExpertConsult.com) (Video V.21.1). Although not documented in his medical history, based on the bronchoscopic findings, we suspected OSA in our patient. This can also contribute to poor outcomes caused by perioperative complications. Indeed, evidence suggests that patients with OSA may have more post-operative hypoxemia, upper airway obstruction, cardiac

treating airway narrowing from both extrinsic compression and direct tumor invasion and have been shown to be useful in the treatment of ERF, if present.[4,17,18] The choice of stent depends on the clinician, the place of practice, financial or health care social policy circumstances, institutional biases, and equipment availability, as well as the particular needs of the individual patient. Clinician factors include personal training, familiarity with rigid and flexible bronchoscopy, and personal preference. Institution-related factors include costs (self-expanding metallic stents [SEMS] are generally more expensive), availability of operating theaters and anesthesiologists for emergency rigid bronchoscopy, and stent availability. In terms of patient factors, one might consider the fitness of the patient for general anesthesia, the risk of provoking complete airway occlusion outside of an operating theater while performing flexible bronchoscopy, and any foreseeable chance that a stent may need to be adjusted or replaced subsequently.[11]

Contraindications

Owing to illness severity, high anesthesia risk, or surgical refusal, patients with advanced esophageal carcinoma may not be candidates for minimally invasive airway procedures, in which case comfort care and placement of a feeding tube, if warranted, may be offered. Except for the high likelihood of OSA, our patient had no obvious pulmonary or cardiac comorbidities that could have increased the risk for perioperative myocardial infarction. Nor did evidence reveal renal or hepatic dysfunction, which, in cases of interventional bronchoscopy under general anesthesia, could make perioperative fluid management difficult and increase risks for bleeding.

Expected Results

Stent insertion in the involved airway of esophageal cancer has been shown to improve the life quality and outcomes of patients with advanced esophageal cancer.[4] In the largest case series to date, 66 airway stents (65 studded silicone stents and 1 Wallstent metal stent) were inserted in 51 patients with airway involvement from esophageal carcinoma. Forty stents were inserted in the trachea, 16 in the left main bronchus, and 10 in the right main bronchus. In 47 patients (92%), improvement in respiratory symptoms was significant. The mean survival was 107.7 days.[8]

Although some might say that bronchoscopic stent insertion is an unwarranted and potentially costly therapeutic alternative with patients with ultimately and rapidly fatal disease, we contend that stent insertion is a palliative intervention that always warrants consideration, not only because it results in greater comfort, even over the short term, but also because it improves quality of life, might allow withdrawal from mechanical ventilation so that patients can communicate more fully with their loved ones, and may result in a reduction in level of care or more rapid discharge from the intensive care or hospital setting. In the Netherlands, where euthanasia is a legal alternative to certain palliative therapies for patients with advanced cancer, 7 out of 12 patients with esophageal cancer who elected to have airway stents inserted were judged by their family physicians to have received "worthwhile" palliation in terms of quality of life during the terminal phase of their disease, despite their relatively short remaining survival time.[19]

Team Experience

In high esophageal tumors and in locally invasive tumors with evidence of ERF, a shared interdisciplinary care approach between gastroenterology and pulmonary teams is recommended.[20] The type of airway stent selected may depend on the level of team experience and training in the technique of rigid bronchoscopy.[21] Bronchoscopic resectional techniques such as laser, electrocautery, cryotherapy, argon plasma coagulation (APC), and photodynamic therapy (PDT), in addition to metal or silicone stent insertion, were available at our institution. Therefore in our case, the choice of treatment was guided by (1) a need for immediate improvement in airway patency to facilitate extubation, (2) a need to maintain airway patency in view of extrinsic compression, and (3) a desire for a stent that could be removed or changed easily in case of changes in clinical illness. Thus we elected to perform our procedure using a resection technique such as Nd:YAG laser for possible hemostasis and photocoagulation of tumor in conjunction with coring out, and to insert a silicone rather than a covered metal stent because of its greater expansile force.[22,23]

Therapeutic Alternatives for Restoring Airway Patency

Alternative therapeutic modalities include insertion of SEMS, radiation therapy, chemotherapy, surgical intervention (esophageal bypass, diversion, and attempted resection), and comfort measures. This patient was not considered a candidate for surgical intervention given his advanced disease, poor functional status, and respiratory failure. Less invasive palliative interventions considered included other palliative bronchoscopic options such as mechanical debridement, dilation, laser ablation, electrocautery, cryotherapy, photodynamic therapy, and brachytherapy alone.[24] Without stent insertion, however, restoration of airway patency may not be immediate or long-lasting. In addition, any remaining extrinsic compression after debulking would require stent placement to maintain patency.

1. *Covered self-expandable metallic stents (SEMS)* have been used to relieve the airway obstruction and seal ERFs to avoid aspiration symptoms.[10,17] Insertion of SEMS in mechanically ventilated patients could be performed via rigid bronchoscopy under general anesthesia (Figure 21-4) or via flexible bronchoscopy under fluoroscopic guidance.[25] Some patients are not suitable for rigid bronchoscopy with a general anesthetic because of the severity of their illness, comorbidities, or refusal to undergo intervention. Fluoroscopy requires special facilities that may not be available in every intensive care unit (ICU). In the absence of ready availability of an operating room, and for those operators not versed in the techniques of rigid bronchoscopy,[21] this procedure can, however, be performed while the patient is on the ventilator in the ICU. Because a significant part of the obstruction was caused by

Figure 21-4   A, Partially covered 14 × 40 mm Ultraflex stent placed in the lower trachea and the right mainstem bronchus in a patient with respiratory failure post esophageal stent placement. **B,** The distal aspect of the stent is just above the right upper lobe takeoff, thus allowing ventilation to the right upper lobe bronchus. **C,** Axial computed tomography (CT) view post stent placement shows a patent but still compressed airway. **D,** Coronal CT view reveals the exact location of the stent with its distal aspect above the right upper lobe takeoff.

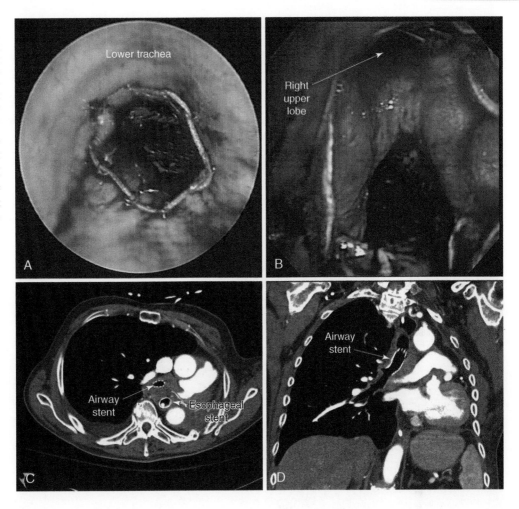

malignant extrinsic compression in our patient, stent insertion could have restored airway patency with or without minimal flexible bronchoscopic debulking of the mass using electrocautery or APC. A technique for placing these stents without fluoroscopy includes the following steps: The bronchoscope is inserted into the mouth through a bite block alongside the endotracheal tube (ETT) and is advanced into the space between the tracheal wall and the endotracheal tube; the scope is then positioned proximal to the lesion; a guidewire is inserted through the bronchoscope and is passed alongside the lesion, after which the bronchoscope is withdrawn, leaving the guidewire in place. The scope is reinserted into the ETT to confirm guidewire location. A stent delivery catheter is advanced over the guidewire, and the stent is deployed under bronchoscopic visualization. The delivery catheter and the guidewire are withdrawn together, with the stent left in position (Figure 21-5). If necessary, the stent can be repositioned by grasping its proximal loop with a flexible alligator forceps (see video on ExpertConsult.com) (Video V.21.2).

2. *Definitive chemo-radiotherapy* has been proposed for patients with esophageal cancer and airway invasion with or without ERF. Radiation therapy

is effective in palliating dysphagia in 34% to 48% of patients with inoperable esophageal cancer.[26] Concurrent chemotherapy with radiotherapy affords even greater benefit in terms of survival and loco-regional control,[1] although it is associated with significant treatment-related morbidity and mortality. Anecdotal evidence suggests a clinical complete response with induction chemotherapy followed by consolidation with concurrent chemo-radiotherapy—an approach that may reduce the morbidity of upfront radiation.[27] Progression to ERF, however, has been reported with radiotherapy; in one case series, the incidence was approximately 10% (9 of 85 patients).[28] This palliative intervention was not considered a first step in our patient given his poor performance status and the presence of respiratory failure.

3. *Double stent insertion* can effectively palliate both dyspnea and dysphagia. Several reports have described the use of "double" stenting of the esophagus and the airway. Results in terms of immediate relief of respiratory and swallowing symptoms appear to be excellent. Esophageal stents, however, are known to compress the adjacent airway, precipitating or exacerbating airway narrowing (see Figure 21-3).[7,29] Acute airway obstruction

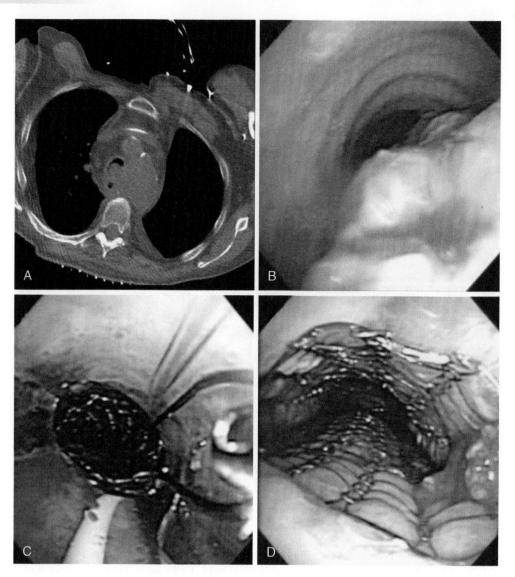

Figure 21-5 A, Computed tomography (axial view) from a different patient with esophageal cancer, respiratory failure, and tracheal obstruction. **B,** Flexible bronchoscopy shows the mixed pattern of obstruction with extrinsic compression and exophytic endoluminal tumor. **C,** The self-expandable metallic stent is adjusted by pulling the proximal loop using a grasping forceps through the flexible bronchoscope introduced through the No. 8 endotracheal tube. **D,** Final view of the stent expanded in the trachea, restoring airway patency and allowing removal of mechanical ventilation.

accompanied by stridor, respiratory failure, and death has been reported after placement of esophageal stents in the proximal one third of the esophagus.[7,30] Double stenting of the esophagus and the airway has been described to manage this complication,[7,8,17] particularly when malignancy obstructs the lumina of the esophagus and the tracheobronchial tree. The incidence of airway obstruction following esophageal stent insertion ranges from about 1% to 10%.[9] Airway stent insertion effectively restores airway patency in this setting.[7] Airway stent insertion should always be considered when the esophagus requires stent placement, and certainly respiratory compromise accompanying or following esophageal stent insertion should raise the possibility of airway obstruction by the stent itself. A multidisciplinary approach including an initial airway evaluation for patients being considered for esophageal stent insertion improves prognosis and decreases airway complications related to the esophageal stent.[31] The double stenting

procedure is not without complications, however. When double stenting is used in combined esophago-airway lesions, massive bleeding is reported in up to 27%.[32] Double stenting is associated with ERF in up to 18% to 38% of patients with esophageal cancer,[29,32] although it is unclear whether fistulas occur as a direct result of stent-related erosion of altered neoplastic infiltration or airway and esophageal mucosa, or if they are a natural result of disease progression.

Pneumothorax may occur in 3% to 4% of esophageal cancer patients receiving airway stents.[8] Patients with previous radiotherapy to the stented area may be especially vulnerable to airway damage.[33] In patients with respiratory symptoms, we prefer to place airway and esophageal stents in stages, inserting the airway stent first. In patients without respiratory symptoms, palliation of the esophageal obstruction takes precedence, and an airway stent is inserted only in case of development or suspicion of airway compromise. Of course, in a patient with an esophageal tumor above the level of the tracheal bifurcation, it is advisable to exclude tracheal stenosis before esophageal stent insertion even if the patient is not dyspneic. Although bronchoscopic inspection of the airway before insertion of an esophageal stent is routine practice in many centers, it is not clear from the literature whether this procedure is absolutely cost-effective. An alternative is to insert an airway stent preventively before esophageal stent placement if significant airway compromise is present on CT scan or bronchoscopic evaluation.[34] Otherwise, airway compromise after esophageal stent insertion can be effectively palliated by airway stents. Colt et al.[7] performed bronchoscopy in 39 patients requiring esophageal stents for esophageal cancer. Airway stents were required in 10 of these patients (26%) because of airway obstruction. Placement of the esophageal prosthesis contributed significantly to airway compromise in 4 of these patients (10% overall). In our patient, we elected to proceed with conversations regarding esophageal stent insertion only after airway patency had been safely established and the patient had been successfully extubated.

4. *Supportive care measures* include intravenous hydration, feeding tubes, antibiotics, analgesics, and comfort care, including medication for sedation and pain control.

Cost-Effectiveness

No formal cost-effectiveness evaluations of these various modalities have yet been published. Emergent bronchoscopic interventions in the setting of central airway obstruction (CAO) favorably affect health care utilization in patients with acute respiratory distress from CAO who require ICU hospitalization.[16] Successful withdrawal from mechanical ventilation and substantial level of care changes from ICU hospitalization to the medical ward in more than 50% of patients, whether for initiation of systemic therapy or for initiation of comfort/supportive care, suggest that consideration should be given to emergent bronchoscopic intervention in cases of CAO resulting in ICU admission. Early intervention probably is justified from both a clinical and an economic standpoint. If mechanical ventilation cannot be discontinued, the long-term prognosis is dismal, and conversations addressing supportive care, including transfer to hospice, should be initiated.

With regard to the placement of metallic stents, bronchoscopic removal, when indicated, has been shown to be associated with significant complications, health care resource utilization, and costs. Their use therefore should be restricted to patients with advanced malignant airway disease with a short life expectancy, in which case long-term complications requiring stent removal are unlikely to occur.[35]

Informed Consent

No learning barriers were identified in our patient, and the patient's wife had good insight into her husband's disease. Expectations were realistic. After she had been advised regarding all of the alternatives, the wife elected to proceed with rigid bronchoscopy under general anesthesia. She was informed of our potential inability to restore airway patency, and she was informed of the risks for bleeding, airway perforation, worsening respiratory failure, prolonged mechanical ventilation, and death.

Techniques and Results

Anesthesia and Perioperative Care

In patients with OSA, the effects of general anesthesia, neuromuscular agents (when used), narcotics, and sedatives may enhance pharyngeal muscle relaxation and depress the arousal response. This results in more frequent and longer apneas postoperatively.[13] Nasal continuous positive airway pressure (CPAP) after extubation may improve outcomes, but only limited data suggest possible benefit.[13]

At our institution, we perform procedures with patients under general anesthesia, usually achieved by intravenous propofol and, when necessary, remifentanil. Neuromuscular blocking drugs are not used because we aim to keep patients breathing spontaneously throughout the procedure. Ideally, the depth of anesthesia should allow spontaneous breathing while preventing excessive body movement in response to rigid bronchoscopy stimulation.[36] We routinely use a local anesthetic, such as 1%, 2%, or 4% lidocaine, sprayed directly to the larynx before insertion of the rigid bronchoscope to prevent laryngospasm, to reduce patient discomfort leading to coughing and bucking during the procedure, and to help avoid throat soreness afterward.

Instrumentation

Selection of a particular stent for an individual patient is often based on the operator's preference and previous experience with a particular stent, evolution in stent technology, and the local availability of various stents. In addition to the geometry (extent, morphology, severity) of the tumor, knowledge of the mechanical properties of the stent is helpful in selecting the appropriate stent.[37] We therefore consider the biomechanical properties of various stents before insertion because the expansile force (physical strength) and ability to withhold angulation (buckling) vary widely among different types. The important attribute of a stent in a case of extrinsic compression is its expansile force because this determines whether the stent is likely to expand fully. However, in a distorted, curved airway, the buckling radius becomes important as well because this determines whether the stent can conform to an acutely angulated tumor and yet remain functional. Stents may differ greatly in their elasticity and resistance to angulation. Available information on this topic for airway stents is unfortunately very limited.* For example, Ultraflex stents (Boston Scientific, Natick, Mass) were shown to withstand angulation, but their expansile force is not very great, and a studded silicone stent

---

*For esophageal stents, on the other hand, methods of measurement under experimental conditions simulating actual stent implantation have been developed, and the test results for various types of metal stents are available (*ASAIO J.* 2001 Nov-Dec;47:646-650).

(Dumon stent, Novatech, Cedex, France) has the opposite behavior.[22,23] In this regard, a recent study evaluating the role of therapeutic bronchoscopy for malignant CAO showed that the stent used most commonly in the trachea and the right mainstem bronchi (relatively straight airways) was the Dumon stent, and the one used most commonly in the left mainstem bronchus (curved, tapered airway; often distorted in the setting of malignancy) was the Ultraflex stent, likely because of its better ability to withhold angulation.[38] In this study, patients with esophageal carcinoma involving the airway most often required only stent placement without laser-assisted debulking, probably because the main problem was extrinsic compression.[38]

Anatomic Dangers and Other Risks

Limited neck mobility as noted in this patient potentially increased the risk for difficult rigid intubation. Therefore, an endotracheal tube had to be readily available to allow prompt intubation of the patient in case rigid bronchoscopy could not be performed (especially once anesthesia induction had occurred). In this patient with significant tumor involvement, risks for airway perforation, hypoxemia, bleeding, and procedure-related death were present.

Results and Procedure-Related Complications

Because of the limited neck mobility, we chose to insert the rigid scope via the corner of the mouth (Figure 21-6). We used a large-diameter tube (13 mm) to facilitate placement of a large stent. The ETT was removed under direct visualization, and the bronchoscope was inserted through the larynx as the endotracheal tube was being removed (see video on ExpertConsult.com) (Video V.21.3). We avoided laser resection of tumor to avoid necrosis and rupture of the posterior membrane of the trachea, which might precipitate ERF formation. Partial resection and coring out of the tumor within the airway were achieved using the beveled edge of the rigid bronchoscope; once tissues were partially removed, significant extrinsic compression remained and extended for 3 cm (see video on ExpertConsult.com) (Video V.21.4). This began at 5 cm below the vocal cords and extended to an area 2.5 cm

above the carina. Flexible bronchoscopy was performed through the rigid tube to remove blood and secretions from the airway. Hemostasis was achieved by using an Nd:YAG laser at 30 W, with 1 second pulse photocoagulation, using a total of 935 joules. We chose to insert a Dumon silicone stent (16 mm × 50 mm) because its advantages include ease of adjustment in cases of migration, as well as protection against tumor invasion. Its main disadvantage is the need for rigid bronchoscopy and general anesthesia, which may be poorly tolerated in malnourished patients or in those with concurrent cardiopulmonary disease. Compared with flexible bronchoscopy, however, rigid bronchoscopy affords superior airway control and the ability to safely ventilate patients during the procedure.

The relative thickness of the stent wall tends to lower the maximum achievable luminal diameter. After stent insertion, the rigid scope was removed, and the patient was intubated with a No. 7 endotracheal tube positioned so that its distal aspect was within the stent itself. No intraoperative or postoperative complications were reported. During rigid bronchoscopy with stent insertion, the airway walls can be traumatized or perforated by instrumentation during stent placement and by pressure exerted onto the walls by the stent itself. Complications such as hemorrhage, fistula formation, pneumothorax, pneumomediastinum, or infection cannot always be avoided. Expected delayed adverse events post silicone stent insertion include migration, obstruction by mucus, and granulation. Migration rates for silicone airway stents placed in esophageal cancer patients are reportedly 8% to 12%.[11] With migration, not only does the stenotic region again become obstructed, but the solid walls of a displaced silicone stent may potentially block off a bronchial orifice. To prevent mucus plugging after stent insertion, we routinely begin chest physiotherapy as soon as the patient can tolerate it, usually later on the day of stent insertion. Inhaled air is moisturized by means of steam inhalation or nebulized saline, and mucolytics can be given occasionally. Pneumonia, which may result from sputum plugging, has been reported in 4% of esophageal cancer patients after airway stent insertion.[8] Granulation tissue overgrowth can be very rapid and can cause

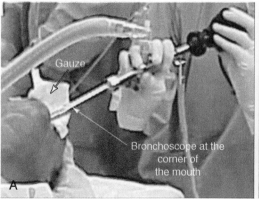
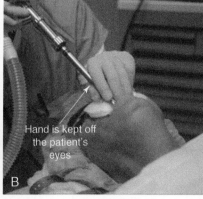
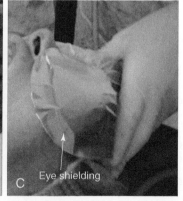

Figure 21-6 The rigid scope is introduced through the corner of the mouth to avoid neck hyperextension. **A,** The teeth are protected by cotton gauze. **B,** The eyes are protected by keeping the hand off the patient's face at all times and **(C)** by applying eye shielding in cases of laser use.

significant obstruction of either or both ends of an airway stent within days or weeks. Excessive pressure from too large a stent or friction of a loose stent rubbing against the airway wall might also enhance granulation tissue formation.[39]

Long-Term Management

Outcome Assessment

The underlying disease, the location of the obstructing lesion, the nature of the lesion (extrinsic, intraluminal, or mixed), and the treatment modality are independent predictors of survival in patients with CAO who undergo therapeutic bronchoscopy.[38] In one study, for instance, the median survival for esophageal carcinoma was 2.5 months versus 5.5 months for lung cancer; the median survival for patients with tracheal and bilateral mainstem bronchial stenosis was 1.6 months versus 4.7 and 4.8 months for patients with left- and right-sided obstruction, respectively. Patients with mixed obstruction had a median survival of 2.3 months versus 5.7 months for patients with purely intraluminal disease.[38] Patients treated with laser and stent had a median survival of 3 months versus 2.7 months for stent only and 10.7 months for laser only treatment. These data do not necessarily imply that one treatment modality is better than another but may simply reflect the nature and severity of the airway obstruction. For example, patients who needed only laser therapy had less severe airway obstruction (e.g., intrinsic exophytic obstructive lesion) and lesions amenable to this modality alone.[38]

Referral

Upon discussion in our multidisciplinary chest conference (cardiothoracic surgery, oncology, critical care, and medical and radiation oncology), a referral to oncology was recommended. Hospice evaluation and home nursing care were also recommended.

Follow-up Tests and Procedures

After stent insertion, a follow-up CXR was performed to confirm its location (see Figure 21-1). Surveillance bronchoscopy is warranted in those patients suspected of having stent-related adverse effects. Secretions, migration, tumor progression, fistula formation, and pneumothorax usually are detected by follow-up bronchoscopy or on chest imaging studies. Complications usually are detected by the onset of new respiratory symptoms and do not necessitate systematic flexible bronchoscopy. Preventive measures such as aerosol therapy, respiratory physiotherapy, and clinical visits[8] are advocated. If patients undergo radiation treatment, bronchoscopy can reveal radiation-induced changes and can help the clinician determine the need for a prolonged indwelling airway stent. In the vast majority of cases of advanced esophageal carcinoma, airway stents are, in fact, permanent once placed. Although this probably reflects the short survival of this group of patients, given the potential for stent-related complications, arguments for removing airway stents in cases of subsequent tumor-specific therapy are valid here, as well as in cases of remission of the airway stenosis.[40] We provided the family with a stent alert card. This document includes the patient's name; indication for stent insertion; type, location, and size of stent inserted; and contact information, as well as instructions for both patients and physicians in case of stent-related complications (Figure 21-7).

The patient was successfully extubated the day after the procedure. He then was transferred back to the referring hospital and was discharged home. Six weeks later, however, he was hospitalized with malnutrition, muscle weakness, and respiratory failure. His airway stent was patent. After a few days of hydration, nutrition, and resting on a ventilator, he was successfully extubated and this time was discharged to home hospice care.

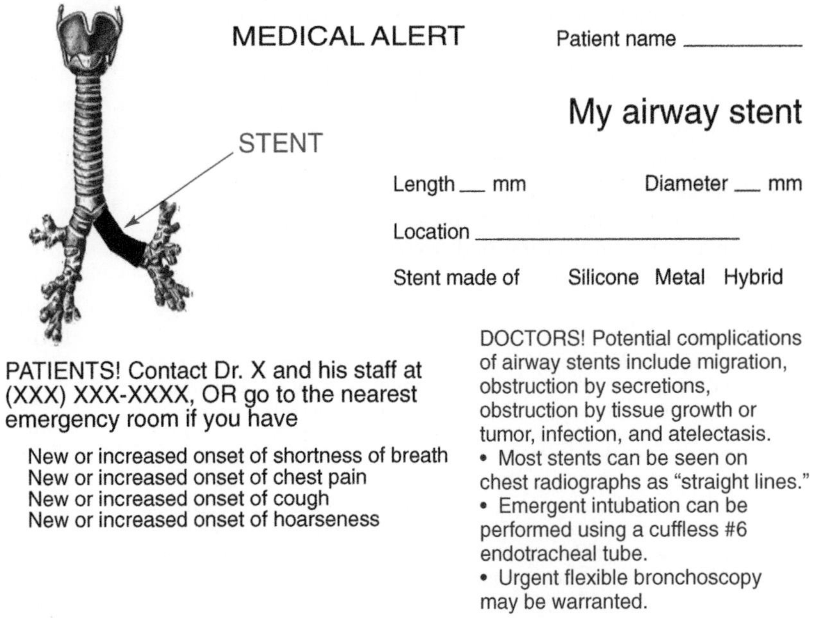

Figure 21-7 The stent alert card provides information both for patients and for physicians who may encounter patients with airway stents. They are informed that even though the stents are not radiopaque, one can identify them on the chest x-ray (CXR) as straight lines. Also, if intubation is necessary, we advise bronchoscopic intubation using a cuffless No. 6 endotracheal tube (ETT) to avoid stent dislodgment or mucosal trauma.

MEDICAL ALERT

STENT

Patient name _____

My airway stent

Length __ mm   Diameter __ mm

Location _____

Stent made of   Silicone Metal Hybrid

PATIENTS! Contact Dr. X and his staff at (XXX) XXX-XXXX, OR go to the nearest emergency room if you have

New or increased onset of shortness of breath
New or increased onset of chest pain
New or increased onset of cough
New or increased onset of hoarseness

DOCTORS! Potential complications of airway stents include migration, obstruction by secretions, obstruction by tissue growth or tumor, infection, and atelectasis.
• Most stents can be seen on chest radiographs as "straight lines."
• Emergent intubation can be performed using a cuffless #6 endotracheal tube.
• Urgent flexible bronchoscopy may be warranted.

Quality Improvement

We did not believe that an earlier bronchoscopy could have altered the outcome in our patient because, after all, he had no diagnosis before the time of his initial hospitalization. The high incidence of airway involvement by esophageal cancer and the difficulty in predicting it accurately with clinical data or other staging procedures, however, argue for the routine use of bronchoscopy in patients with known tumor located at or above the level of the tracheal bifurcation. Excluding airway invasion is warranted, especially in patients with esophageal tumors longer than 8 cm, or in those for whom CT findings suggest airway invasion. A multivariate logistic regression model indicated, for example, that suspect CT findings (odds ratio, 4.4) and maximal tumor length greater than 8 cm (odds ratio, 3.7) were associated independently with airway invasion.[41] Although esophageal ultrasound and CT are considered the best means of assessing the local extent of esophageal cancer, bronchoscopy is best to identify invasion of the cancer into the airways. If patients have previously undergone chemoradiotherapy, interpreting bronchoscopic findings is more difficult than at baseline; the positive predictive value of macroscopic abnormalities without microscopic proof of cancer is low, and even with extensive sampling for histology and cytology, the false-negative rate is 9.4%.[42]

DISCUSSION POINTS

1. Describe three patient-related factors associated with difficult rigid bronchoscopic intubation.
   - *Anatomy factors:* In addition to the Mallampati score,* one should evaluate for obesity, short or thick neck, face or neck trauma, teeth integrity, dentures, large tongue, and micrognathia or macrognathia.
   - *Evaluate the 3-3-2 rule because successful laryngoscopy is predicated by relative normal anatomy:* three fingers in the mouth opening; three fingers from the front of the chin to the hyoid, and two fingers from the hyoid to the thyroid cartilage.
   - *Evaluate neck mobility:* This is reduced in neck trauma, cervical spine arthritis, osteoporosis, bone metastases, ankylosing spondylitis, and burns, as well as post neck surgery.
2. Explain the rationale for stent insertion after tumor debulking in this patient.

   In patients with CAO, stents are placed for extrinsic compression and combined extrinsic and intrinsic obstruction, and in patients with intrinsic obstruction,

they are placed when more than 50% of the lumen is obstructed after debulking or when involvement and instability of the airway wall (malacia) are significant.[43]

The physiologic rationale for the "50%" cutoff rests on several facts:
   - In a simulation study of tracheal stenosis, the effect of glottic narrowing was of the same order as that of 50% constriction; therefore in theory, an airway narrowing of 50% or less may not significantly affect airflow.[44]
   - A significant pressure increase (which correlates with the work of breathing and dyspnea) was observed well beyond 70% narrowing in a characteristic pattern that was similar for 15 and 30 L/min flows; at 50% narrowing, an increase in pressure was seen only at 30 L/min.[44]
   - These data may provide physiologic justification for the practice of increasing the size of the airway lumen to less than 50% narrowing when treating tracheal obstruction (by stent insertion if necessary).

3. List at least three strategies to prevent airway perforation and hemorrhage during rigid bronchoscopy.
   - To prevent airway perforation during laser treatment, the operator should:
     - Avoid aiming the laser directly into the airway wall.
     - Aim parallel to the wall.
     - Use appropriate settings depending on the goal (vaporization or coagulation).
     - Use laser sparingly, before mechanical dilation and resection.
     - Always find the correct axis and identify airway anatomy distal to the stenosis.
   - To prevent hemorrhage, the bronchoscopist should:
     - Correct coagulopathy.
     - Perform devascularization (deep coagulation) by observing tissue blanching using laser at low power density and before vaporization of tissues.
     - Use the suction catheter frequently to remove debris, blood, and secretions and to palpate necrosing tissues.
     - Be knowledgeable of regional vascular anatomy.
4. Describe five ways to avoid complications of rigid bronchoscopy.
   - Protect the eyes (see Figure 21-6).
     - Place tape over eyelids.
     - Avoid laser-induced eye injury by using protective eye shielding.
     - Keep the bronchoscopist's fingers and palm off the eyes of the patient during the procedure.
   - Protect the teeth.
     - Avoid breaking the teeth or lacerating the gums by carefully inserting the rigid bronchoscope and using a mouth guard or gauze to protect the teeth, lips, and gums (see Figure 21-6).
   - Protect the neck.
     - Intubate through the corner of the mouth rather than at midline to avoid hyperextension, especially in a patient with known limited cervical range of motion.

---

*The Mallampati rule states that there is a relationship between what is seen on direct peroral pharyngeal visualization and what is seen with laryngoscopy. To perform a Mallampati evaluation, with the patient seated, have the patient extend his neck, open his mouth fully, protrude his tongue, and say "ah." Visualize the airway, looking for the tongue, soft and hard palate, uvula, and tonsillar pillars. In patients with a Mallampati score of 1, the entire posterior pharynx is easily visualized; with a 4, no posterior structures can be seen. Patients with a higher Mallampati grade tend to have poorer visualization during direct laryngoscopy. The examination can be approximated in supine and comatose patients using a tongue blade.

- If the patient cannot be intubated with the rigid bronchoscope, the patient should be intubated with the flexible bronchoscope using an ETT. A resectional technique can then be used in conjunction with expandable metal stent insertion.
- Protect the larynx.
  - Provide sufficient medication during induction so that muscles are relaxed and alignment of the mouth, larynx, and trachea is possible.
  - Decrease risk for laryngospasm by providing sufficient laryngotracheal analgesia with lidocaine.
- Protect the cardiovascular and respiratory systems.
  - Avoid hypoxemia.
  - Avoid complete airway collapse by keeping the patient spontaneously breathing.
  - Avoid vomiting and reflux by inserting a nasogastric tube in selected instances (e.g., patients with known aspiration history or gastroesophageal reflux disease [GERD]).

Expert Commentary

provided by Norihiko Ikeda, MD, PhD

As a thoracic surgeon, I would like to focus on issues pertaining to procedural strategies as they apply to this patient. In my analysis of the case using the four-box approach, I will focus on indications and results, team experience, and risk-benefit/alternative therapeutic modalities.

From indications, contraindications, and expected results perspectives, we know that two main types of airway stents are in use today: silicone stents and expandable metallic stents. The Dumon-type studded stent, a silicone tube, is well established, especially for the treatment of stenosis caused by intraluminal growth of tumors. Expandable metallic airway stents are used most often in patients with airway stenosis caused by extramural compression. Silicone and expandable metallic stents have different indications and advantages, which should be considered when the interventional bronchoscopist (whether a pulmonologist or a thoracic surgeon) selects the most appropriate stent for the lesion.

We speculate that the management of mixed malignant tracheal obstruction caused by esophageal cancer may be different depending on whether the case has already been treated by chemotherapy or radiotherapy, or both. For treatment-naive cases, similar to the present case, tumor debulking using rigid bronchoscopy followed by silicone stent insertion should be standard practice. If the tumor responds to chemotherapy or radiotherapy, and increased airway patency is obtained, the silicone stent could be removed. Similar tracheal stenosis occurs in patients with esophageal cancer who have been treated previously, in which case the insertion of an expandable covered metal or hybrid stent is recommended. Particularly in such cases of previous treatment, as the tracheal stenosis tends to get worse because of persistent tumor growth, it is possible that the silicone stent will not maintain airway patency.

Cases of esophago-respiratory fistula (ERF) are good indications for metallic (or covered expandable metal and hybrid) stent insertion to the airway because stent insertion into the esophagus can be problematic. Frequently, the esophageal stent causes external compression to the airway, which worsens the airway stenosis. The effect of an esophageal stent on the airway should be predicted by preoperative CT scanning. I personally am not happy with the results of double stent insertion because ERF frequently occurs as the result of poor local blood circulation. Once ERF occurs, the patient seldom takes nourishment orally even if the esophageal stent is inserted successfully. We consider that for these reasons, esophageal stenting is not a complete solution for ERF.

Regarding the issue of operator and team experience and expertise, we need experienced anesthetists to enable us to perform interventions for severe airway stenosis. In patients with severe airway stenosis, obstruction by hemorrhage, secretion, and edema occur easily; therefore certain measures should be taken for the operation, and various precautions are required during the perioperative period. For example, anesthesia usually is maintained with propofol (2.0 to 4.0 mg/kg/hr) and fentanyl citrate (0.1 to 0.2 mg/body weight) for therapeutic rigid bronchoscopy.[45] In select cases of severe tracheal stenosis, it is our custom to ensure percutaneous cardiopulmonary support (PCPS) via the femoral artery and vein before induction of anesthesia. Figure 21-3 shows a patient who has had a left pneumonectomy. In such cases, pulmonary reserve is limited, and the shift of the trachea may hinder insertion of rigid bronchoscopy. This is an example in which we find preparation by PCPS extremely helpful, especially if less-experienced operators are performing the procedure.

With regard to risk-benefit analysis and therapeutic alternatives, it is true that a standard method of operation would consist of tumor debulking and silicone stent insertion under rigid bronchoscopy in cases such as that described. This is probably the most effective way to improve the caliber of the severely restricted airway diameter. Patients can receive chemotherapy and radiotherapy after performance status and respiratory condition improve.[46] However, we should explain ERF may develop as an effect of the treatment. Fistula formation prompted by the treatment itself will probably adversely affect the patient's quality of life and survival. Therefore alternatives should be considered and possibly offered to the patient during or before the informed consent process. An expandable metallic stent may be inserted by using a rigid bronchoscope or a flexible bronchoscope. When the flexible bronchoscope is used, intubation with an endotracheal tube is necessary in patients with poor respiratory condition. Advantages of intubation include the ability to maintain sufficient ventilation; the ability to control airway bleeding by compressing the bleeding area or tumor with the inflated cuff of the endotracheal tube; and the possibility for unilateral intubation to protect the contralateral airway in case of massive bleeding. To provide a safeguard against any surprises that might be found during intervention, I insist on performing an inspection flexible bronchoscopy before proceeding with therapeutic procedures, especially if deviation of the proximal airway is suspected on chest x-ray or CT. Doing so allows me to prepare equipment and my team for any otherwise unexpected events, thereby enhancing patient safety and building team confidence.

REFERENCES

1. Herskovic A, Martz K, Al-Sarraf M, et al. Combined chemotherapy and radiotherapy compared to radiotherapy alone in patients with cancer of the esophagus. *N Engl J Med.* 1992;326:1593-1598.
2. Nelson DB, Axelrad AM, Fleischer DE, et al. Silicone-covered Wallstent prototypes for palliation of malignant esophageal obstruction and digestive-respiratory fistulas. *Gastrointest Endosc.* 1997;45:31-37.
3. Cheng SL, Wang HC, Lee YC, et al. The role of bronchoscopic assessment in esophageal cancer—clinical and survival analysis in 153 patients. *J Formos Med Assoc.* 2005;104:168-173.
4. Alexander EP, Trachiotis GD, Lipman TO, et al. Evolving management and outcome of esophageal cancer with airway involvement. *Ann Thorac Surg.* 2001;71:1640-1644.
5. Altorki NK, Migliore M, Skinner DB. Esophageal carcinoma with airway invasion. *Chest.* 1994;106:742-745.
6. Kato H, Tachimori Y, Watanabe H, et al. Thoracic esophageal carcinoma above the carina: a more formidable adversary? *J Surg Oncol.* 1997;65:28-33.
7. Colt HG, Meric B, Dumon JF. Double stents for carcinoma of the esophagus invading the tracheo-bronchial tree. *Gastrointest Endosc.* 1992;38:485-489.
8. Belleguic C, Lena H, Briens E, et al. Tracheobronchial stenting in patients with esophageal cancer involving the central airways. *Endoscopy.* 1999;31:232-236.
9. Chan KP, Eng P, Hsu AA, et al. Rigid bronchoscopy and stenting for esophageal cancer causing airway obstruction. *Chest.* 2002;122:1069-1072.
10. Takamori S, Fujita H, Hayashi A, et al. Expandable metallic stents for tracheobronchial stenoses in esophageal cancer. *Ann Thorac Surg.* 1996;62:844-847.
11. Sihoe AD, Wan IY, Yim AP. Airway stenting for unresectable esophageal cancer. *Surg Oncol.* 2004;13:17-25.
12. Murgu SD, Colt HG. Interventional bronchoscopy from bench to bedside: new techniques for central and peripheral airway obstruction. *Clin Chest Med.* 2010;31:101-115.
13. Gupta RM, Parvizi J, Hanssen AD, et al. Postoperative complications in patients with obstructive sleep apnea syndrome undergoing hip or knee replacement: a case-control study. *Mayo Clin Proc.* 2001;76:897-905.
14. Finkel KJ, Searleman AC, Tymkew H, et al. Prevalence of undiagnosed obstructive sleep apnea among adult surgical patients in an academic medical center. *Sleep Med.* 2009;10:753-758.
15. Leon AM, Knapp S. Involving family systems in critical care nursing: challenges and opportunities. *Dimens Crit Care Nurs.* 2008;27:255-262.
16. Colt HG, Harrell JH. Therapeutic rigid bronchoscopy allows level of care changes in patients with acute respiratory failure from central airways obstruction. *Chest.* 1997;112:202-206.
17. Freitag L, Tekolf E, Steveling H, et al. Management of malignant esophagotracheal fistulas with airway stenting and double stenting. *Chest.* 1996;110:1155-1160.
18. Sihoe AD, Wan IY, Yim AP. Airway stenting for unresectable esophageal cancer. *Surg Oncol.* 2004;13:17-25.
19. Vonk-Noordegraaf A, Postmus PE, Sutedja TG. Tracheobronchial stenting in the terminal care of cancer patients with central airways obstruction. *Chest.* 2001;120:1811-1814.
20. Gottlieb J, Wedemeyer J. Endoscopic palliation of esophageal and bronchial carcinomas. *Internist (Berl).* 2010;51:237-245.
21. Colt H, Prakash U, Offord K. Bronchoscopy in North America: survey by the American Association for Bronchology, 1999. *J Bronchol.* 2000;7:8-25.
22. Freitag L, Eicker R, Donovan TJ, et al. Mechanical properties of airway stents. *J Bronchol.* 1995;2:270-278.
23. Hautmann H, Rieger J, Huber RM, et al. Elastic deformation properties of implanted endobronchial wire stents in benign and malignant bronchial disease: a radiographic in vivo evaluation. *Cardiovasc Intervent Radiol.* 1999;22:103-108.
24. Stephens KE Jr, Wood DE. Bronchoscopic management of central airway obstruction. *J Thorac Cardiovasc Surg.* 2000;119:289-295.
25. Lee KE, Shin JH, Song HY, et al. Management of airway involvement of oesophageal cancer using covered retrievable nitinol stents. *Clin Radiol.* 2009;64:133-141.
26. Petrovich Z, Langholz B, Formenti S, et al. Management of carcinoma of the esophagus: the role of radiotherapy. *Am J Clin Oncol.* 1991;14:80-86.
27. Ku GY, Goodman KA, Rusch VW, et al. Successful treatment of esophageal cancer with airway invasion with induction chemotherapy and concurrent chemoradiotherapy. *J Thorac Oncol.* 2009;4:432-434.
28. Lewinsky BS, Annes GP, Mann SG, et al. Carcinoma of the esophagus. *Radiol Clin Biol.* 1975;44:192-196.
29. Nomori H, Horio H, Imazu Y, et al. Double stenting for esophageal and tracheobronchial stenoses. *Ann Thorac Surg.* 2000;70:1803-1807.
30. Dasgupta A, Jain P, Sandur S, et al. Airway complications of esophageal self-expandable metallic stent. *Gastrointest Endosc.* 1998;47:532-535.
31. Paganin F, Schouler L, Cuissard L, et al. Airway and esophageal stenting in patients with advanced esophageal cancer and pulmonary involvement. *PLoS One.* 2008;3:e3101.
32. Yamamoto R, Tada H, Kishi A, et al. Double stent for malignant combined esophago-airway lesions. *Jpn J Thorac Cardiovasc Surg.* 2002;50:1-5.
33. Yorozu A, Dokiya T, Ogita M, et al. Complications of esophageal stenting after radiotherapy and brachytherapy. *Jpn J Clin Radiol.* 1997;42:1579-1585.
34. Neuhaus H. The use of stents in the management of malignant esophageal strictures. *Gastrointest Endosc Clin North Am.* 1998;8:503-519.
35. Alazemi S, Lunn W, Majid A et al. Outcomes, health-care resources use, and costs of endoscopic removal of metallic airway stents. *Chest.* 2010;138:350-356.
36. Wong AYC, Lawmin JC, Irwin MG. Anaesthetic management of a patient with low tracheal obstruction requiring placement of a T-Y stent. *Anaesth Intensive Care.* 2000;28:196-198.
37. Chan AC, Shin FG, Lam YH, et al. A comparison study on physical properties of self-expandable esophageal metal stents. *Gastrointest Endosc.* 1999;49:462-465.
38. Chhajed PN, Somandin S, Baty F, et al. Therapeutic bronchoscopy for malignant airway stenoses: choice of modality and survival. *J Cancer Res Ther.* 2010;6:204-209.
39. Cotran RS, Kumar V, Robbins SL. *Robbins Pathologic Basis of Disease.* 4th ed. Philadelphia, Pa: WB Saunders; 1989:73-76.
40. Witt C, Dinges S, Schmidt B, et al. Temporary tracheobronchial stenting in malignant stenoses. *Eur J Cancer.* 1997;33:204-208.
41. Riedel M, Stein HJ, Mounyam L, et al. Predictors of tracheobronchial invasion of suprabifurcal oesophageal cancer. *Respiration.* 2000;67:630-637.
42. Riedel M, Stein HJ, Mounyam L, et al. Influence of simultaneous neoadjuvant radiotherapy and chemotherapy on bronchoscopic findings and lung function in patients with locally advanced proximal esophageal cancer. *Am J Respir Crit Care Med.* 2000;162:1741-1746.
43. Bolliger CT. Multimodalities treatment of advanced pulmonary malignancies. In: *Interventional Bronchoscopy: Progress in Respiratory Research.* Vol 30. Basel, Switzerland: S. Karger AG; 2000.
44. Brouns M, Jayaraju ST, Lacor C, et al. Tracheal stenosis: a flow dynamics study. *J Appl Physiol.* 2007;102:1178-1184.
45. Furukawa K, Ishida J, Yamaguchi G, et al. The role of airway stent placement in the management of tracheobronchial stenosis caused by inoperable advanced lung cancer *Surg Today.* 2010;40:315-320.
46. Saji H, Furukawa K, Tsutsui H, et al. Outcomes of airway stenting for advanced lung cancer with central airway obstruction. *Interact Cardiovasc Thorac Surg.* 2010;11:425-428.

Chapter 22

Rigid Bronchoscopy with Laser and Stent Placement for Bronchus Intermedius Obstruction from Lung Cancer Involving the Right Main Pulmonary Artery

This chapter emphasizes the following elements of the Four Box Approach: risk-benefit analyses and therapeutic alternatives; and anatomic dangers and other risks.

CASE DESCRIPTION

A 50-year-old female with a 30–pack-year history of smoking developed wheezing and worsening shortness of breath, limiting her daily activities. Right lateral decubitus position worsened her symptoms, and she could not sleep on her right side. She was admitted to an outside hospital, where flexible bronchoscopy showed complete obstruction of the right upper lobe bronchus and severe obstruction ($\approx$80%) of the bronchus intermedius (BI). She was transferred for bronchoscopic restoration of airway patency. The patient had a history of stage III squamous cell carcinoma of the lung diagnosed 18 months previously. Her pulmonary function test at that time showed a vital capacity of 2.94 L (80% predicted) and FEV_1 of 2.39 L (85% predicted). She received neoadjuvant chemotherapy and radiation therapy followed by right lower lobectomy and mediastinal node dissection; all nodes were negative. The primary tumor measured $2.5 \times 2 \times 2$ cm and extended to the parenchymal resection margins; evidence showed peritumoral lung consolidation related to the secondary effects of radiation therapy. Shortly after undergoing treatment, the patient lost her insurance coverage and was unable to pursue clinical or imaging surveillance. Comorbidities included rheumatoid arthritis (RA) requiring methotrexate and prednisone 20 mg/day and bipolar disorder treated with valproic acid. She was unemployed and divorced and lived with her children. Her physical examination was remarkable for expiratory wheezing noted in the right lung field. No limitation of cervical spine mobility was detected, but she had ulnar deviation of her hands and swan neck deformities of her fingers. She had significant functional impairment with a KPS score of 30 and was scored ECOG 3. Chest radiography showed a prominent hilar mass and right middle lobe atelectasis (Figure 22-1, A). Chest CT revealed a mass measuring $4 \times 7 \times 3$ cm that invaded the BI and encased the right pulmonary artery (Figure 22-1, B). Repeat flexible bronchoscopy showed a near complete mixed pattern of obstruction (by exophytic tumor and extrinsic compression) of the BI, but right middle lobe

bronchial segments were patent. The right upper lobe bronchus was occluded by extrinsic compression (Figure 22-1, C and D), but the flexible bronchoscope could be passed beyond the occluded airway, noting patent anterior and apical segmental bronchi (see video on ExpertConsult.com) (Video V.22.1). Echocardiogram showed a systolic pulmonary artery pressure of 60 mm Hg and a moderately dilated right atrium but normal bilateral ventricular size and function.

DISCUSSION POINTS

1. Enumerate four anesthesia considerations during rigid bronchoscopic laser resection in this patient in light of severe bronchial obstruction and pulmonary artery involvement.
2. Enumerate three different types of stents that could be inserted in this patient with incomplete obstruction of the bronchus intermedius and right upper lobe bronchus.
3. Explain differences in tissue penetration and coagulation effects of neodymium-doped yttrium aluminum garnet (Nd:YAG), CO_2, and potassium-titanyl-phosphate (KTP) lasers, and describe pertinent clinical implications for treating obstructive airway lesions.
4. Describe the principle of power density and its effect on tissues when the Nd:YAG laser is used.

CASE RESOLUTION

Initial Evaluations

Physical Examination, Complementary Tests, and Functional Status Assessment

This patient's focal wheezing on auscultation of the right chest suggests airflow obstruction distal to the carina.[1] Positional wheezing suggests a component of dynamic obstruction such as excessive dynamic airway collapse, malacia, or, as in our patient, positional worsening in an already narrowed airway. When localized to a bronchus, these processes will be worsened in the lateral decubitus position.

The hand-joint deformities seen in this patient are characteristic of advanced rheumatoid arthritis (RA) and may predict involvement of the axial skeleton,[2] of which the cervical spine joints are the most clinically important,

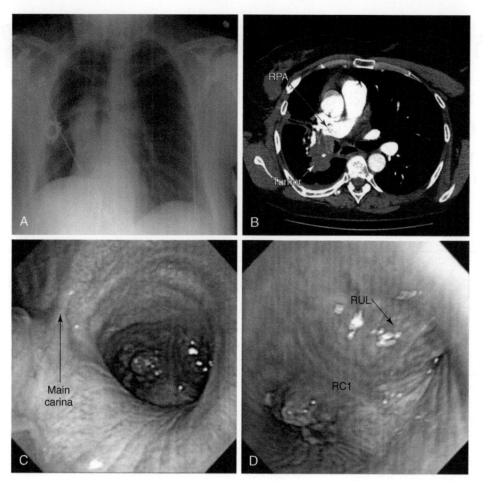

Figure 22-1 A, Chest radiograph reveals a prominent right hilar mass. **B,** Chest computed tomography confirmed the mass and reveals encasement of the right pulmonary artery (RPA). **C,** Bronchoscopy shows a patent right main bronchus. **D,** Near complete obstruction of bronchus intermedius (BI) and the right upper lobe bronchus (RUL) with significant enlargement of the carina between the RUL and BI (RC1).

with a prevalence of involvement ranging from 15% to 86%.[3] This patient had no symptoms of instability related to atlantoaxial (C1-C2) or subaxial (below C1-C2) subluxation. These include neck pain, stiffness, and radicular pain, all of which should be explored in cases of rigid bronchoscopy or endotracheal intubation. During these procedures, the cervical spine is hyperextended to align the mouth, larynx, and trachea. In one study, preoperative cervical spine assessment with cervical spine films in asymptomatic patients with RA before elective surgery revealed an incidence of unsuspected C1-C2 subluxation of 5.5%.[4] Subluxations can vary over time, may be unrecognized, and can be fatal in up to 10% of patients because of spinal cord or brainstem compression.[5] Because of the dangers of neck movements required for intubation, and because subluxation is not always symptomatic, radiographic evaluation of the cervical spine probably should be considered for all patients with RA scheduled to undergo procedures requiring cervical manipulation.[6]

The cricoarytenoid joint may be involved in 30% of patients with RA. Hoarseness and stridor in patients with RA suggest laryngeal involvement and are present in 75% of patients,[7] but those with chronic cricoarytenoid arthritis may be relatively asymptomatic. Any disease process leading to hyperventilation, increased airflow (exertion, acidosis, infection), or reduction in the diameter of the airway (upper respiratory infection) can precipitate symptoms.[8] In addition, patients with cricoarytenoid arthritis

are at risk both during intubation and after extubation. Intubation may be difficult if the airway is narrow and, even if atraumatic and of short duration, can prompt mucosal edema and further compromise of airway caliber, leading to airway obstruction and stridor following extubation.[9] Systemic glucocorticoids are often effective in reversing the obstruction caused by acute cricoarytenoid arthritis, and local periarticular steroid injections have been shown to improve cricoarytenoid function. In chronic cricoarytenoid arthritis, the degree of airflow limitation dictates the need for laser cordotomy or arytenoidectomy.[10] Other potential manifestations of RA that could interfere with airway management include limited temporomandibular joint (TMJ) mobility (<4.5 cm), which is present in approximately 66% of patients with long-standing RA. Most of these patients experience pain and tenderness in the TMJ. Upper airway obstruction can occur because of pharyngeal obstruction, as in patients with micrognathia or obstructive sleep apnea. Furthermore, a small mouth opening from TMJ disease may preclude rigid bronchoscopic intubation. In our patient, upper airway anatomy was normal, and no signs of RA-related laryngeal involvement or TMJ disease were noted.

Comorbidities

This patient had been diagnosed with bipolar disorder. Although possibly attributable to higher unmeasured severity of illness in patients with psychiatric comorbidity, existing psychiatric disease has been found to be associated with a modestly increased risk of death among patients undergoing surgery.[11] Our patient had been taking prednisone 20 mg/day for many years. The equivalent of 15 mg/day of prednisone for longer than 3 weeks should raise suspicion for hypothalamic-adrenal axis suppression,[12] warranting increased glucocorticoid supplementation associated with possible adrenal insufficiency related to medical and surgical stress.[12] In this regard, one must recall that supplemental corticosteroids can induce or exacerbate manic or depressive episodes, potentially interfering with postoperative care.[13]

Support System

An assessment of the support system is particularly important in this patient for the following reasons:

1. Mental illness is associated with higher case-fatality rates in patients with cancer, in part because of the challenges of drug interactions, lack of capacity, and difficulties in coping with treatment regimens as a result of psychiatric symptoms. A multidisciplinary approach that includes members of mental health services is warranted to ensure effective treatment and to avoid inequalities of care that might result from physician biases or mismanagement of patient behaviors and treatment choices.[14]
2. Nonoperative non–small cell lung carcinoma (NSCLC) trials showed that marital status was not independently predictive of overall survival; however, single females had significantly better overall survival than both single and married males.[15]
3. Socioeconomically disadvantaged patients with NSCLC may receive less intensive cancer-specific care. Differences in access to care, comorbidities, and lifestyle may contribute to these inequalities.[16]

Patient Preferences and Expectations

This patient wished to improve her shortness of breath, which caused significant emotional and physical distress. Results from studies show that more than 50% of patients with inoperable lung cancer report breathing difficulty, pain, and fatigue as the symptoms most associated with physical and emotional distress.[17]

Procedural Strategies

Indications

The main reasons to address this patient's bronchial obstruction were to relieve her dyspnea and to potentially improve her performance status. Her severe bronchus intermedius (BI) obstruction impeded ventilation only to the middle lobe because she had previously undergone right lower lobectomy. Restoring function to the right middle lobe (RML) was expected to improve symptoms and prevent post obstructive pneumonia. The right upper lobe (RUL) bronchial obstruction was incomplete, characterized by extrinsic compression and mucosal infiltration. Stents usually are not placed in the RUL lobar or segmental bronchi. Furthermore, this type of obstruction was not amenable to stent insertion

or other bronchoscopic interventions because no exophytic endoluminal disease was present. We elected to proceed with rigid bronchoscopic laser resection and silicone stent insertion with the patient under general anesthesia.

Contraindications

The lack of functional lung distal to the obstruction would preclude bronchoscopic interventions. In this patient, however, flexible bronchoscopy showed a patent RML bronchus. No absolute contraindications to rigid bronchoscopy were noted, nor did concerns arise regarding RA-related upper airway obstruction. The cervical spine range of motion was normal, and dynamic (flexion-extension) magnetic resonance imaging (MRI) showed no evidence of cord compression. Entrapment of the right pulmonary artery by the tumor (see Figure 22-1) could result in hemodynamic instability during general anesthesia owing to high risk for acute cor pulmonale.

Expected Results

Relief of BI obstruction was expected to improve her lung function and potentially her dyspnea by restoring ventilation to the right middle lobe. A vast majority of patients with malignant central airway obstruction (CAO) improve their dyspnea and performance status if the CAO is palliated. The modality used to restore airway patency (i.e., laser, stent, photodynamic therapy [PDT], electrocautery, or brachytherapy) depends on tumor characteristics (i.e., extrinsic, endoluminal, or mixed) and severity and type of obstruction (i.e., critical, compromising respiratory status), operator preference, and availability of specific technologies.[18] The modality used to restore airway patency might not make a difference in terms of outcome, suggesting that it is restoration of airway patency per se that counts, not the method used to achieve it.[19] Survival may also be improved, especially if further systemic therapy can be initiated post procedure. Overall, the median survival of patients with untreated malignant CAO can be as low as 1 to 2 months.[20] If interventional bronchoscopy is successful in relieving airway obstruction, survival is similar to that in patients without CAO.[21] Stent insertion results in significant improvement in Medical Research Council Dyspnea Scales (MRC)-measured dyspnea and Eastern Cooperative Oncology Group (ECOG) performance status, although in one study, a significant survival advantage was seen only in the intermediate performance group (ECOG ≤3, MRC ≤4) when compared with historic controls. Perhaps improved survival is noted if airway patency is restored before the development of complications such as post obstructive pneumonia, irreversible atelectasis, or loss of ventilatory function from malignant CAO.[22]

Team Experience

Rigid bronchoscopy with laser resection and stent insertion warrant a team familiar with the technical and anesthesia-related issues that might arise in patients undergoing this procedure. Patient safety should be addressed at all times, and the team must be ready to respond promptly to procedure- or disease-related complications.

Risk-Benefit Analysis

We considered that the potential benefits of a broncho-scopic procedure in relieving dyspnea, avoiding post obstructive pneumonia and respiratory failure, and improving survival outweighed the risks of the intervention, all of which were shared with the patient during the informed consent process.

Therapeutic Alternatives

- *External beam radiation therapy (EBRT)* for recurrent locally advanced NCSLC previously treated with radiation therapy is a feasible, noninvasive therapeutic alternative.[23] However, when associated severe airway obstruction results in atelectasis, the response rate is 20% to 50% in studies involving more than 50 patients.[24] Smaller studies showed that bronchial obstruction could be relieved in up to 74% of patients, resulting in complete or partial re-expansion of the collapsed lung. The time to initiation of treatment matters because 71% of patients irradiated within 2 weeks after radiologic evidence of atelectasis had complete re-expansion of their lungs, compared with only 23% of those irradiated after 2 weeks.[25] In our patient, EBRT was potentially limited by evidence of radiation-induced toxicity from previous radiotherapy. Improvements in imaging and treatment planning using three-dimensional (3D) conformational radiation and respiratory gating can precisely target radiotherapy, and by decreasing the normal tissue margins included to account for uncertainties in position, can diminish the risk of clinically significant pneumonitis and esophagitis.[26]
- *Endobronchial brachytherapy (EBB)* has proven efficacy in patients with endoluminal tumor and a substantial extrabronchial component. For palliation of NSCLC symptoms, EBB alone appears to be less effective than EBRT. For this patient previously treated with EBRT, who was symptomatic from recurrent endobronchial CAO, EBB is a reasonable alternative.[27] Success rates vary between 53% and 95%,[28] but the overall incidence of fatal hemoptysis is 10% (range, 0% to 42%). Irradiation in the vicinity of major vessels, in this case the right pulmonary artery, increases bleeding risk.[29] In fact some authors suggest that patients with tumors involving the major vessels should be excluded from EBB.[30] Squamous cell pathology and tumor located in the mainstem bronchus or upper lobe represent additional risk factors for hemoptysis.[31] Patients with poor performance status may be at higher risk for periprocedural complications such as cough, bronchospasm, and pneumothorax caused by catheter placement.
- *Photodynamic therapy (PDT)* could be provided, but because of the severe nature of the airway obstruction, the sloughed tissue resulting from PDT could occlude the airway and cause complete obstruction, resulting in worsening symptoms and post obstructive pneumonia.[32] This patient's previous surgery, chemotherapy, and radiation therapy did not represent contraindications to PDT, and in fact this therapy can be offered to patients who become unresponsive to chemotherapy or radiation therapy.[33] PDT is most effective when obstruction from mucosal disease is greater than 50% and in patients with good performance status.[34] Hemorrhage has been reported in 0 to 2.3% of patients, but the risk may be greater when the disease involves major blood vessels.
- *Cryotherapy* would address only the endoluminal component of the obstructing airway lesion. It can be combined with EBRT to enhance its efficacy.[35] The effect is delayed, and initially sloughed tissue resulting from vasoconstriction and necrosis might worsen airway obstruction. Cryotherapy is reportedly effective in up to 75% of patients with lung cancer with endoluminal obstruction,[36] but it is not the therapy of choice when extrinsic compression is present.
- *Argon plasma coagulation (APC) and electrocautery* allow removal of exophytic disease.[18] Systemic, life-threatening APC-related gas embolism has been reported.[37] Risks may be increased when highly vascularized lesions are treated and in proximity of large blood vessels. Depth of penetration and distribution of thermal-induced necrosis within tissues are not as predictable as they are with lasers because electrical current follows the path of least electrical resistance within different tissue types.
- *Metal stents* are more costly than silicone stents, but procedures can be performed via flexible bronchoscopy with or without fluoroscopy.[38] Therefore it is an appropriate alternative, especially in patients with significant comorbidities precluding general anesthesia.
- *Silicone Y stent insertion at the right primary carina (RC1)* was shown to improve symptoms in a small published case series of three patients with malignant disease. The bronchial limbs of the stent saddled the involved carina between the bronchus to the right upper lobe and the bronchus intermedius.[39] The very wide RC1 and the near complete obstruction in the RUL bronchus precluded this approach in our patient.
- *Comfort care without palliative bronchoscopic intervention* is not an unreasonable approach to treating this patient with poor quality of life and a grim prognosis. A palliative care consultation and potential initiation of hospice care, especially if quality of life continues to deteriorate, should be considered, regardless of other therapeutic alternatives.

Cost-Effectiveness

To our knowledge, no formal cost-effectiveness evaluations of these various modalities have yet been published, but investigators report potential cost savings by implementing an airway program and timely (at diagnosis) bronchoscopic palliation of malignant CAO.[22] Long hospitalizations and sojourns on mechanical ventilation are often avoided by rapidly initiating bronchoscopic palliation of airway obstruction or, in case palliative treatments are not selected, by referring patients for best supportive care and hospice.

Informed Consent

The patient showed understanding of her disease process and the planned procedure. We discussed the clinical issue (dyspnea due to malignant CAO) and described the procedure in detail. We discussed the risks and potential benefits of the procedure and informed the patient of therapeutic alternatives and potential consequences of choosing those alternatives. She was informed of the risks for bleeding, perforation, respiratory failure, and death. Using feedback communication techniques, we assessed the patient's understanding of her disease and discussed her preference to proceed with rigid bronchoscopy under general anesthesia.

Techniques and Results

Anesthesia and Perioperative Care

In patients with RA, rigid bronchoscopic intubation can be difficult and may result in loss of the airway. If the patient with RA is known to have upper airway obstruction, immediate tracheostomy may be necessary. Depending on physician biases, credentialing, and competencies, surgical standby may be warranted. Intubation should be as gentle as possible to avoid even minimal trauma because of the risk for mucosal edema and post extubation respiratory insufficiency. In cases of post extubation airway difficulties, the work of breathing can be reduced and airflow improved with the use of 80:20 helium/oxygen mixtures. Racemic epinephrine (2.25% solution) can be delivered via nebulization for stridor; the onset of action is 1 to 5 minutes, so if no improvement is noted, noninvasive positive-pressure ventilation or, if necessary, awake, flexible bronchoscopic intubation can be considered in those already moved to the recovery area.

Because cervical entrapment is common even without signs or symptoms, the anesthesiologist and the bronchoscopist should assume that patients with RA are at increased risk for neurologic injury from cervical manipulation. Precautionary measures include assessing for possible cervical spine involvement by dynamic (flexion-extension) MRI, avoiding hyperextension, and maintaining the cervical spine in midline without extension before, during, and after the procedure. One might resort to awake flexible bronchoscopic intubation or reintubation rather than rigid laryngoscopic intubation.

This patient was at risk for hemodynamic instability during general anesthesia because of right pulmonary artery compression from tumor and pulmonary hypertension documented on echocardiogram. In fact, pulmonary artery compression by lung cancer, lymphoma, and benign tumors is well recognized and can have serious implications during interventions because any reduction in preload may significantly reduce cardiac output.

When lasers are used via rigid bronchoscopy, airway fires are rare if all flammable objects (e.g., suction catheter, stent) are removed from the laser path, the laser fiber tip is kept clean, the fraction of inspired oxygen (FiO$_2$) is kept at less than 0.4, and laser pulses are of short duration (0.5 to 1 second) and are delivered at 40 W or less. Of course, in a patient with poor lung reserve (previous lobectomy), hypoxemia could occur from the use of low FiO$_2$ and from bleeding and debris occluding the airway.

Both hypoxemia and hypoventilation could exacerbate pulmonary hypertension, resulting in right heart failure and hypotension.

Instrumentation

We chose an 11 mm and a 12 mm Efer-Dumon rigid bronchoscope (Bryan Corp., Woburn, Mass) and the Nd:YAG laser in case of bleeding or for tumor coagulation and debulking. Various types and sizes of silicone stents were readily available because stent insertion was likely, given the presence of extrinsic compression.

Anatomic Dangers and Other Risks

The proximal BI is surrounded by the right inferior pulmonary artery at the lateral wall and the right inferior pulmonary vein at the medial wall. In this patient, however, anatomy was distorted by her previous lobectomy, and the right main pulmonary artery was adjacent to the anterolateral wall of BI (see Figure 22-1). Displacement of anatomic structures must be expected in planning and performing bronchoscopic intervention, especially when lasers are being used. Deep Nd:YAG laser photocoagulation of tumor in the proximal BI is dangerous, given the proximity of the pulmonary artery already involved with tumor. Overly aggressive coring out, or inadvertent deep photocoagulation with resultant necrosis, could lead to perforation, uncontrollable hemorrhage, and death, even many days after the procedure.

Results and Procedure-Related Complications

The patient was intubated initially with an 11 mm Efer-Dumon rigid ventilating bronchoscope. The tumor was seen obstructing the BI and the RUL bronchus (see Figure 22-1). The flexible bronchoscope was advanced through the rigid scope, and inspection of the distal airways was attempted. Because the RML segments were patent (see video on ExpertConsult.com) (Video V.22.1), we decided that stent insertion in the BI was warranted. The RUL bronchial tumor, characterized by extrinsic compression, was not addressed because of concern for airway perforation and major bleeding in view of pulmonary artery involvement. The Nd:YAG laser was used at 30 W power and 1 second pulses for a total of 100 Joules, and high-power density was used to vaporize the exophytic component of the tumor before the rigid bronchoscope was advanced in the distal BI. Using the bevel edge of the bronchoscope, a small amount of necrotic tumor was cored out from the BI, thereby restoring airway patency. The bronchoscope was removed, and the patient was reintubated using a 12 mm Efer-Dumon rigid ventilating bronchoscope. With the rigid scope in the distal BI, a 12 × 30 mm studded silicone stent was deployed (Figure 22-2). Saline washes performed through the flexible bronchoscope confirmed the absence of pus or excess necrotic material within the BI and the RML bronchus. The case lasted 60 minutes with no bleeding or hemodynamic instability. Extubation was well tolerated, and the patient was kept in the intensive care unit (ICU) for 24 hours, during which no complications were noted. She returned to the referring facility shortly thereafter.

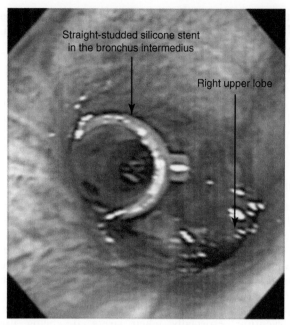

Straight-studded silicone stent
in the bronchus intermedius

Right upper lobe

Figure 22-2 Bronchoscopic view immediately after stent insertion: The bronchus intermedius is open, and the right upper lobe continues to show severe narrowing owing to extrinsic compression from an enlarged primary right carina (the carina between the upper lobe and the bronchus intermedius).

Long-Term Management

Outcome Assessment

Airway patency to the RML was successfully restored and dyspnea subjectively improved. The focal wheeze was no longer present. Objective tools such as ECOG, the Karnofsky Performance Scale (KPS), and MRC were not used postoperatively to assess the patient's functional status. Stent care instructions and a medical alert bracelet were provided before discharge to patients with indwelling stents.

Referral

We did not recommend additional radiation therapy to her referring physician but suggested consultation with radiation oncology, oncology, and palliative medicine specialists.*

Follow-up Tests and Procedures

The patient was transferred to the care of the referring physician, who performed a surveillance outpatient flexible bronchoscopy 1 month later. Although it is usually our practice to avoid routine surveillance bronchoscopy, in this case the patient had chosen to undergo additional radiation therapy, which, if effective, might have resulted

---

*Following life-prolonging procedures, it is common for patients to request continued care at the tertiary institution providing the procedure. This obviously creates an ethical dilemma: Should the performing physician continue to provide care to the patient at his/her institution, at the patient's request, or should he or she insist on continued care from the referring health care providers? The answer depends on the capability of the referring facility to provide comprehensive cancer care.

in increased airway patency, making the stent unnecessary. The stent was found to be patent and to show no evidence of migration or mucus plugging.

Quality Improvement

We reflected on quality practice in this case. After airway patency had been restored, the patient improved subjectively and was promptly transferred to the care of her physicians at the outside hospital. We did not recommend additional external beam radiation therapy because we were aware that the role of postoperative radiotherapy in patients with completely resected stage III NSCLC is uncertain and may be influenced by the extent of nodal involvement and the use of adjuvant chemotherapy. Results from studies suggest that although postoperative radiotherapy may prevent loco-regional recurrence, it may not significantly alter survival because this is often limited by the development of distant metastatic disease. Retrospective Surveillance, Epidemiology, and End Results (SEER) database analysis and the Adjuvant Navelbine International Trialist Association (ANITA) trial subset analysis suggest that postoperative radiotherapy may improve survival in patients with N2 lymph node involvement.[40] Our patient did not have N2 involvement on pathologic staging, but postoperative radiotherapy could have been offered, given her positive resection margins.

DISCUSSION POINTS

1. Enumerate four anesthesia considerations during rigid bronchoscopic laser resection in this patient in light of severe bronchial obstruction and pulmonary artery involvement.
   - Avoid combustible gases such as halothane.[41]
   - Keep the FiO_2 below 40%.[42]
   - Beware of severe hypoxemia and potential death from massive bleeding due to accidental laser perforation of the right pulmonary artery.[43]
   - Beware of hemodynamic instability due to pulmonary hypertension caused by right pulmonary artery tumor compression.[44]
2. Enumerate three different types of stents that could be inserted in this patient with incomplete obstruction of the bronchus intermedius and RUL bronchus.
   - Bifurcated silicone stent (Y-stent technique on RC1)
   - Straight silicone stent with a side-hole for RUL ventilation
   - Covered metal stent in the bronchus intermedius
3. Explain differences in tissue penetration and coagulation effects of Nd:YAG, CO_2, and KTP lasers, and describe pertinent clinical implications for treating obstructive airway lesions.

   Laser selection requires an understanding of the reflective, absorptive, scattering, and transmissive properties of the target tissue (Figure 22-3).*

---

*However, several nonlinear events may occur with very short pulses (nanoseconds or picoseconds): multiphoton absorption, plasma formation, and ionization.

- Reflection occurs when radiation is returned by the surface (reflective surfaces are bright or humid).
- Absorption is the transfer of energy from photons to molecules (also referred to as *pigments*) within the tissue that is to be altered. Absorption depends on the power and the color of the tissue (which also

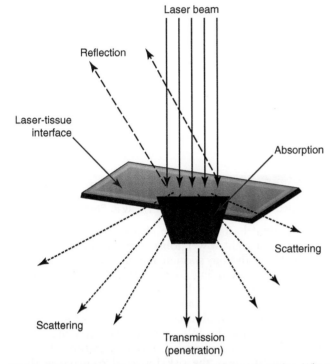

Figure 22-3 Light energy response in laser-tissue interaction. When a laser light is directed to a tissue, it may be reflected back to the source or to another undesired surface. When it enters the tissue, it is absorbed to effect tissue change via heat, photochemistry, fluorescence, or ionization. The tissue itself can scatter the light or may transmit it through the tissue. Reflective, scattering, and transmission properties are tissue dependent. The quantity of energy absorbed by tissue is dependent on the incident power and the absorption coefficient, which is tissue dependent: The higher the absorption coefficient, the greater is the energy deposited in a volume or depth of tissue, and the lower the absorption, the greater is the penetration.

depend on vascular supply). The more colored the tissue, the greater the absorption (darker tissues show preferential absorption for Nd:YAG) (Table 22-1).
  - KTP laser has strong absorption in hemoglobin but very weak absorption in water.
  - Nd:YAG has low absorption in both hemoglobin and water and in other body pigments; this is why it will penetrate more deeply into tissues compared with other lasers.
  - The CO_2 laser has weak absorption in hemoglobin but strong absorption in water, which is why it has shallow penetration compared with other lasers.
- Transmission (penetration), the passage of radiation through a medium, is governed by the law of inverse absorption. The paler the tissue, the greater is the transmission (a white tissue will transmit the laser completely).
- *Clinical implications* (Table 22-2): Physicians who use lasers should acquire the ability to differentiate laser-induced tissue changes (Figure 22-4) visually, so that the heating process and its consequences can be stopped at the desired point. If the wavelength does not penetrate sufficiently (too heavily absorbed), it will not reach the vessels to control the bleeding, and it will not be able to destroy a sufficient volume of tumor by photocoagulation; in contrast, if a laser penetrates too deeply, it will create too much damage, resulting in delayed healing, edema, and possibly perforation of a vessel or an airway wall.

4. Describe the principle of power density and its effect on tissues when the Nd:YAG laser is used.
  - Power represents the time rate at which energy is expended, transmitted, or converted (Power = Energy/time) and is expressed in joules per second. The concept of laser power is important because physical, chemical, and biologic systems have certain rates at which energy can be produced or absorbed. Values of power in excess of these limits

Table 22-1 Characteristics of Lasers Commonly Used for Airway Disorders

Type	Wavelength	Spectrum	Scattering	Absorption	Penetration	Coagulation	Cutting Precision
Nd:YAG	1064 nm	Near-infrared (invisible)	Significant	Proteins of any opaque tissue	Deep (4 to 6 up to 10 mm)	+++	+
CO_2	10,600 nm	Far-infrared (invisible)	Insignificant	Water	Shallow (0.1 mm)	+	+++
KTP	532 nm	Visible band (green)	Average	Hemoglobin	Average (1 to 2 mm)	++	+

CO_2, Carbon dioxide; *KTP*, potassium-titanyl-phosphate; *Nd:YAG*, neodymium-doped yttrium aluminum garnet.

Table 22-2 Thermal Effects of Laser on Tissues and Expected Visible Changes

	TEMPERATURE (° C)				
	37 to 60	60 to 90	90 to 100	Several Hundreds	Several Hundreds
Biologic effect	Heating	Coagulation and denaturation of proteins	Evaporation of water	Carbonization/burning	Vaporization/burning
Visual change in the tissue	None	Blanching/whitening (due to increased scattering)	Shrinkage/drying (constant scattering)	Blackening/charring (increased absorption)	Smoke and gas generation
Mechanical change	None	Disintegration of structures	Shrinkage of tissues	Serious tissue damage	Tissue ablation

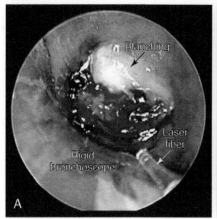
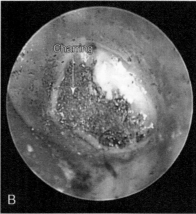

Figure 22-4 Visual changes on a tumor completely occluding the bronchus intermedius during laser application. **A,** Blanching (from coagulation and denaturation of proteins) is seen after a neodymium-doped yttrium aluminum garnet (Nd:YAG) laser was used at low power density. **B,** After laser use at high power density, part of the tumor shows charring (burning) as the result of carbonization effects.*

can cause malfunction, disruption, or destruction of the system.[45]

- Power density represents the power per unit of volume or per unit area within which energy is released, transmitted, or absorbed (Power density = Power/volume or Power/area). The power density required in tissues for each of these functions is different. Power density is different at different levels because of scattering.

- *Clinical use of power density:* (1) For cutting, a small spot (area) is desirable at high power density (see video on ExpertConsult.com) (Video V.22.2). (2) For coagulation and gentle ablation, a large spot at low power density is used (see video on ExpertConsult.com) (Video V.22.3); the wider the spot, the less the energy density. Spot size can be controlled by changing the distance of the distal tip of the delivery system from the target.[†] Parameters that determine the total energy density are controlled by the operator and include the setting in watts, the length of time the beam is fired, and the spot size on the tissue. At low power density, the fiber usually is placed 1 cm away from the lesion for coagulation. At high power density, the fiber is placed close to the lesion ($\approx$0.3 cm) for vaporization (see video on ExpertConsult.com) (Video V.22.4). Coagulation usually is obtained at 8 to 20 W/cm^2 without vaporization; power density in excess of this value will cause the temperature to rise to 100° C, and boiling of tissue water will occur. The high power density that cannot be removed by thermal conduction will cause rapid vaporization of tissues.

---

*The conversion of organic substances into carbon or carbon-containing residue through thermochemical decomposition at elevated temperatures (aka pyrolysis).

†This would not be the case for an insignificant divergence of a truly collimated laser beam (effectively, a parallel beam of light with very low divergence or convergence), but through multiple internal reflections of a laser fiber, the transmitted beam loses its collimation and emerges with a 10 to 12 degree spread of divergence.

Expert Commentary

provided by Suresh Senan, MRCP, FRCR, PhD

This patient had undergone chemo-radiotherapy followed by a right lower lobectomy 18 months previously. The pathology specimen revealed an R1 resection with tumor extending to the parenchymal resection margins, but no nodal metastases were found. The preoperative dose of radiation was not specified, but most published studies have used a dose of 45 Gy in this setting, not the full curative doses ranging from 66 to 74 Gy as reported in recent literature. An R1 resection increases the risk for local recurrence; this was the first site of treatment failure because this patient had no nodal metastases. However, the benefit of administering additional focal irradiation during the immediate postoperative period is unclear because of the difficulty involved in identifying a radiation target volume in the lung parenchyma on postoperative computed tomography (CT) scans, increased risks of radiation toxicity, which in turn depend on prior radiation dose, and the reduced radiobiologic effect caused by the "gap" in radiation delivery from the time of surgery and postoperative recovery.

The patient now presents with a symptomatic local recurrence measuring 4 × 7 × 3 cm, invading the bronchus intermedius and encasing the right pulmonary artery. In addition to exophytic tumor seen in the BI, a major component of extrinsic compression of the BI and the right upper lobe bronchus was observed. The patient expresses a strong wish to undergo treatment to improve her shortness of breath, which has caused significant emotional and physical distress.

I agree with using an approach that provides endobronchial therapy because this can achieve faster palliation than is possible, for example, with the use of external beam radiotherapy in this particular case. However, failure to address extrabronchial tumor may not lead to durable palliation and may not offer the possibility of cure. Progression of extrabronchial disease can rapidly lead to complete atelectasis and/or decreased perfusion to the right lung. Therefore after initial endobronchial treatment has been completed, and some palliation has been achieved, I would recommend a staging positron emission tomography (PET)-CT scan and an MRI scan of the brain to exclude occult metastatic disease, before external beam irradiation is considered.

External bean irradiation is a curative treatment option in patients who develop loco-regional recurrence after surgical resection.[46] If disease extent is limited to the right hilum, external beam irradiation planned using a four-dimensional CT scan and delivered using intensity-modulated radiotherapy will allow for high-dose repeat irradiation, while limiting doses to the spinal cord, esophagus, and lung parenchyma.[47] The risks of radiation-induced toxicity, including risks for pulmonary hemorrhage and late bronchial stenosis, will depend in part on the prior radiation dose received. If a dose of 45 Gy was administered, additional high-dose radiotherapy may be given, considering that a dose of 74 Gy is currently being evaluated in the experimental arm of the RTOG 0617 phase III trial in North America.[48] Older literature has reported on outcomes after high-dose re-irradiation for recurrences after previous radiotherapy; long-term disease control with acceptable acute and late toxicity has been described.[23,49,50] The risk-benefit ratio of delivering a dose of up to 60 Gy is expected to be better with the use of currently available techniques.

Because this patient has a centrally located tumor invading mediastinal structures (i.e., a possible T4 lesion), chemotherapy should be considered if a choice for curative options has not been excluded. This will depend on the patient's performance score following endobronchial palliation and on an assessment of her motivation and ability to tolerate the more toxic chemo-radiotherapy approach. Platinum-based chemoradiation generally should be considered in this setting only for patients with an ECOG performance score of 0 to 1. If the previous dose of radiation administered was 50 Gy or more, then sequential administration of chemotherapy and high-dose radiotherapy to 60 Gy may represent a less toxic approach.

Finally, one must be cognizant of the purely palliative nature of endobronchial brachytherapy in patients who present with bulky extra-bronchial disease. The rapid fall-off in radiation doses to peribronchial regions implies that the entire tumor volume will not receive a curative radiation dose. Attempting to encompass the patient's peribronchial disease by means of brachytherapy would result in administration of prohibitively high doses to the bronchial wall, creating high risk for radiation-induced necrosis and perforation. For this reason, the combination of endobronchial debulking with or without stent insertion, followed by external beam radiotherapy, has become a widespread therapeutic palliative approach in recent years.

In summary, I believe that it is important that curative nonsurgical salvage treatments be considered in patients who present with a loco-regional recurrence, and to inform patients that re-irradiation is feasible with the use of newer delivery techniques and dose-response strategies, even after prior thoracic radiotherapy. Therefore a multidisciplinary approach to lung cancer management, even in cases where initial bronchoscopic palliation of airway obstruction is planned, can benefit patients and may result in better outcomes.

REFERENCES

1. Hollingsworth HM. Wheezing and stridor. *Clin Chest Med.* 1987;8: 231-240.
2. Winfield J, Young A, Williams P, et al. Prospective study of the radiological changes in hands, feet, and cervical spine in adult rheumatoid disease. *Ann Rheum Dis.* 1983;42:613-618.
3. Bland JH. Rheumatoid subluxation of the cervical spine. *J Rheumatol.* 1990;17:134-137.
4. Campbell RS, Wou P, Watt I. A continuing role for pre-operative cervical spine radiography in rheumatoid arthritis? *Clin Radiol.* 1995;50:157-159.
5. Mikulowski P. Sudden death in rheumatoid arthritis with atlantoaxial dislocation. *Acta Med Scand.* 1975;198:445-451.
6. Neva MH, Hakkinen A, Makinen H, et al. High prevalence of asymptomatic cervical spine subluxation in patients with rheumatoid arthritis waiting for orthopaedic surgery. *Ann Rheum Dis.* 2006;65:884-888.
7. Geterud A, Bake B, Berthelsen B, et al. Laryngeal involvement in rheumatoid arthritis. *Acta Otolaryngol.* 1991;111:990-998.
8. Geterud A, Ejnell H, Mansson I, et al. Severe airway obstruction caused by laryngeal rheumatoid arthritis. *J Rheumatol.* 1986;13: 948-951.
9. Wattenmaker I, Concepcion M, Hibberd P, et al. Upper-airway obstruction and perioperative management of the airway in patients managed with posterior operations on the cervical spine for rheumatoid arthritis. *J Bone Joint Surg Am.* 1994;76:360-365.
10. Bandi V, Munnur U, Braman SS. Airway problems in patients with rheumatologic disorders. *Crit Care Clin.* 2002;18:749-765.
11. Abrams TE, Vaughan-Sarrazin M, Rosenthal GE. Influence of psychiatric comorbidity on surgical mortality. *Arch Surg.* 2010;145: 947-953.
12. Jung C, Inder JW. Management of adrenal insufficiency during the stress of medical illness and surgery. *Med J Aust.* 2008;188: 409-413.
13. Naber D, Sand P, Heigl B. Psychopathological and neuropsychological effects of 8-days' corticosteroid treatment: a prospective study. *Psychoneuroendocrinology.* 1996;21:25-31.
14. Howard LM, Barley EA, Davies E, et al. Cancer diagnosis in people with severe mental illness: practical and ethical issues. *Lancet Oncol.* 2010;11:797-804.
15. Siddiqui F, Bae K, Langer CJ, et al. The influence of gender, race, and marital status on survival in lung cancer patients: analysis of Radiation Therapy Oncology Group trials. *J Thorac Oncol.* 2010; 5:631-639.
16. Berglund A, Holmberg L, Tishelman C, et al. Social inequalities in non-small cell lung cancer management and survival: a population-based study in central Sweden. *Thorax.* 2010;65:327-333.
17. Tishelman C, Petersson LM, Degner LF, et al. Symptom prevalence, intensity, and distress in patients with inoperable lung cancer in relation to time of death. *J Clin Oncol.* 2007;25:5381-5389.
18. Ernst A, Feller-Kopman D, Becker HD, et al. Central airway obstruction. *Am J Respir Crit Care Med.* 2004;169:1278-1297.
19. Santos RS, Raftopoulos Y, Keenan RJ, et al. Bronchoscopic palliation of primary lung cancer: single or multimodality therapy? *Surg Endosc.* 2004;18:931-936.
20. Macha HN, Becker KO, Kemmer HP. Pattern of failure and survival in endobronchial laser resection: a matched pair study. *Chest.* 1994;105:1668-1672.
21. Chhajed PN, Baty F, Pless M, et al. Outcome of treated advanced non-small cell lung cancer with and without central airway obstruction. *Chest.* 2006;130:1803-1807.

22. Razi SS, Lebovics RS, Schwartz G, et al. Timely airway stenting improves survival in patients with malignant central airway obstruction. *Ann Thorac Surg.* 2010;90:1088-1093.
23. Okamoto Y, Murakami M, Yoden E, et al. Reirradiation for locally recurrent lung cancer previously treated with radiation therapy. *Int J Radiat Oncol Biol Phys.* 2002;52:390-396.
24. Slawson RG, Scott RM. Radiation therapy in bronchogenic carcinoma. *Radiology.* 1979;132:175-176.
25. Reddy SP, Marks JE. Total atelectasis of the lung secondary to malignant airway obstruction: response to radiation therapy. *Am J Clin Oncol.* 1990;13:394-400.
26. Decker RH, Wilson LD. Advances in radiotherapy for lung cancer. *Semin Respir Crit Care Med.* 2008;29:285-290.
27. Cardona AF, Reveiz L, Ospina EG, et al. Palliative endobronchial brachytherapy for non-small cell lung cancer. *Cochrane Database Syst Rev.* 2008;2:CD004284.
28. Scarda A, Confalonieri M, Baghiris C, et al. Out-patient high-dose-rate endobronchial brachytherapy for palliation of lung cancer: an observational study. *Monaldi Arch Chest Dis.* 2007;67:128-134.
29. Hara R, Itami J, Aruga T, et al. Risk factors for massive hemoptysis after endobronchial brachytherapy in patients with tracheobronchial malignancies. *Cancer.* 2001;92:2623-2627.
30. Khanavkar B, Stern P, Alberti W, Nakhosteen JA. Complications associated with brachytherapy alone or with laser in lung cancer. *Chest.* 1991;99:1062-1065.
31. Macha HN, Wahlers B, Reichle C, et al. Endobronchial radiation therapy for obstructing malignancies: ten years' experience with iridium-192 high-dose radiation brachytherapy afterloading technique in 365 patients. *Lung.* 1995;173:271-280.
32. Moghissi K, Dixon K. Is bronchoscopic photodynamic therapy a therapeutic option in lung cancer? *Eur Respir J.* 2003;22:535-541.
33. Moghissi K, Dixon K, Stringer M, et al. The place of bronchoscopic photodynamic therapy in advanced unresectable lung cancer: experience of 100 cases. *Eur J Cardiothorac Surg.* 1999;15:1-6.
34. Edell ES, Cortese DA. Photodynamic therapy: its use in the management of bronchogenic carcinoma. *Clin Chest Med.* 1995;16:455-463.
35. Vergnon JM, Schmitt T, Alamartine E, et al. Initial combined cryotherapy and irradiation for unresectable non-small cell lung cancer: preliminary results. *Chest.* 1992;102:1436-1440.
36. Vergnon JM, Huber RM, Moghissi K. Place of cryotherapy, brachytherapy and photodynamic therapy in therapeutic bronchoscopy of lung cancers. *Eur Respir J.* 2006;28:200-218.
37. Reddy C, Majid A, Michaud G, et al. Gas embolism following bronchoscopic argon plasma coagulation: a case series. *Chest.* 2008;134:1066-1069.
38. Alazemi S, Lunn W, Majid A et al. Outcomes, health-care resources use, and costs of endoscopic removal of metallic airway stents. *Chest.* 2010;138:350-356.
39. Oki M, Saka H, Kitagawa C, et al. Silicone Y-stent placement on the carina between bronchus to the right upper lobe and bronchus intermedius. *Ann Thorac Surg.* 2009;87:971-974.
40. Douillard JY, Rosell R, De Lena M, et al. Adjuvant vinorelbine plus cisplatin versus observation in patients with completely resected stage IB-IIIA non-small-cell lung cancer (Adjuvant Navelbine International Trialist Association [ANITA]): a randomised controlled trial. *Lancet Oncol.* 2006;7:719-727.
41. Ramser ER, Beamis JF Jr. Laser bronchoscopy. *Clin Chest Med.* 1995;16:415-426.
42. Colt HG. Laser bronchoscopy. *Chest Surg Clin N Am.* 1996;2:277.
43. Vanderschueren RG, Westermann CJ. Complications of endobronchial neodymium-YAG (Nd:YAG) laser application. *Lung.* 1990;168:1089.
44. Mackie AM, Watson CB. Anaesthesia and mediastinal masses: a case report and review of the literature. *Anaesthesia.* 1984;39:899-903.
45. Fisher JC. The power density of a surgical laser beam: its meaning and measurement. *Lasers Surg Med.* 1983;2:301-315.
46. Jeremic B, Shibamoto Y, Milicic B, et al. External beam radiation therapy alone for loco-regional recurrence of non-small-cell lung cancer after complete resection. *Lung Cancer.* 1999;23:135-142.
47. Haasbeek CJ, Slotman BJ, Senan S. Radiotherapy for lung cancer: clinical impact of recent technical advances. *Lung Cancer.* 2009;64:1-8.
48. Radiation Therapy Oncology Group. RTOG clinical trials listed by study number. www.rtog.org/ClinicalTrials/ProtocolTable.aspx. Accessed February 12, 2012.
49. Wu KL, Jiang GL, Qian H, et al. Three-dimensional conformal radiotherapy for locoregionally recurrent lung carcinoma after external beam irradiation: a prospective phase I-II clinical trial. *Int J Radiat Oncol Biol Phys.* 2003;57:1345-1350.
50. Tada T, Fukuda H, Matsui K, et al. Non-small-cell lung cancer: reirradiation for loco-regional relapse previously treated with radiation therapy. *Int J Clin Oncol.* 2005;10:247-250.

Chapter 23

Photodynamic Therapy for Palliation of Infiltrative Endoluminal Obstruction at Left Secondary Carina and Left Lower Lobe Bronchus

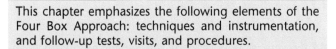

This chapter emphasizes the following elements of the Four Box Approach: techniques and instrumentation, and follow-up tests, visits, and procedures.

CASE DESCRIPTION

This patient was a 75-year-old man with stage IIIA squamous cell carcinoma who presented with worsening dyspnea, hemoptysis, and wheezing. A bronchoscopy performed by his pulmonologist showed near complete left lower lobe bronchial obstruction. He had undergone three cycles of chemotherapy, which were poorly tolerated. He refused further chemotherapy but agreed to receive external beam radiation therapy (EBRT), which unfortunately was complicated by radiation pneumonitis. Repeat bronchoscopy several weeks later showed recurrence of the tumor, prompting high-dose brachytherapy (dose and fractions unknown) at an outside facility. Follow-up bronchoscopy showed diffuse infiltrative tumor at the left secondary carina (LC2) nearly completely occluding the left lower lobe (LLL) bronchus. The segments in the left upper lobe (LUL) were infiltrated but patent, and the LLL bronchus was circumferentially narrowed by inflamed, necrotic, and friable mucosa, which was likely responsible for his hemoptysis and wheezing (Figure 23-1). His limited pulmonary function test (PFT) performed several months before showed FVC (forced vital capacity) of 2.26 L (69% of predicted), FEV_1 (forced expiratory volume in one second) of 1.73 L (74% of predicted), and DLCO (diffusing capacity of the lungs for carbon monoxide) 68% of predicted. He was on no medications. On examination, the patient was cachectic, weighed 118 lbs, and had localized wheezes on the left side. After discussing various treatment alternatives, the patient decided to proceed with photodynamic therapy (PDT) to attempt restoration of LLL bronchial patency (see Figure 23-1).

DISCUSSION POINTS

1. List three indications for PDT in this patient.
2. List three potential contraindications to PDT.

3. Describe the instructions to be provided to a patient who has undergone PDT.
4. Describe the clinical indications and the physics of brachytherapy as compared with PDT.

CASE RESOLUTION
Initial Evaluations

Physical Examination, Complementary Tests, and Functional Status Assessment

This patient had lobar obstruction due to endobronchial involvement from squamous cell carcinoma. Central airway obstruction from locally advanced lung cancer is seen in approximately 30% of patients previously treated with radiotherapy or chemoradiotherapy. This patient's prior systemic chemotherapy and external beam radiation therapy (EBRT) did not preclude the use of photodynamic therapy (PDT) because PDT causes no direct injury to lung parenchyma. In one series, 85% of patients treated with PDT had received prior chemoradiotherapy.[1] This patient's previous brachytherapy did not preclude PDT either, and evidence indicates that the two modalities can be safely administered together or sequentially.[2,3]

Although bronchoscopy is essential in planning PDT, the response to PDT does not seem to correlate with the degree of airway obstruction or with tumor pathology. Preoperatively, the patient's chest radiograph showed left lower lobe consolidation (see Figure 23-1); however, during initial evaluation of these patients, a computed tomography (CT) of the chest is probably preferable because CT may provide information regarding the extent of peribronchial involvement and airway distortion, which can be underestimated by bronchoscopy alone. Ventilation-perfusion studies may show absence or reduction of regional perfusion out of proportion to ventilation in the involved lung zone—a finding usually associated with extensive peribronchial involvement and poor outcome.[4] Identification of significant peribronchial disease on CT has therapeutic implications because this is not treated using debulking techniques, and even if the airways are reopened, gas exchange may not improve if a reduction in local perfusion is due to tumor infiltration of the pulmonary vasculature.

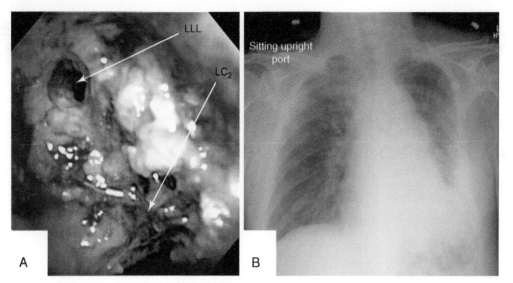

Figure 23-1 A, Pre–photodynamic therapy (PDT) bronchoscopic view of the left lower lobe (LLL) bronchus and the secondary left carina (LC2); note circumferential narrowing of the bronchus due to significant mucosal neoplastic infiltration. **B,** Chest radiograph before PDT shows prominent left hilum and LLL consolidation.

Comorbidities

When considering PDT, physicians should be aware that patients with hepatic or renal impairment may need greater preventive measures for photosensitivity* because the commonly used photosensitizer, photofrin, is retained in the skin and in the reticuloendothelial system as well. In addition, interaction between photofrin† and other drugs is possible, and concomitant use of other photosensitizing agents such as tetracyclines, sulfonamides, phenothiazines, sulfonylurea hypoglycemic agents, thiazide diuretics, griseofulvin, and fluoroquinolones can increase the risk of photosensitivity reactions. Our patient had no evidence of hepatic or renal dysfunction and was on no medications.

Support System

The patient lived by himself but had two daughters who were very supportive. They were willing to spend a couple of days with him after the procedure. Patient and family education is extremely important after PDT to reduce the risk of complications. Constant reinforcement of information may be necessary because of transient memory impairment after use of sedatives or anesthetic drugs, and because patients are often reluctant to avoid sun exposure.

Patient Preferences and Expectations

During the interview process, the patient wondered whether another treatment would be necessary, and if this could be safely repeated. We explained that during the cleanup bronchoscopy, performed a day or two after PDT, we could use the laser light to re-illuminate the lesion if persistent obstructing disease was present. In addition, two administrations of photofrin‡ within 30 to

---

*Patients should be informed that the period requiring precautionary measures for photosensitivity may sometimes be longer than 90 days.

†Photofrin is, at present, the most frequently used photosensitizer. Other variants of purified hematoporphyrin derivatives are marketed (e.g., Photosan in Germany).

‡The usual dose is 2 mg/kg as slow intravenous injection over 3 to 5 minutes.

45 days apart is possible if subsequent follow-up bronchoscopies continue to reveal symptomatic bronchial obstruction.

Procedural Strategies

Indications

Described indications for PDT in the treatment of central airway obstruction include palliation of advanced malignant airway obstruction (especially chemoradiation-resistant lesions), tumor ingrowth through stents (Figure 23-2), and, rarely, benign disorders such as granulation tissue growth or papillomas.[5,6] Accepted selection criteria for patients with locally advanced lung cancer consist of the following: (1) patients have inoperable or unresectable tumor with existing or impending related symptoms; (2) patients still have good performance status (Karnofsky Performance Status [KPS] index >50% or World Health Organization [WHO] scale ≤3); and (3) patients have no extrathoracic metastasis.[7]

PDT should be applied only to patients with intraluminal airway obstruction. Among these, the best response involves patients with mucosal involvement. Results from studies show that the mean duration of complete response was 22 weeks if more than 50% of the obstruction was due to mucosal disease, compared with only 7 weeks if the tumor was submucosal or extraluminal.[4] In addition to the type of obstruction, the morphology (shape) of the treatment area leads to variations in response rates. In this regard, debulking and stent insertion add uniformity to the field of treatment by providing a more consistent shape and diameter of the obstructed airway. Although this could amplify PDT effect, airway stents may attenuate it by reducing light penetration.

Contraindications

Patients suffering from porphyria should not be given photofrin because this drug could exacerbate their disease. PDT is also contraindicated in patients with known or high risk for esophagorespiratory fistula because necrosis induced by PDT can enlarge these processes. Tumors eroding or suspected to involve major blood vessels are

Figure 23-2 Other potential applications for photodynamic therapy (PDT). **A,** Tumor ingrowth through the uncovered portion of an Ultraflex stent in the left main bronchus. **B,** Granulation tissue partially occluding the distal aspect of a straight silicone stent.

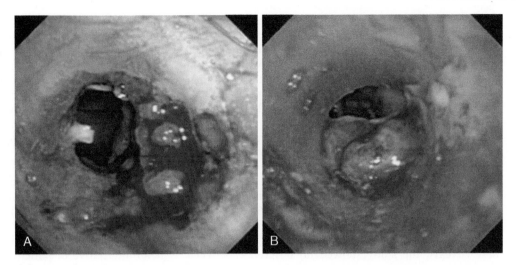

considered contraindications to PDT because they may lead to bronchoarterial fistulas and fatal hemoptysis. PDT is contraindicated for emergency treatment of patients with critical airway obstruction and severe acute respiratory distress caused by an obstructing endobronchial or endotracheal lesion because at least 40 to 50 hours is required between photofrin injection and laser light exposure, and because PDT-induced tumor necrosis is delayed for several days. Careful review of a patient's records and current medications should identify drugs such as nonsteroidal anti-inflammatory drugs (NSAIDs), steroids, and strong antioxidants that may diminish the efficacy of PDT. Photofrin is considered a pregnancy risk C (toxicity, no malformation) medication and is nondialyzable.

Expected Results

In a review of 12 articles that describe a total of more than 600 patients with advanced lung cancer,[8] bronchoscopic PDT was considered safe and effective for malignant endobronchial obstruction, providing symptomatic relief in all patients and a survival benefit for those without metastatic disease and with good performance status. Palliation of symptoms occurs in 74% to 100% of patients.[5] Regardless of the pathology of the malignant obstruction (primary lung cancer, metastases), several factors influence the response to PDT. These include different optical properties of tissues that will influence the absorption of light and the depth of penetration (pigmentation, bleeding, and necrosis), extent of the lesion (superficial vs. "bulky" obstruction), and location of the lesion (large or small airways). Effects are less predictable with tumors located at acute angles, such as those noted in our case.

The basic principle of PDT is that the injected chemical (i.e., photofrin) accumulates more in rapidly growing tissues than in normal tissues. These molecules absorb light and produce cytotoxic oxygen species upon illumination with light of appropriate wavelength (600 to 800 nm).* This photochemical reaction leads to

formation of reactive oxygen species, direct cell injury, and induction of apoptosis and vascular effects such as congestion, red cell extravasation within the tumor, and ischemic necrosis through neovascular shutdown mediated in part by thromboxane A2 release.[9,10] The variability in clinical response noted in studies occurs when the interactions are inconsistent.

Results from randomized controlled studies* of patients with advanced-stage disease presented in abstract form show no survival advantage for PDT compared with neodymium-doped yttrium aluminum garnet (Nd:YAG) laser therapy, or PDT combined with radiotherapy compared with radiotherapy alone, but an advantage for PDT with radiotherapy was noted with respect to symptom control.[11,12] One study randomized 211 patients to PDT or Nd:YAG laser therapy and found that the response was significantly greater 1 month after treatment with PDT than after treatment with Nd:YAG laser (55% vs. 30%).[11] In another trial, the bronchial lumen was completely opened with no evidence of gross tumor in 14 of 20 patients receiving PDT plus radiotherapy compared with 2 of 21 patients receiving radiotherapy alone.[12] Three of 20 patients experienced massive and fatal hemoptysis at 67, 187, and 567 days after treatment with PDT and radiotherapy,[12] potentially suggesting that the addition of radiation after PDT may increase the risk for bronchoarterial fistula formation.

Noncontrolled studies have reported post-PDT reductions in dyspnea, hemoptysis, cough, or bronchial obstruction and atelectasis.[13-16] One of these studies included 68 men and 32 women (mean age, 62.5 years) with advanced inoperable bronchogenic carcinoma and endobronchial obstruction; 43 patients had a functional WHO class of 2 or less, and 54 had a WHO class of greater than 2. Patients were followed and were re-treated on an as-needed basis every 6 to 8 weeks for 1 year, and then every 3 to 6 months until death; average PDT treatments per person numbered 1.47. Mean and median survival times

---

*The absorption spectrum in the 600 to 800 nm range facilitates depth of penetration, which is 3 to 5 mm.

*Neither paper reported whether assessment of response was blinded, and the response was not clearly defined.

for WHO of 2 or less were 17.8 and 14 months, respectively; for WHO of greater than 2, they were 6.9 and 4 months, respectively, potentially suggesting that PDT treatments should be offered to patients who are still functional with a reasonable performance status.[16] When compared with Nd:YAG laser, PDT may offer a more durable response, and more patients may be symptom-free at 1 month in the PDT group.[5]

At least one study has shown that PDT may be better than Nd:YAG laser for symptom palliation in patients with central airway obstruction caused by non–small cell lung carcinoma (NSCLC).[17] However, the two groups were unbalanced in terms of staging or severity of illness. This study included 31 patients (mean age, 65 years; KPS >40), and 57% of the PDT group had advanced NSCLC (IIIA, IV) versus 88% in the Nd:YAG laser group. Given these caveats, the study showed no difference between groups at 1 week in terms of symptoms or degree of obstruction, but the median time to treatment failure was 50 days for PDT versus 38 days for the Nd:YAG group ($P = .03$). Overall survival in this study favored the PDT group (265 vs. 95 days; $P = .007$), but again, this might be explained by the more advanced stage of disease in the Nd:YAG group.[17]

Expected complications after PDT include photosensitivity* ($\approx21\%$), which can be prolonged. Patients must avoid sun exposure for approximately 4 to 6 weeks after injection. Within days after treatment, however, airway obstruction may result from necrotic tissue, so a cleanup bronchoscopy† within 24 to 72 hours post intervention may be necessary when large obstructing lesions are treated. Other potential complications include dyspnea 30%, hemoptysis 16%, fever 16%, coughing 15%, pneumonia 12%, and bronchitis 10%.

Team Experience

Decisions about PDT probably should result from deliberations of a multidisciplinary lung cancer conference or clinic, including surgery, radiation oncology, pulmonary, and oncology subspecialties. An institution that offers PDT should have a readily available bronchoscopy team because PDT may require salvage bronchoscopies performed within 48 hours post illumination for tumor slough removal.‡ The bronchoscopy team should also be readily available during the treatment period because the risk of fatal hemoptysis is increased, especially in patients who have undergone multiple endobronchial procedures, previous radiation therapy, or metal stent placement.

The most common adverse effect related to PDT is skin photosensitivity, with an incidence between 5% and 28%. Lesser rates were reported from centers that had a dedicated member of the team assigned to provide counseling and information to patients.[8] Great value is derived from having a dedicated PDT nurse to offer patient education and to explain the importance of adhering to protection from sunlight strategies.*

Therapeutic Alternatives

For patients with malignant obstruction, apart from traditional surgical resection, radiotherapy, and chemotherapy, several bronchoscopic options are available. Nd:YAG laser, brachytherapy, and cryotherapy have been used alone or in combination for symptom palliation. Rigid bronchoscopy with laser photocoagulation and coring out of the tumor is especially useful for tracheal or mainstem bronchial disease and when hemoptysis is present. In our patient, the lobar obstruction caused by mucosal disease was not appropriate for laser treatment because of a substantial infiltrative rather than endoluminal exophytic component. In addition, although stent insertion is an alternative in patients with malignant obstruction, our patient had a distal lobar location of disease (LLL) that was not ideal for stent placement because the LLL bronchus is both short and narrow. Cryotherapy usually preserves airway cartilage and was an alternative for this patient[18]; however, it was not ideal because of the absence of substantial exophytic disease. Further high-dose brachytherapy was not warranted because it had already been attempted without success.

Cost-Effectiveness

Since 1988, PDT has been approved by the U.S. Food and Drug Administration for palliative treatment of central airway lesions due to NSCLC.[19] In 2004, the National Institute for Clinical Excellence stated, "Current evidence on safety and efficacy of PDT for advanced bronchial carcinoma is adequate to support its use to treat patients with inoperable NSCLC."[20]

Informed Consent

The patient understood the risks and benefits of PDT for advanced bronchial carcinoma. His fears pertaining to photosensitivity were alleviated by an educational session provided by our nurses.

Techniques and Results

Anesthesia and Perioperative Care

Studies report flexible bronchoscopic PDT with patients under moderate sedation. Some studies have used general anesthesia and rigid bronchoscopy or endotracheal tube

---

*Mild to moderate erythema, but also includes swelling, itching, and burning sensation; occasionally induces pseudoporphyria state.

†This may not be necessary when PDT is used to treat early lung cancer.

‡Appropriate equipment for slough removal should be available and may include large-channel bronchoscopes and cryotherapy probes.

---

*All patients who receive photofrin will be photosensitive and must observe precautions to avoid exposure of skin and eyes to direct sunlight or to bright indoor light (from examination lamps, including dental lamps, operating room lamps, and unshaded light bulbs at close proximity) for at least 30 days, but some may remain photosensitive for up to 90 days or more. However, exposure of the skin to ambient indoor light is beneficial because the remaining drug will be inactivated gradually and safely through a photobleaching reaction. Before any area of skin is exposed to direct sunlight or bright indoor light, the patient should test it for residual photosensitivity. A small area of skin should be exposed to sunlight for 10 minutes. If no photosensitivity reaction (erythema, edema, blistering) occurs within 24 hours, the patient can gradually resume normal outdoor activities. If some photosensitivity reaction occurs with the limited skin test, the patient should continue precautions for another 2 weeks before retesting.

Figure 23-3 A, The 2.5 cm cylindrical diffuser is advanced in the distal left main bronchus and lower lobe bronchus. **B,** Post photodynamic therapy (PDT) after 8 minutes and 20 seconds application.

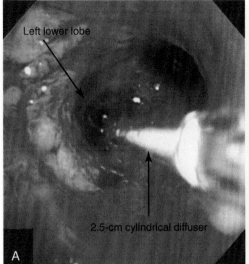
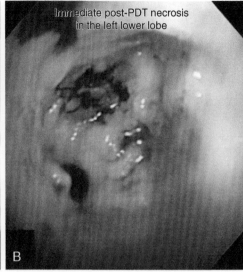

Left lower lobe

2.5-cm cylindrical diffuser

Immediate post-PDT necrosis in the left lower lobe

for ventilation, through which operators place the flexible instrument for tumor location and illumination. Use of general anesthetic and the rigid bronchoscope in patients with bronchial obstruction undergoing PDT allows good access for debridement, thereby achieving a thorough cleaning of the bronchial tree and ample room to maneuver in case of complications.[8] In the opinion of many PDT experts, combined rigid and flexible instruments under general anesthesia are best for patients with obstructive tumors of the trachea and mainstem bronchi, but for other cases, the method depends on the experience of the operator and a patient's comorbidities and personal choice.[7] We decided to perform this particular procedure on our patient while under general anesthesia to allow better control of the diffuser in the distal left main and lower lobe bronchi and to have a secure airway in case the patient's hemoptysis worsened during the procedure.

Technique and Instrumentation

Light is delivered to the tumor by cylindrical fiberoptic diffusers passed through the working channel of the bronchoscope (Figure 23-3). The fiber may be positioned alongside the tumor when it is relatively flat, or it can be implanted within the tumor when it is bulky and exophytic. Cylindrical diffusers are commonly used for central airway obstruction and are available in several lengths; the choice of diffuser tip length* depends on the length of the tumor to be treated. Diffuser length should be properly sized to avoid exposure of nonmalignant tissue to light and to prevent overlapping of previously treated malignant tissue. Therefore, before light administration, the length of the tumor is assessed with bronchoscopy, and a suitable light fiber length is selected to transilluminate the tumor. Within lung and tumor tissue,

630 nm light will penetrate to a depth of 5 to 10 mm from the point of origin, depending on the power density and the length of the fiber.[21] Argon-pumped dye laser and diode-based systems have been used as a light source. We used a compact diode-based laser (Diomed Ltd., Andover, Mass) that was available at our institution. This is a nonthermal laser, so no risks of airway fire are present. Photoactivation of photofrin is controlled by the total light dose delivered. In the treatment of endobronchial cancer, a light dose of 200 J/cm of diffuser length should be delivered. The total power output at the fiber tip is set to deliver the appropriate light dose using exposure times of 8 minutes and 20 seconds.[21]

A step-by-step approach to bronchoscopic PDT proceeds as follows: First, the *treatment plan* is developed by performing diagnostic flexible bronchoscopy, during which time the length of the tumor is assessed and the diffuser length is selected (see Figure 23-1). Then, in the *presensitization* phase, photofrin is injected; after a latent period of 2 to 3 days (which permits optimal differential concentration between tumor and healthy surrounding tissue), some investigators measure drug levels by point spectroscopy; others proceed straight to the *illumination* (irradiative) phase* using laser light of appropriate wavelength (630 nm) (see Figure 23-3). Light doses of 200 J/cm of diffuser length are used in endobronchial cancer for both palliation of obstructing cancer and treatment of superficial lesions.[22] One to three days later, *debridement* is usually necessary when obstructing lesions are treated (Figure 23-4); before a second laser light treatment is provided, any residual tumor should be debrided, which may cause bleeding if performed vigorously. In fact, debridement of necrotic tissue should be discontinued if the volume of bleeding increases; this may indicate

---

*Fibers for the treatment of endobronchial cancer are generally 1, 2, and 2.5 cm tip lengths and in general are adequate for tumor necrosis within the central airways.

---

*It is important to realize that an appropriate wavelength of laser light is one that interacts with the particular photosensitizer used for photosensitization of the target. It is also relevant that the duration of the latent period is dependent on the chemical structure of the photosensitizing agent and its handling by tumor and normal cells.

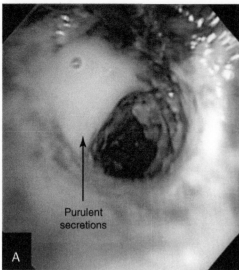 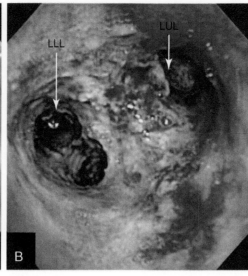

Figure 23-4 A, Twenty-four hours after photodynamic therapy (PDT), bronchoscopy reveals necrotic debris and purulent secretions in the left lower lobe. **B,** Once debridement was performed, patency to the left lower lobe segments was re-established. *LLL,* Left lower lobe; *LUL,* Left upper lobe.

that debridement has gone beyond the zone of the PDT effect. *Re-illumination* can then be performed if residual obstruction remains, usually within 96 to 120 hours after the initial injection, but no further injection of photofrin should be given for such re-treatment with laser light. In fact, most patients receive two treatments during their hospitalization, and many return several weeks later for *repeated treatments.*[23]

Anatomic Dangers and Other Risks

PDT can completely destroy malignant tissues that have been adequately dosed with the photosensitizer and exciting light. This may result in necrosis that may not be apparent during the irradiative phase of treatment, when the full cross-sectional extent of the tumor may not be obvious to the bronchoscopist (see video on ExpertConsult.com) (Video V.23.1). In addition, further necrosis of the tumor develops hours to days after treatment. Thus when performed in hollow organs such as the airway or the esophagus, PDT can lead to fistula formation. Increased airway inflammation increases the effects of PDT and may lead to damage of adjacent nonmalignant but inflamed mucosa. Tissue sloughing can cause severe lobar and segmental airway obstruction and respiratory failure. Salvage bronchoscopy may be necessary as soon as 6 hours after treatment, and when main central airway treatment is performed, postprocedure intensive care unit (ICU) admission is probably warranted. Having ready access to flexible bronchoscopy, as well as a good grasping forceps or cryotherapy unit available, can be lifesaving. Local edema and formation of mucus from adjacent normal tissues may result in transient bronchitis, which may exacerbate coexisting chronic obstructive pulmonary disease (COPD) or asthma.

Results and Procedure-Related Complications

After administration of general anesthesia with propofol, our patient was intubated with a No. 8.0 endotracheal tube. Flexible bronchoscopy showed again circumferential neoplastic infiltration in the distal left mainstem bronchus (LMB) with near total occlusion of the left lower lobe (LLL) and involvement of the left secondary carina (LC2) and the left upper lobe (LUL) (see Figure 23-1). The 2.5 cm cylindrical diffuser was inserted, and a total of 300 joules (480 seconds) of light energy was applied using a 630 nm diode laser to treat the distal LMB and the LLL bronchus (see Figure 23-2). At the end of the procedure, the patient was extubated without difficulty. He was treated as an inpatient given the fact that he was very frail and lived 150 miles away from the hospital. The next day, he underwent a flexible bronchoscopy under moderate sedation, at which time the LLL bronchus was found to be occluded by necrotic debris. Pus was noticed in the distal segmental airways (see Figure 23-4).* Abundant saline washes were performed to rid the area of the obstructing material. Once this had been performed, we noted that patency to the LLL segmental bronchi had been restored (see Figure 23-4). Two days later, rigid bronchoscopy was performed because additional necrotic material had to be removed from the LLL bronchus (Figure 23-5). Patency to the left lower lobe was thus established (see video on ExpertConsult.com) (Video V.23.2). A small piece of cartilage that had likely been destroyed by tumor was noted, although this might have resulted from PDT-induced bronchial wall and mucosal necrosis (see video on ExpertConsult.com) (Video V.23.3).

When light of two to three times the recommended dose (aka light overdose) has been administered to patients with superficial endobronchial tumors, increased symptoms and damage to normal tissue can be expected. Occasionally local edema and mucous formation from surrounding normal tissues may result in transient bronchitic symptoms, including cough and dyspnea. Necrotic

---

*Prevention of infection is relevant for patients with significant lobar or segmental tumor obstruction. In such patients, post-PDT necrosis creates a culture medium for microorganisms. Chest physiotherapy, deep breathing exercises, incentive spirometry, and antibiotics may be needed.

Figure 23-5 Second cleanup bronchoscopy at 72 hours post photodynamic therapy (PDT). **A,** Sloughing of tissue and thick mucus were completely occluding the left lower lobe (LLL) bronchus. **B,** After saline lavage was used, the segmental airways in the LLL were open, although evidence of necrosis and inflammation of the mucosa was noted. **C,** Chest radiograph 1 week later shows improved aeration to the left lower lobe but residual retrocardiac consolidation.

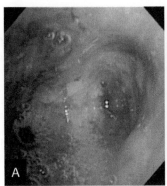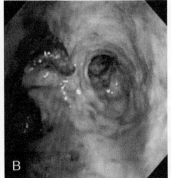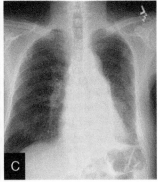

tumor slough and secretions from bulky tumors may potentially cause respiratory distress, atelectasis, or pneumonia. Although rapid tumor vascular stasis is observed, cytotoxicity and cellular death of tumor cells are delayed in such a way that necrotic debris eventually forms at the site of treatment over the next 48 hours. This debris is tenacious and can be difficult or impossible to expectorate (see Figure 23-5), prompting the need for repeated bronchoscopic intervention.

Long-Term Management

Outcome Assessment

A clinic appointment a week later after bronchoscopy improved aeration in the LLL on chest radiograph, improved symptoms, and resolved airway obstruction (see Figure 23-5). Four weeks after the intervention, during a sunny day, the patient went outside of his house and developed sunburn with significant erythema, pain, and itching around the eyes. He went to the local emergency department, where he was diagnosed with PDT-induced sunburn and was given local anesthetic to be applied to the affected area for pain. When we discussed this issue with him, he told to us that a home health nurse had instructed him that he could leave the house after 4 weeks post intervention. He had neglected to call our nursing team to inform us of this recommendation.

Follow-up Tests and Procedures

When compared with electrocautery, more airway scarring and more subepithelial fibrosis may be seen after treatment with PDT or Nd:YAG laser. Prominent scar tissue formation and significant stenosis were found in four of six (67%) patients treated with PDT in one series—a finding that contrasts with the assumption that PDT is highly selective for tumor tissue. In the treatment of early lung cancer, normal airway mucosa is exposed more than in patients with advanced disease; however, the fact that normal mucosa can be affected, resulting in scar tissue formation, is important in the choice of diffuser length.[24] A follow-up bronchoscopy is almost always warranted, not only to explore the need for additional bronchoscopic interventions, but also to rule out potential strictures in the treated area. If subsequent radiotherapy is planned, it is advisable to allow 2 to 4

weeks between PDT and radiation to ensure that the inflammatory response* produced by the PDT has subsided. Patients should be carefully evaluated for tumor erosion into a major blood vessel. If on follow-up bronchoscopy, evidence of tumor recurrence and obstruction is apparent, patients may receive a second course of PDT a minimum of 30 days after the initial therapy.† Our patient was not a candidate for further radiotherapy but could have undergone PDT again.

The interaction between PDT and radiation, chemotherapy, and stent insertion is important when multimodality treatments are planned for these patients with advanced-stage lung cancer. Certain chemotherapy drugs such as Adriamycin and mitomycin can enhance the PDT effect.[25] Ionizing radiation has a synergistic effect and has been given before, after,[26] or during the PDT treatment period.[27] PDT in lung cancer is compatible when used in conjunction, or in sequence, with other standard systemic or endobronchial treatment methods.[28] PDT can be combined with brachytherapy concomitantly or sequentially, as was done in our case.[3] Also, PDT can be applied in sequence with Nd:YAG laser; in one series, Nd:YAG laser was used to debulk endobronchial obstructing tumors. The addition of PDT by its specific action resulted in long periods of local remission and provided an apparent survival benefit.[28] When our patient was seen during follow-up, he informed us that he did not wish to undergo further bronchoscopic treatment. We chose to respect his decision, and we did not inquire as to his reasons.

Referrals

After PDT, the patient was referred back to his oncologist for consideration for further systemic treatment. In patients with advanced lung cancer, local control and distant control are not independent factors, and quality of life may not improve if only local or distal control has been achieved.[29] Because medical treatments had been exhausted, we thought that palliative care consultation was appropriate. This recommendation was accepted by the patient and his family.

---

*The inflammatory response from PDT will depend on tumor size and the extent of surrounding normal tissue that receives light.

†In general, up to three courses of PDT (each separated by a minimum of 30 days) can be given.

Quality Improvement

We assumed responsibility for not clarifying discharge instructions regarding post-PDT care and for not communicating this to the patient's home health nurse, who had been arranged by his previous caregivers. Sunburn due to cutaneous hypersensitivity may be completely prevented with careful instruction and patient compliance with sunlight avoidance.[5] Indeed, after 4 weeks, our patient should have tested his skin for photosensitivity. We apologized for our lack of satisfactory communication and shared our misgivings with the patient and with his family. Patients and surrogate decision makers need to know and fully understand the status of their health so they can make fully informed decisions regarding their care. Health care providers must not hesitate to advocate for patients in this regard. Often, problems of communication and other follow-up care issues can be resolved if an interventional team has the appropriate personnel and other resources necessary to provide telephone, computer-based, and in-person follow-up. This is not always the case, particularly in institutions that have not yet perceived the importance of an interventional service, or in institutions where administrators do not recognize the spectrum of disease and the substantial comorbidities often present in patients with central airway obstruction.

If a patient has been injured during medical treatment, full participation in subsequent informed consent processes is possible only if the details that led to an injury are fully understood.[30] Because many patients with central airway obstruction may require repeated bronchoscopic or other treatments, withholding information relevant to the patient's health care could be interpreted as dishonest and could severely undermine a physician's relationship with the patient,[30] drastically altering the patient's ability to make an informed and correct decision regarding further intervention.

An adverse event is defined as "harm that is the result of the process of health care rather than the patient's underlying disease." This is different from a medical error in that it refers to a specific outcome (sunburn in this case) rather than to a breakdown in the process of care (lack of proper patient education). In general, patients want to be told about medical errors. They want to hear an explicit statement that an error occurred and the reasons for its occurrence. They also wish to be told about the implications that the adverse event might have for their health and their ongoing health care. Disclosure of medical errors is considered one component of a culture of accountability. However open communication and transparency do entail some risks. A patient may lose confidence in a physician, a health care team, or an institution and may not fully understand that some adverse events are "expected" and cannot always be avoided. At other times, a patient may not understand that errors may be human or system related, and that although preventive measures may be instituted, 100% success in avoiding errors is not always possible. As a result, patients may refuse further potentially beneficial treatment, especially if communication with the patient by health care providers, hospital administration, ethics committee members, or representatives of risk management services is mishandled. In our case, the adverse event was, in our opinion, minor. However, for our patient, who had after all originally voiced concerns regarding the effect that sun avoidance might have on his quality of life, transient sunburn and the additional time that he needed to spend indoors served as a substantial nuisance. Fortunately, our patient understood the reasons why this had happened and 2 weeks after the event, after proper testing, was able to resume his limited outdoor activities without further evidence of photosensitivity.

DISCUSSION POINTS

1. List three indications for PDT in this patient.
   - The patient was a nonsurgical candidate owing to his advanced-stage disease.
   - Lobar airway obstruction was characterized by mucosal involvement.
   - Associated symptoms of dyspnea and hemoptysis were evident.
2. List three potential contraindications to PDT.
   - Central airway obstruction with impending respiratory failure
   - Tumors invading the mediastinal vasculature
   - Esophagorespiratory fistulas
3. Describe the instructions to be provided to a patient who has undergone PDT.
   - After administration of photofrin, the skin and the eyes will be very sensitive to direct sunlight and bright lights for 30 days or longer.
   - If outdoor activities are performed, advise the patient to wear dark sunglasses (<4% light transmittance), gloves, a wide-brimmed hat, long-sleeved shirts, slacks, and socks.
   - Advise patients to avoid direct sunlight or bright light such as a reading light; although normal indoor light is not harmful, direct skylight should be avoided by having draped windows or shades.
   - After 30 days, advise patients to test for photosensitivity by putting their hand in a paper bag with a 2 inch hole in it and exposing it to direct sunlight for 10 minutes; if swelling, redness, or blistering occurs within 24 hours, the patient should continue to take precautions for another 2 weeks before retesting; if no reaction occurs within 24 hours, the patient may gradually increase exposure to sunlight.[31]
4. Describe the clinical indications and the physics of brachytherapy as compared with PDT.
   - High dose rate endobronchial brachytherapy (HDREB)* is the most common brachytherapy

---

*This technique is usually performed in the following steps: the tumor location and length are identified on bronchoscopy and chest x-ray; one or more catheters are implanted next to the lesion via the working channel of the bronchoscope. The bronchoscope is then removed and the catheter(s) are fixed to the nose. Orthogonal films are taken after a phantom is positioned in the catheter(s). The target volume is then drawn on the films with a 1 to 2 cm safety margin with respect to the bronchoscopy image. The dose is usually prescribed to be delivered at 1 cm from an iridium-192 source.

technique applied endobronchially because it is performed through the flexible bronchoscope on an outpatient basis. Similar to PDT, the indications for HDREB in patients with symptomatic advanced predominantly intraluminal disease include palliation of hemoptysis, cough, and dyspnea; lobar or segmental atelectasis; and recurrent infection. However, results from a systematic review of the literature suggest that external beam radiation (EBRT) alone is more effective than HDREB for symptom palliation in previously untreated patients with endobronchial non–small cell lung carcinoma. When brachytherapy is performed, HDREB with EBRT seems to provide better symptom relief than EBRT alone.[32] Because its tissue effects are deeper than those of PDT (1 to 2 cm vs. 0.5 to 1 cm), HDREB has been used successfully in patients with endobronchial and peribronchial disease. Similar to probes used in PDT, brachytherapy catheters can be placed into the upper lobe bronchi, as well as into segmental bronchi—areas typically difficult to access with relatively stiff laser fibers. Also, because of its delayed effect and dose fractionations, HDREB is usually offered to patients with a life expectancy greater than 3 months. Similar to PDT, HDREB is contraindicated in patients with massive post obstructive atelectasis owing to complete airway obstruction (the catheter cannot be passed through the lesion) and critical airway obstruction (resulting tumor debris can worsen the degree of obstruction).[7] Treatment of tumors in the right and left upper lobes has the highest incidence of treatment-related hemoptysis, probably because of proximity of the great vessels. Indeed, results of one study found a 32% rate of massive hemoptysis in patients with recurrent tumors in the right upper lobe, right mainstem, and left upper lobe bronchus.[33] One study reported fatal hemoptysis in 9.5% of patients undergoing HDREB, and the only factor related to this was the larger irradiated volume.[34] In this regard, if previous laser treatment has been provided, it is probably wise to wait longer than 3 days before initiating brachytherapy treatment to avoid the potential development of broncho-arterial fistula.[7]

- The physics of brachytherapy is different from that of PDT. Although PDT relies on photochemical reactions to cause cell damage and apoptosis, HDREB uses ionizing radiation to cause single chain breaks of DNA, resulting in apoptosis and a decrease in cell proliferation. The visible effects of brachytherapy with iridium-192 HDREB are delayed, with maximum visible and histologic changes taking place 3 weeks after application (vs. several days after PDT). Therefore a follow-up bronchoscopy is usually performed 3 to 6 weeks after the end of a planned treatment series. The primary radiation produced for HDREB consists of gamma rays using iridium-192 as a radiation source. In the past, radium was the primary isotope used in brachytherapy, but because of its long half-life (1.6 years) and high energy output (0.83 MeV), radium has been replaced with isotopes that have shorter half-lives and can be shielded easily because of their lower energies (i.e., iridium [Ir]: half-life 74.2 days, energy 0.38 MeV). The physical characteristics of these radioactive isotopes are characterized by the inverse square law, which means that the dose rate decreases as a function of the inverse square of the distance to the source center.* Because the gamma ray beam travels in straight but divergent directions, radiation intensity in a three-dimensional structure (i.e., tracheobronchial tree) dictates that radiation intensity will decrease with the inverse square of the distance. The law is particularly important in radiotherapy treatment planning; for example, the dose at 2 cm will be one fourth the dose at 1 cm.

- Prescription point, dose, and fractionation for HDREB: The International Commission of Radiation Units defines high dose rate (HDR) as the application of more than 20 cGy•min^{-1}, which means a delivery of more than12 Gy•h^{-1}, with the dose per session (fraction) varying from approximately 300 to 1000 cGy (calculated at 10 mm from the source axis).[35,36] The reference point from which doses should be calculated is the source axis. The treatment dose is usually prescribed at 10 mm from the source center, but given the variability in the tracheobronchial lumen diameter, larger doses will affect the bronchial mucosa to a greater extent than the tracheal one.[35,36] Therefore alternative methods have been described. These include prescribing the dose at various distances from the center of the catheter based on the diameter of the trachea or bronchus at the treatment point.[37] The dose varies according to tumor location, the percentage of lumen occlusion, and the length of airway involvement; for the length, a safety margin of 1 to 2 cm at each end usually adequately covers the tumor in case of catheter movement. Dose fractionation varies among institutions, ranging from 15 Gy in one fraction to 4 Gy × 5 fractions; however, one study showed that when prescribed at 1 cm, a dose of 2 × 7.2 Gy at 3 week intervals was equivalent to a 4 × 3.8 Gy dose given on a weekly basis.[38] The American Brachytherapy Society suggests the use of one of the following regimens: 7.5 Gy 3 times per week, two fractions of 10 Gy twice a week, or four fractions of 6 Gy when HDR is the only measure for palliation. Doses are smaller when HDR is used as a boost to palliative EBRT.[35-37]

---

*Because the surface area of a sphere ($4\pi r^2$) is proportional to the square of the radius, as the emitted radiation gets farther from the source, it must spread out over an area that is proportional to the square of the distance from the source. Therefore, radiation passing through any unit area is inversely proportional to the square of the distance from the source.

PROCEDURE TODAY: PDT RECIPE

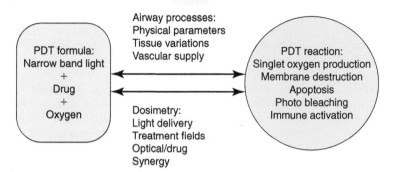

Figure 23-6 Photodynamic therapy (PDT) reaction within the airway and key factors effecting responses.

Expert Commentary

provided by Gordon H. Downie, MD, PhD

PDT for endobronchial carcinoma has been used with varying degrees of success since first attempted and reported by Dr. Kato in the late 1980s. More than 30 years of basic science, clinical science, and clinical reports, as well as expert user reviews, support PDT use in the airway. The authors provide a practical case that demonstrates many classic features of PDT use in the airway, and their review of the literature highlights the key concepts required when one is contemplating the use of PDT to treat cancer in the airway.

Most institutions have minimal experience with PDT and do not have the clinical physics support to adapt to the nuisances that individual cases can generate. Because of this, PDT is often left as a last hope intervention when other approaches have failed. In my opinion, this approach maximizes the possibility of clinical response variation and unwanted side effects. Furthermore, the inertia to use PDT as a last resort does the technology a disservice. The authors outlined several sources of clinical variation and included some important but little considered interactions. In my opinion, an approach using frontline PDT in this patient might have lessened potential side effects but still may have provided the upside palliative effect.

Two non-PDT features of this case deserve review: the choice to treat the cancer systemically with chemotherapy then locally with radiation before offering direct treatment for the partial airway obstruction, and the diagnostic options used to assess the functional parameters of the left lower lobe airway obstruction. Marasso et al. reviewed 98 patients with advanced lung cancer and an obstructive airway component. Fifty patients were treated with chemotherapy and radiation first, followed by direct local airway manipulation; 48 patients had local airway treatment first followed by chemotherapy and radiation. The mean survival rates in the two groups were 5 and 14 months, respectively.[39] He argued that optimizing airway function improved performance status, lessened post obstructive airway pathophysiology, and subsequently allowed better tolerance of chemotherapy and radiation. In my opinion, the discussion of airway intervention prior to chemotherapy/radiation is one that every

multidisciplinary thoracic oncology team should have before providing any treatment for advanced lung cancer. The authors made an excellent point about CT scanning and how it provides key in-depth information about the left lower lobe consolidation not provided by the chest x-ray. In a similar manner, selective bronchography of the left lower lobe bronchial tree would add functional information that CT scan does not. Selective bronchography has been shown to be superior to the 4 week rule* or CT scans of the chest in predicting the reversibility of lobar or lung atelectasis caused by neoplastic bronchial obstruction.[40] Selective bronchography provides functional information that still life imaging cannot address, and the procedure itself is low-cost, safe, and technically simple.

Because PDT involves the unique interaction of a device (laser) and a drug (photosensitizer) to create a clinical response, PDT users must intimately understand the photodynamic reaction and must perceive where individual cases can potentially result in unexpected responses. Figure 23-6 is a depiction of the PDT reaction within the airway and the key factors effecting responses. It will be useful to review this case point by point from Figure 23-6 to appreciate how variations can be minimized and the clinical response can be more predictable.

Airways can affect the PDT reaction in three major ways: the physical parameters of the airway/tumor presentation, neoplastic tissue characteristics, and vascular supply. Airway/tumor presentation includes the percentage of luminal obstruction, the diameter of the native airway, and the length of the tumor, as well as shadowing caused by irregular tumor shape and viscous secretions. Neoplastic tissue characteristics include reflectance, necrosis, inflammation, bleeding, and pigmentation. Vascular supply will affect the delivery of the drug to the site, the kinetics of drug

---

*The 4 week rule refers to the duration of collapse that is sometimes used by bronchoscopists to predict a response to bronchoscopic intervention in the setting of malignant central airway obstruction; identifying patients who meet the 4 week criteria can be unreliable because in clinical practice, definitive symptoms or imaging studies that can pinpoint duration of collapse are seldom found. In addition, the 4 week rule has not been studied in randomized clinical trials and is most often recommended on the basis of expert opinion rather than evidence-based data.

washout, and the delivery of oxygen necessary for singlet oxygen production.

The authors commented that the degree of obstruction does not correlate with the PDT response; however, the degree of obstruction does dramatically affect dosimetry considerations, which in turn directly determine the PDT response. The first PDT dosimetry question a clinician should answer is whether the obstruction should be treated with interstitial or superficial catheter placement. Interstitial catheter placement requires a separate physics calculation that is independent of the airway's area because the impaled tumor receives 100% of the delivered light energy. Superficial catheter placement light delivery is affected by shadowing, luminal area, percentage of tumor occupancy, and amount/type of secretions.[41] Weighing the pros and cons of catheter placement to optimize the predictability of response is, in my opinion, underutilized.

This case presents several challenges related to the patient's airway physical parameters: significant luminal diameter change over a very short length of airway, bloody secretions, irregular tumor edges with shadowing, and distal airway location affected by respiration movements. Tumor shape in this case would not allow an interstitial catheter placement, so the author's discussion of stent placement before treatment with PDT is very relevant. An uncovered stent can resolve much of airway/tumor irregularity; bleeding would be better tamponaded, thus reducing secretions and causing the treatment area to become easier to define.[42] Use of a 1 centimeter long catheter in this case would have lessened luminal diameter variation; the 2.5 cm catheter used appears to be treating totally different airway calculated areas with the same light/energy delivery at its proximal versus distal ends. Finally, strongly filtered fiberoptic bronchoscopy will allow real-time observation of catheter movement that digital scopes often cannot follow when the digital camera is super saturated with light. Tissue variations were well addressed by the authors, but strict airway toilet before light delivery must be emphasized.

Vascular supply in this case may have been affected by chemotherapy, radiation therapy (external beam or HDR), and stenting. Unfortunately a strong theoretical argument can be made for an augmented or reduced vascular supply. In my opinion, confirming significant drug uptake at the treatment site would answer the practical question of vascular supply and drug and oxygen delivery. This could have been accomplished by employing point spectrometric measurements just before the time of treatment. Additionally, taking measurements before and after treatment allows confirmation that an adequate photodynamic reaction has taken place by demonstrating drug consumption.[43]

Dosimetry cannot be calculated by a one size fits all approach. Dosimetry recommendations quoted by the authors were generated by trials for FDA approval of photofrin and reflect the understanding of the field 15 to 20 years ago. Preset diode laser options also encourage a nonadaptable approach to airway dosimetry. Programs that are employing PDT as a

BIOENERGETICS AND TISSUE OPTICS

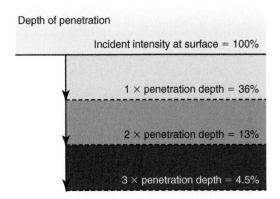

Approximate values of incident intensity at various penetration depths

Figure 23-7 Effect of tissue on light delivery.

frontline oncologic treatment are universally customizing dosimetry to the individual's clinical presentation. Customization takes into account light delivery variations, treatment field plasticity, tissue interference with light absorption, drug uptake variations, and synergistic effects of patient medications and previous oncologic treatments.[43]

Figure 23-7 presents unpublished data from Dr. Tom Mang's laboratory at the University of Buffalo and depicts the effects of tissue on light delivery. For airway tissue, one penetration depth is approximately 8 mm, and the assumption that a significant clinical PDT response can be seen to a depth of 8 mm comes from basic science information such as this. However, in our program, we have seen a significant tumoricidal response with 90% attenuation of light intensity and apoptosis within cells with 95% light intensity attenuation. This suggests that tumor cell death can occur out to 2.4 cm from the light source. Pre-PDT external beam radiation to the treatment field would have dramatically lowered this patient's cellular sensitivity to singlet oxygen damage and would have changed significantly the predicted response depth. Drug uptake, oxygen delivery, HDR, current medications, stent placement, and previous chemotherapy also affect PDT response. This case presents so many variables that a truly predictable PDT response in my opinion was not possible. A positive outcome does not change how unpredictable PDT really was in this setting; however, the balancing factors included upfront full disclosure of risk benefits and limited available treatment options.

REFERENCES

1. Moghissi K, Bond MG, Sambrook RJ, et al. Treatment of endotracheal or endobronchial obstruction by non-small cell lung cancer: lack of patients in an MRC randomized trial leaves key questions unanswered. Medical Research Council Lung Cancer Working Party. *Clin Oncol (R Coll Radiol)*. 1999;11:179-183.
2. Weinberg BD, Allison RR, Sibata C, et al. Results of combined photodynamic therapy (PDT) and high dose rate brachytherapy

(HDR) in treatment of obstructive endobronchial non-small cell lung cancer (NSCLC). *Photodiagn Photodyn Ther.* 2010;7:50-58.

3. Freitag L, Ernst A, Thomas M, et al. Sequential photodynamic therapy (PDT) and high dose brachytherapy for endobronchial tumour control in patients with limited bronchogenic carcinoma. *Thorax.* 2004;59:790-793.

4. Lam S, Müller NL, Miller RR, et al. Predicting the response of obstructive endobronchial tumors to photodynamic therapy. *Cancer.* 1986;58:2298-2306.

5. Loewen GM, Pandey R, Bellnier D, et al. Endobronchial photodynamic therapy for lung cancer. *Lasers Surg Med.* 2006;38:364-370.

6. Shikowitz MJ, Abramson AL, Steinberg BM, et al. Clinical trial of photodynamic therapy with meso-tetra (hydroxyphenyl) chlorin for respiratory papillomatosis. *Arch Otolaryngol Head Neck Surg.* 2005;131:99-105.

7. Vergnon JM, Huber RM, Moghissi K. Place of cryotherapy, brachytherapy and photodynamic therapy in therapeutic bronchoscopy of lung cancers. *Eur Respir J.* 2006;28:200-218.

8. Moghissi K, Dixon K. Is bronchoscopic photodynamic therapy a therapeutic option in lung cancer. *Eur Respir J.* 2003;22:535-541.

9. Edell ES, Cortese DA. Photodynamic therapy: its use in the management of bronchogenic carcinoma. *Clin Chest Med.* 1995;16:455-463.

10. Maziak DE, Markman BR, MacKay JA, et al; Cancer Care Ontario Practice Guidelines Initiative Lung Cancer Disease Site Group. Photodynamic therapy in nonsmall cell lung cancer: a systematic review. *Ann Thorac Surg.* 2004;77:1484-1491.

11. Wieman TJ, Diaz-Jimenez JP, Moghissi K, et al. Photodynamic therapy (PDT) with photofrin is effective in the palliation of obstructive endobronchial lung cancer: results of two randomized trials [abstract]. *Proc Am Soc Clin Oncol.* 1998;17:464a.

12. Lam S, Grafton C, Coy P, et al. Combined photodynamic therapy (PDT) using photofrin and radiotherapy (XRT) versus radiotherapy alone in patients with inoperable obstructive non-small cell bronchogenic carcinoma. *SPIE.* 1991;1616:20-28.

13. Vincent RG, Dougherty TJ, Rao U, et al. Photoradiation therapy in advanced carcinoma of the trachea and bronchus. *Chest.* 1984;85:29-33.

14. Hugh-Jones P, Gardner WN. Laser photodynamic therapy for inoperable bronchogenic squamous carcinoma. *Q J Med.* 1987;243:565-581.

15. LoCicero J, Metzdorff M, Almgren C. Photodynamic therapy in the palliation of late stage obstructing non-small cell lung cancer. *Chest.* 1990;98:97-100.

16. Moghissi K, Dixon K, Stringer M, et al. The place of bronchoscopic photodynamic therapy in advanced unresectable lung cancer: experience of 100 cases. *Eur J Cardiothorac Surg.* 1999;15:1-6.

17. Diaz-Jiménez JP, Martínez-Ballarín JE, Llunell A, et al. Efficacy and safety of photodynamic therapy versus Nd-YAG laser resection in NSCLC with airway obstruction. *Eur Respir J.* 1999;14:800-805.

18. Homasson JP. Bronchoscopic cryotherapy. *J Bronchol.* 1995;2:145-153.

19. Johnson JR, Williams G, Pazdur R. End points and United States Food and Drug Administration approval of oncology drugs. *J Clin Oncol.* 2003;21:1404-1411.

20. National Institute for Clinical Excellence. Photodynamic therapy for advanced bronchial carcinoma. http://guidance.nice.org.uk/nicemedia/live/11101/31032/31032.pdf. Accessed May 6, 2011.

21. Dougherty TJ, Marcus SL. Photodynamic therapy. *Eur J Cancer.* 1992;28:1734-1742.

22. Mang TS. Dosimetric concepts for PDT. *Photodiagn Photodyn Ther.* 2008;5:217-223.

23. Minnich DJ, Bryant AS, Dooley A, et al. Photodynamic laser therapy for lesions in the airway. *Ann Thorac Surg.* 2010;89:1744-1749.

24. van Boxem AJ, Westerga J, Venmans BJ, et al. Photodynamic therapy, Nd-YAG laser and electrocautery for treating early-stage intraluminal cancer: which to choose? *Lung Cancer.* 2001;31:31-36.

25. Baas P, van Geel IP, Oppelaar H, et al. Enhancement of photodynamic therapy by mitomycin C: a preclinical and clinical study. *Br J Cancer.* 1996;73:945-951.

26. Schaffer M, Schaffer PM, Corti L, et al. Photofrin as a specific radiosensitizing agent for tumors: studies in comparison to other porphyrins, in an experimental in vivo model. *J Photochem Photobiol B.* 2002;66:157-164.

27. Madsen SJ, Sun CH, Tromberg BJ, et al. Effects of combined photodynamic therapy and ionizing radiation on human glioma spheroids. *Photochem Photobiol.* 2002;76:411-416.

28. Moghissi K, Dixon K, Hudson E, et al: Endoscopic laser therapy in malignant tracheo-bronchial obstruction using sequential Nd: YAG laser and photodynamic therapy. *Thorax.* 1997;52:281-283.

29. Sutedja TG. Photodynamic therapy in advanced tracheobronchial cancers. *Diagn Ther Endosc.* 1999;5:245-251.

30. Loren DJ, Gallagher T. Disclosure of harmful medical errors: the verdict. In: Colt HG, Quadrelli S, Friedman L, eds. *The Picture of Health: Medical Ethics and the Movies.* New York: Oxford University Press; 2011.

31. Pinnacle Biologics. PDT with photofrin. www.photofrin.com. Accessed May 6, 2011.

32. Ung YC, Yu E, Falkson C, et al; Lung cancer disease site group of Cancer Care Ontario's Program in Evidence-Based Care. The role of high-dose-rate brachytherapy in the palliation of symptoms in patients with non-small-cell lung cancer: a systematic review. *Brachytherapy.* 2006;5:189-202.

33. Bedwinek J, Petty A, Bruton C, et al. The use of high dose rate endobronchical brachytherapy to palliate symptomatic endobronchial recurrence of previously irradiated bronchogenic carcinoma. *Int J Radiat Oncol Biol Phys.* 1991;22:23-30.

34. Carvalho Hde A, Gonçalves SL, Pedreira W Jr, et al. Irradiated volume and the risk of fatal hemoptysis in patients submitted to high dose-rate endobronchial brachytherapy. *Lung Cancer.* 2007;55:319-327.

35. Nag S, Dally M, de la Torre M, et al. Recommendations for implementation of high dose rate 192Ir brachytherapy in developing countries by the Advisory Group of International Atomic Energy Agency. *Radiother Oncol.* 2002;64:297-308.

36. Nag S, Abitbol AA, Anderson LL, et al. Consensus guidelines for high dose rate remote brachytherapy in cervical, endometrial, and endobronchial tumors. Clinical Research Committee, American Endocurietherapy Society. *Int J Radiat Oncol Biol Phys.* 1993;27:1241-1244.

37. Nag S, Kelly JF, Horton JL, et al. Brachytherapy for carcinoma of the lung. *Oncology.* 2001;15:371-381.

38. Huber RM, Fischer R, Hautmann H, et al. Palliative endobronchial brachytherapy for central lung tumors: a prospective, randomized comparison of two fractionation schedules. *Chest.* 1995;107:463-470.

39. Marasso A, Bernardi V, Gai R, et al. Radiofrequency resection of bronchial tumours in combination with cryotherapy: evaluation of a new technique. *Thorax.* 1998;53:106-109.

40. Downie GH, Childs JH, Landucci DL, et al. The use of selective bronchography in predicting reversal of neoplastic obstructive atelectasis. *Chest.* 2002;123:828-834.

41. Downie GH, Cuenca RE, Allison RR, et al. A comparison of interstitial and superficial light delivery for photodynamic therapy of intraluminal neoplasms. *J Bronchol.* 2002;9:193-196.

42. Allison R, Sibata C, Sarma K, et al. High-dose-rate brachytherapy in combination with stenting offers a rapid and statistically significant improvement in quality of life for patients with endobronchial recurrence. *Cancer J.* 2004;10:368-373.

43. Downie GH. Clinical considerations for airway photodynamic therapy. In: *Report of the 13th World Congress for Bronchology (WCB) and 13th World Congress for Bronchoesophagology (WCBE). Medimond International Proceedings* 2005;1-9.

Chapter 24

Rigid Bronchoscopy with Y Stent Insertion at Left Secondary Carina

This chapter emphasizes the following elements of the Four Box Approach: risk-benefit analysis and therapeutic alternatives, techniques and instrumentation, and referrals to medical, surgical, or palliative/end-of-life subspecialty care.

CASE DESCRIPTION

A 75-year-old man with a 120–pack-year history of smoking and COPD (FEV_1 52% predicted, DLCO 39% predicted) developed progressive dyspnea, a weak and hoarse voice, and hemoptysis. His usual exertional dyspnea had progressed to the point that he now required assistance with activities of daily living. Chest CT showed a $6 \times 5 \times 7$ cm left infrahilar mass involving the distal left main bronchus (LMB) and the entrance to the left upper and lower lobe bronchi (Figure 24-1, A and B). In addition, mediastinal lymphadenopathy was significant in stations 7 (subcarinal) and 4 L (left lower paratracheal). Flexible bronchoscopy showed an immobile left vocal cord and near complete obstruction in the distal LMB characterized by extrinsic compression and exophytic endoluminal tumor with hypervascular mucosa (Figure 24-1, C). Examination of the airways distal to the tumor was possible using forced saline lavage and showed patent distal segments but significant involvement of the left secondary carina (LC2). Rigid bronchoscopy was performed under general anesthesia with spontaneous assisted ventilation. Endobronchial needle aspiration (EBNA) with rapid on-site evaluation (ROSE) revealed non–small cell lung cancer (NSCLC). Nd:YAG laser photocoagulation and bronchoscopic debulking partially restored patency to left upper and lower lobe bronchi. However, tumor infiltration, cartilaginous collapse, and extrinsic compression required insertion of a large Y silicone stent (16 mm diameter tracheal limb, 12 mm bronchial limbs) placed within the left main bronchus (Figure 24-1, D and E).

DISCUSSION POINTS

1. Describe two techniques to deploy a Y stent.
2. Describe the indications for stent insertion before initiation of systemic therapy in this particular patient.
3. List three potential complications resulting from stent insertion at the left secondary carina.

CASE RESOLUTION

Initial Evaluations

Physical Examination, Complementary Tests, and Functional Status Assessment

This patient required considerable assistance at home. His functional impairment was consistent with a Karnofsky Performance Scale score (KPS) of 50. At the time of hospitalization, however, KPS was only 20 (severely disabled, where hospitalization was necessary but death was not imminent).[1] His Eastern Cooperative Oncology Group (ECOG) performance scale, which may be a better predictor of prognosis than KPS,[2,3] was 3 (i.e., the patient was capable of only limited self-care and was confined to bed or chair for more than 50% of waking hours). Assessment of this patient's performance status is essential for guiding therapeutic interventions because this degree of impairment, due to lung cancer or comorbid conditions (e.g., chronic obstructive pulmonary disease [COPD]), may preclude resection or, alternatively, chemoradiotherapy.[4] In fact, this patient was not operable based on his pulmonary function tests and functional status. Relevant to his case, however, is that the combination of interventional bronchoscopy and external beam radiation therapy (EBRT) might improve survival, symptoms, and quality of life, as has been previously shown in patients with lung cancer, central airway obstruction, and KPS less than 50.

The patient's weak voice and hoarseness are explained by unilateral (left) vocal cord immobility as noted on bronchoscopy (see video on ExpertConsult.com) (Video V.24.1). This was likely due to unilateral recurrent laryngeal nerve (RLN) injury, which caused the affected vocal fold to rest in the paramedian position. The contralateral vocal fold may or may not provide adequate glottic closure during phonation. If closure is not achieved, the residual glottal gap results in air escape with a weak voice secondary to a "leaky valve" phenomenon.[5] In unilateral RLN injury, the glottic aperture is usually adequate, and related dyspnea and stridor are rare. Glottal incompetence, however, increases the risk for aspiration, particularly with thin liquids. Cough, which requires transient tight glottic closure, may also be affected; this is important in cases of airway stent insertion with risk for mucus plugging and difficulty raising secretions. Associated sensory loss from RLN involvement may also cause dysphagia, a symptom not seen in our patient. With regard

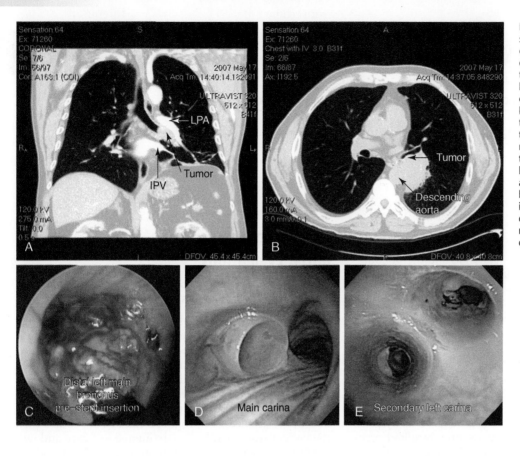

Figure 24-1 **A,** Tumor extension in the distal left main bronchus (LMB). The lung parenchyma distal to the obstruction is functional. **B,** Tumor extension in the left upper lobe bronchus and occlusion of the left lower lobe bronchus. **C,** Distal LMB obstruction caused by a highly vascular tumor invading the posterior and medial walls. **D,** Main carina shows the proximal aspect of the tracheal limb of the Y stent. **E,** Restored airway patency to the upper and lower lobe bronchi after Y stent insertion at the left secondary carina (LC2). *IPV,* Inferior pulmonary vein; *LMB,* left main bronchus; *LPA,* left pulmonary artery.

to staging, RLN involvement is consistent with T4 disease. In conjunction with N2 disease on computed tomography (CT) scan (involvement of stations 7 and 4 L), this patient's clinical stage is at least IIIB, and estimated median survival time is 10 months and 5 years for 7% despite multimodality treatment.[6]

Comorbidities

This patient had moderate, Global Obstructive Lung Disease (GOLD) stage II COPD. Although no other comorbidities were reported, careful examination and review of systems are warranted because COPD is associated with hypertension, coronary heart disease, stroke, obstructive sleep apnea, depression, anxiety, and cognitive dysfunction, which could preclude or complicate interventions under general anesthesia.[4]

Support System

The patient had good social support from his daughter and his wife. Early discussions about quality of life and symptom concerns are warranted because patients suffering from cancer will commonly develop pain, dyspnea, cough, and fatigue during the course of their illness.[7] These conversations took place with the patient and his family because a diagnosis of cancer has a significant psychological and emotional impact on family members and caregivers as well.[8]

Patient Preferences and Expectations

This gentleman had expressed his desire for diagnosis and was ready to consider all available treatment options. He was very clear, however, that he did not want to live

"being dependent on machines," and he wanted to make all decisions regarding his care. In the United States, most patients diagnosed with cancer want a shared or active role in the decision-making process, usually with greater participation than what actually occurs. Role preferences (active vs. passive), however, vary greatly during decision making, and repeated assessments are required to meet patients' expectations and improve their satisfaction with treatment decisions.[9]

Procedural Strategies

Indications

This patient required tissue diagnosis. We elected to proceed with rigid bronchoscopy under general anesthesia to restore airway patency with laser and silicone stent insertion and to diagnose the airway lesion using endobronchial biopsy, bronchial washing, and/or endobronchial needle aspiration. Chemoradiotherapy currently constitutes the standard of care for patients with inoperable locally advanced non–small cell lung cancer (NSCLC).[10] This treatment, however, is usually restricted to patients who maintain a good performance status.[11]

Central airway obstruction (CAO) in the setting of NSCLC is associated with a very poor prognosis. In one study, median and 1 year survival of patients with malignant CAO were reportedly as low as 3.4 months and 15%, respectively.[12] However, patients with advanced NSCLC with locally treated CAO combined with systemic chemotherapy might have survival rates similar to those patients without CAO treated with chemotherapy alone.[13] Interventional bronchoscopic procedures in this

Figure 24-2 Main carinal tumor in different patient **(A)** before and **(B)** after Y stent insertion. Y stents are shaped with **(C)** a long tracheal and left main bronchial limbs and a shorter right main bronchial limb. Models with and without external studs are available.

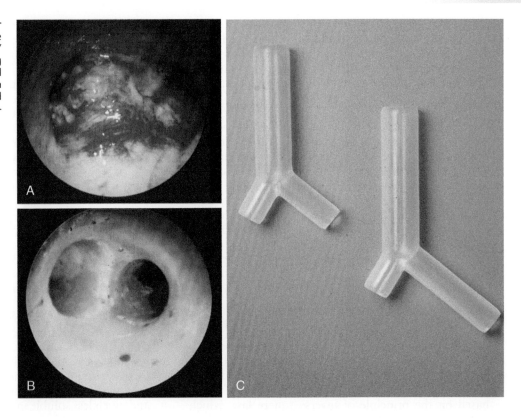

patient with inoperable disease are expected to restore airway patency and improve lung function, dyspnea, and functional status, thus allowing initiation of systemic therapy, which could improve his survival.[14]

Contraindications

No absolute contraindications to rigid bronchoscopy were noted. Although COPD treatment should be optimized before elective interventions to reduce perioperative complications, our patient had stable disease at the time of evaluation and was being treated with short-acting β_2-agonists and long-acting anticholinergic agents in accordance with international guidelines.[15]

Expected Results

For diagnosis, endobronchial needle aspiration (EBNA) with rapid on-site evaluation (ROSE) was performed. In patients with visible endobronchial lesions such as this, the diagnostic yield increases from 76% with conventional procedures alone to 96% with EBNA in addition to conventional procedures (washings, brushings, and biopsy).[16]

For restoring airway patency in our patient with near complete obstruction in the distal left main bronchus (LMB), left secondary carina (LC2) involvement, and a mixed pattern of obstruction (extrinsic and endoluminal exophytic), a straight metal or silicone stent would not have restored patency to the obstructed lobar bronchi. Therefore we decided to insert a silicone Y stent. This type of stent can be used for patients with fixed or dynamic CAO from benign or malignant disease, but the most common uses are to restore airway patency, to improve dyspnea and quality of life for patients with malignant

CAO involving the mainstem bronchi and the lower trachea (Figure 24-2), and to reduce recurrent infection in patients with tracheoesophageal or bronchoesophageal fistulas.[17-20] Y stents are also effective in restoring airway patency, and they improve symptoms in patients with severe diffuse tracheobronchomalacia, but with a high rate of nonfatal complications.[21,22] In our patient, a Y silicone stent insertion was planned to restore and maintain LMB and left upper lobe (LUL) and left lower lobe (LLL) airway patency, which would allow the following:

1. *Initiation of systemic therapy:* By improving functional status, this patient could become a candidate for systemic treatment; in fact, evidence suggests that patients with advanced NSCLC and CAO who undergo successful interventional bronchoscopy to relieve airway obstruction might have survival similar to that of patients without CAO.[13]

2. *Improved exercise capacity and dyspnea:* A significant improvement in symptoms in up to 94% of patients undergoing central airway stent insertion has been reported, although 40% of patients required multiple procedures. This raises questions about the costs per quality of life-years in patients with advanced disease.[14]

Team Experience

Studies reporting an association between results of interventional bronchoscopy, procedure-related complications, and the required level of technical expertise have not yet been performed. It is known, however, that survival and complications after such procedures are worse for malignant than for benign CAO, and it was suggested that these patients should be considered distinct populations to be analyzed and reported separately.[23] One can only hypothesize that referral to an experienced bronchoscopist and oncologic team will result in reduced complications, more rapid diagnosis, greater restoration of airway patency, and earlier discharge from the hospital.

Risk-Benefit Analysis

For diagnosis, we chose to perform EBNA before proceeding with laser photocoagulation. In our experience, EBNA has a lower risk of bleeding and provides immediate diagnosis when ROSE is available. In contrast with endobronchial biopsy, however, tissue architecture is not seen.[16] With regard to restoring airway patency, the risks of further physiologic compromise and massive bleeding were considered to be outweighed by the benefit of restoring airway patency, the ability to diagnose the lesion, and improved functional status and the offer of systemic therapy. Alternatives to our approach should be considered on a case-by-case basis.

Therapeutic Alternatives for Restoring Airway Patency

These include endobronchial and systemic therapies.

- *Endobronchial brachytherapy (EBB):* This technique has proven efficacy in patients with endoluminal tumor and a substantial extrabronchial component. It is based on the principle of inverse square law, which states that dose rate decreases as a function of the inverse square of the distance to the source center, making it possible to achieve a high irradiation dose in the center of the irradiation source with a fast decrease toward the periphery. EBB offers significant palliation with rates of recanalization ranging from 60% to 90%, and symptomatic improvement is seen in 70% to 80% of patients. The variability in reported results is explained by patient selection, different treatment schemata, and the use of additional treatments. For palliation of NSCLC symptoms, however, a Cochrane meta-analysis concluded that EBB alone was less effective than EBRT. For patients previously treated by EBRT who are symptomatic from recurrent CAO, however, EBB may be considered.[24] EBB is usually performed via flexible bronchoscopy. Effects are delayed, and complications include hemoptysis, which could be fatal in up to 21% of patients, as well as fistula formation, radiation bronchitis (10%), and bronchial stenosis. This modality was not considered optimal for our patient because of his severe airway obstruction and marginal pulmonary function. Furthermore, EBB for this tumor would have to be extensive, including the LMB along with the LUL and the LLL. Treatment in the upper lobes is associated with the highest incidence of hemoptysis, probably because of the proximity of great vessels.
- *Photodynamic therapy (PDT):* This treatment can be performed via flexible bronchoscopy and is approved for local regional palliation for advanced NSCLC. This modality is most effective when more than 50% narrowing results from mucosal disease.[25] The outcome of PDT seems to be best, however, when patients have a relatively good performance status.[26] In addition, associated risks of phototoxicity for approximately 4

weeks post intervention ($\approx$20%) and a therapeutic effect that is delayed for at least 48 hours make it less than ideal in our patient. PDT might actually worsen airway obstruction during the initial post-treatment period because of sloughing of airway mucosa and retained tumor debris. Similar to EBB, PDT is contraindicated in patients at high risk for fatal massive hemoptysis.

- *Cryotherapy:* This approach causes thrombosis and necrosis of tumor tissues and could have been used for the exophytic, endobronchial component of this patient's CAO. No risk for airway fire or perforation is present, but cryotherapy can cause cold-induced bronchospasm—a matter of particular risk in our patient with COPD. Cryotherapy has been shown to be most effective when performed in combination with EBRT.[27] Similar to PDT and EBB, the effect is delayed and initially might worsen airway obstruction, causing post obstructive pneumonia due to sloughed necrotic tissue.
- *Electrocautery and argon plasma coagulation (APC):* These techniques remove the exophytic endoluminal component and provide superficial cauterization (3 to 6 mm), which may not suffice to stop large airway bleeding. APC has a risk for gas embolization, which is relevant in our patient because of the vascular pattern of his airway tumor. Argon gas is heavy, inert, and much less soluble in the body than carbon dioxide. As gas is forced into the airway wall, causing perforation, it collects in a blood vessel and passes into the systemic circulation, causing embolism.[28] Erosion from tumor also presents a risk to major vessels. Systemic, life-threatening gas embolism has been reported as a complication of endobronchial APC.[29]
- *Fully or partially covered metal stent insertion:* This alternative may be used in cases of malignant CAO. In patients with significant comorbidities precluding general anesthesia, it is a suitable alternative in that stents can be placed via flexible bronchoscopy with or without fluoroscopy.[30] Metal stents are more costly than silicone stents and can be difficult to remove. Furthermore, a straight stent would not palliate this patient's lobar bronchial obstruction.
- *Flexible bronchoscopy using laser:* This procedure could be performed but would be very time-consuming in this patient because of his extensive intraluminal disease. Furthermore, this would only assist with management of the endobronchial component, and stent insertion would still be necessary to palliate extrinsic obstruction. Because of severe bleeding or bronchial obstruction from tissue debris, pulmonary hygiene may be difficult in this patient with COPD.
- *Systemic therapies such as EBRT and systemic chemotherapy:* These treatments might be appropriate once a final tissue diagnosis is available. If NSCLC is confirmed, this tumor would be a clinical stage IIIB.[6] Current evidence shows that for individuals with unresectable disease, a good performance score, and minimal weight loss, treatment with combined chemoradiotherapy results in better survival than radiotherapy alone. Concurrent chemoradiotherapy seems to be associated with improved survival compared with sequential chemoradiotherapy.[31] Restoration of airway

patency could improve the performance score and accelerate appropriate initiation of systemic therapy. Initiation of EBRT as a primary treatment without attempts to restore airway patency is of doubtful benefit in this patient. EBRT is only variably effective for cancer-induced CAO, especially when CAO results in atelectasis. In a study of 330 patients, EBRT palliated hemoptysis in 84% of patients and superior vena cava syndrome in 86% of patients, but atelectasis in only 23%.[32] EBRT after effective laser treatment, however, could potentially improve survival.[33] A factor that limits most EBRT treatments is unwanted exposure of the normal lung parenchyma, heart, spine, and esophagus.

Cost-Effectiveness

The costs of interventional procedures providing immediate palliation of airway patency are probably small compared with the costs of repeated systemic therapies, but these economic factors might be institution, insurer, and country specific. Silicone stent insertion requires rigid bronchoscopy under general anesthesia in an operating theater, which increases costs. Risk is associated with general anesthesia, especially in patients with significant cardiopulmonary disorders. After taking into account the type of CAO (mixed extrinsic compression and exophytic endoluminal), indications, contraindications, tissue interactions, response time, and expected results of various bronchoscopic interventions, we thought that neodymium-doped yttrium aluminum garnet (Nd:YAG) laser therapy followed by silicone stent insertion would offer rapid improvement in symptoms, so that systemic therapy could be initiated. A multimodality bronchoscopic approach is likely to be more effective than a single modality for symptomatic palliation of lung cancer–related CAO. In a study comparing Nd:YAG laser, stent insertion, PDT, or brachytherapy alone versus a combination of bronchoscopic interventions such as laser and stent insertion, or versus laser and stent insertion closely followed by brachytherapy, significant improvement in survival was noted in the multimodality group. One-year and 3-year cumulative survival rates for the two groups were 51.3% versus 50% and 2.3% versus 22%, over 14 months' follow-up.[34]

Informed Consent

The patient and his family had good insight into his disease. Expectations were realistic. After they had been advised of all alternatives, the family elected to proceed with rigid bronchoscopy under general anesthesia. They were informed of potential failure to restore airway patency and were told about the risks for bleeding, perforation, respiratory failure, temporary mechanical ventilation, and death. Prolonged mechanical ventilation was declined by the patient.

Techniques and Results

Anesthesia and Perioperative Care

Concern for hypoxemia and hypoventilation during induction exists because of the already critical bronchial narrowing.[35] If possible, induction should be cautious and preferably provided without neuromuscular blockers, which might cause complete loss of muscular tone in the posterior membrane and may worsen an already critically narrowed airway.[36] Spontaneous-assisted ventilation can be provided through an open circuit during the rigid bronchoscopic procedure.[37] In case of a large air leak resulting in an inability to ventilate and oxygenate satisfactorily, the mouth and the nose can be packed with gauze. In case of bleeding from the large tumor in the distal LMB, the patient should be quickly turned toward his left lateral decubitus. A large tamponade balloon may have to be inserted into the LMB to protect the contralateral bronchial tree. Because Nd:YAG laser is used, fire safety precautions are followed and the fraction of inspired oxygen (FiO_2) is reduced to less than 0.4 before and during laser activation.

Instrumentation

We chose a 13 mm Efer-Dumon rigid ventilating bronchoscope (Bryan Corp., Woburn, Mass) and an Nd:YAG laser on standby in case of bleeding and for tumor coagulation and debulking. Various sizes of silicone Y stents were readily available. These stents have a smooth internal surface and could have a studded external to prevent migration. The bronchoscopist can trim the stent using scissors or a scalpel. In general, the largest stent possible should be used to avoid migration.

Anatomic Dangers and Other Risks

The left pulmonary artery is anterior, the descending aorta is posterior, and the inferior pulmonary vein and left atrium are medial to the distal LMB (see Figure 24-1). Therefore, laser treatment should be performed carefully in this area to avoid direct application onto the posterior and medial walls. In hypervascular tumors, the absorption of laser energy is high for Nd:YAG laser, and perforation risk is present. Airway obstruction from blood and tumor debris may cause hypoxemia. Technical considerations during stent insertion include concern for (1) perforation of the medial wall of the main bronchus, resulting in bronchomediastinal fistula and possible mediastinal misplacement of the stent; (2) perforation of the posterior membrane, which may cause aortic laceration; and (3) hypoventilation and hypoxemia, which occur when the large stent does not unfold satisfactorily.

Results and Procedure-Related Complications

After induction of general anesthesia, the patient was intubated with a 13 mm Efer-Dumon rigid ventilating bronchoscope. Inspection of the trachea and the right bronchial tree was unremarkable. On the left side, the tumor was highly friable, invading the posterior wall and obstructing the distal LMB, as well as the entrance to the left upper and lower lobes (see Figure 24-1). Once the blood clot covering the tumor was removed, we performed EBNA to the submucosal tumor. Bleeding after EBNA stopped after instillation of 60 mL of saline. ROSE revealed NSCLC. Nd:YAG laser photocoagulation was followed by rigid bronchoscopic debulking in the distal LMB. The tumor involved the LC2 and lobar bronchi. Airway patency to the LUL was restored, but the tumor extended into the LLL bronchus. Once passed, the basal segments were open. Because of the tumor's location in the distal LMB and its extension to the LC2 and lobar bronchi, a large Y silicone stent was inserted within the LMB, so that its bronchial limbs extended into the LUL and LLL. The stent had a 16 mm diameter tracheal limb and 12 mm diameter bronchial limbs. The more vertical limb entered the LLL, and the more horizontal limb was shortened to less than 2 cm so that it would enter the LUL (see Figure 24-1). Silicone Y stents are usually deployed into the trachea and LMB and RMB using the "push" technique or the "pullback" technique. With the push technique, the stent is ejected from the bronchoscope above the carina and then is pushed down with an open rigid grasping forceps placed at stent bifurcation. With the pullback technique, both bronchial limbs are placed within one bronchus (usually the one most involved with disease) then are pulled back slowly until the shorter limb pops out. The stent can then be adjusted using forceps. In our patient, both bronchial limbs were simultaneously present at the entrance to the LUL bronchus. The stent was pulled proximally to deploy the vertical (right) limb into the relatively straight LLL bronchus. The tracheal limb of the Y stent was now in the LMB (see video on ExpertConsult.com) (Video V.24.2). No perioperative complications were noted; the patient was extubated, recovered, and was discharged home the next day.

Long-Term Management

Outcome Assessment

Final cytology confirmed squamous cell carcinoma of the lung. Diagnosis and relief of airway obstruction had been achieved simultaneously; dyspnea improved and hemoptysis ceased. The patient became able to care for himself but was unable to carry on normal activities or to actively work, consistent with KPS 70 and ECOG 2.

Referral

The optimal treatment for stage IIIB NSCLC depends on several variables, including extent of disease, patient age, comorbidities, performance scores, and weight loss.[31] Because of this, a thorough evaluation is warranted before patients are committed to potentially toxic treatments. After discussion in our multidisciplinary chest conference, given his lack of weight loss and improved performance status, concurrent chemoradiotherapy therapy was offered.

Follow-up Tests and Procedures

Complete staging included a whole body positron emission tomography (PET)/CT scan and brain magnetic resonance imaging (MRI) showing no extrathoracic disease. He was started on concurrent chemoradiotherapy. Follow-up bronchoscopies at 4 and 6 months post stent insertion revealed patent airways and no evidence of stent migration or obstruction by mucus or granulation. Stent insertion does not have to be permanent. In one report, airway stents were removed in 50% of patients with malignant CAO after a median of 31.7 days after successful systemic therapy.[38] In cases where systemic therapy is unsuccessful, stent insertion maintains airway patency, relieves dyspnea, and improves quality of life.

Quality Improvement

We discussed whether our patient should undergo routine surveillance flexible bronchoscopy to identify stent-related complications or progression of tumor. Although evidence against this practice has been found,[39] because of the particular location of this stent at LC2 and its unknown long-term consequences, we chose to perform surveillance bronchoscopy every 3 months and as needed on the basis of symptoms. In general, the risk of stent migration is rare, with an estimated incidence of 1% to 5%,[12] and such migration may be even less common with Y stents. Impairment in mucociliary clearance may promote retained secretions and stent obstruction in about a third of cases. No published experience has described the use of Y stents for LMB/LUL/LLL obstruction.

In general, flexible bronchoscopies are reportedly necessary to remove secretions in up to 40% of patients with indwelling stents.[14] Additional rigid bronchoscopic procedures, however, are seldom required in patients with malignant CAO, in part because of limited survival.[12] We recognized the risk of stent revision in this patient because of his increased risk for fistula, in part secondary to tumor involvement, but also related to radiation therapy.

DISCUSSION POINTS

1. Describe two techniques used to deploy a Y stent.
   - *The "push" technique:* The stent is ejected from the bronchoscope above the carina and then is pushed down with an open rigid grasping forceps placed at stent bifurcation.
   - *The "pullback" technique:* Both bronchial limbs are placed within one bronchus (usually the one most involved with disease), then the stent is pulled back slowly until the shorter limb pops out.
2. Describe the indications for stent insertion before initiation of systemic therapy in this particular patient.
   - Ability to initiate systemic therapy that will be better tolerated
   - Improvement in exercise capacity and dyspnea
   - Prevention of post obstructive pneumonia and loss of lung function
3. List three potential complications resulting from stent insertion at the left secondary carina.
   - Perforation of the medial wall of the LMB, resulting in bronchomediastinal fistula and possible mediastinal misplacement of the stent
   - Perforation of the posterior membrane, which may cause laceration of the descending aorta and fatal hemorrhage
   - Hypoventilation or hypoxemia caused when the stent does not unfold satisfactorily

Expert Commentary

provided by James R. Jett, MD

This 75-year-old male had moderate COPD but was severely debilitated, with an ECOG performance score of 3 due to a stage IIIB non–small cell lung cancer in the left infrahilar area with complete obstruction of the distal left main bronchus. He also had left vocal cord paralysis. CT scan noted lymph node metastases in stations 4 L (left lower paratracheal) and 7 (subcarinal). If we assume that the vocal cord paralysis is due to direct extension of the primary cancer, then the lesion would be T4, and the clinical stage would be T4N2M0 (assuming no distinct metastases) or stage IIIB. If vocal cord paralysis was due to N2 lymph node metastases, the clinical stage would be T3N2M0, stage IIIA.[6] With IIIA or IIIB, the patient is inoperable owing to poor performance status, borderline pulmonary function, and multiple-station mediastinal nodal involvement.

The severity of the patient's illness and deterioration in performance status necessitated immediate treatment with the potential for rapid response. In my opinion, endobronchial treatment with the Nd:YAG laser, debulking, and stent placement were appropriate and successful, with immediate improvement in ECOG performance status to 2. Further staging with MRI of the brain and PET scan demonstrated no distinct metastases.

We are told that the initial biopsy (EBNA) was called non–small cell lung cancer (NSCLC). Although this was adequate to proceed with endobronchial treatment, it is not adequate for optimal decision making regarding chemotherapy. Sufficient tissue is needed to determine whether the NSCLC is squamous cell, adenocarcinoma, or large cell because histology dictates optimal chemotherapy choices.[40]

One of the most exciting advances in lung cancer in the past few years has been the identification of sensitizing mutations, or so-called driver mutations. These have been most commonly identified in adenocarcinoma.[41] Currently, the most important mutations to be elucidated are the tyrosine kinase domain of epidermal growth factor receptor (EGFR) and anaplastic lymphoma kinase (ALK).

Sensitizing mutations in EGFR (exon 19 deletion or exon 21 transition) and ALK are associated with an excellent clinical response to therapy with specific tyrosine kinase inhibitors and improvement in overall survival compared with standard chemotherapy.[42,43] Accordingly, it is now the responsibility of the bronchoscopist to obtain adequate tissue samples for both histologic diagnosis and molecular testing. A simple aspiration cytology demonstrating NSCLC is inadequate and unacceptable as of this writing. Obtaining appropriate tissue specimens at the time of bronchoscopy is the responsibility of the bronchoscopist and provides an opportunity to make a significant contribution to the multidisciplinary management of the patient with lung cancer.

The large majority of centrally located NSCLC is of squamous cell histology and seldom contains the sensitizing mutations previously mentioned. However, mutations and gene amplifications are being identified and are likely to influence future treatment decisions. The usual treatment for unresectable stage IIIA and IIIB disease consists of concurrent chemotherapy and radiotherapy if the patient has a performance status of 0 or 1* and minimal weight loss (≤5%) over the previous 3 months.[31] This patient had a performance status of 2 after endobronchial treatment. In this situation, treatment would have to be decided on an individual basis. Endobronchial disease is best treated with concurrent therapy rather than with radiation or chemotherapy alone or sequentially. However, concurrent therapy is more toxic than sequential therapy, especially in terms of esophageal toxicity. External beam radiotherapy is considered the standard method of irradiation rather than endobronchial brachytherapy (EBB), especially when combined with chemotherapy. In this patient with N2 disease in stations 4R and 7, EBB would not be appropriate for treating the nodal disease. Recent trials with concurrent chemoradiotherapy for definitive treatment of stage IIIA/B disease have reported a median survival time of 20 to 24 months, 2 year survival of 40% to 50%, and 5 year survival of approximately 20%.[44,45] The patient under discussion was deemed suitable for concurrent chemoradiotherapy.

In summary, from an oncologic perspective, I would emphasize the following three points: (1) Optimal treatment for NSCLC is based on precise histologic classification—efforts should therefore be made to avoid labeling disease as NSCLC-NOS (not otherwise specified); (2) sufficient tissue should be obtained at the time of bronchoscopy to provide histologic typing and molecular testing for a variety of potential molecular sensitizing mutations (e.g., EGFR, ALK) because these findings may affect treatment choices and prognosis; and (3) optimal treatment for unresectable stage IIIA/B NSCLC of any cell type consists of concurrent chemoradiotherapy in patients with a good performance score and minimal weight loss.

REFERENCES

1. Schag CC, Heinrich RL, Ganz PA. Karnofsky performance status revisited: reliability, validity, and guidelines. *J Clin Oncol.* 1984;2: 187-193.
2. Oken MM, Creech RH, Tormey DC, et al. Toxicity and response criteria of the Eastern Cooperative Oncology Group. *Am J Clin Oncol.* 1982;5:649-655.
3. Buccheri G, Ferrigno D, Tamburini M. Karnofsky and ECOG performance status scoring in lung cancer: a prospective, longitudinal study of 536 patients from a single institution. *Eur J Cancer.* 1996; 32A:1135-1141.

---

*The ECOG score, also called the World Health Organization (WHO) or Zubrod score, runs from 0 to 5, with 0 denoting perfect health and 5 death; 0—asymptomatic (fully active, able to carry on all predisease activities without restriction), 1—symptomatic but completely ambulatory (restricted in physically strenuous activity but ambulatory and able to carry out work of a light or sedentary nature).

4. Sin DD, Man SF. Chronic obstructive pulmonary disease as a risk factor for cardiovascular morbidity and mortality. *Proc Am Thorac Soc.* 2005;2:8-11.

5. Havas T, Lowinger D, Priestley J. Unilateral vocal fold paralysis: causes, options and outcomes. *Aust N Z J Surg.* 1999;69:509-513.

6. Goldstraw P, Crowley J, Chanksy K, et al. The IASLC Lung Cancer Staging Project: proposals for the revision of the TNM stage groupings in the forthcoming (seventh) edition of the TNM classification of malignant tumours. *J Thorac Oncol.* 2007;2:706-714.

7. Podnos YD, Borneman TR, Koczywas M, et al. Symptom concerns and resource utilization in patients with lung cancer. *J Palliat Med.* 2007;10:899-903.

8. Duhamel F, Dupuis F. Guaranteed returns: investing in conversations with families of patients with cancer. *Clin J Oncol Nurs.* 2004;8:68-71.

9. Tariman JD, Berry DL, Cochrane B, et al. Preferred and actual participation roles during health care decision making in persons with cancer: a systematic review. *Ann Oncol.* 2010;21:1145-1151.

10. Trodella L, D'Angelillo RM, Ramella S, et al. Multimodality treatment in locally advanced non-small cell lung cancer. *Ann Oncol.* 2006;17:ii32-ii33.

11. Spira A, Ettinger DS. Multidisciplinary management of lung cancer. *N Engl J Med.* 2004;350:379-392.

12. Lemaire A, Burfeind WR, Toloza E, et al. Outcomes of tracheobronchial stents in patients with malignant airway disease. *Ann Thorac Surg.* 2005;80:434-438.

13. Chhajed PN, Baty F, Pless M, et al. Outcome of treated advanced non-small cell lung cancer with and without central airway obstruction. *Chest.* 2006;130:1803-1807.

14. Wood DE, Liu YH, Vallières E, et al. Airway stenting for malignant and benign tracheobronchial stenosis. *Ann Thorac Surg.* 2003;76:167-174.

15. Global Initiative for Chronic Obstructive Pulmonary Disease, Executive Summary: Global strategy for the diagnosis, management, and prevention of COPD, 2006. www.goldcopd.com. Accessed September 5, 2010.

16. Mazzone P, Jain P, Arroliga AC, et al. Bronchoscopy and needle biopsy techniques for diagnosis and staging of lung cancer. *Clin Chest Med.* 2002;23:137-158.

17. Cavaliere S, Venuta F, Foccoli P, et al. Endoscopic treatment of malignant airway obstructions in 2,008 patients. *Chest.* 1996;110:1536-1542.

18. Mitchell JD, Mathisen DJ, Wright CD, et al. Resection for bronchogenic carcinoma involving the carina: long-term results and effect of nodal status on outcome. *J Thorac Cardiovasc Surg.* 2001;121:465-471.

19. Dutau H, Toutblanc B, Lamb C, et al. Use of the Dumon Y-stent in the management of malignant disease involving the carina: a retrospective review of 86 patients. *Chest.* 2004;126:951-958.

20. Shiraishi T, Kawahara K, Shirakusa T, et al. Stenting for airway obstruction in the carinal region. *Ann Thorac Surg.* 1998;66:1925-1929.

21. Murgu SD, Colt HG. Complications of silicone stent insertion in patients with expiratory central airway collapse. *Ann Thorac Surg.* 2007;84:1870-1877.

22. Ernst A, Majid A, Feller-Kopman D, et al. Airway stabilization with silicone stents for treating adult tracheobronchomalacia: a prospective observational study. *Chest.* 2007;132:609-616.

23. Ernst A, Simoff M, Ost D, et al. Prospective risk-adjusted morbidity and mortality outcome analysis after therapeutic bronchoscopic procedures: results of a multi-institutional outcomes database. *Chest.* 2008;134:514-519.

24. Cardona AF, Reveiz L, Ospina EG, et al. Palliative endobronchial brachytherapy for non-small cell lung cancer. *Cochrane Database Syst Rev.* 2008;(2):CD004284.

25. Edell ES, Cortese DA. Photodynamic therapy: its use in the management of bronchogenic carcinoma. *Clin Chest Med.* 1995;16:455-463.

26. Moghissi K, Dixon K, Stringer M, et al. The place of bronchoscopic photodynamic therapy in advanced unresectable lung cancer: experience of 100 cases. *Eur J Cardiothorac Surg.* 1999;15:1-6.

27. Vergnon JM, Schmitt T, Alamartine E, et al. Initial combined cryotherapy and irradiation for unresectable non-small cell lung cancer: preliminary results. *Chest.* 1992;102:1436-1440.

28. Kono M, Yahagi N, Kitahara M, et al. Cardiac arrest associated with use of an argon beam coagulator during laparoscopic cholecystectomy. *Br J Anaesth.* 2001;87:644-646.

29. Reddy C, Majid A, Michaud G, et al. Gas embolism following bronchoscopic argon plasma coagulation: a case series. *Chest.* 2008;134:1066-1069.

30. Saad CP, Murthy S, Krizmanich G, et al. Self expandable metallic airway stents and flexible bronchoscopy: long-term outcomes analysis. *Chest.* 2003;124:1993-1999.

31. Jett JR, Schild SE, Keith RL, et al; American College of Chest Physicians. Treatment of non-small cell lung cancer, stage IIIB: ACCP evidence-based clinical practice guidelines (2nd edition). *Chest.* 2007;132:266S-276S.

32. Slawson RG, Scott RM. Radiation therapy in bronchogenic carcinoma. *Radiology.* 1979;132:175-176.

33. Eichenhorn MS, Kvale PA, Miks VM, et al. Initial combination therapy with YAG laser photoresection and irradiation for inoperable non-small cell carcinoma of the lung. *Chest.* 1986;89:782.

34. Santos RS, Raftopoulos Y, Keenan RJ, et al. Bronchoscopic palliation of primary lung cancer: single or multimodality therapy? *Surg Endosc.* 2004;18:931-936.

35. McMahon CC, Rainey L, Fulton B, et al. Central airway compression: anaesthetic and intensive care consequences. *Anaesthesia.* 1997;52:158-162.

36. Pullerits J, Holzman R. Anaesthesia for patients with mediastinal masses. *Can J Anaesth.* 1989;36:681-688.

37. Perrin G, Colt HG, Martin C, et al. Safety of interventional rigid bronchoscopy using intravenous anesthesia and spontaneous assisted ventilation: a prospective study. *Chest.* 1992;102:1526-1530.

38. Witt C, Dinges S, Schmidt B, et al. Temporary tracheobronchial stenting in malignant stenoses. *Eur J Cancer.* 1997;33:204-208.

39. Matsuo T, Colt HG. Evidence against routine scheduling of surveillance bronchoscopy after stent insertion. *Chest.* 2000;118:1455-1459.

40. Scagliotti GV, Parikh P, von Pawel J, et al. Phase III study comparing cisplatin plus gemcitabine with cisplatin plus pemetrexed in chemotherapy-naïve patients with advanced non-small-cell lung cancer. *J Clin Oncol.* 2008;26:3543-3551.

41. Travis WD, Brambilla E, Noguchi M, et al. International Association for the Study of Lung Cancer/American Thoracic Society/European Respiratory Society International multidisciplinary classification of adenocarcinoma. *J Thorac Oncol.* 2011;6:244-285.

42. Mok T, Wu YL, Throngprasert S, et al. Gefitinib or carboplatin—paclitaxel in pulmonary adenocarcinoma. *N Engl J Med.* 2009;361:947-957.

43. Kwak EL, Bang YJ, Camidge DR, et al. Anaplastic lymphoma kinase in non-small-cell lung cancer. *N Engl J Med.* 2010;363:1693-1703.

44. Hanna N, Neubauer M, Yiannoutsos C, et al. Phase III study of cisplatin, etoposide and concurrent chest radiation with or without consolidation docetaxel in patients with inoperable stage III non-small-cell lung cancer: the Hoosier Oncology Group and US Oncology. *J Clin Oncol.* 2008;26:5755-5760.

45. Albain KS, Swann RS, Rusch V, et al. Radiotherapy plus chemotherapy with or without surgical resection for stage III non-small-cell lung cancer: a phase III randomized controlled trial. *Lancet.* 2009;374:379-386.

SECTION 6

Practical Approach to Other Central Airway Disease Processes

Chapter 25

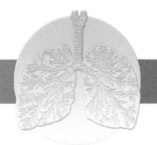

Rigid Bronchoscopy for Removal of a Foreign Body Lodged in the Right Lower Lobe Bronchus

This chapter emphasizes the following elements of the Four Box Approach: physical examination, complementary tests, and functional status assessment; indications, contraindications, and expected results; respect for persons (informed consent); techniques and instrumentation; and results and procedure-related complications.

CASE DESCRIPTION

A 14-year-old male with a past medical history of asthma developed acute cough and wheezing immediately following an episode of intense laughter. Actually, he was holding a thumbtack between his teeth when his brother made a funny comment. Bursting into laughter, he suddenly aspirated the thumbtack. He did not tell his parents. Several days later, his intractable cough prompted his parents to bring him to the hospital, where he told physicians about the accident. Flexible bronchoscopy revealed the foreign object in the distal left main bronchus, but despite multiple attempts, it could not be removed and was inadvertently dropped over and into the right bronchial tree. He was transferred to our facility a few days later. His vital signs showed a BP of 150/85, HR of 110, RR of 22, temperature of 100.5° F, and O_2 sat of 94% on room air. On examination, he had no wheezing, but air entry at the right base was diminished. The child was a nonsmoker and had no significant family history. His asthma was well controlled on inhaled fluticasone 110 mcg twice a day, with which he was usually noncompliant. Laboratory data were normal, except for a WBC of 18,000. Chest radiograph showed a radiopaque object projecting over the right lower lung field (Figure 25-1). During rigid bronchoscopy, a thumbtack surrounded by inflamed mucosa and granulation tissue was found and was causing complete obstruction of the right lower lobe bronchus (see Figure 25-1).

DISCUSSION POINTS

1. List five accessory instruments that can be used to remove a foreign body from the airway.
2. List three complications that might occur during attempts to remove a sharp or pointed object from a lower lobe bronchus.
3. Describe the advantages and disadvantages of flexible bronchoscopy and rigid bronchoscopy for removing aspirated foreign bodies.

CASE RESOLUTION

Initial Evaluations

Physical Examination, Complementary Tests, and Functional Status Assessment

This patient's presentation was classic for foreign body aspiration (FBA), defined as the inhalation of an organic or inorganic foreign object into the larynx and respiratory tract.[1] The object was in the right lower lobe, but when a foreign body is in the trachea, patients may have a brassy cough, with or without loss of voice, and bidirectional (during inspiration and expiration) stridor. Complete airway obstruction and asphyxia can develop when a large object is lodged in the trachea or larynx.[2] Cyanosis, stridor, and altered level of consciousness are ominous signs and predict impending respiratory arrest.

Most patients with FBA present after an acute episode of choking followed by intractable cough (aka choking crisis). The sensitivity of this syndrome for the diagnosis of FBA varies from 13% to 88% because symptoms of FBA depend on the size, shape, and nature of the object, the age of the patient, and the duration, degree, and location of the obstruction. Children, in particular, may present with a history of choking while eating or playing or may have cough and wheezing that do not improve despite medical treatment for asthma or bronchitis. Very young and very old patients might not be able to provide a history for FBA, and certainly nonspecific symptoms such as cough, wheeze, and shortness of breath may be caused by coexisting illnesses such as asthma, pneumonia, chronic obstructive pulmonary disease (COPD), or congestive heart failure. In children, in elderly patients, and in individuals with impaired neurologic function, swallowing disorders, vocal cord dysfunction, or psychiatric histories, a high index of suspicion for FBA should be maintained and confirmatory studies performed promptly.

As in this case, signs predictive of bronchial FBA include radiopaque objects seen on chest x-ray (CXR), a history of FBA associated with unilaterally decreased breath sounds, localized wheezing, focal hyperinflation, and atelectasis (this is usually a later finding, which occurs after air has been resorbed). Prompt diagnosis is essential, especially in children, because results from studies show that complication rates are twofold higher in patients who receive medical attention 2 or more days after the aspiration, compared with patients cared

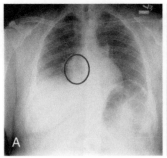 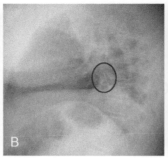 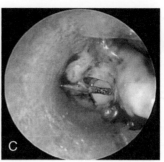

Figure 25-1 A and **B**, Chest radiographs (posteroanterior [PA] and lateral views) show the radiopaque object projecting over the right lower lobe lung field. **C**, During rigid bronchoscopy, a thumbtack is seen. It completely occludes the right lower lobe bronchus, and the surrounding mucosa is inflamed and friable.

for sooner.[3] Physical examination in patients with bronchial FBA may reveal unilateral wheezing, which suggests partial airway obstruction distal to the carina.[4,5] By the time our patient came to our institution, wheezing had ceased, probably complete obstruction had developed, and there was no longer any airflow to the right lower lobe (RLL) bronchus.

Chest radiograph is a commonly performed imaging modality for suspected FBA in a stable patient. Standard frontal and lateral views can help locate the object (see Figure 25-1).[4] Lateral soft tissue views of the neck are performed if upper airway involvement is suspected clinically. If the patient is critical and suspicion for FBA is high based on the history and physical examination, CXR is not absolutely necessary, and airway management should take priority. Characteristic findings on CXR depend on the density of the aspirated object and on the duration of symptoms. Radiopaque materials such as coins, thumbtacks, metallic nails, toys, bones, teeth, and dental appliances usually can be detected on radiographs. Radiopaque foreign bodies, however, are seen in only 2% to 19% of patients with FBA because most aspirated objects are radiolucent. Furthermore, radiopaque material seen on x-ray may actually represent calcifications of mucoid impaction or a broncholith, and thus could be a false-positive finding. In fact, the sensitivity of CXR performed in the emergency department for FBA is reportedly only 22.6%. False-negative rates vary between 5% and 30% in children and between 8% and 80% in adults, probably because of differences in physical properties of aspirated materials. For example, organic materials such as meat and vegetables are difficult to visualize because they are not radiopaque.[6,7] When the aspirated material is radiolucent and is not identified on chest x-ray, nonspecific CXR findings that suggest FBA include atelectasis, pneumonia, air trapping, and pneumomediastinum. Air trapping is an early radiographic finding that results from obstruction of the airway by the foreign body, which acts as a ball valve, allowing air to enter the bronchus but not to exit during expiration. Expiratory and inspiratory chest x-rays, when feasible, may help detect any air trapping.[8] In children with aspirated foreign bodies, the absence of air trapping was found to have a negative predictive value of 70%.[9] However, because overall sensitivity is low, a normal CXR, does not preclude additional diagnostic studies such as chest computed tomography (CT), which can detect foreign bodies not visualized on CXR in up to 80% of cases.[10] This

modality is particularly useful in patients with chronic respiratory symptoms or with recurrent pneumonia. False-negative CT scans, especially with 10 mm slice thickness, may occur because CT can miss small objects, and because image quality is compromised by motion artifacts in patients with severe dyspnea.[4] CT findings include visualizing the foreign body in the airway lumen and observing indirect findings such as atelectasis, hyperlucency, bronchiectasis, lobar consolidation, tree-in-bud opacities, ipsilateral pleural effusion, ipsilateral lymphadenopathy, and thickening of the bronchial wall adjacent to the foreign body.

In children, low-dose multidetector CT (MDCT) scanning and virtual bronchoscopy (VB) (Figure 25-2) have a sensitivity of 92% to 100% and a specificity of 80% to 85%.[11,12] False-positives occur because of secretions and endobronchial tumors. Therefore MDCT and VB, if available and when feasible, can be used as noninvasive tools to confirm FBA and to determine the exact location of the obstruction before bronchoscopy. Some authors suggest that in the presence of a positive clinical diagnosis and a negative CXR, VB should be considered in all children with suspected FBA to avoid a potentially unwarranted rigid bronchoscopy.[12]

In stable adults, flexible bronchoscopy should be used to confirm suspected cases of FBA and to attempt removal of the foreign body.[4] This is also true for victims of cervicofacial trauma (Figure 25-3). Rigid bronchoscopy usually is not indicated in these patients because of neck immobilization. In addition to allowing removal of the FB, bronchoscopy determines the exact nature of the foreign body, its location and degree of airway obstruction, and associated mucosal abnormalities such as surrounding mucosal edema and granulation tissue (see Figure 25-3). In patients presenting with acute asphyxia, flexible bronchoscopy or rigid bronchoscopy can be performed, depending on availability. In stable children with suspected FBA, flexible bronchoscopy has been shown to safely confirm the diagnosis and has been used to extract foreign objects[5]; it provides rapid and definitive diagnosis of FBA in approximately 12% of children who present with persistent wheezing (lasting longer than 6 weeks and not responding to bronchodilators and inhaled corticosteroids).[13] Controversy continues, however, because some authorities recommend rigid bronchoscopy in children younger than 12 years of age when there is a strong suspicion of FBA, arguing that rigid bronchoscopy permits better control and visualization of the pediatric airway.[14]

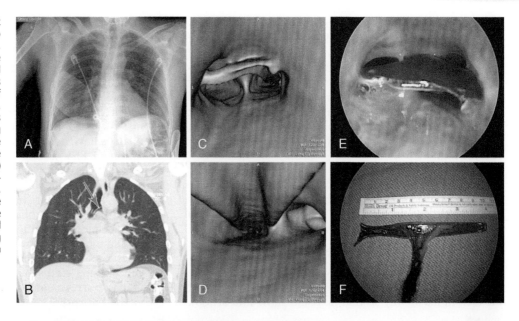

Figure 25-2 **A,** A portable chest radiograph from a patient who aspirated a piece of a plastic spoon. The radiograph appears to be normal. **B,** Coronal computed tomography (CT) image suggests that the proximal aspect of the object is above the carina. **C,** Virtual bronchoscopy confirms the location of the object, showing its proximal aspect against the airway wall. **D,** The handle of the object (a broken plastic spoon) extends into the bronchus intermedius and the right lower lobe. **E,** During rigid bronchoscopy, the object is seen in exactly the same location as is visualized by virtual bronchoscopy. **F,** The 10 cm long shaft of a broken plastic spoon after removal.

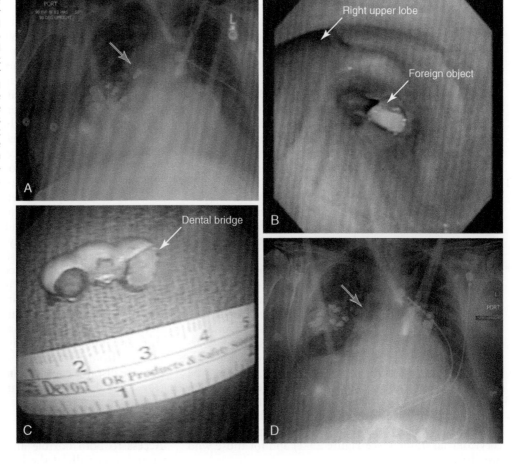

Figure 25-3 **A,** A radiopaque object is seen along with other opacities adjacent to several screws used to stabilize a halo brace in this patient with cervical spine injury; atelectasis is evident in the right middle and lower lobes. **B,** The object is seen during bronchoscopic inspection of the bronchus intermedius. **C,** The three-unit dental bridge was removed using a basket. **D,** Chest radiograph after the procedure confirms the absence of the foreign object and shows improved aeration to the middle and lower lobes.

Comorbidities

Our patient had controlled asthma on inhaled corticosteroids. Although acute asthma exacerbation was in the differential diagnosis, wheezing in asthma is usually paroxysmal, intermittent, and diffuse and improves after bronchodilators. Symptoms are triggered by exercise, cold, sleep, and allergens, and the CXR usually shows peribronchial cuffing and bilateral hyperinflation. The presence of these findings, however, would not rule out FBA.[15] Indeed, dyspnea alters the coordination between deglutition and respiration, increasing the risk for aspiration.[16]

Our patient had no evidence of dysphagia or impaired cough reflex.[4] These conditions are usually seen in the elderly, especially in cases of cerebrovascular or degenerative neurologic disease. More than one third of patients with acute stroke have radiologic evidence of aspiration.[17] Patients with dysphagia have delayed triggering of the pharyngeal motor response and decreased laryngeal elevation, resulting in poor coordination and timing of oral, pharyngeal, and laryngeal movement during swallowing.[18] Anticholinergics, antipsychotics, and anxiolytics also impair the cough reflex and/or swallowing.

Support System

The patient lived at home with his parents and was financially dependent on his father. His parents, as well as a group of friends and siblings, were very supportive.

Patient Preferences and Expectations

Initially, our patient was most concerned about his image among his peers. Later, however, he requested photos of the tack in his airway so that he could show it at school.

Procedural Strategies

Indications

Although some controversy continues, most clinicians agree that rigid bronchoscopy is indicated in patients with FBA associated with stridor or asphyxia, as well as in children with radiopaque objects seen on CXR (because the diagnosis is obvious), a history of FBA associated with localized wheezing, obstructive hyperinflation, atelectasis, or unilaterally decreased breath sounds suggesting mainstem bronchial obstruction. Large, round, or smooth foreign bodies probably are best approached with the rigid bronchoscope (see video on ExpertConsult. com) (Video VI.25.1).

In other cases, flexible bronchoscopy should be performed to confirm the diagnosis and attempt removal. Although this procedure is safe, effective, and cost-effective, dislodgment and unsuccessful retrieval of the object are possible.[14] Potential complications of attempting to remove large foreign bodies with a fiberoptic bronchoscope include displacement or impaction of the foreign body in a lobar or mainstem bronchus, shearing off of the foreign body in the narrow subglottic area, and acute asphyxia from subglottic or laryngeal obstruction.[19] If flexible bronchoscopy fails, rigid bronchoscopy is warranted.[9] Advantages of rigid bronchoscopy include the ability to function as an endotracheal tube, securing the airway and providing a conduit through which the foreign body can be removed using a variety of larger instruments. As mentioned earlier, however, flexible bronchoscopy remains the method of choice for patients with cervicofacial trauma (see Figure 25-1) and for those who are already intubated.[4]

Contraindications

This patient's asthma was not a contraindication to bronchoscopy, but optimal control before the intervention is warranted; studies have shown that even patients with mild asthma have a more pronounced post bronchoscopy decrease in forced expiratory volume in 1 second (FEV_1) compared with normal subjects.

Reductions in FEV_1 and forced vital capacity (FVC) are especially greater after bronchioloalveolar lavage and biopsies.[20] Bronchoscopy is safe in asymptomatic asthmatic patients with FEV_1 >60% predicted.[21] Premedication with bronchodilators was associated with no fall in post procedure FEV_1.[22] This is different from COPD, in which premedication with an inhaled short-acting agonist is not routinely recommended (in COPD, bronchodilators have not been shown to affect post procedure reduction in FEV_1).[23]

If patients have active diffuse wheezing, premedication with nebulized bronchodilators is warranted, and in elective cases, the procedure might have to be postponed until bronchospasm is controlled. One large study found that bronchoscopic interventions in asthmatic patients were associated with significantly higher rates of procedure- or anesthesia-related complications such as laryngospasm or bronchospasm, status asthmaticus, severe hypoxemia, and cardiac arrest, compared with interventions in non-asthmatic patients.[24]

Expected Results

Both flexible and rigid bronchoscopy can be performed for removal of foreign bodies, but overall, flexible bronchoscopy seems to be an efficient initial method in both children and adults, with a success rate greater than 90%.[5,25] Repeated bronchoscopic examination may be necessary to remove a foreign body completely in 1% to 3% of patients, especially if the foreign body is a peanut or another material that breaks easily.[9,14] When flexible bronchoscopy fails, rigid bronchoscopy should be performed,[9] as was done in this case. Open surgical interventions are very rarely necessary and are reserved for repeatedly unsuccessful bronchoscopic interventions.

Complications of FBA are usually prevented by prompt removal of the object. A retained object can lead to prolonged atelectasis and lung destruction, occasionally requiring thoracotomy and resection. Early complications of FBA include asphyxia, cardiac arrest, laryngeal edema, and pneumomediastinum. Organic objects, especially those with high oil content such as peanuts, may cause significant mucosal inflammation and bulky granulation tissue growth within a few hours, eventually causing complete bronchial obstruction. Late complications include bronchiectasis, hemoptysis, bronchial stricture, and inflammatory polyps. Objects can change sides, moving from left to right or from right to left, or can migrate distally, causing complete obstruction and atelectasis.[14] Table 25-1 summarizes potential complications associated with FBA.

Team Experience

Access to both flexible and rigid bronchoscopy is warranted, especially if the bronchoscopist is inexperienced or unskilled in flexible foreign body retrieval. Consultation with a rigid bronchoscopist, who may be a pulmonologist, a thoracic surgeon, or an otorhinolaryngologist, can help in developing a management strategy. Care should always be taken to avoid inadvertently pushing foreign objects more distally into the airway because this will make subsequent retrieval more difficult. Communication among team members is essential. For example,

Table 25-1 Potential Complications Due to Foreign Body Aspiration and Its Bronchoscopic Removal

Complication	Comments
Asphyxia	Aspiration of a foreign body is the fifth most common cause of mortality from unintentional injury in the United States, and it is the leading cause of mortality from unintentional injury in children younger than 1 year.
Pneumonia	Seen in 20% of patients who present days or weeks after FBA.[7] The incidence may be higher with delayed presentation.
Atelectasis	Complete obstruction from the foreign body or associated secretions and granulation tissue can cause atelectasis, seen in approximately 20% of patients on CXR and in approximately 60% on chest CT scan.[4]
Bronchiectasis	On chest CT, this is a late complication that can be seen in about 30% of patients with FBA; occasionally, severe and recurrent infections may require thoracotomy and pulmonary resection.
Pneumomediastinum	A rare acute finding on CXR in approximately 3% of patients with FBA.[7]
Subglottic edema related to rigid bronchoscopy	Between 2% and 4% of patients requiring rigid bronchoscopy for foreign body extraction develop laryngeal edema that requires brief intubation and admission to intensive care.[9]
Bronchoscopy-related bronchospasm	More than 4% of children who require rigid bronchoscopy for foreign body extraction develop bronchospasm.[9]
Bronchial stricture	Aspiration of iron or potassium-chloride pills can cause airway inflammation, resulting in fibrosis and bronchial strictures.

CT, Computed tomography; CXR, chest x-ray; FBA, foreign body aspiration.

several different foreign body removal accessory instruments should be available, and one should not assume that simple grasping forceps will suffice. If procedures are being performed with the patient under general anesthesia, it may be necessary to cease ventilation to avoid blowing the object away from the grasping instrument. Wedging the foreign object into the rigid bronchoscope or endotracheal tube before removal may be necessary to avoid laryngeal or airway wall injury; sometimes, it is preferable to remove the tube and foreign body en bloc, rather than attempt to remove the foreign body alone. At other times, if the bronchoscopist is taking too long to grasp the object in a distal airway and ventilation is inadequate, a momentary retreat to the mid-trachea is warranted, so the anesthesiologist can ventilate the lungs adequately.[26] If a forceps and a bronchoscope are removed en bloc, along with the foreign body, the bronchoscopist should ask the anesthesiologist to deepen the level of anesthesia to avoid bucking or coughing, which may result in dropping of the foreign body back into the airway or inadvertent traumatizing of a closing glottis. Care must also be taken to avoid losing the foreign body in the oral pharynx once the vocal cords have been passed.

The foreign object should always be kept in view and grasped firmly. One should be ready to remove the object from the oral cavity using one's fingers, a Magill forceps, a rigid laryngoscope, or the rigid bronchoscope. It may be necessary to pull the tongue outward (using a gauze to hold the tip of the tongue firmly between one's index finger and thumb) to create more space in the oropharynx. A retrieval strategy should be shared with the team. For example, we have seen (1) foreign bodies removed by flexible bronchoscopy performed through the nares; once the foreign body is grasped, it is discovered that it is too large to be removed through the nares and thus must be dropped into the oral cavity and extracted, spit out, or accidentally swallowed; (2) foreign bodies grasped with forceps, only to be wedged within the subglottis, causing acute asphyxia; (3) sharp objects stabbing the inferior aspect of the glottis because the object is removed tangentially to the airway in an unprotected fashion; and (4) flexible bronchoscopes being broken because the foreign body is released into the oropharynx. During retrieval, the bite block was loosened and retracted proximally, which exposed the scope to a patient's teeth during a violent cough.

Therapeutic Alternatives for Foreign Body Removal

Other than rigid bronchoscopy, two methods may be used to retrieve foreign objects with specific indications, advantages, and disadvantages that should be discussed with patients and their families.

1. Flexible bronchoscopy is the method of choice in a patient with cervicofacial trauma because rigid bronchoscopy would be impossible in such a patient, and the only alternative is open thoracotomy. Flexible bronchoscopy is also a reasonable first therapeutic choice in a patient with a foreign body lodged in the distal airways.[4] Because patient cooperation facilitates foreign body retrieval by flexible bronchoscopy, this method may not be ideal in very young children.

2. Surgery is indicated if repeated flexible *and* rigid bronchoscopic attempts fail. Thoracotomy with pulmonary resection is usually reserved for cases of a destroyed pulmonary segment or lobe, or damage to the entire lung.[27]

Cost-Effectiveness

Rigid bronchoscopy is commonly performed even as a diagnostic approach in children.[9,28] However, in cases of suspected but not confirmed FBA, the high rate of negative initial rigid bronchoscopies (11% to 46%) may not justify this approach. The American Thoracic Society considers flexible bronchoscopy a cost-effective alternative in cases of equivocal airway foreign body, avoiding unnecessary rigid bronchoscopy and general anesthesia.[29] In children with confirmed radiopaque foreign bodies in the presence of associated unilateral decreased breath sounds and atelectasis, rigid bronchoscopy is often recommended.[9] It is reasonable from a cost-effectiveness and a patient comfort/safety perspective to proceed with an attempt at rigid bronchoscopic extraction before considering open thoracotomy.

Informed Consent

This 14-year-old patient had a clear understanding of the risks, benefits, and alternatives to treatment. He was able to describe the procedure, its potential associated complications, and the consequences of not undergoing the procedure. We believed he had the decision-making capacity for health care. Regarding treatment of minors, the recurrent question is whether they should give informed consent, or if this should be provided by parents or legal guardians, who may be seen as more capable of making a knowledgeable decision on a subject as important as a medical intervention. In our society, a trend beyond setting an arbitrary "age of consent" has been noted, with many preferring instead a movement that entertains respect for each individual child's reflective abilities, in part because a child's overall life experience is usually more relevant than age with regard to ascertaining a child's capacity for decision making. The statutory age of consent to treatment varies considerably between countries from 12 to 19 years, illustrating the arbitrary nature of these criteria.[30]

In our case, both the patient and his family were provided with a verbal description and justification for our management strategy. Written informed consent was obtained from the parents (patient's father had actually signed the form). To our knowledge, although no state or court in the United States has authorized minors younger than age 12 to make medical decisions for themselves, after the minor becomes a teenager, states begin to digress in terms of decision-making responsibilities.[31] In California, "a minor may consent to the minor's medical care if *all* of the following conditions are satisfied: (1) The minor is 15 years of age or older; (2) the minor is living separate and apart from the minor's parents or guardian, whether with or without the consent of a parent or guardian, and regardless of the duration of the separate residence; and (3) the minor is managing his or her own financial affairs, regardless of the source of the minor's income."[32]

In California, an emancipated minor* may consent to medical, dental, and psychiatric care.[33] This is a relatively new legal concept. The "mature minor" doctrine allows minors to give consent to medical procedures if they can show that they are mature enough to make a decision on their own. The mature minor doctrine takes into account the age, the situation, and proof of conduct of the minor in determining maturity. Usually, the doctrine has been applied in cases where minors are 16 years of age or older, where they show understanding of the medical procedure in question, and where the procedure is not considered "serious."†

---

*A person younger than 18 years is an emancipated minor if any of the following conditions is satisfied: (1) The person has entered into a valid marriage, whether or not the marriage has been dissolved; (2) the person is on active duty with the Armed Forces of the United States; or (3) the person has received a declaration of emancipation from the court. (Cal. Family Code §7002) (National Center for Youth Law; www.youthlaw.org; revised January 2003).

†Outside of reproductive rights, the U.S. Supreme Court has never ruled on applicability to medical procedures (http://www.enotes.com/everyday-law-encyclopedia/treatment-minors).

Techniques and Results

Anesthesia and Perioperative Care

Before the procedure is begun, administration of corticosteroids and antibiotics may lead to better outcomes in children with FBA, and 1 to 2 mg/kg prednisolone for 12 to 24 hours may be useful in reducing inflammation and facilitating FB extraction.[34] During this period, spontaneous dislodgment of the FB is possible. The FB may be expectorated or swallowed, or it may migrate to a different airway, causing further mucosal injury. Prophylactic use of corticosteroids to reduce the incidence of subglottic edema probably is not warranted. If evidence reveals post procedure laryngeal edema, steroids (dexamethasone, 0.5 to 1 mg/kg to a maximum dose of 20 mg), aerosolized epinephrine (0.5 mL of 2.25% solution diluted 1:6), or inhalation of a helium-oxygen mixture should be considered. The length of stay in the hospital after surgery depends on the patient's general condition and need for continuing antibiotics or other medications.

If the patient develops bronchospasm during the perioperative period, bronchodilators should be administered promptly, especially in patients with a previous diagnosis of asthma. Given our patient's history, we administered nebulized albuterol 2.5 mg with ipratropium 0.5 mg before beginning the procedure. If bronchospasm develops during the procedure, these medications can be delivered via metered dose inhaler (MDI) or may be directly instilled into the airway.

Ideally, patients should fast from solids for 4 to 6 hours and from clear liquids for 2 hours to prevent aspiration of gastric contents during the perioperative period. In cases of aspiration of gastric contents, which can occur spontaneously, can result from violent coughing or stress-related vomiting, or can be anesthesia related, the operating table should be immediately tilted to a 30 degree head-down position, thus positioning the larynx at a higher level than the pharynx. This allows gastric contents to drain externally. Once the mouth and the pharynx are suctioned, the airway is secured by endotracheal intubation if necessary. Endotracheal suctioning before initiation of positive-pressure ventilation is essential to avoid forcing aspirated material deeper into the lungs.[4,35] Bronchoscopy may be useful if performed promptly to suction the aspirated fluid still present in the central airways or to remove any solid material.[36] A nasogastric tube should be inserted to empty the stomach once the airway is secured. Positive-pressure ventilation with positive end-expiratory pressure (PEEP) can be applied to prevent atelectasis and improve the ventilation-to-perfusion ratio.[35] Antibiotics might be necessary in cases of confirmed or suspected infection.

The actual anesthetic management of bronchoscopic FB removal can be challenging.[2] During induction for rigid bronchoscopy, spontaneous ventilation can be maintained until it is evident that the patient can be ventilated under anesthesia.[28] Spontaneous-assisted ventilation is favored by some anesthesiologists because it allows continuous ventilation during removal of the foreign body. However, foreign bodies may migrate distally during a patient's deep, spontaneous inspiration. On the other hand, positive-pressure ventilation can

Figure 25-4 **A,** Flexible electrocautery probe is used to remove granulation tissue formed proximal to the foreign object before its retrieval. **B,** A rigid electrocautery catheter is used to remove granulation tissue following removal of an aspirated plastic spoon. **C,** During rigid bronchoscopic removal, the shaft of the spoon remains wedged between the vocal cords. **D,** Magill forceps is used to remove the shaft of the spoon that is lodged in the larynx.

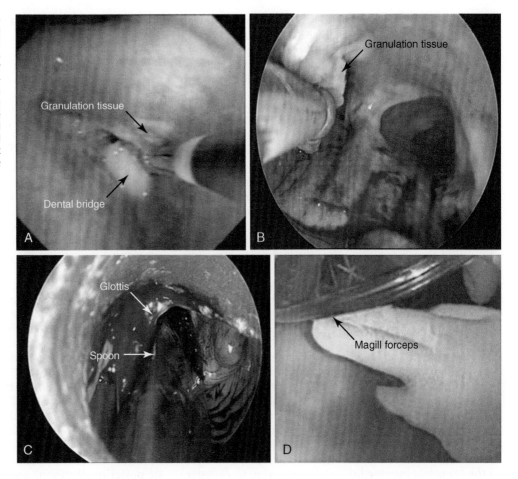

push the foreign object distally. Intubation or the use of positive-pressure ventilation combined with muscle relaxants allows for a still airway that facilitates retrieval of the foreign body. However, this technique may result in distal movements of the foreign body, which can make removal more difficult and may lead to ball-valve obstruction.[28] Overall, the reported outcomes of these two techniques are similar.[37] Jet ventilation-assisted anesthesia has been reported for removal of foreign bodies in adults but is not widely advocated in children, perhaps because clinicians have less experience in using this technique in children, or because jet ventilation is more likely to dislodge the foreign body and cause barotrauma.[38,39]

Technique and Instrumentation

Resuscitation equipment should be readily available in case clinical decompensation occurs as the result of accidental dislodgment of the FB and obstruction of the trachea or larynx. Instruments available for FB extraction include forceps, snares, baskets, suction catheters, Fogarty balloons, and cryotherapy probes. Fogarty balloons are useful for completely lodged objects. The Fogarty catheter can be passed distal to the foreign body. The balloon is inflated and is gently withdrawn until the object is brought up into a larger proximal airway, from which it can be removed with the use of other accessory instruments

(see video on ExpertConsult.com) (Video VI.25.2). A magnet accessory can be used for metal objects such as nails and pins. Cryotherapy is particularly useful for organic materials that contain water; furthermore, cryotherapy avoids maceration of very friable foreign objects. The object, the probe, and the scope are then removed en masse[40] (see video on ExpertConsult.com) (Video VI.25.3). Laser and endobronchial electrosurgery may be used to free an embedded foreign body from the airway wall or to remove associated granulation tissue (Figure 25-4). Sometimes it may be necessary to break the object before removal. This can occasionally be done using neodymium-doped yttrium aluminum garnet (Nd:YAG) laser, usually at high power density. For example, metal can be cut. In one case, we were unable to grasp a slippery olive pit; we used the laser to make several small incisions in the pit, which could then be used as a hold for grasping forceps.

We advise that if the nature of the object is known before intervention, the bronchoscopist can obtain an identical object and practice removal in vitro, thus determining the best instrument and technique to use during the actual procedure.[5] If the object is not small enough to fit through the rigid bronchoscope or an endotracheal tube, the object and the scope or endotracheal tube should be removed en bloc with the accessory instrument holding the object (see video on ExpertConsult.com)

(Video VI.25.2). If the foreign body is lost during retrieval, usually in the narrow subglottis space, the object should be pushed down into a mainstem bronchus to allow sufficient ventilation and oxygenation before retrieval is reattempted. If the object is large or is very long, and if it is lost in the larynx, it can be promptly removed with Magill forceps applied under direct laryngoscopy (see Figure 25-4).

Anatomic Dangers and Other Risks

Our patient met the criteria for sepsis given his vital signs and the presence of RLL infiltrate/atelectasis. Typically, anesthesiologists do not like to perform general anesthesia in patients with ongoing sepsis because of concerns for hemodynamic instability. In this case, treatment of the patient's acute post obstructive pneumonia included removal of the obstruction. Thus the intervention may in fact facilitate secretion clearance and recovery. Given the sharp nature of this object, the risk for possible airway perforation, resulting in bleeding, pneumothorax, or pneumomediastinum, was present.

Results and Procedure-Related Complications

After administration of general anesthesia, the patient was intubated with an 11 mm ventilating Efer-Dumon rigid bronchoscope (Bryan Corp., Woburn, Mass). Flexible bronchoscopy was performed through the rigid tube, revealing granulation tissue formation at the distal aspect of the left main bronchus, likely due to the previous presence of the FB in that location. The object was seen in the RLL bronchus. With the rigid bronchoscope wedged in the bronchus intermedius, we used suction to dislodge the object before removal. Because of the metallic and sharp nature of the object, we decided to customize our grasping forceps to avoid loss of the object during retrieval. Nasal cannula tubing was cut, and two short pieces were placed over the jaws of a grasping forceps. The forceps was then advanced carefully under direct visualization. Great care was necessary to avoid pushing the object downward. Both the forceps and the thumbtack were pulled up and were removed en bloc from the airway into the rigid tube (see video on ExpertConsult. com) (Video VI.25.4). Rather than remove the tack through the rigid tube, we preferred to extubate the patient, removing the forceps, the tack, and the tube en bloc. Once the object had been removed, the patient was reintubated with the rigid scope, and the airways were carefully re-examined. From the right side, granulation tissue and significant amounts of pus were removed, and washings were performed for microbiologic analysis. No bleeding was noted, but had it occurred, epinephrine (0.25 mg) was available to instill directly onto the airway as an initial step. Flexible bronchoscopy was repeated through the rigid scope and showed patent segmental airways in the RLL. Laser photocoagulation (Nd:YAG 30 Watts power, 1 second pulses) was performed to coagulate a polypoid granulation tissue structure obstructing 40% of the distal left main bronchus (LMB). This was subsequently removed with the use of rigid forceps (Figure 25-5). The patient was extubated and was transferred to the recovery area, where no bronchospasm, laryngospasm, or laryngeal edema was noted.

Long-Term Management

Outcome Assessment

The patient's cough improved post intervention. CXR showed improved aeration to the RLL, and the diaphragm was now visualized (see Figure 25-5). The patient was discharged home on antibiotics (amoxicillin/clavulanic acid 875 mg q 12 hr) for a total of 10 days post intervention.

Follow-up Tests and Procedures

No universally accepted monitoring protocol is available for patients with a history of FBA. Follow-up bronchoscopy may be warranted to document resolution of inflammatory changes after the foreign body has been removed, and to ascertain the absence of airway strictures. A bronchoscopy performed by the referring physician 1 month after our intervention showed normal airways.

Quality Improvement

We thought that it was appropriate to educate the patient and the family before the time of discharge about the risks of FBA. We informed them that the risk of FBA is usually higher in older people, especially during and after the seventh decade, probably because of a higher prevalence of aging-associated degenerative neurologic and cerebrovascular disorders that can cause dysphagia and/or impaired cough reflex.[4,19] We were aware of studies showing that more than 50% of patients with acute food asphyxiation* are between 71 and 90 years old.[41] Young children are at high risk as well because of poor chewing ability, a tendency to put objects in their mouths, and lack of posterior dentition, and because of vigorous inspirations when laughing or crying.[9] Risk is greater in children with developmental delay or swallowing difficulties and in males, for whom the risk is almost twice that noted in females.[9] This risk is probably a result of the more boisterous behavior of children.[9] In the elderly, increased risk is probably caused by higher rates of neurologic and cardiovascular disorders in men.[19] Alcohol or sedative use and head trauma are also leading causes of FBA in adults.[19] Decreased level of consciousness associated with trauma, use of sedatives or alcohol, general anesthesia, and neurologic disorders such as brain tumor, seizures, Parkinson's disease, and cerebrovascular accidents impairs airway protection mechanisms and increases aspiration risk.[4,19] Aspiration of dental debris, appliances, or prostheses can complicate facial trauma or dental procedures.[42] Elderly and neurologically impaired people should eat or be fed small meals of appropriate consistency at a slow pace to prevent choking or regurgitation. The importance of good oral hygiene is also emphasized. Nonrestorable teeth should probably be extracted.

Primary prevention of FBA is important. In the United States, strategies to prevent aspiration of toys and food-related choking among children include (1) efforts by the Consumer Product Safety Commission (CPSC) to ensure that toys sold in retail store bins, through vending

---

*The syndrome of fatal or near fatal food asphyxiation is also referred to as *café coronary*; for practical purposes, it is important to remember that the foreign material is in a supraglottic position in about one third of cases.

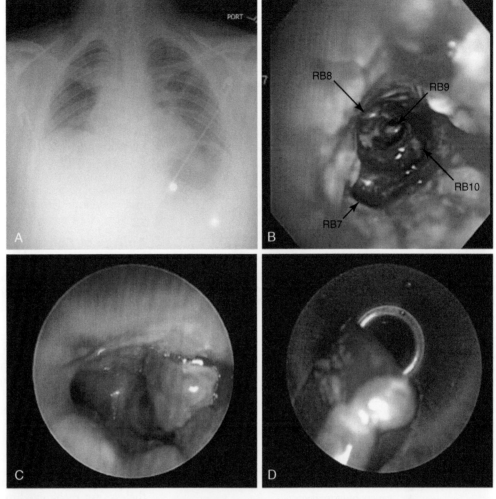

Figure 25-5 A, Chest radiograph after the procedure shows improved aeration to the right lower lobe and interval disappearance of the radiopaque object. **B,** Flexible bronchoscopy image of the now patent right lower lobe segments after removal of the thumbtack. **C,** Granulation tissue is noticed on the medial wall of the distal left main bronchus. **D,** After laser-assisted debulking, the granulation tissue is removed using a rigid suction catheter through the rigid bronchoscope.

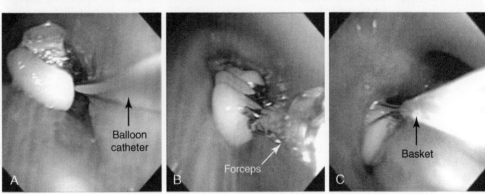

Figure 25-6 A, An angioplasty balloon is passed distal to the foreign object and is inflated, then pulled back into a more proximal airway (i.e., right mainstem bronchus). **B,** A grasping forceps is used to remove the object (a broken tooth), but its slippery nature led to its drop within the right mainstem bronchus. **C,** A basket is used, and the dental bridge, the basket, and the scope are removed en masse.

machines, and on the Internet have appropriate choking-hazard warnings, and (2) establishment by the U.S. Food and Drug Administration of surveillance, hazard evaluation, enforcement, and public education activities to prevent food-related choking among children.[43] More than 50% of cases of foreign body aspiration occur under the supervision of adults. This suggests that the number and the severity of injuries could be reduced by educating both parents and children.*[44]

DISCUSSION POINTS

1. List five accessory instruments that can be used to remove a foreign body from the airway.
   - Forceps, baskets, suction catheters, angioplasty balloons, and cryotherapy probes (Figure 25-6)
2. List three complications that might occur during attempts to remove a sharp or pointed object from a lower lobe bronchus.
   - Bleeding from mucosal trauma or airway perforation
   - Pneumomediastinum/pneumothorax from airway perforation and rupture of mediastinal pleura

---

*We had a patient who aspirated a coin while he was showing his 10-year-old son how easy it was to flip a coin into the air and catch it in his mouth. This "money-catcher" became the talk of his child's school.

Table 25-2 Advantages and Disadvantages of Flexible and Rigid Bronchoscopy for Foreign Body Removal

Technique	Advantages	Disadvantages
Flexible bronchoscopy	• Commonly available • Of choice in patients with cervicofacial trauma and in patients on mechanical ventilation • Of choice for diagnosis in stable patients with suspected but not confirmed FBA • Performed under moderate sedation	• Does not offer a secure airway • May not be tolerated in children because of their small airway and potential lack of cooperation • Limits the number of accessory instruments that can be used • May result in dislodgment but unsuccessful retrieval
Rigid bronchoscopy	• Offers a secure airway • Preferred in patients with stridor or asphyxia • May be the initial diagnostic and therapeutic test in children with radiopaque foreign body, or in the presence of associated unilateral decreased breath sounds, localized wheezing, hyperinflation, or atelectasis • Allows the use of a variety of instruments for foreign body extraction	• Limited availability • Contraindicated in patients with cervicofacial trauma • Requires general anesthesia and its associated risks • Small increased risk of laryngeal edema

FBA, Foreign body aspiration.

• Failure to extract the foreign body, resulting in post obstructive pneumonia, bronchiectasis, or the need for a thoracotomy

3. Describe the advantages and disadvantages of flexible bronchoscopy and rigid bronchoscopy for removing aspirated foreign bodies.
   • These are summarized in Table 25-2.

Expert Commentary

provided by Priscilla Alderson, BA, PhD

The preceding chapter provides a valuable example of the challenges that complex treatment poses for informed consent. These can be further complicated when the patient is a legal minor. The clinical knowledge and skills required for locating and retrieving an inhaled object need to be complemented by ethical knowledge and skill in attaining valid consent.

Definitions of Consent

Meanings of *consent* have developed through international codes on health care research,[45,46] which have been extended to apply also to health care treatment. Informed consent includes understanding the nature, duration, and purpose of the intervention, the methods, any risks and inconveniences, the likely effects, and the alternatives. Consent should be voluntary[45] and free from constraint or coercion, apart from the inevitable pressures of the problem that requires treatment. The legal origins of consent to health care treatment are comparable with those of consent to marriage, with the aims of respecting free choice and preventing force and coercion. Patients therefore need to know that consent is a choice, not a duty.

An Age of Consent?

The legal age of consent to medical treatment varies between states and countries from 12 to 21 years.[30,31] Some American states allow older minors to consent, mainly for three pragmatic reasons: (1) when parents or guardians cannot be contacted during an emergency; (2) when the minor has left home or is married or otherwise independent; (3) when the minor needs treatment for drug, alcohol, sexual, and other problems and does not want the parents to know. Paradoxically, deviant, risk-taking "mature minors" could be seen as more mature than their law-abiding, often better-educated peers, whose consent may not be recognized in law.

Assent is a vague term that ranges from the nonrefusal of young children, to tacit agreement, to the competent consent of minors, whose views are, nevertheless, not recognized in law. Assent lacks the important history, definition, and legal status of consent.[47-49]

In contrast to the United States, the 54 British Commonwealth countries share the common law *Gillick ruling,*[50] which respects the competence of minors in making decisions and giving informed, voluntary, legally valid consent, without stating a minimum "age of consent." English law respects the consent of minors if the child's doctors deem the child to be competent. The law defines *competence* as having the ability to understand what is involved and the discretion to make a wise choice in the best interests of the child.[50] Adults can make any decision for themselves, including self-destructive ones, whereas decisions made by and for minors have to be in their best interests. *Best interests* are usually defined by the child's doctors and parents or guardians. However, some children's independent views are respected and, at times, children understand more about their clinical problems and treatments than their parents do.[30,47,51] For example, some very short children give cogent personal reasons for requesting or refusing leg lengthening treatment.[51] Surgeons have reported that they will correct a mild case of scoliosis, which they would not usually treat, or that they will withhold or delay treatment for more severe cases, depending on young patients' strongly reasoned preferences.[51] Besides these cosmetic and lifestyle decisions, clinicians respect the decisions of certain minors about attempts to prolong life. At the heart-lung transplant unit in the main children's hospital in London, after lengthy informed discussion, some children do not consent to join the transplant waiting list.[51] Their decision is respected because staff consider that the child's willing commitment to having a transplant is essential for successful treatment, although they assure children that they can change their mind and return for treatment. Pain, illness, and depression may confuse the decision making of both child and adult patients, which is why careful discussions between doctors and families are vital to analyze flaws and strengths in the patient's reasoning. Experiences of illness or disability are not entirely negative. They can deepen children's understanding of complex problems and treatments, and can inform and strengthen their values and aspirations.[50,51] To see that illness can have positive aspects connects with another insight, which is essential if patients' consent is to be understood and respected. This is to move beyond the model of the active informed doctor versus the passive ignorant patient and to recognize how patients too can be informed and active. Much of their health care and well-being is in their hands, as can be seen in daily decisions about the use of inhalers to treat asthma or of physiotherapy to treat cystic fibrosis.[47,51]

Children who have long-term problems and undergo repeated treatments have time to acquire and reflect on experience and knowledge; this enables them to weigh risks and benefits and to make informed competent decisions.[51] This can be harder for unprepared healthy children who suddenly need an urgent intervention such as a bronchoscopy. They may feel too ignorant and shocked, frightened and bewildered, and perhaps too guilty or foolish after inhaling an object, to be able to make a reflective competent decision. Yet skillful clinicians can help young people to overcome these problems, as is shown by the 14-year-old in this chapter, who was assessed by his doctors as able to give informed consent.

Lawyers advise clinicians to involve the parents or guardians of minors and to request their consent, whenever possible, to support or to substitute for the minor's decision. High standards in pediatric care entail informing and involving all children, competent to consent or not, as far as they are willing and able to take part. Skillful practitioners use the consent process as a teaching and learning dialogue, exploring with children how they can learn and become involved—not simply as a test, which can easily underestimate the child's capacity. Practitioners who are convinced that children should be warned about risks, in case the intervention fails or damages the child, find that young patients can understand and come to terms with serious risks, at least in nonemergency cases.[50,51] If parents want to protect children by keeping them in ignorance, practitioners have to decide who the primary patient is, what obligations they owe to the child, and how much the child already knows and secretly worries about. Risky medical and surgical interventions expose children, who usually are so carefully protected, to exceptional dangers. Clinicians therefore may have to discuss with parents how best to give support as well as honest information to the child during this novel daunting experience.

Managing Time

Clinicians can examine and treat patients in emergencies without information giving or consent if they need to save a life or prevent lasting serious injury. However, apart from extreme emergencies, practitioners have to use time effectively, not only to provide explanations, but also to enable patients and/or parents to absorb and come to terms with unfamiliar details.

Four Partially Conflicting Purposes of Consent

Attention to informed and voluntary consent increased over the 20th century.[47] Consent serves several purposes. First, respect for their consent or informed refusal expresses principled respect for patients' human dignity, integrity of mind and body, and right to make personal decisions. Laws protect people from unauthorized touching and intrusion to reduce risks and prevent harms. Ethical standards in medical research[45,46] to prevent abuse or neglect have gradually spread and now influence routine standards of respect for consent or refusal in medical treatment.

Second, and pragmatically, patients who are informed and committed to the treatment, in terms of believing that it really is the best option, tend to be more willing and able to cooperate with medical regimens and advice.[51-53] When clinicians give clear and detailed information, listen, work through patients' objections and misunderstandings, and encourage patients' active cooperation, beyond passive or reluctant compliance, then this consent process becomes part of effective therapy. To force interventions on resisting children is sometimes necessary, but it undermines trusting partnerships between children and doctors on which effective longer-term care depends.

Third, legal standards to protect patients increasingly serve also to protect clinicians and their institutions. Consent is a device that is used to transfer responsibility for risk from the doctor to the informed patient, who signs the statement of knowing acceptance of the risks of unwanted side effects or of ineffective treatment. If patients sue doctors for not giving them adequate information and warning of risk, the signed consent form is a necessary although not sufficient part of doctors' defense.[49] This third purpose potentially sets practitioners against patients, besides exposing patients to responsibility for risk, and this partially conflicts with the first two more protective purposes.

Fourth, legal standards may require immensely detailed accounts of risks and alternatives, to forestall subsequent allegations of medical negligence or assault through inadequate information leading to invalid consent. The information may all be relevant, but many details can confuse rather than inform patients, both children and adults, undermining the first two purposes. Practitioners have to ensure that the parents at least are informed to a level that satisfies legal standards.

Managing Information

Skillful clinicians respond to patients' varying needs. Some people want to hear many details, others want few. Many will ask for help with making sense of the information, sifting major from minor concerns, ordering priorities, and relying on clinicians' experience and judgment. Impersonal information giving can merge toward more personal advice giving, which can be valuable but risky if legal standards regard this as distorting the information, or favoring the physician's personal bias, or exerting pressure on patients to make certain decisions. Essential core information can be supplemented with details for each specific patient.

Managing Emotions

Patients and parents may feel anxious and afraid, and at first may fear the dangers of proposed treatment more than the untreated problem. The voluntary consent process involves making an emotional, and often rapid, journey from fear and doubt toward trust and confidence in the treatment and the clinical team.[54] Therefore while they increase patients' doubts through complicated warnings of risk, clinicians simultaneously have to encourage patients to trust and hope.

When patients ask for details about their illness or problem and about the treatment, they imply trust, respect, and reliance on practitioners' knowledge. Yet if patients ask about complications and risks, if they question or disagree with practitioners, or if they are reluctant or refuse treatment and advice, this seeming mistrust can lead to tense, distressing, and possibly angry interactions. Disagreements about children's health care arouse extra tensions if adults are perceived to be dangerously negligent in refusing or withholding treatment, or dangerously invasive in trying to impose unwanted, unnecessary, or very risky treatment on the child. Anxious although misleading assumptions that minors must always be given all the relevant treatment, or that their refusal is always irrational and must be overridden, increase the tensions.

Research observations of hundreds of consultations between doctors, parents/guardians, and children in England[51,54] found that, apart from emergencies in which it might be necessary to proceed without consent, skillful doctors were compassionate (which means "feeling with") and were also calm and firm. They were confident enough not to feel too threatened by challenging questions. They saw that valid consent involves real hard knowledge about risks, which they explained. They knew that respect for informed consent includes respect for informed refusal. Therefore, to ensure that refusal, if it was expressed, was informed, they listened to objections and discussed misunderstandings. They could accept that, occasionally, children refused treatment because of deeply held values about their quality of life, or their wish to live the final stage of terminal illness at home.

These doctors dexterously managed their own less positive emotions when they felt challenged, as well as the feelings of their young patients and the parents/guardians. Allowing time for patients to change their minds, when possible, could encourage eventual consent. A surgeon and a mother worked for a year to persuade a severely learning disabled girl, aged 12 years, until she felt ready to undergo a series of operations.[51] A nurse found that a girl with cystic fibrosis who had been refusing a heart-lung transplant changed her mind "because you listened."[51] In rare cases of irresolvable disputes, doctors apply to courts of law to make the decision to provide or withhold treatment.

Summary

Consent is often reviewed in terms of correct/incorrect standards at opposite ends of the ethical/unethical, legal/illegal spectrum. It can, however, be more useful to think of working toward a central balance between giving too much or too little information; warning of risk while encouraging confidence; respecting parents but primarily treating the child; underestimating children's abilities and overestimating them; and neither overprotecting children by excluding them from being informed and involved nor increasing anxiety or confusion by overinvolving them. Much depends on the personal skill and judgment of each clinician.

REFERENCES

1. Marik PE. Aspiration pneumonitis and aspiration pneumonia. *N Engl J Med.* 2001;344:665-671.
2. Verghese ST, Hannallah RS. Pediatric otolaryngologic emergencies. *Anesthesiol Clin North Am.* 2001;2:237-256.
3. Shlizerman L, Mazzawi S, Rakover Y, et al. Foreign body aspiration in children: the effects of delayed diagnosis. *Am J Otolaryngol.* 2010;31:320-324.
4. Boyd M, Chatterjee A, Chiles C, et al. Tracheobronchial foreign body aspiration in adults. *South Med J.* 2009;102:171-174.
5. Swanson KL, Prakash UB, Midthun DE, et al. Flexible bronchoscopic management of airway foreign bodies in children. *Chest.* 2002;121:1695-1700.
6. Paintal HS, Kuschner WG. Aspiration syndromes: 10 clinical pearls every physician should know. *Int J Clin Pract.* 2007;61:846-852.
7. Pinto A, Scaglione M, Pinto F. Tracheobronchial aspiration of foreign bodies: current indications for emergency plain chest radiography. *Radiol Med.* 2006;111:497-506.
8. Kavanagh PV, Mason AC, Müller NL. Thoracic foreign bodies in adults. *Clin Radiol.* 1999;54:353-360.
9. Righini CA, Morel N, Karkas A, et al. What is the diagnostic value of flexible bronchoscopy in the initial investigation of children with suspected foreign body aspiration? *Int J Pediatr Otorhinolaryngol.* 2007;71:1383-1390.
10. Zissin R, Shapiro-Feinberg M, Rozenman J, et al. CT findings of the chest in adults with aspirated foreign bodies. *Eur Radiol.* 2001;11:606-611.
11. Adaletli I, Kurugoglu S, Ulus S, et al. Utilization of low-dose multidetector CT and virtual bronchoscopy in children with suspected foreign body aspiration. *Pediatr Radiol.* 2007;37:33-40.
12. Bhat KV, Hegde JS, Nagalotimath US, et al. Evaluation of computed tomography virtual bronchoscopy in paediatric tracheobronchial foreign body aspiration. *J Laryngol Otol.* 2010;124:875-879.
13. Cakir E, Ersu RH, Uyan ZS, et al. Flexible bronchoscopy as a valuable tool in the evaluation of persistent wheezing in children. *Int J Pediatr Otorhinolaryngol.* 2009;73:1666-1668.

14. Martinot A, Closset M, Marquette CH, et al. Indications for flexible versus rigid bronchoscopy in children with suspected foreign-body aspiration. *Am J Respir Crit Care Med.* 1997;155:1676-1679.
15. Martinati LC, Boner AL. Clinical diagnosis of wheezing in early childhood. *Allergy.* 1995;50:701-710.
16. Warner MA, Warner ME, Warner DO, et al. Perioperative pulmonary aspiration in infants and children. *Anesthesiology.* 1999;90:66-71.
17. Smith Hammond CA, Goldstein LB. Cough and aspiration of food and liquids due to oral-pharyngeal dysphagia: ACCP evidence-based clinical practice guidelines. *Chest.* 2006;129(suppl 1):154S-168S.
18. Lundy DS, Smith C, Colangelo L, et al. Aspiration: cause and implications. *Otolaryngol Head Neck Surg.* 1999;120:474-478.
19. Limper AH, Prakash UB. Tracheobronchial foreign bodies in adults. *Ann Intern Med.* 1990;112:604-609.
20. Djukanovic R. The safety aspects of fiberoptic bronchoscopy, bronchoalveolar lavage, and endobronchial biopsy in asthma. *Am Rev Respir Dis.* 1991;143:772-777.
21. Summary and recommendations of a workshop on the investigative use of fiberoptic bronchoscopy and bronchoalveolar lavage in asthmatics. *Am Rev Respir Dis.* 1985;132:180-182.
22. Rankin J. Bronchoalveolar lavage: its safety in subjects with mild asthma. *Chest.* 1984;85:723-728.
23. Stolz D, Pollak V, Chhajed PN, et al. A randomized, placebo-controlled trial of bronchodilators for bronchoscopy in patients with COPD. *Chest.* 2007;131:765-772.
24. Lukomsky GI, Ovchinnikov AA, Bilal A. Complications of bronchoscopy: comparison of rigid bronchoscopy under general anesthesia and flexible fiberoptic bronchoscopy under topical anesthesia. *Chest.* 1981;79:316-321.
25. Debeljak A, Sorli J, Music E, et al. Bronchoscopic removal of foreign bodies in adults: experience with 62 patients from 1974-1998. *Eur Respir J.* 1999;14:792-795.
26. Verghese ST, Hannallah RS. Pediatric otolaryngologic emergencies. *Anesthesiol Clin North Am.* 2001;19:237-256.
27. Lundy DS, Smith C, Colangelo L, et al. Aspiration: cause and implications. *Otolaryngol Head Neck Surg.* 1999;120:474-478.
28. Farrell PT. Rigid bronchoscopy for foreign body removal: anaesthesia and ventilation. *Paediatr Anaesth.* 2004;14:84-89.
29. Green CG, Eisenberg J, Leong A, et al. Flexible endoscopy of the pediatric airway. *Am Rev Respir Dis.* 1992;145:233-235.
30. Alderson P. Competent children? Minors' consent to health care treatment and research. *Soc Sci Med.* 2007;65:2272-2283.
31. E Notes. Treatment of minors. http://www.enotes.com/everyday-law-encyclopedia/treatment-minors. Accessed January 28, 2011.
32. Cal. Fam. Code §6922(a) .National Center for Youth Law. www.youthlaw.org, revised January 2003. Accessed January 28, 2011.
33. Cal. Fam. Code §7050(e). National Center for Youth Law. www.youthlaw.org. Accessed January 28, 2011.
34. Steen KH, Zimmermann T. Tracheobronchial aspiration of foreign bodies in children: a study of 94 cases. *Laryngoscope.* 1990;100:525-530.
35. Vaughan GG, Grycko RJ, Montgomery MT. The prevention and treatment of aspiration of vomitus during pharmacosedation and general anesthesia. *J Oral Maxillofac Surg.* 1992;50:874-879.
36. Dines DE, Titus JL, Sessler AD. Aspiration pneumonitis. *Mayo Clin Proc.* 1970;45:347-360.
37. Litman RS, Ponnuri J, Trogan I. Anesthesia for tracheal or bronchial foreign body removal in children: an analysis of ninety-four cases. *Anesth Analg.* 2000;91:1389-1391.
38. Baraka A. Oxygen enrichment of entrained room air during Venturi jet ventilation of children undergoing bronchoscopy. *Paediatr Anaesth.* 1996;6:383-385.
39. Eyrich JE, Riopelle JM, Naraghi M. Elective transtracheal jet ventilation for bronchoscopic removal of tracheal foreign body. *South Med J.* 1992;85:1017-1019.
40. Swanson KL. Airway foreign bodies: what's new? *Semin Respir Crit Care Med.* 2004;25:405-411.
41. Wick R, Gilbert JD, Byard RW. Café coronary syndrome—fatal choking on food: an autopsy approach. *J Clin Forensic Med.* 2006;13:135-138.
42. Weber SM, Chesnutt MS, Barton R, et al. Extraction of dental crowns from the airway: a multidisciplinary approach. *Laryngoscope.* 2005;115:687-689.
43. Committee on Injury VaPP. Prevention of choking among children. *Pediatrics.* 2010;125:601-607.
44. Göktas O, Snidero S, Jahnke V, et al. Foreign body aspiration in children: field report of a German hospital. *Pediatr Int.* 2010;52:100-103.
45. Nuremberg Code, 1947. http://www.cirp.org/library/ethics/nuremberg/. Accessed March 15, 2011.
46. Declaration of Helsinki, World Medical Association, 1964/2004. http://ohsr.od.nih.gov/guidelines/helsinki.html. Accessed March 15, 2011.
47. Alderson P. Children's consent and 'assent' to healthcare research. In: Freeman M, ed. *Childhood and the Law.* Oxford: Oxford University Press; 2011.
48. Gillick v. Wisbech and West Norfolk Area Health Authority and the Department of Health and Social Security. http://www.bailii.org/uk/cases/UKHL/1985/7.html. Accessed March 15, 2011.
49. Faden R, Beauchamp T. *A History and Theory of Informed Consent.* New York: Oxford University Press; 1986.
50. Alderson P, Sutcliffe K, Curtis K. Children's consent to medical treatment. *Hastings Centre Report.* 2006;36:25-34.
51. Alderson P. *Children's Consent to Surgery.* Buckingham: Open University Press; 1993.
52. Alderson P. *Choosing for Children: Parents' Consent to Surgery.* Oxford: Oxford University Press; 1990.
53. Dose adjustment for normal eating. www.dafne.uk.com. Accessed March 16, 2011.
54. Lansdown G, Goldhagen J, Waterston T. Children's rights and child health: a course for health professionals, American Academy of Pediatrics and Royal College of Paediatrics and Child Health, 2010. http://labspace.open.ac.uk/mod/oucontent/view.php?id=425620&printable=1. Accessed March 16, 2011.

Chapter 26

Treatment of Critical Left Main Bronchial Obstruction and Acute Respiratory Failure in the Setting of Right Pneumonectomy

This chapter emphasizes the following elements of the Four Box Approach: patient preferences and expectations (also includes family); and referrals to medical, surgical, or palliative/end-of-life subspecialty care.

CASE DESCRIPTION

The patient was a 69-year-old Hispanic male who 6 days before arrival in our facility was admitted to an outside hospital with hypercapnic respiratory failure requiring endotracheal intubation and mechanical ventilation. He had a history of COPD, atrial fibrillation, and asbestos exposure. Non–small cell lung cancer was diagnosed 5 years earlier, for which he underwent right pneumonectomy followed by systemic treatment with chemotherapy and radiation therapy. His medications included digoxin, Cardizem, Protonix, and albuterol and Atrovent nebulization. On examination, he had diffuse coarse breath sounds in the left lung field and diminished breath sounds on the right. The chest radiograph showed complete opacification of the right hemithorax consistent with his previous right pneumonectomy (Figure 26-1). Laboratory markers were normal, except for sodium of 128 mEq/L and albumin of 2.3 g/dL. Bronchoscopy showed a mass protruding from the medial wall of the distal left main bronchus, obstructing it by approximately 90% (see Figure 26-1). The patient's wife and daughter were very involved in his care and stated that his goals were to be at home and not on life support.

DISCUSSION POINTS

1. List two treatment alternatives that will fit this patient's goals of care.
2. List four reasons for bronchoscopic intervention in a patient with malignant central airway obstruction and respiratory failure.
3. Describe three risks of bronchial stent insertion in this patient.

---

*The prioritization model used for this purpose defines those patients who will benefit most from the ICU (priority 1) versus those who will not benefit at all (priority 4) from ICU admission.

CASE RESOLUTION

Initial Evaluations

Physical Examination, Complementary Tests, and Functional Status Assessment

In a critically ill patient with malignant central airway obstruction (CAO) who requires ventilatory assistance, interventional bronchoscopic procedures may be lifesaving, may allow extubation and time for additional therapies to be initiated, and may prolong survival.[1-6] Reported overall median survival rates of critically ill patients with malignant CAO vary between 2 and 38 months post bronchoscopic interventions,[1,6,7] and 1 year survival reportedly has been as low as 15%.[8] This wide variability in results is probably explained by inclusion of patients at various stages of their disease, with those with various types of malignancies undergoing various treatments before and after interventions, and receiving different degrees of respiratory support. These critically ill patients are often admitted emergently to the intensive care unit (ICU) only when respiratory failure develops. According to Society of Critical Care Medicine (SCCM) guidelines on ICU triage, admissions, and discharge, patients with advanced cancer should be admitted to the ICU when a reversible cause (e.g., pulmonary embolism, tamponade, airway obstruction) is identified.* Patients with advanced malignancy complicated by airway obstruction are given priority 3, which is defined as "unstable patients who are critically ill but have a reduced likelihood of recovery because of underlying disease or nature of their acute illness."[9] According to these guidelines, patients "may receive intensive treatment to relieve acute illness, however, limits on therapeutic efforts may be set, such as no intubation or cardiopulmonary resuscitation." In practice, patients with acute respiratory failure usually are intubated, placed on mechanical ventilation, and transferred to the ICU. Patients with non–small cell lung cancer (NSCLC) and respiratory failure from CAO, such as our patient, therefore may warrant invasive mechanical ventilatory support and admission to the ICU, pending evaluation for palliative bronchoscopic interventions.[10] If the bronchoscopic intervention is successful and the patient's physiologic status has stabilized, ICU monitoring and care may no longer be necessary, and the patient can be transferred to a unit that provides a lower level of

Figure 26-1 **A,** Portable antero-posterior chest radiograph shows complete opacification of the right hemithorax and the indwelling endotracheal tube. **B,** Image obtained during rigid bronchoscopy shows near complete closure of the distal left main bronchus by a mixed type of obstructing lesion (endoluminal exophytic and extrinsic compression).

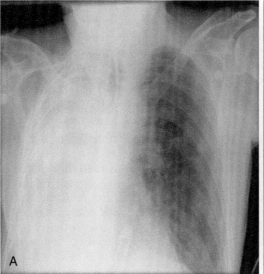
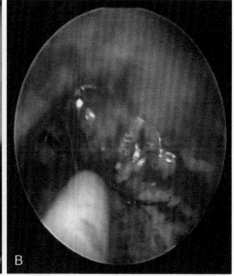

care. If, on the other hand, airway interventions are not successful, or if a patient's physiologic status has deteriorated and active interventions are no longer planned, discharge to a lower level of care, including withdrawal of life support or referral to hospice, is a reasonable consideration. Families and referring physicians can be comforted by knowing that bronchoscopic intervention was not indicated, or that is was performed but was unsuccessful in alleviating the airway obstruction.

Many patients and their families may wonder whether all possible therapeutic alternatives are being considered, especially when the patient is possibly in the terminal stages of disease. Truthful disclosure by physicians is crucial in these instances to avoid compromising a physician-patient relationship built on trust. Although some patients and families are averse to truthfulness, most want their doctors to be honest and forthcoming in their communications about diagnosis and prognosis, even when it means announcing the likelihood of death. In addition to other factors, such as age and disease diagnosis, ethnicity may play an important role in a patient's perceptions regarding truth telling and availability of therapeutic interventions. For example, approximately one in five deaths in the United States occurs in or shortly after a stay in the ICU,[11] where evidence of disparities in end-of-life care has been found. In the United States, racial minorities apparently have been subjected to lower quality of care than whites,[12] and although these findings are not consistent,*[13,14] some studies report that African American patients receive fewer medical interventions, have shorter lengths of stay, and use fewer resources. One large study, however, evaluated the medical charts of patients who died in 15 intensive care units (3138 patients, of whom 2479 [79%] were white and 659 [21%] were nonwhite [e.g., African American, Asian, Pacific Islander, American Indian, Hispanic]). Logistic regression adjusted for socioeconomic factors measured by education, income, and insurance status showed that nonwhite patients were less likely to have living wills, were more likely to die with full support including cardiopulmonary resuscitation (CPR), and were more likely to die in a setting of full support than were white patients. In addition, nonwhites were more likely to have undergone medical interventions during their ICU stay, including dialysis, vasopressors, and mechanical ventilation.*[15] Although all patients are and should be treated as VIPs (very important persons), consideration and respect for patient and family perceptions regarding therapy and truth telling are warranted, particularly if factors known to affect perceptions and behaviors are present.

The patient's laboratory tests revealed hypoalbuminemia and moderate hyponatremia. The latter was likely due to the syndrome of inappropriate antidiuretic hormone (SIADH) secretion†[16] because the patient was euvolemic, and no signs of hypovolemic hyponatremia, such as gastrointestinal losses, excessive diuresis or adrenal insufficiency, or salt wasting nephropathy or cerebral salt wasting, were noted. Other laboratory tests revealed a blood urea nitrogen (BUN) level less than 10 mg/dL and urine osmolarity greater than 100 mOsm/kg of water—findings consistent with the diagnosis of SIADH.

---

*This discrepancy appears to be largely due to the fact that the studies showing nonwhite patients receiving more life-sustaining measures focused on patients dying in the ICU and, therefore, reflect life-sustaining treatments provided during end-of-life care.

*Nonwhite patients were also more likely to have documentation that the prognosis was discussed and that physicians recommended withdrawal of life support, and were more likely to have discord documented among family members or with clinicians, but the socioeconomic status did not modify these associations and was not a consistent predictor of end-of-life care. With regard to truth telling, at least one study in the United States suggests that in case of serious illness, elderly European Americans and African Americas were more likely to believe they should be told the truth about diagnosis and prognosis than were Korean Americans and Mexican Americans (Blackhall L. Should patients always be told the truth? *AORN J.* 1988;47:1306-1310).

†SIADH is seen in 1% to 2% of patients with lung cancer (usually caused by small cell carcinoma). Signs and symptoms of SIADH (gait disturbances, falls, headaches, muscle cramps, confusion, lethargy, seizure, and even respiratory failure and coma) usually occur with acute and more severe hyponatremia (sodium <125 mEq/L).

Comorbidities

This patient had chronic obstructive pulmonary disease (COPD) and atrial fibrillation, increasing the risks for postoperative pulmonary and cardiovascular complications, respectively, in cases of interventions performed under general anesthesia.

Support System

The patient had no medical insurance. The family expressed their frustration that before this event of respiratory failure, the patient's access to care had been very limited and, they believed, suboptimal; they mentioned to us that urgent care centers on two occasions prescribed a 5 day antibiotic course but had not performed imaging studies or other tests, even though health care providers had been told about his prior history of lung cancer. One hates to think that differences in insurance status might contribute directly to different outcomes of patients suffering from lung cancer. Surely, few patients understand the complexities of the health insurance system in the United States, where copayments of various types, a mixture of health maintenance organization/preferred provider organization (HMO/PPO) plans, and constantly changing rules regarding deductibles and the need for authorizations can trouble the consumer, especially when illness strikes. Few patients understand that virtually all health plans provide for coverage in case of an emergency, regardless of geographic location, and that patients have a right to request and advocate for laboratory tests and imaging studies if they believe these will be important for their care.

In addition, differences in race, ethnicity, income, and education may have an effect on processes of care and outcomes. In the United States, results of studies show that patients with Medicaid* or no insurance had worse outcomes than other patients suffering from lung cancer. Although some of these disparities may have been secondary to confounding factors such as smoking and other health behaviors, available data suggest that patients with lung cancer without insurance do poorly because access to care is limited, and/or because they present with more advanced disease that is less amenable to treatment.[17] On the other hand, the risk for Medicare† patients has been found to be similar to that for patients with private insurance; for those with Medicare disability insurance, no differences in stage were noted when a fee-for-service status was compared with a health maintenance organization or combination insurance status.[18]

Patient Preferences and Expectations

This patient with a known lung cancer had health care advance directives with regard to a Do Not Resuscitate (DNR) order in case of terminal irreversible disease. In general, published evidence reveals a low rate of completion of these documents among Hispanics.[19] In addition to lack of trust in the health care system, health care disparities, and cultural perspectives on death and suffering, lack of acceptance of advance directives among Hispanics may originate from a view of collective family responsibility.[20] In many Latin American countries, in fact, illness is viewed as a family affair rather than as a struggle of individual suffering. Before his respiratory failure, our patient had expressed his wish to not be on "breathing machines" if the disease process became irreversible. Therefore a DNR had been placed in his medical record upon his admission to the outside facility. One might recall that cardiopulmonary resuscitation (CPR) was originally designed for the prevention of sudden, unexpected death—not necessarily to prolong the life of an irreversibly terminally ill person.[21] At the same time, the quality and duration of life-related value judgments should be avoided, and sanctity of life arguments can be made to justify CPR in virtually any setting.

In making decisions about code status orders, physicians and patients must communicate effectively, so that patients can receive informed and compassionate care that respects their wishes. Communication between physicians and patients (or their surrogates) about code status orders, however, is difficult, especially if matters are being discussed emergently at the time of a medical crisis. Misunderstandings about code status and overall goals of care preferences may lead to unwanted medical interventions or withholding/withdrawing of desired interventions. Results of studies show that patients in the ICU and their surrogates have insufficient knowledge about in-hospital CPR and its likelihood of success, such as whether CPR will result in preservation of life, preservation of organ function, discharge from an intensive care unit, or discharge alive from the hospital. In general, it appears that many patients, families, and physicians probably share an excessively positive estimation of the outcomes of CPR.[22]

A patient's code status preferences may not always be reflected in code status orders, and assessments may differ between patients, their surrogates, family members, and physicians about what goal of care is most important.[22] In our case, the patient's family was particularly concerned that any de-escalation of the patient's care, including proceeding with extubation or removal from mechanical ventilation, would constitute euthanasia. They also expressed firm disagreement with a proposed strategy of palliative sedation.* Oftentimes, when

---

*Medicaid is a joint federal-state program designed to provide financial assistance to eligible low-income low-asset persons (people with disabilities, children, parents of eligible children, pregnant women, elderly nursing home residents, and those with certain diseases such as human immunodeficiency virus [HIV]/acquired immunodeficiency syndrome [AIDS] and minimal assets based on percentage of the Federal Poverty Level). Currently, more than 50 million persons in the United States, including millions of children and more than 60% of nursing home residents, are covered by Medicaid programs.

†Medicare is a federal health insurance program that covers people age 65 and older and those younger than 65 with certain disabilities, such as permanent kidney failure. Legal residence in the United States for at least 5 years is mandatory for eligibility. Medicare Part A covers inpatient hospital stays, residence in skilled nursing facilities, and hospice or home care and may be premium free. Medicare Part B covers required outpatient and some preventive services and has a monthly premium. Medicare prescription coverage can be purchased, and Medigap coverage (Medicare supplement insurance) is available to pay for uncovered costs such as deductibles and copayments.

---

*Palliative sedation refers to the use of medications to induce decreased or absent awareness to relieve otherwise intractable suffering.

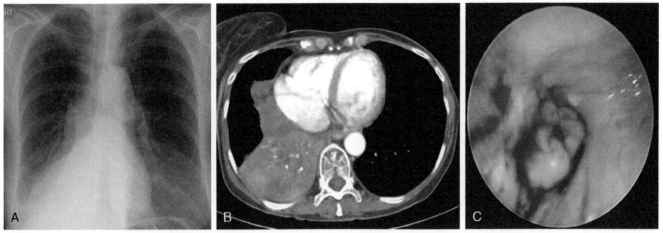

Figure 26-2 Images obtained from a different patient show the right lower lobe and middle lobe atelectasis **(A)** on chest radiograph and **(B)** on chest computed tomography, as well as **(C)** complete closure of the bronchus intermedius by a mucosal infiltrating tumor.

disagreements occur, an ethics consultation can help clarify terminology and avoid adversarial encounters between the treating team and the family. Anyone may request the assistance of ethics consultants, including family members and even health care providers not involved in the care of a particular patient if they sense impending difficulties in the medical encounters or in their own dealings with conflict. The involvement of other disciplines, including palliative care medicine, chaplaincy, and a social worker to address the family's concerns, is a reasonable first step. In our case, physicians explained to the family that euthanasia is completely different from palliative sedation or withdrawal of life-sustaining treatment based on its intent and outcome. In euthanasia, the intent is deliberate termination of a patient's life (which is illegal in the United States), and palliative sedation is designed to relieve symptoms or the effects of burdensome interventions (i.e., mechanical ventilation). This is ethically justified and legal, even when sedation might cause, from its double effect, a hastened demise.[23]

Procedural Strategies

Indications

Relieving central airway obstruction could prevent post obstructive pneumonia, sepsis, and septic shock; allow extubation and a change in the level of care; permit initiation of systemic therapy; and potentially improve survival. Evidence suggests that bronchoscopic therapies often provide acute relief of the obstruction, improve quality of life, and serve as a therapeutic bridge until systemic treatments become effective.[1,4,7] Subsequent systemic treatments (chemotherapy and/or radiotherapy) were shown to increase disease-free survival during the first year after restoration of airway patency.[1,8]

In patients with CAO (lobar or mainstem), assessing the functionality of the lung parenchyma distal to the obstruction is useful when interventions meant to establish airway patency are considered. Functionality of the lung distal to the obstruction may not be restored in

patients who have had chronic complete obstruction and lack of ventilation (Figure 26-2). Determining whether there is functional airway and lung beyond an obstruction is essential for any successful bronchoscopic intervention,* in part because significant friability of bleeding from thin infiltrated bronchial mucosa, or lack of lung perfusion despite restored airway patency, might preclude intervention. In one study, 71% of patients who initiated radiation therapy within 2 weeks after radiologic evidence of atelectasis had complete re-expansion of their lungs, compared with only 23% of those irradiated after 2 weeks.[24] Studies pertaining to successful bronchoscopic treatment and time to treatment are lacking.

One way to assess the perfusion status of lung parenchyma distal to an airway obstruction is to attempt bypass of the stenosis using a high-resolution endobronchial ultrasonography (EBUS) radial probe. For instance, the perfusion to one lobe could be completely shut down in a case of complete bronchial obstruction simply because of the Euler-Liljestrand reflex,† not because of pulmonary artery involvement. In cases of frank pulmonary artery occlusion, however, establishing airway patency could result in increased dead space ventilation. This finding should probably annul further intervention.[25] Our patient had a critical distal left main bronchial obstruction in the setting of right pneumonectomy, but lobar and segmental airways in the left lung were patent bronchoscopically, and distal lung parenchyma appeared functional on the chest radiograph (see Figure 26-1).

---

*Other conditions include experienced bronchoscopist and team; experienced anesthesiologist; control of patient's overall performance status; whether additional systemic or local therapy is still possible; and control of comorbidities.

†The Euler–Liljestrand reflex describes the relation between ventilation and perfusion in the lung. If the ventilation in a part of the lung decreases, this leads to local hypoxia and to vasoconstriction in that particular lung region. This adaptive mechanism is beneficial because it diminishes the amount of blood that passes the lung without being oxygenated, thus avoiding ventilation-perfusion mismatch and hypoxemia.

Contraindications

No absolute contraindications to bronchoscopic interventions performed under moderate sedation or general anesthesia were identified.

Expected Results

Patients with advanced NSCLC and CAO who undergo successful interventional bronchoscopy to relieve airway obstruction might have a survival similar to those without CAO.[26] Studies also show that patients with respiratory failure and malignant CAO palliated by bronchoscopic intervention who underwent additional definitive therapy survived longer (median, 38.2 months; range, 1.7 to 57.0 months) than those who did not (median, 6.2 months; range, 0.1 to 33.7 months; $P < .001$).[7] Successful removal from mechanical ventilation in patients with CAO due to malignancy has been reported in 50% to 100% of patients in several small case series[2,4] and, in some, prolonged survival was documented when systemic treatment was also administered (98 vs. 8.5 days).[1]

Team Experience

Rigid bronchoscopic interventions with laser and/or stent placement are performed on a weekly basis at this institution by a dedicated interventional bronchoscopy team with enough expertise and experience to perform a procedure in a patient in poor general condition and with only one insufficiently ventilated lung.

Therapeutic Alternatives

Withdrawal of mechanical ventilation and initiation of palliative sedation can be considered in patients with respiratory failure requiring mechanical ventilation in the setting of advanced malignant CAO and for whom no additional systemic or local (including bronchoscopy) therapies are indicated or feasible. These interventions, however, are used in patients who warrant aggressive symptom control and still have severe suffering (most commonly physical symptoms such as delirium, dyspnea, and pain) related to their underlying disease or therapy-related adverse effects.[23] The effectiveness* of palliative sedation is in the range of 70% to 90%. In our patient, we decided to attempt relief of the airway obstruction using bronchoscopic techniques; had this been unsuccessful, we would have consulted palliative care medicine and discussed with the patient's family withdrawal of life-sustaining treatments.[23†]

Cost-Effectiveness

The costs of interventional bronchoscopic procedures such as laser resection and stent insertion are probably small compared with the costs of repeated external beam radiation therapy, palliative chemotherapy, or prolonged ICU stays for already advanced and refractory disease. These economic factors are obviously institution, insurer, and country specific.

Informed Consent

The patient was sedated and was on mechanical ventilation. We discussed the indications, risks, benefits, and alternatives of bronchoscopic intervention with the patient's wife and family during ICU family meetings. Using certified interpreters, we assessed their understanding of the proposed interventions and options—essential for an autonomous decision. Although it may seem paradoxical, patients and their surrogates benefit from the help of others to make truly autonomous decisions because they require accurate and comprehensive information. They may also need someone to help them relate the information they have to what they care about. Furthermore, because most people do not have a clear rank of priorities ready at hand for all situations, most need help identifying what they care about most and how this relates to the current health care encounter.[27]

Techniques and Results

Anesthesia and Perioperative Care

In the perioperative setting, anesthesiologists and surgeons may need to reconsider and re-evaluate standing DNR orders, which may need to be temporarily suspended during the intraoperative and immediate postoperative periods. Anesthesiologists may be skeptical of what they read in the patient's chart, especially because it is possible that up until the time of the procedure, they usually know very little about the patient.* The surgeon may not be the patient's primary physician and may not know the details of the circumstances in which the DNR decision was made. It is nearly impossible for advance directives to address adequately the multitude of clinical situations that may be encountered during the operative setting. CPR, if needed during the operative and immediate postoperative periods, includes not only chest compressions or electrical shocks, but also what could be viewed as excessive vasopressor usage or an inappropriate duration of resuscitation. Therefore it is important that all such patients be seen by the anesthesiologist and the surgeon preoperatively, and that a strategy be mutually agreed upon in case of the patient's "death." Although logistically difficult, a multidisciplinary discussion is warranted and might include the patient and/or the patient's representative surrogate, the anesthesiologist, the surgeon, and the intensivist, who may be called upon postoperatively.[28] A palliative care specialist or medical ethicist can also

---

*Defined as the patient's, family's, or physician's perceived relief of refractory physical symptoms.

†With this end-of-life decision making, the cause of death is the underlying disease, but the intent is to remove burdensome interventions (e.g., mechanical ventilation); this is a legal practice in United States, but several states limit the power of surrogate decision makers regarding life-sustaining treatment.

---

*The ability of anesthesiologists to re-evaluate the DNR order is also hampered by the lack of a system that allows early notification of pending cases, which would give the anesthesiologist ample time to discuss these issues with the patient, family caregivers, the surgeon, and other health care providers.

provide helpful insights. Multidisciplinary discussions may allow time to address the complex ethical and practical issues often present in these situations. For example, in the United States, patients who do not speak English fluently generally are less likely than more fluent English speakers to be actively engaged in end-of-life decision making, even in less hurried situations.[29] Language barriers can be considerable, and working through translators, although necessary, is not always easy. Perioperative DNR orders also raise many issues of special concern. The DNR discussion with the patient or appropriate surrogate should include information about the characteristics of a possible resuscitation during the perioperative period; the risks, the benefits, and the likely outcome; and the reasons why resuscitation during the perioperative period might be determined by the patient, the surrogate, or the health care provider to be more or less burdensome than beneficial. If a surrogate is making the decision, the medical record should note the surrogate's relationship to the patient (e.g., health care agent, spouse, guardian) and the basis on which the surrogate's decision is made (e.g., "patient's prior wishes," "best interests").

The DNR order should be written in detail and signed by one of the treating physicians. If the DNR order is cancelled preoperatively, as is often the case, then the time period and circumstances under which it is to be re-enacted should be specified.[30] Interviews with terminally ill patients about perioperative resuscitative orders have revealed that some patients wanted their preoperative DNR orders revoked, some wanted to use procedure-directed perioperative DNR orders, and others wanted to redefine their goals for the procedure and postoperative outcome. This requires that the anesthesiologist and the surgeon decide about appropriate means for resuscitation during the procedure,[31] and certain limits may be set. For example, we have seen patients with advanced illness having a respiratory arrest at the end of a procedure, who are responsive to intubation and ventilation but who never require chest percussion or vasopressors. We have also seen cardiac arrest rapidly reversible by defibrillation and not requiring reintubation or pressors. Special attention should be paid to issues related to the response to any iatrogenic arrest.[32] Surrogates can be good decision makers for others when they know specifically what the person would have wanted, or when they have a strong general impression of that person's values and beliefs. In some cases, however, surrogate decision making will be an approximation, subject to conscious and unconscious biases, concerns, and conflicts; in studies assessing agreement between a patient and surrogate regarding the use of CPR, the percent of agreement ranged from only 53% to 90%, with the frequency of agreement least in sicker patients.[33]

With regard to our patient's preoperative physiologic optimization, fluid restriction (<1000 mL/day) was initiated during the ICU stay. Twenty-four hours later, his sodium had improved from 128 to 132 mEq/L. Had this not shown improvement, demeclocycline (300 to 600 mg orally twice daily), conivaptan (20 to 40 mg/day intravenously), tolvaptan (10 to 60 mg/day orally), or even hypertonic (3%) saline at less than 1 to 2 mL/kg/hr[16]* could have been used to correct hyponatremia preoperatively.

Instrumentation

We selected a ventilating rigid bronchoscope (Bryan Corp., Woburn, Mass) because the tumor was in the distal left main bronchus, and nonventilating bronchoscopes would have been too short to reach this region. These stainless steel tubes have a length of 36 cm and have exterior diameters of 7, 8, 10, 12, and 13.2 mm and internal diameters of 6.5, 7, 9.2, 11, and 12.2 mm, respectively. A neodymium-doped yttrium aluminum garnet (Nd:YAG) laser was set up for photocoagulation and potential vaporization of the tumor.

Anatomic Dangers and Other Risks

The descending aorta is posterior and the inferior pulmonary vein and left atrium are medial to the distal left main bronchus (LMB), where this patient's tumor was located. Laser photocoagulation must be performed carefully in this area to avoid direct application onto the posterior and medial walls, which may result in high absorption of laser energy due to a hypervascular, hemorrhagic pattern of mucosal disease in this area and potential airway wall perforation. This is especially true in patients with pneumonectomy because normal anatomic relationships in the mediastinum have changed as a result of a postsurgical mediastinal shift. This also changes the alignment of bronchial structures in the chest—an important consideration when proceeding with rigid bronchoscopic debulking. Airway obstruction from blood and tumor debris in a patient with pneumonectomy may be fatal owing to severe impairment in gas exchange and refractory hypoxemia, and of course any obstruction of distal airways during resection will further compromise ventilatory and eventually hemodynamic status. Priority during resection in patients with only one lung should be given to ventilation and oxygenation, with recognition that in case of bleeding, it may be necessary to move the rigid tube beyond the obstruction, compressing the bleeding site with the tube itself, while ensuring ventilation through the distal patent segmental airways. Depending on the location of the bleed, one may wish to place the patient in a slightly head-down position so that blood moves proximally, protecting the distal airway, and if, for example, bleeding is coming from tumor along the medial wall of the left main bronchus, one might want to place the patient in the right lateral decubitus position, so that the rigid tube may more easily compress the bleeding site while maintaining ventilation of more distal bronchi.†

Results and Procedure-Related Complications

After administration of general anesthesia, the patient's endotracheal tube (ETT) was removed under direct visualization, and he was intubated with a 13 mm

---

*Rapid correction can occur with hypertonic saline, and this can lead to water egress, brain dehydration, and central pontine and extrapontine myelinolysis, characterized by lethargy, dysarthria, spastic quadriparesis, and pseudobulbar palsy; therefore the correction rate should not be faster than 0.5 to 1 mmol/L/hr.

†Note that in this situation, the adage of "bleeding side down" applies to the medial wall of the bronchus, not to the right or left hemithorax.

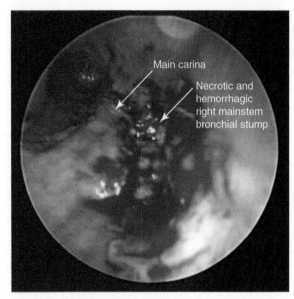

Figure 26-3 Rigid bronchoscopy picture taken at the level of the main carina showing neoplastic infiltration and a necrotic right pneumonectomy stump.

Efer-Dumon rigid ventilating bronchoscope (see video on ExpertConsult.com) (Video VI.26.1). Once inside the airways, a necrotic and infiltrated right bronchial stump was seen, suggesting recurrence of tumor, which posed a high risk for dehiscence (Figure 26-3); tumor was invading the main carina and the distal aspect of the right tracheal wall. In the distal left main bronchus, tumor extended for 1.5 cm, compressing and invading the airway and narrowing the lumen by 90% (see video on ExpertConsult.com) (Video VI.26.2). Flexible bronchoscopy performed through the rigid tube showed patent distal airways in the left upper and lower lobes. We decided to not insert a stent, but instead proceeded with bronchoscopic resection of the tumor. We initially performed laser photocoagulation of the right stump and carina to stop bleeding from the mucosal tumor. We then photocoagulated tumor in the distal left main bronchus by using a total of 442 Joules, applying 1 second 30 Watt Nd:YAG laser pulses. Tumor was partially debulked using the beveled edge of the rigid bronchoscope, and large pieces of tumor were removed and sent for histopathologic analysis. Abundant saline washings were performed to remove bloody secretions, tissue fragments, and small pieces of destroyed cartilage. At the end of the procedure, left bronchial patency had been restored (see video on ExpertConsult.com) (Video VI.26.3). We noted that tumor was extending distally all the way to the secondary left carina; therefore straight stent insertion would not have been ideal. The procedure was terminated, the rigid bronchoscope was removed, and the patient was reintubated as planned with a 7.5 ETT. He was transferred back to the medical ICU uneventfully.

Long-Term Management

Outcome Assessment

Flexible bronchoscopy was performed the next day to remove mucus plugs and blood clots in the airways before

a planned extubation was begun. The patient had been off narcotics and major sedatives and was fully awake but comfortable. The airways were patent, and no evidence of active bleeding was noted. We proceeded with the weaning protocol. Weaning parameters were not precluding extubation; however, the cuff leak volume was 100 mL. Testing for a cuff leak before endotracheal tube removal is a method commonly used to determine whether airway patency may be decreased. In this patient, the risk factors* for post extubation laryngeal edema included prolonged intubation (≥6 days) and the presence of a nasogastric tube that had been placed in the ICU.[34] Normally, a cuff leak represents normal airflow around the ETT after the cuff of the ETT is deflated. Its absence suggests that space is reduced between the ETT and the supraglottic, glottis, or subglottic laryngeal structures. A pooled analysis found a sensitivity and specificity of only 56% and 92%, respectively, however, for predicting upper airway obstruction in adults.[35] This may be due to the fact that reduced cuff leak volumes are explained not only by laryngeal edema, but also by secretions, or by the presence of an ETT that is large for that particular patient's larynx. Cuff leak volume can be detected qualitatively† and quantitatively. Quantitative assessment is performed by deflating the ETT cuff and measuring the difference between inspired and expired tidal volumes of ventilator-delivered breaths during volume-cycled mechanical ventilation.‡[36] Cuff leak volumes less than 110 mL (or <12% to 24% of the delivered tidal volume) have been suggested as thresholds for determining whether airway patency may be diminished. Even though many patients are safely extubated despite an absent cuff leak,[37] it is reasonable to delay extubation if cuff leak is reduced and other risk factors for laryngeal edema are present. If a cuff leak is absent, management strategies include a course of glucocorticoid therapy,§[38] extubation under bronchoscopic guidance, extubation over an airway exchange catheter, or extubation in a controlled environment with an anesthesiologist or other airway specialist at the bedside or in the operating room.[39]

In our patient, we chose to delay extubation for another day. The patient was administered a mild anxiolytic and was assured a good night's sleep. The following day, a weaning trial was again performed, after which the patient was extubated over the flexible bronchoscope and

---

*Other risk factors for laryngeal edema include age greater than 80 years, female gender, an elevated Acute Physiology and Chronic Health Evaluation (APACHE) II score, a Glasgow Coma Scale (GCS) score less than 8, a large endotracheal tube (>8 mm in men, >7 mm in women), a ratio of ETT to laryngeal diameter greater than 45%, a small ratio of patient height to ETT diameter, traumatic intubation, excessive tube mobility due to insufficient fixation, insufficient or lack of sedation, and aspiration.
†The qualitative assessment is done by deflating the ETT cuff and listening for air movement around the ETT using a stethoscope placed over the upper trachea after deflating the ETT cuff.
‡The lowest three expired tidal volumes obtained over six breaths are averaged and then subtracted from the inspired tidal volume to obtain the cuff leak volume.
§One potential regimen in patients with reduced cuff leak volume and with risk factors for post extubation stridor includes administration of methylprednisolone 20 mg intravenously every 4 hours for a total of four doses before extubation.

placed on bilevel positive-pressure ventilation (settings 12/5 cm H_2O). He was successfully weaned from bilevel positive airway pressure (BiPAP) over the next 10 hours. Evidence suggests that noninvasive positive-pressure ventilation may prevent post extubation respiratory failure if it is applied immediately after extubation in patients requiring more than 48 hours of mechanical ventilation and considered at risk for developing post extubation respiratory failure. This includes patients with hypercapnia, congestive heart failure, ineffective cough and excessive tracheobronchial secretions, more than one failure of a weaning trial, multiple comorbidities, and upper airway obstruction.[40] In our opinion, prolonged intubation in a poorly conditioned patient with respiratory failure, one lung, a history of lung cancer, recent general anesthesia, and successful debulking of an obstructing main bronchial obstruction also fits into this category.

Follow-up Tests and Procedures

The final diagnosis after microscopy showed invasive squamous cell carcinoma, moderately differentiated with necrosis. The patient's functional status (Eastern Cooperative Oncology Group [ECOG] 4) was too compromised for him to undergo chemotherapy at that time, and his previous external beam radiation barred further radiation. Local control of the tumor in the left main bronchus after patency was re-established using Nd:YAG laser–assisted rigid debulking could have been possible with the use of high-dose brachytherapy. One of the main advantages of endobronchial brachytherapy (EBT) is its potentially longer-lasting effect and greater tissue penetration when compared with other endobronchial therapies. The effects of brachytherapy extend beyond the airway wall cartilage into the peribronchial tissues.[41] In one study, the median time to symptom relapse was 4 to 8 months for all symptoms, and the median time to symptom progression was 6 to 11 months.[41] EBT was shown to palliate dyspnea, hemoptysis, and cough in patients with poor performance status with a success rate of 53% to 95%[42] and can be used in patients who have already received external beam radiation therapy,* as in our case.[41,43]

High response rates, however, are not consistent among studies. For example, one prospective study evaluated patients who had completed external irradiation at least 1 month before entry into the study. Outpatient bronchoscopic placement of one to three HDR brachytherapy catheters for delivery of 750 to 1000 cGy of intraluminal irradiation was performed every 2 weeks on one to three occasions. Only 5 of 18 patients had radiographic improvement in the extent of atelectasis, and response rates ranged from 25% for signs and symptoms related to pneumonitis to 69% for hemoptysis; performance status improved in only 24% of patients.[43] In another series, on the other hand, when treatment was performed weekly and consisted of three to four 8 to 10 Gy fractions at a radius of 10 mm from the center of the

source, symptomatic relief was obtained for hemoptysis in 74% and for dyspnea and cough in 54%, and a complete bronchoscopic response was noted in 54% of cases. Median survival was 7 months for the entire group.[44] In a review of 11 studies using HDR, overall symptomatic improvement was seen in 60% to 90%, and better rates were reported for controlling hemoptysis.[45] Patients who undergo brachytherapy should be carefully monitored for hemoptysis, which may be fatal in approximately 10% of patients. Although squamous cell pathology may be better controlled locally as compared with other histologic types,[46] bleeding risks are increased.*[47] Regardless of pathology, radiation bronchitis and stenosis ($\approx$10%) may occur weeks to months after treatment, especially in patients who have undergone concurrent external beam radiation therapy or have had prior laser resection.[48]

Another justification for brachytherapy in this patient is that a multimodality bronchoscopic approach may be more effective than a single-modality approach for symptomatic palliation of lung cancer–related CAO. In one study comparing Nd:YAG laser, stent insertion, photodynamic therapy (PDT), or brachytherapy alone with a combination of bronchoscopic interventions such as laser and stent insertion, or laser and stent insertion closely followed by brachytherapy, significant improvements in survival were noted in the multimodality group ($P = .04$). One and 3 year cumulative survival rates for the two groups were 51.3% versus 50%, and 2.3% versus 22%, respectively, during the course of a 14 month follow-up.[49] The type of modality used among patients from the single-modality group had no impact on survival, suggesting that it is restoration of airway patency that counts, not the method used to achieve it. Indeed, one might immediately remove a severe endoluminal exophytic obstruction using Nd:YAG laser–assisted debulking, for instance, and follow that with the use of a delayed effect therapy such as PDT or EBT. Using HDR brachytherapy as part of this strategy has been studied by several investigators[50] and was shown to lessen disease progression and potentially reduce the cost of treatment when compared with repeated Nd:YAG laser treatments alone in advanced NSCLC.†[50]

Referrals

This patient was referred to our institution for the purpose of undergoing rigid bronchoscopic intervention. Once this was performed and the patient was successfully extubated, he was transferred back to his referring hospital. There, he was hospitalized for 1 additional week, during which time he became weaker and had complete loss of appetite. The decision was made to send the patient home with hospice care. Before the time of his transfer, we

---

*Other risk factors for hemoptysis when brachytherapy is used include tumors located in the mainstem or upper lobe bronchi, irradiation in the vicinity of a large vessel, and doses greater than 10 Gy/fraction.

†Results of this study show that the symptom-free period was 2.8 months for the Nd:YAG laser group and increased to 8.5 months for the combination modality group ($P < .05$). The progression-free period of the disease increased from 2.2 months to 7.5 months ($P < .05$), and the number of additional endoscopic treatments was reduced from 15 to 3 ($P < .05$).

---

*In previously nonirradiated patients with a good performance status, high-dose-rate (HDR) brachytherapy cannot be offered as the only modality in primary palliative treatment.

shared additional concerns with the patient and the family. We feared that he was severely malconditioned and depressed. He had lost muscle mass and had been poorly nourished. We suggested an aggressive regimen of bedside physical therapy, placement of a long-term feeding tube to provide enteral nutrition, and use of antidepressants. All were refused.

A few words are warranted with regard to interfacility transportation. In a health care system that comprises tertiary care facilities, regional referral centers, and both community and specialty hospitals, there is a need to practice patient transfers. Movement of patients between facilities is a process that can easily compromise a patient's health, safety, and well-being, in addition to having financial and legal implications.[51] Patient transfers occur for a variety of medical and nonmedical reasons. Certain diagnostic or therapeutic interventions may be unavailable at a transferring facility, for example, or a patient and family may request transfer to another hospital for personal reasons, for convenience (e.g., location), or for insurance reasons (e.g., hospital insurance contracts, network considerations).

Before transfer of a patient like ours is initiated, several parameters must be considered, including distance of travel, the cost-benefit ratio, logistics, specialized equipment needs, and, most important, safety for the patient and for transport personnel. Some authors suggest that ground systems be used for unstable patients when travel distance is less than 30 miles and for stable patients when the distance is less than 100 miles.[52] Ground services may be provided by local Emergency Medical Services or by the transferring or receiving hospital. The decision to transfer our patient to our institution was made expediently once the diagnosis of airway obstruction was made. In many cases, however, patients can lie for days in a hospital bed while families, physicians, and insurers debate the costs and benefits of transfer. Direct communication between physicians at the referral center and accepting physicians at the place of transfer can be helpful. This ensures that clinical information is not lost or misunderstood by intermediaries.[51] To optimize the transfer of an unstable patient, the referring (transferring) physician has the following obligations: (1) Document and discuss with the patient (or surrogates) that the benefits of transfer outweigh the risks, which include delayed care, further injury, disability, and death; (2) obtain informed consent from the patient or family, or implied consent if applicable; (3) arrange for the appropriate mode of transport with qualified personnel and equipment; (4) provide any treatments within the referring physician's scope of practice and hospital capability that minimize the risk involved with the transfer; (5) arrange for a receiving hospital; and (6) deliver all applicable medical records, including diagnostic tests (e.g., imaging studies), to the receiving facility.[53]

Before the transfer occurs, the patient usually has already received the maximum amount of clinical care available from the referring institution. Those hospitals with the capability and capacity to care for patients requiring specialized tests or procedures such as interventional bronchoscopy, which are not available at a transferring facility, must accept the transfer, regardless of the

reason,* including the patient's inability to pay or lack of approval of the transfer by a managed care organization or an insurance provider.[51] Depending on individual state laws, the accepting party does not have to be a physician and may be a hospital administrator, a nurse from a regional referral phone line, or another hospital designee. In our practice, direct communication with the referring physician is routine both before the patient is accepted and post intervention, before the patient's transfer back to the referring facility. However, the actual transfer of the patient is sometimes impeded by lack of financial clearance due to specific health care insurance contracts.

Quality Improvement

We had not consulted the palliative care medicine team on this patient even though published evidence suggests that early referral to this service improves comfort and possibly survival.[54] There is no doubt that it is preferable to have such teams involved because of their familiarity with palliative sedation strategies.[23]

With regard to this patient's family's perceptions of care in the ICU, a moral judgment might have been made by our ICU staff. Sociologic studies show no discretion in reflecting ascribed social and/or moral worth of patients. It is possible, however, that people are valued more or less on the basis of various social characteristics such as age, skin color, ethnicity, level of education, occupation, family status, social class, beauty, personality, talent, and accomplishments.[55,56]

Relevant to this case is that sometimes patients acquire labels even before they arrive at the hospital, potentially by manifesting excessively pessimistic behavior in the setting of respiratory failure. We have seen this in frail older persons with advanced lung cancer, but also in persons dealing with the anger of having become ill or the frustrations of loss of autonomy and independence. This provides an extra argument for individual ICUs to create admission policies that are specific to their unit. We believe that criteria for ICU admission of patients with NSCLC and CAO in respiratory failure requiring mechanical ventilatory support should be explicitly described. This might lead to the selection of patients who are most likely to benefit from ICU care,[9] including those patients who might benefit from palliative or curative bronchoscopic interventions. Relevant to our patient is that as of this writing, the SCCM recommends ICU admission for patients with acute respiratory failure requiring ventilatory support and for patients with airway obstruction, but these patients are given a priority 3, and it has been suggested that limits on therapeutic efforts such as no intubation or cardiopulmonary resuscitation should be set. Given the available evidence, we propose that these guidelines should be revised, and that many patients with acute respiratory failure due to central airway obstruction, whether or not they are already intubated, are very likely to benefit from expert bronchoscopic intervention.

---

*42 USC 1395dd, The Emergency Medical Treatment and Active Labor Act.

DISCUSSION POINTS

1. List two treatment alternatives that will fit the patient's goals.
   - *Palliative bronchoscopic intervention:* Given a patient's desire to be at home and not on the ventilator, one may argue that immediate effect bronchoscopic modalities are more appropriate for this patient. These may include Nd:YAG laser (as done in this case) as well as electrocautery, argon plasma coagulation, and airway stent placement.[42]
   - *Palliative sedation and withdrawal of life-sustaining support:* This is a reasonable alternative in a patient like this, particularly if the patient is not a candidate for further chemoradiotherapy or for bronchoscopic interventions (such as those with endobronchial obstruction and lack of distal lung functionality).
2. List four reasons for bronchoscopic intervention in a patient with malignant central airway obstruction and respiratory failure.
   - Wean off of mechanical ventilation
   - Improve functional status
   - Allow initiation of systemic chemotherapy and external beam radiation
   - Improve survival
3. Describe three risks of bronchial stent insertion in this patient.
   - Perforation of the medial wall of the distal left main bronchus, resulting in broncho-mediastinal fistula, massive hemorrhage, and potentially mediastinal misplacement of the stent
   - Perforation of the posterior membrane, which may cause the complications just listed, along with potentially descending aorta laceration and fatal hemorrhage
   - Hypoventilation and hypoxemia caused by the large stent not unfolding satisfactorily or by occlusion of the stent with mucus or blood after the intervention

Expert Commentary

provided by Solomon Liao, MD, FAAHPM

This case illustrates how a thoughtful review of patient management strategies might help improve care for future patients. I agree, therefore, with the quality improvement statement made by the health care providers, who concluded that palliative medicine could have been consulted earlier in this case. The growing literature suggests that in patients such as the one discussed, palliative care consultation improves not only the quality but also potentially the quantity of the patient's life. The literature also suggests that patient and family satisfaction improves, and that communication in the intensive care unit also improves. Ideally, this consultation could have occurred at the referring hospital to assist both the patient and the patient's family in deciding whether to proceed with bronchoscopic interventions. However, such consultation services may not be available in community hospitals, although their availability is increasing.

The approach of a palliative medicine consultant can be divided into two broadly distinct but related categories. One domain of the palliative medicine consultant is to assist the patient and the family in decision making. The other consists of pain and symptom management. In assisting with decision making, the palliative care team explores with the patient and family their goals of care. The palliative medicine consultant guides the patient and family through the informed decision-making process. The goal is not to tell them what to do, but instead to help them arrive at an answer that fits their priorities. Therefore we are more concerned about the validity of the process rather than the outcome, trusting that if the process is valid, the outcome too will be valid. True informed consent for any procedure requires that all alternatives (and their potential consequences) be explained, including that of not undergoing invasive or minimally invasive procedures. In my opinion, in cases such as the one described, all options are of palliative intent. Therefore a palliative medicine consultant is particularly well suited to assist the patient and family. We discuss a spectrum of care options with patients and their families, from the most aggressive or invasive to the most comfortable, supportive, and natural. As a general rule, I also offer one or two "middle of the road" alternatives because most people can handle only three or four options. We then discuss the advantages and disadvantages of each, always keeping in mind the primary goal of care. An example is provided in the accompanying Table 26-1, in which the primary goal of care is for the patient to be discharged from the hospital and return home.

When alternatives are described, it is essential to avoid confusion and to define carefully terms frequently used by health care providers in end-of-life settings. In this respect, a palliative care consultation can prove to be extremely beneficial. Palliative sedation, for example, must be distinguished from euthanasia* or physician-assisted death,† in that the intended outcome is comfort, not death. Palliative sedation is legal in every state in the United States. Several studies have shown that palliative sedation is effective in relieving symptoms and does not change the survival of end-stage patients.[57,58] Because of these study results, many palliative medicine experts have argued that the ethical principle of double effect is no longer needed to justify the use of palliative sedation. The ethical principle of double effect argues that an intervention intended for good, such as high-dose opioids for the relief of pain, is appropriate, even if it runs the risk of harm, such as shortening a patient's life.

---

*This intervention is used by the physician with the goal of terminating a patient's life and is not legal in the United States.

†This intervention is prescribed by the physician and is used by the patient with the goal of terminating the patient's life. In the United States, physician-assisted death is presently legal only in Oregon, Washington, and Montana.

Table 26-1 Spectrum of Care Options to Achieve the Goal of Going Home

Level of Care	Most Invasive	Middle of the Road	Least Invasive
Care options	Interventional bronchoscopy	Noninvasive ventilation and opioid ± anxiolytic	Palliative sedation
Advantages	Will likely improve quality of life and survival	No procedural risks Still awake and interactive	Ensures complete comfort
Disadvantages	Risk of complications that might prolong hospitalization, leading to dying in the hospital or other severe symptoms	May not be as comfortable	Unable to interact or communicate

Investigators have described several effective pharmacologic agents and approaches to palliative sedation.[59] In practice, the choice of medications depends on the setting of care and other practical considerations. Short-acting benzodiazepines such as midazolam or lorazepam, for example, are generally the first choice in the ICU. My personal approach is to select a benzodiazepine that the patient has been given before. This approach reduces exposure of the patient to a new medication at the end of life, so as to minimize the risk for drug allergies or reactions. We certainly do not want the family's last memory of their loved one to be that of the patient breaking out in a diffuse red rash. If discharge home or transfer to a medical ward is anticipated, then lorazepam is preferred because most nurses outside of the ICU are not comfortable with the use of midazolam. In addition, lorazepam can be administered as a subcutaneous infusion at home. Older patients are more likely to have a "paradoxical" response to benzodiazepines, especially at the middle range of the titration. Because benzodiazepines are frontal lobe disinhibitors, they trigger agitation in older patients and in patients with central nervous system disease before the sedation effect. To avoid this response, an antipsychotic can be given prophylactically, or the benzodiazepine can be rapidly titrated to deep sedation.

Outside of the ICU, barbiturates such as phenobarbital or pentobarbital may be preferred, especially in the geriatric population. These longer-acting medications have the advantage, however, of not wearing off during transportation or when parenteral access is lost, but they are more difficult to titrate. They can also be administered enterally through a feeding tube or rectally. Propofol is the agent of last resort, after standard palliative sedation agents have failed.[60] In many hospitals, propofol is restricted to intubated patients already on ventilators because of its high risk of respiratory depression. Because of the need for close monitoring, its use is limited to the ICU, and it is not practical for patients to use at home.* Ketamine, when used for sedation, is generally restricted to use by anesthesiologists.

Clear titration parameters and goals should be given to nursing staff and pharmacists to distinguish palliative sedation from euthanasia. A sedation scale such as the Richmond Agitation Sedation Scale can be used in the ICU. For non-ICU settings, the degree of sedation should be specified, such as "unresponsive to pain." For patients with respiratory failure, deep sedation is generally warranted, although the degree of sedation may be adjusted according to the goals of care. Various protocols for palliative sedation and ventilator withdrawal have been published.[61] For benzodiazepines in the ICU setting, my personal approach is to give a loading dose double that of the maximum dose the patient had been given previously. We then start an infusion at the same dose per hour as the loading dose and titrate every hour until the sedation goal is achieved—up to 5 times the starting dose. Intravenous barbiturates can be titrated every 4 to 6 hours, using a loading dose of 60 to 100 mg and an initial rate of 30 to 60 mg per hour, depending on the age and size of the patient. A typical therapeutic dose ranges between 50 and 100 mg per hour. Rarely is 120 mg an hour or more needed. Conversion from intravenous to enteral administration is 1:1. Maintenance enteral administration is provided every 8 hours.

Although artificial* hydration and nutrition can be administered during palliative sedation, this generally is not recommended at the end of life. Administration of artificial hydration and nutrition in patients with advanced cardiopulmonary conditions can, in fact, worsen their symptoms. Furthermore, hydration and nutrition have not been shown to prolong survival in end-stage patients.

A final point I would like to mention is that regardless of the palliative care option selected, home care possibilities should be discussed with the patient if possible and of course with the family. These are not always easy conversations, and they must be quite detailed to avoid misunderstandings and to ensure that the appropriate level of care and support is being provided. Consultation with case management and palliative medicine is therefore important. In the United States, it is often necessary to discuss financial matters, such as insurance coverage, possible out-of-pocket expenses for uncovered services, or costs of medications.† In no way should the patient or

---

*Artificial nutrition and/or hydration is an intervention that delivers nutrition and/or fluids by means other than taking something in the mouth and swallowing it.

†Both Medicare and Medicaid provide hospice care and home palliative care. Home palliative care is covered as a skilled need for pain and symptom management. Under Medicare, hospice can provide 24 hour home care if an uncontrolled problem exists that needs continued monitoring and intervention, such as palliative sedation. Hospice pays for all comfort-related measures such as medications, oxygen, and durable medical equipment. Home palliative care does not. On the other hand, while on palliative care, patients may continue to receive interventions such as chemotherapy and radiation and may undergo diagnostic and interventional procedures or blood transfusions, or they may receive parenteral nutrition; these are services that hospice does not cover. Patients can move back and forth between hospice and home palliative care without penalties.

---

*As evidenced by the Michael Jackson case, albeit for a different indication.

the patient's family feel as if they have been abandoned. In my opinion, the patient presented in this chapter could have been discharged directly to hospice without returning to the referring hospital. A direct home discharge, with the approval of the referring physician, would have maximized home time for the patient and family and would have decreased costs to the health care system.

REFERENCES

1. Stanopoulos IT, Beamis JF Jr, Martinez FJ, et al. Laser bronchoscopy in respiratory failure from malignant airway obstruction. *Crit Care Med.* 1993;21:386-391.
2. Colt HC, Harrell J. Therapeutic rigid bronchoscopy allows level of care changes in patients with acute respiratory failure from central airways obstruction. *Chest.* 1997;112:202-206.
3. Shaffer JP, Allen JN. The use of expandable metal stents to facilitate extubation in patients with large airway obstruction. *Chest.* 1998;114:1378-1382.
4. Lo CP, Hsu AA, Eng P. Endobronchial stenting in patients requiring mechanical ventilation for major airway obstruction. *Ann Acad Med Singapore.* 2000;29:66-70.
5. Wood DE, Liu YH, Vallières E, et al. Airway stenting for malignant and benign tracheobronchial stenosis. *Ann Thorac Surg.* 2003;76:167-174.
6. Vonk-Noordegraaf A, Postmus PE, Sutedja TG. Tracheobronchial stenting in the terminal care of cancer patients with central airways obstruction. *Chest.* 2001;120:1811-1814.
7. Jeon K, Kim H, Yu CM, et al. Rigid bronchoscopic intervention in patients with respiratory failure caused by malignant central airway obstruction. *J Thorac Oncol.* 2006;1:319-323.
8. Lemaire A, Burfeind WR, Toloza E, et al. Outcomes of tracheobronchial stents in patients with malignant airway disease. *Ann Thorac Surg.* 2005;80:434-438.
9. Guidelines for intensive care unit admission, discharge, and triage, Task Force of the American College of Critical Care Medicine, Society of Critical Care Medicine. *Crit Care Med.* 1999;27:633-638.
10. Murgu SD, Langer S, Colt HG. Success of bronchoscopic intervention in patients with acute respiratory failure and inoperable central airway obstruction from non small cell lung carcinoma. *Chest.* 2010;138(suppl 4):720A.
11. Angus DC, Barnato AE, Linde-Zwirble WT, et al.; Robert Wood Johnson Foundation ICU End-of-Life Peer Group. Use of intensive care at the end of life in the United States: an epidemiologic study. *Crit Care Med.* 2004;32:638-643.
12. Loggers ET, Maciejewski PK, Paulk E, et al. Racial differences in predictors of intensive end-of-life care in patients with advanced cancer. *J Clin Oncol.* 2009;27:5559-5564.
13. Williams JF, Zimmerman JE, Wagner DP, et al. African-American and white patients admitted to the intensive care unit: is there a difference in therapy and outcome? *Crit Care Med.* 1995;23:626-636.
14. Degenholtz HB, Thomas SB, Miller MJ. Race and the intensive care unit: disparities and preferences for end-of-life care. *Crit Care Med.* 2003;31:S373-S378.
15. Muni S, Engelberg RA, Treece PD, et al. The influence of race/ethnicity and socioeconomic status on end-of-life care in the ICU. *Chest.* 2011;139:1025-1033.
16. Pelosof LC, Gerber DE. Paraneoplastic syndromes: an approach to diagnosis and treatment. *Mayo Clin Proc.* 2010;85:838-854.
17. Slatore CG, Au DH, Gould MK; American Thoracic Society Disparities in Healthcare Group. An official American Thoracic Society systematic review: insurance status and disparities in lung cancer practices and outcomes. *Am J Respir Crit Care Med.* 2010;182:1195-1205.
18. Roetzheim RG, Chirikos TN, Wells KJ, et al. Managed care and cancer outcomes for Medicare beneficiaries with disabilities. *Am J Manag Care.* 2008;14:287-296.
19. Blackhall LJ, Murphy ST, Frank G, et al. Ethnicity and attitudes toward patient autonomy. *JAMA.* 1995;274:820-825.
20. Morrison RS, Zayas LH, Mulvihill M, et al. Barriers to completion of healthcare proxy forms: a qualitative analysis of ethnic differences. *J Clin Ethics.* 1998;9:118-126.
21. American Heart Association. Standards and guidelines for cardiopulmonary resuscitation (CPR) and emergency cardiac care (ECC): medicolegal considerations and recommendations. *JAMA.* 1974;227(suppl):864-866.
22. Gehlbach TG, Shinkunas LA, Forman-Hoffman VL, et al. Code status orders and goals of care in the medical ICU. *Chest.* 2011;139:802-809.
23. Olsen ML, Swetz KM, Mueller PS. Ethical decision making with end-of-life care: palliative sedation and withholding or withdrawing life-sustaining treatments. *Mayo Clin Proc.* 2010;85:949-954.
24. Reddy SP, Marks JE. Total atelectasis of the lung secondary to malignant airway obstruction: response to radiation therapy. *Am J Clin Oncol.* 1990;13:394-400.
25. Shirakawa T, Ishida A, Miyazu Y, et al. Endobronchial ultrasound for difficult airway problems. In: Bolliger CT, Herth FJF, Mayo PH, et al., eds. *Clinical Chest Ultrasound: From the ICU to the Bronchoscopy Suite.* Basel: Karger; 2009:189-201.
26. Chhajed PN, Baty F, Pless M, et al. Outcome of treated advanced non-small cell lung cancer with and without central airway obstruction. *Chest.* 2006;130:1803-1807.
27. Hawkins J. Making autonomous decisions: million dollar baby. In: Colt HG, Quadrelli S, Friedman L, eds. *The Picture of Health: Medical Ethics and the Movies.* New York: Oxford University Press; 2011.
28. Waisel DB, Truog RD. The end-of-life sequence. *Anesthesiology.* 1997;87:676-686.
29. Thompson BL, Lawson D, Croughan-Minihane M, et al. Do patients' ethnic and social factors influence the use of do not resuscitate orders? *Ethn Dis.* 1999;9:132-139.
30. Walker RM. DNR in the OR: resuscitation as an operative risk. *JAMA.* 1991;266:2407-2412.
31. Truog RD, Waisel DB, Burns JP. DNR in the OR: a goal-directed approach. *Anesthesiology.* 1999;90:289-295.
32. Waisel DB, Burns JP, Johnson JA, et al. Guidelines for perioperative do-not-resuscitate policies. *J Clin Anesth.* 2002;14:467-473.
33. Seckler AB, Meier DE, Mulvihill M, et al. Substituted judgment: how accurate are proxy predictions? *Ann Intern Med.* 1991;115:92-98.
34. Kriner EJ, Shafazand S, Colice GL. The endotracheal tube cuff-leak test as a predictor for postextubation stridor. *Respir Care.* 2005;50:1632-1638.
35. Ochoa ME, Marín Mdel C, Frutos-Vivar F, et al. Cuff-leak test for the diagnosis of upper airway obstruction in adults: a systematic review and meta-analysis. *Intensive Care Med.* 2009;35:1171-1179.
36. Miller RL, Cole RP. Association between reduced cuff leak volume and postextubation stridor. *Chest.* 1996;110:1035-1040.
37. Engoren M. Evaluation of the cuff-leak test in a cardiac surgery population. *Chest.* 1999;116:1029.
38. Epstein SK. Preventing postextubation respiratory failure. *Crit Care Med.* 2006;34:1547.
39. Mort TC. Continuous airway access for the difficult extubation: the efficacy of the airway exchange catheter. *Anesth Analg.* 2007;105:1357-1362.
40. Nava S, Gregoretti C, Fanfulla F, et al. Noninvasive ventilation to prevent respiratory failure after extubation in high-risk patients. *Crit Care Med.* 2005;33:2465-2470.
41. Mallick I, Sharma SC, Behera D. Endobronchial brachytherapy for symptom palliation in non-small cell lung cancer—analysis of symptom response, endoscopic improvement and quality of life. *Lung Cancer.* 2007;55:313-318.
42. Vergnon JM, Huber RM, Moghissi K. Place of cryotherapy, brachytherapy and photodynamic therapy in therapeutic bronchoscopy of lung cancers. *Eur Respir J.* 2006;28:200-218.
43. Hernandez P, Gursahaney A, Roman T, et al. High dose rate brachytherapy for the local control of endobronchial carcinoma following external irradiation. *Thorax.* 1996;51:354-358.
44. Taulelle M, Chauvet B, Vincent P, et al. High dose rate endobronchial brachytherapy: results and complications in 189 patients. *Eur Respir J.* 1998;11:162-168.
45. Michailidou I, Becker HD, Eberhardt R. Bronchoscopy high dose rate brachytherapy. In: Strausz J, Bolliger CR, eds. *Interventional Pulmonology.* Lausanne, Switzerland: European Respiratory Society; 2010:173-189.
46. Huber RM, Fischer R, Hautmann H, et al. Does additional brachytherapy improve the effect of external irradiation? A prospective,

randomized study in central lung tumors. *Int J Radiat Oncol Biol Phys.* 1997;38:533-540.

47. Hara R, Itami J, Aruga T, et al. Risk factors for massive hemoptysis after endobronchial brachytherapy in patients with tracheobronchial malignancies. *Cancer.* 2001;92:2623-2627.

48. Speiser B, Spratling L. Intermediate dose rate remote afterloading brachytherapy for intraluminal control of bronchogenic carcinoma. *Int J Radiat Oncol Biol Phys.* 1990;18:1443-1448.

49. Santos RS, Raftopoulos Y, Keenan RJ, et al. Bronchoscopic palliation of primary lung cancer: single or multimodality therapy? *Surg Endosc.* 2004;18:931-936.

50. Chella A, Ambrogi MC, Ribechini A, et al. Combined Nd-YAG laser/HDR brachytherapy versus Nd-YAG laser only in malignant central airway involvement: a prospective randomized study. *Lung Cancer.* 2000;27:169-175.

51. Blackwell TH. Interfacility transports. *Semin Respir Crit Care Med.* 2002;23:11-18.

52. Brink LW, Neuman B, Wynn J. Air transport. *Pediatr Clin North Am.* 1993;40:439-456.

53. Bitterman RA. EMTALA. In: Henry GL, Sullivan DJ, eds. *Emergency Medicine Risk Management: A Comprehensive Review.* 2nd ed. Dallas, Tex: American College of Emergency Physicians; 1997: 103-123.

54. Temel JS, Greer JA, Muzikansky A, et al. Early palliative care for patients with metastatic non-small-cell lung cancer. *N Engl J Med.* 2010;363:733-742.

55. Glaser BG, Strauss AL. The social loss of dying patients. *Am J Nurs.* 1964;64:119-121.

56. Hill TE. How clinicians make (or avoid) moral judgments of patients: implications of the evidence for relationships and research. *Philos Ethics Humanit Med.* 2010;5:11.

57. Mercadante S, Intravaia G, Villari P, et al. Controlled sedation for refractory symptoms in dying patients. *J Pain Symptom Manage.* 2009;37:771-779.

58. Maltoni M, Pittureri C, Scarpi E, et al. Palliative sedation therapy does not hasten death: results from a prospective multicenter study. *Ann Oncol.* 2009;20:1163-1169.

59. Cherny NI, Radbruch L; Board of the European Association for Palliative Care. European Association for Palliative Care (EAPC) recommended framework for the use of sedation in palliative care. *Palliat Med.* 2009;23:581-593.

60. Treece PD, Engelberg RA, Crowley L, et al. Evaluation of a standardized order form for the withdrawal of life support in the intensive care unit. *Crit Care Med.* 2004;32:1141-1148.

61. Dalal S, Del Fabbro E, Bruera E. Is there a role for hydration at the end of life? *Curr Opin Support Palliat Care.* 2009;3:72-78.

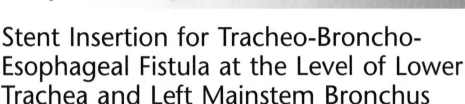

Chapter 27

Stent Insertion for Tracheo-Broncho-Esophageal Fistula at the Level of Lower Trachea and Left Mainstem Bronchus

This chapter emphasizes the following elements of the Four Box Approach: techniques and instrumentation; results and procedure-related complications; and outcome assessment.

CASE DESCRIPTION

A 74-year-old male with a 25–pack-year smoking history developed hoarseness and dysphagia to solid and semisolid foods. Symptoms progressed to intractable cough and pneumonia. He had a 40 pound weight loss over the last few months before admission to the hospital. Flexible bronchoscopy showed an immobile left vocal cord and a mass penetrating the posterior wall of the left main bronchus (LMB). Biopsy revealed squamous cell carcinoma of the esophagus. Initially, the patient declined treatment, but when he became unable to swallow at all and developed a severe productive cough, a percutaneous gastrostomy tube was placed. Flexible bronchoscopy this time showed a large tracheo-broncho-esophageal fistula, prompting transfer to our institution for further care. Vital signs revealed HR of 115/min, RR of 23/min, temperature of 100° F, and blood pressure of 100/60 mm Hg. Coarse rhonchi were heard bilaterally, as was a focal wheeze on the left during forced exhalation, accompanied by decreased breath sounds at the base of the left lung. Laboratory markers were significant for albumin 1.6, WBC 14, and hemoglobin 11. Chest radiograph showed patchy bilateral infiltrates, dense left lower lobe opacification, and a left suprahilar mass. A repeat flexible bronchoscopy at our institution revealed a 3 cm fistula at the junction of the posterior and lateral walls of the LMB, extending proximally to the lower trachea (see video on ExpertConsult. com) (Video VI.27.1). Associated compression of the LMB and a distorted main carina were noted. A silicone Y stent was placed at the main carina via rigid bronchoscopy (Figure 27-1).

DISCUSSION POINTS

1. What is the expected survival in this patient with and without treatment of the malignant esophago-respiratory fistula?
2. List three therapeutic alternatives for occluding an esophago-respiratory fistula.
3. List three expected benefits derived from stent insertion in this patient.

CASE RESOLUTION

Initial Evaluations

Physical Examination, Complementary Tests, and Functional Status Assessment

Most adults with esophago-respiratory fistulas (ERFs) have the acquired form of disease comprising tracheo-esophageal, broncho-esophageal, or tracheo-broncho-esophageal fistulas. Their prognosis and management depend on whether the fistula is the result of a benign process or a malignancy, with the latter usually due to primary esophageal cancer. In one series of 264 patients with malignant ERF, 243 (92%) had esophageal cancer, 19 (7%) had lung cancer, and 2 (1%) had mediastinal tumor.[1] Results from studies show an overall frequency of ERF in patients with esophageal cancer of 5% to 10%, but fistulas may be more common toward the terminal stage of the disease.[1] Compared with patients without ERF, those with esophageal cancer and ERF present at a more advanced stage of disease, have more frequent involvement of the upper to mid-thoracic esophagus, and have a longer segment of tumor. Although the median time from diagnosis of esophageal cancer to the development of a fistula is approximately 8 months, our patient was diagnosed with ERF only 2 months after his initial diagnosis. ERF can be the presenting manifestation of cancer in approximately 6% of cases.[1] The median survival time after diagnosis of ERF is only 8 weeks.[2]

During initial evaluation of these patients, a thorough oncologic treatment history is important because the use of some antiangiogenesis drugs such as bevacizumab, along with radiation therapy, has been linked to the development of malignant ERF.[3] Nonmalignant causes of ERF include complications of mechanical ventilation or indwelling tracheal or esophageal stents, complications from prior tracheal or esophageal surgery, granulomatous mediastinal infection (tuberculosis, syphilis, histoplasmosis), trauma (blunt or penetrating), and ingestion of caustic or foreign bodies. A large study from the Mayo Clinic found that esophageal surgery was the most common cause of nonmalignant ERF.[4]

Regardless of its origin, ERF is a life-threatening condition with severe pulmonary complications consisting of ongoing tracheobronchial bacterial contamination and impaired nutrition.[4] Patients present with intractable cough, recurrent respiratory infections, rapid deterioration, and death, if left untreated.[2,5,6] In a study of 207

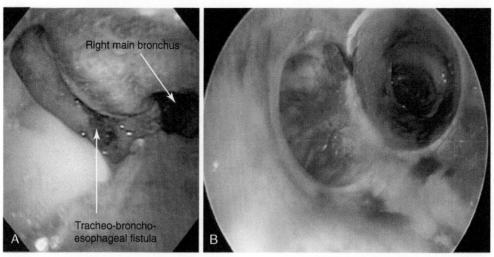

Figure 27-1 A, Flexible bronchoscopy revealed the fistula at the junction of the posterior and lateral walls of the left main bronchus (LMB), extending proximally to the lower trachea. **B,** Rigid bronchoscopy shows the silicone Y stent placed at the main carina.

malignant trachea-esophageal fistulas (TEFs), symptoms and signs included cough in 116 (56%), aspiration in 77 (37%), fever in 52 (25%), dysphagia in 39 (19%), pneumonia in 11 (5%), hemoptysis in 10 (5%), and chest pain in 10 (5%).[7] Our patient's aspiration probably was worsened by his left recurrent laryngeal nerve palsy, causing an immobile left vocal cord (see video on ExpertConsult. com) (Video VI.27.2). Seen in approximately 10% of patients with ERF, this finding contributes to swallowing difficulties and periodic or constant aspiration.[1]

Comorbidities

This patient had pneumonia, was hospitalized, and had a poor performance status (Eastern Cooperative Oncology Group [ECOG]/Zubrod 4).* His pneumonia resulted in sepsis, but no evidence was found of other organ dysfunction that could have interfered with anesthesia and perioperative care. He was severely malnourished, as manifested by his anemia and hypoproteinemia. Wound healing, in particular healing of the anastomosis in case surgery is performed, would be expected to be poor. Muscle wasting reduces respiratory reserve and the patient's ability to breathe, cough, and clear secretions.[8]

Support System

This gentleman had a supportive wife. Married patients have been shown to have a lower risk of death than unmarried patients, independent of socioeconomic status.[9] In addition, relevant to this case, married patients suffering from esophageal carcinoma report higher baseline quality of life with regard to legal concerns (e.g., having a will, advance directives) and friend and family support compared with single patients. Over time, married patients may have a decrease in pain frequency compared with single patients.[10]

*Completely disabled; cannot carry out any self-care; totally confined to bed or chair.

Patient Preferences and Expectations

Our patient showed understanding of the gravity of his diagnosis. Patients with ERF have a poor prognosis, and many patients die from respiratory infection and malnutrition within a month of diagnosis.[11] Control of pulmonary contamination provides an opportunity for secondary treatment, as well as for improved survival and quality of life. Therefore treatment should include closure of the fistula and re-establishment of oral intake in a timely and cost-efficient manner, while minimizing the need for secondary medical interventions. Our patient wished he could eat and breathe better during the time he had left to live, but he did not want to be a burden to his wife. A significant proportion of caregivers of patients with esophageal cancer experience high levels of strain and psychological distress. Support and services targeted specifically at reducing the considerable strain of caring for patients with esophageal cancer are necessary, particularly for caregivers of patients from lower socioeconomic groups.[12]

Procedural Strategies

Indications

Treatment must correct the two problems of airway contamination and poor nutrition. Reflux of gastric contents is diminished by placement of a gastrostomy tube, and adequate nutrition is sometimes facilitated by insertion of a jejunostomy tube. Treatment depends on whether the patient is resectable and medically fit for surgical therapy. Like our patient, most patients have advanced disease and can be treated only with palliative measures, which involve restoration of the swallowing mechanism and prevention of aspiration. The current standard of palliative therapy for patients with malignant ERF is endoscopic or radiologic placement of esophageal-covered self-expanding metallic stents (SEMS), allowing closure of the fistula. Less common treatment options for selected patients with malignant ERF include chemotherapy and

Figure 27-2 A, Flexible bronchoscopy shows severe tracheal obstruction from esophageal carcinoma and associated tracheoesophageal fistula (TEF). **B,** Rigid bronchoscopy immediately after the TEF is covered with a straight, studded silicone stent.

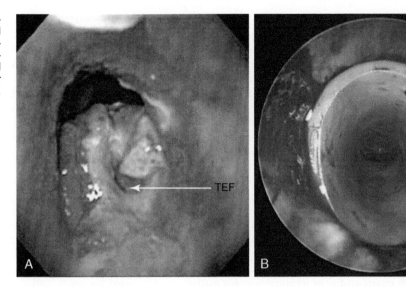

radiation, surgical bypass, esophageal exclusion, and fistula resection and repair.[13] Our patient's functional status and concurrent aspiration pneumonia precluded surgical treatment, chemotherapy, or radiotherapy. We chose to proceed first with silicone airway stent insertion with the goal of palliating left main bronchial patency and covering the fistula, followed by esophageal stent insertion to help prevent aspiration and facilitate oral food intake.

Contraindications

No absolute contraindications to stent insertion or general anesthesia were noted. Given the patient's age and extensive smoking history, a cardiology evaluation was requested before intervention. He was considered to be at intermediate risk (1% to 5%) for cardiac death or nonfatal myocardial infarction. Blood gas analysis showed a partial pressure of oxygen in arterial blood (PaO_2) of 55 mm Hg and an arterial carbon dioxide tension ($PaCO_2$) of 60 mm Hg on room air. The risk associated with this degree of $PaCO_2$ elevation is not prohibitive for a necessary intervention, although it should lead to reassessment of the indication for the proposed procedure and aggressive preoperative preparation. Although preoperative hypoxemia and postoperative pulmonary complications may be associated in patients undergoing surgery,[14] hypoxemia generally has not been identified as a significant independent predictor of complications after adjustment for potential confounders.

Expected Results

Palliation for malignant ERF is usually achieved with endoscopic placement of esophageal, airway, or parallel (dual) stent insertion (in the esophagus and airway). Dual stent insertion appears to work better than a single prosthesis. Particular attention should be paid to airway compression or erosion caused by esophageal stents, prompting some authorities to initially place an airway stent before placing the esophageal one, especially if significant tracheobronchial obstruction is a matter of concern (Figure 27-2). Results from small case series show that respiratory distress can occur from severe airway

obstruction caused by extrinsic compression after esophageal stent insertion.[15] Silicone or covered metallic stents may be preferred for the airway to prevent recurrence of airway narrowing by growth of tumor between the wires of metal stents. For instance, one study evaluated the clinical benefits and complications of studded silicone stent insertion in 35 patients, of whom 6 had ERF. Three of 6 patients showed resolution of the fistula, and 3 other patients improved symptomatically.[16] Symptoms of ERF usually improve after double stent insertion. ERF symptoms may recur as the result of stent-induced pressure necrosis of tracheal and esophageal walls. In addition to fistula enlargement, other complications described with stents placed in the esophagus, in the airway, or after dual stent insertion include pain, reflux, stent migration or fracture, restenosis, massive bleeding, aspiration, airway obstruction, tumor overgrowth, and food impaction.[1,17]

Team Experience

A multidisciplinary approach involving the gastroenterologist, the interventional pulmonologist, the oncologist, and the thoracic surgeon may be helpful. Patients with ERF are prone to develop worsening wall perforation and erosion because of the nature of malignant infiltration, stent-induced necrosis, or concurrent or previously applied radiotherapy and chemotherapy. Locations, the number of stents, and their type and size should be discussed.[18] Some prefer to insert an esophageal stent, an airway stent, and a percutaneous endoscopic gastrostomy tube at the same time, during a single session with the patient under general anesthesia.[19] Others perform procedures sequentially. Interventions performed by different services need to be coordinated, so good communication among treating teams is necessary.

Therapeutic Alternatives

Treatment is individualized and may include esophageal stenting, tracheobronchial stenting, simultaneous stenting of the trachea and esophagus, esophageal exclusion, esophageal bypass, fistula resection, and repair and radiation therapy.[18] Direct surgical fistula closure or resection does not yield satisfactory results in this population. In general, surgical esophageal bypass can resolve respiratory contamination and allow fairly normal swallowing, but it should be reserved for patients who can tolerate a major operation. Esophageal stent insertion helps prevent aspiration and allows swallowing. This procedure can be offered to nearly all patients, regardless of their physiologic condition. The most effective reported treatments are esophageal bypass and esophageal stent insertion. When performed promptly after diagnosis, these treatments may improve survival and quality of life.[13] Discussion of available treatment modalities is warranted among treating team members, and specific indications, contraindications, advantages, and disadvantages of each should be shared with patients and their families.

1. *Surgical treatment:* Surgical procedures carry high morbidity and mortality with relatively poor results.[7] Possible treatments for malignant ERF include resection of the esophagus, collar esophagostomy with gastrostomy or jejunostomy for nutrition, and esophageal bypass.[1] Given the patient's short life expectancy and poor state of health, reconstructive surgical interventions usually are not considered. Studies from centers with access to experienced thoracic and esophageal surgeons have shown that in selected patients, palliation and prolonged survival are obtained with surgical bypass, the hallmark of which is leaving the ERF in place while diverting oral intake retrosternally with the stomach or the colon. In 21 patients with malignant ERF, gastric bypass with lower esophageal exclusion (aka Kirschner operation)* provided a beneficial palliative effect despite a high risk of operative mortality. An overall 30 day mortality of 38% prompted authors to recommend this procedure for patients who do not tolerate stents or in whom stent deployment was unsuccessful, as well as for patients who are in good general health and without respiratory complications that might compromise surgery.[20] Median survival of 55 days, median length of stay in the ICU of 6 days, and hospitalization duration of 17 days raise concerns regarding the quality of life of these terminally ill patients. Furthermore, the very high mortality rate might be considered unacceptable from a health care economics perspective. In another case series of 207 patients with malignant ERF, the percentage of patients alive at 3, 6, and 12 months was 13%, 4%, and 1% in case of supportive care (n = 104); 17%, 3%, and 0%, respectively, for esophageal exclusion (n = 29); 21%, 14%, and 0% for esophageal prosthesis (n = 14); 30%, 15%, and 5% for radiation therapy (n = 20); and 46%, 20%, and 7% for esophageal bypass. Patients treated with radiation therapy and esophageal bypass had prolonged survival compared with patients treated by other means.[7] Based on these data, it seems that esophageal bypass probably offers the best palliation for operable patients.* In general, surgical bypass is reserved for patients with a very large fistula and for those in whom permanent stent placement is unsuccessful or inadvisable, provided patients are in good physical condition, and that general anesthesia and orotracheal intubation are technically feasible.[21]

2. *DJ fistula stent:* This cufflink-shaped prosthesis (Bryan Corp., Woburn, Mass) is designed exclusively for closure of malignant ERF secondary to esophageal or lung cancer. It can be sized to the fistula diameter to occlude the abnormal communication.[18] The stent consists of a top portion, which seals the tracheal defect; a vertical axis, which blocks the passage between the trachea and the esophagus; and a lower ellipse-shaped portion, which anchors the stent in position in the esophageal lumen.[22]

3. *Esophageal stent insertion:* A covered expandable esophageal stent (SEMS) can relieve symptoms in more than 80% of patients with malignant ERF.[18,23] Placement of an SEMS is emerging as a superior alternative to the use of nonexpandable esophageal prostheses and other treatment methods such as percutaneous gastrostomy or surgical esophageal bypass, in terms of successful treatment of malignant dysphagia and associated complications.[24] Fistula occlusion was shown to be more successful with SEMS (92%) than with conventional nonexpanding stents (77%). Reintervention was required more commonly with SEMS[21] but without the frequency of complications such as perforation, hemorrhage, pressure necrosis, obstruction, dislodgment, and migration, which occur in approximately 15% to 40% of patients with nonexpandable esophageal prostheses.[25] Successful closure of ERF by esophageal stent placement improved survival and quality of life in a case series of 264 patients; procedure-related mortality was 0.5%. Mean survival for all patients was 2.8 months, but it was 3.4 months in patients with an implanted endoprosthesis† and less than 2 months in those with only supportive therapy.[1] Stents with barbed covered metallic anchors to the mucosa were used successfully to prevent stent migration in a case series of 20

---

*The Kirschner operation was carried out in all patients with retrosternal tubulization of the stomach and exclusion of the lower end of the esophagus using a Roux-en-Y loop or ligature. This procedure could be proposed to patients with fistula located in the thoracic esophagus, even in the upper third. Obviously, patients with fistula involving the cervical esophagus could not benefit from this technique.

---

*This management is different than management for nonmalignant TEFs, for which several differing approaches have been proposed but the optimal management strategy remains controversial. Direct suture closure of both tracheal and esophageal defects, segmental tracheal resection and primary anastomosis with direct esophageal closure, tracheal closure using an esophageal patch, closure of the defects with soft tissue flaps, a combined surgical and endoscopic approach, and a two-stage approach with esophageal diversion and primary closure of the tracheal defect have all been advocated. In one of the largest published series, 35 patients underwent surgical repair of acquired nonmalignant fistula between the airway and the esophagus. In this population, single-stage primary repair of airway and esophageal defects with tissue flap interposition was performed successfully in most patients, with an overall surgical mortality of 5.7%.[4]

†Stents used were covered and included mainly a steel wire–armored Haring endoprosthesis (Rusch), Wilson-Cook tubes (Wilson-Cook Medical), and Ultraflex self-expanding stents (Boston Scientific).

patients.[26] Esophageal stents can be inserted with the patient under general anesthesia via rigid esophagoscopy, or via flexible esophagoscopy with moderate sedation.[27,28]

4. *Dual stent insertion (esophagus and airways):* This approach has been proposed when fistula occlusion is not achieved by the esophageal or airway prosthesis alone.[29-31] This technique has yielded better results than stents in the airway or the esophagus alone. In such cases, as with our patient, the airway stent should be placed before the esophageal one to prevent airway compression secondary to the esophageal prosthesis.[17,24,32] Some experts consider early double stent insertion when the location, volume, and extent of esophageal and respiratory disease predispose to erosion and further rupture of the airway or esophageal wall.[23,30,33]

5. *Supportive care:* This consists of operative gastrostomy, percutaneous endoscopic gastrostomy, parenteral nutrition, intravenous rehydration, and antibiotic and analgesic therapy. In one of the largest series reviewing the outcomes of 207 patients with malignant ERF, patients who received supportive care alone survived a median of only 22 days.[7]

Cost-Effectiveness

One comparative study evaluated the survival time and quality of life of patients who received different treatments for malignant ERF.[17] Thirty-five patients diagnosed with malignant ERF secondary to esophageal cancer were nonrandomly divided into three groups: (1) 17 patients who received esophageal self-expandable Nitinol stents, (2) 9 patients who received laparoscopic gastrostomy, and (3) a control group of 9 patients who refused both stent insertion and gastrostomy. Authors found no statistically significant difference in survival time, but palliation of respiratory symptoms was best achieved in the stent group versus the gastrostomy group or controls. Patients in the stent group had better quality of life as graded by a quality-of-life questionnaire, particularly with regard to dyspnea, dysphagia, eating problems, dry mouth, cough, and hypersalivation. Dual stent insertion (esophagus and airways) is widely accepted when fistula occlusion is not achieved by esophageal or airway stent alone.[30,31,33]

Informed Consent

The patient and his wife were told that the goal of intervention was purely palliative. They showed understanding of the indications, alternatives, and potential associated complications. Both were able to describe the planned procedure and had realistic expectations regarding its results. They agreed to proceed with rigid bronchoscopy under general anesthesia with silicone stent placement.

Techniques and Results

Anesthesia and Perioperative Care

Several anesthesia-related problems are seen in patients with ERF. If face mask ventilation is not possible, spontaneous ventilation should be maintained until the rigid bronchoscope has been positioned successfully. We prefer employing spontaneous ventilation, but this may be difficult because the stimulation produced by the rigid bronchoscope is sometimes such that it is difficult to have a spontaneously breathing patient sufficiently anesthetized to tolerate the bronchoscope. Although the rigid bronchoscope has a port for ventilation, establishment of controlled ventilation is expected to be somewhat compromised because oxygen delivered through the bronchoscope can be diverted through the large fistula to the esophagus, instead of to the lungs.[34] Theoretically, this could also increase the size of the fistula and decrease tidal volume, resulting in an inability to ventilate the lungs effectively. Massive loss of tidal volume is uncommon in clinical practice, but the patient's spontaneous ventilation probably should not be abolished until it has been demonstrated that it is possible to inflate the lungs by gentle manual ventilation.[8] The amount of gas lost through the fistula depends on airway pressure and lung compliance, in addition to the size of the defect. The lung on the side of the fistula is likely to be contaminated and therefore less compliant than the contralateral lung; thus the contralateral lung tends to be ventilated preferentially. If the patient does not already have an esophageal stent, the expected difficulty of ventilation can be solved by partially sealing the fistula from the esophageal side with an esophageal balloon. In this regard, use of high-frequency jet ventilation might be considered because it offers the theoretical advantage of potentially reducing gas loss through the fistula.

The presence of the fistula presents two additional problems: First, vigorous manual ventilation should be avoided before intubation because this tends to force gas through the fistula and may produce intestinal distention. When severe, this can lead to gastric rupture, hypotension, and cardiac arrest.[8] The marked increase in intra-abdominal and intrathoracic pressures may affect venous return, producing cardiovascular depression. Second, most patients with ERF suffer from pulmonary aspiration of esophago-gastric contents. It is possible that further contamination of the less affected lung may occur before isolation of the fistula. Gentle ventilation with avoidance of gastric distention should minimize this risk. Frequent bronchial hygiene may be necessary to remove secretions during and after anesthesia.

Instrumentation

We had available a variety of large-channel ventilating bronchoscopes but planned on intubating the patient with a 13 mm Efer-Dumon bronchoscope (Bryan Corp.) to allow deployment of a large silicone Y stent (16 mm × 13 mm × 13 mm) at the level of the main carina. These stents were shown to reduce dyspnea and recurrent infection in patients with airway fistulas.[35]

Anatomic Dangers and Other Risks

Enlargement of the fistula is possible during airway stent insertion and manipulation. Inadvertent mediastinal insertion or migration of airway stents has been reported (Figure 27-3).[36] Other risks associated with dual stent insertion include massive bleeding, uncontrollable esophago-airway fistula, mediastinitis, pneumothorax, and vascular fistulas.[37,38]

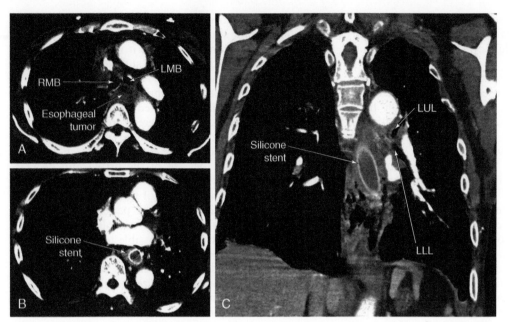

Figure 27-3 A, Axial chest computed tomography (CT) view from a patient with esophago-respiratory fistula resulting from esophageal cancer. **B,** After silicone stent insertion, the stent had migrated into necrotic mediastinal tumor tissues adjacent to the descending aorta. **C,** The coronal chest CT image shows the stent in the mediastinum and distant from the normal airway. *LMB,* Left main bronchus; *LLL,* left lower lobe; *LUL,* left upper lobe; *RMB,* right main bronchus.

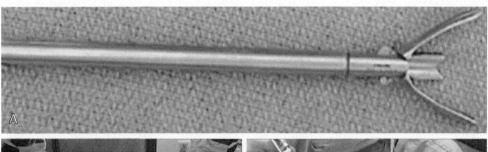

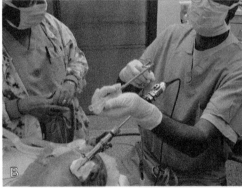

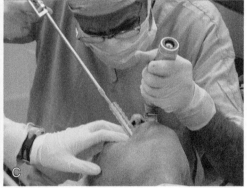

Figure 27-4 A, The Rusch forceps. **B,** Grasping of the Y stent with the Rusch forceps. **C,** Placement of the Y stent using Rusch forceps under direct laryngoscopy.

Results and Procedure-Related Complications

With the patient under general anesthesia with spontaneous-assisted ventilation, a 13 mm Efer-Dumon ventilating bronchoscope was inserted without difficulty into the patient's trachea. Bronchial hygiene was performed using the flexible scope. The fistula was seen in the lower trachea and the proximal left main bronchus (LMB), extending for 3 cm at the junction between the posterior and lateral walls of the LMB. The esophagus could be seen herniating into and obstructing the LMB (see video on ExpertConsult.com) (Video VI.27.1). The Y stent was tailored to extend 5 cm into the LMB and 1 cm into the right main bronchus (RMB) because the orifice of the right upper lobe (RUL) was only 1 cm

below the carina. Y stents are usually deployed using a pullback or a push technique. When the pullback technique is used, the stent can be deployed in its entirety into the ipsilateral bronchus using the stent pusher or even the rigid telescope. The tracheal limb then is grasped with forceps and pulled back gently until the contralateral limb of the stent deploys into the contralateral bronchus (see video on ExpertConsult.com) (Video VI.27.3).

In our patient, a Y stent could not be loaded because the specially designed introducer system had been lost that morning in sterile processing. Instead, the rigid bronchoscope was removed, and a Rusch forceps was used to promptly insert the stent via direct laryngoscopy (Figure 27-4). Once the stent was inside the airway, the patient was reintubated with an 11 mm Efer-Dumon rigid bronchoscope, and forceps was used to ensure that the stent was securely in position, and that the fistula was entirely covered (see Figure 27-1). The patient was extubated uneventfully and was transferred to the ICU for monitoring.

Long-Term Management

Outcome Assessment

The patient's dyspnea and secretions improved immediately after intervention. During the same hospitalization, he underwent endoscopy and placement of an 18 mm × 90 mm fully covered metallic esophageal stent 4 days later. On day 5, he was able to tolerate oral food intake, and discharge was planned in the next 48 hours. In view of his poor prognosis, hospice care was addressed with the patient and his wife.

Follow-up Tests and Procedures

After stent placement, bronchoscopy can be performed to evaluate occlusion of the fistula by the stent. If the stent completely seals the fistula, the patient is allowed a soft diet 2 hours after the procedure and is encouraged to resume a tolerable diet as soon as possible. Esophagography can be performed within 7 days after stent placement and every 1 to 2 months thereafter to evaluate ERF occlusion and stent position.[39]

Three days after esophageal stent placement, however, our patient developed massive hemoptysis and acute respiratory failure requiring emergent intubation with a No. 6 cuffless endotracheal tube. Emergent bronchoscopy showed a large amount of blood flowing from the left main bronchus and spilling into the trachea and right bronchial tree (see video on ExpertConsult.com) (Video VI.27.4). The patient was immediately turned toward the left lateral decubitus position, and continuous suction of bright red blood was performed while we actively commenced resuscitation. The bleeding was emerging from the distal left main bronchus, but the exact location could not be visualized bronchoscopically. Given the nature of the massive active hemorrhage, a bronchovascular fistula was the likely cause. The bleeding was stopped by insertion of an endobronchial blocker; the patient regained consciousness, and the next day he was extubated, but because he was not a candidate for surgical interventions, supportive care was provided. Two days later, massive hemoptysis recurred and the patient expired. Autopsy was offered but was declined by his wife.

Quality Improvement

We did not use existing validated tools to assess this patient's quality of life. One such instrument (QLQ-OG25), designed for patients with esophageal cancer, has six scales pertaining to dysphagia, eating restrictions, reflux, odynophagia, pain, and anxiety. These scales have good reliability and are able to distinguish quality of life differences among different tumor sites and disease stages.[40] Given our patient's dismal prognosis, we probably should have involved palliative care and hospice services earlier during his hospitalization. Although our goal was to eliminate dysphagia and improve quality of life, it is possible that in view of his very poor general health status,

an indwelling percutaneous feeding tube and general palliative measures should have been offered instead of endoscopic and bronchoscopic interventions. Continuity of health and life might have been enhanced through a hospice home care program and appropriate comfort measures to alleviate terminal symptoms that would have allowed our patient to die with dignity and without suffering the effects of cardiopulmonary resuscitation.[41]

DISCUSSION POINTS

1. What is the expected survival in this patient with and without treatment of the malignant esophago-respiratory fistula?
   - The mean survival period of all patients with ERF was 2.8 months in one study, but in patients with esophageal stents it was 3.4 months. With only supportive therapy, it was 1.3 months.[1] Overall median survival time after diagnosis of ERF is only 8 weeks.[2]
2. List three therapeutic alternatives for occluding an esophago-respiratory fistula.
   - Esophageal stent insertion
   - Dual airway and esophageal stent insertion
   - Surgical esophageal bypass
3. List three expected benefits dervived from stent insertion in this patient.
   - Improved quality of life and potentially survival[13]
   - Improved dyspnea
   - Reduced aspiration and recurrent pulmonary infections[31-33,35]

Expert Commentary

provided by Heinrich D. Becker, MD, FCCP

In their treatment of this complex problem, the authors covered many essential diagnostic and therapeutic considerations based on their personal experience and evidence from the literature. From my personal experience, I would like to add a few comments pertaining to the following strategic considerations: (1) type of pathology and its cause, (2) urgency for treatment, (3) prognosis and quality of life, (4) bronchoscopic treatment alternatives, (5) considerations about invasiveness and risk, and (6) cost-effectiveness.

Types and Cause of Fistulas

Aerodigestive fistulas can be connatal, when the septum between the trachea and the esophagus is incomplete or perforated. The most frequent type is the so-called Vogt IIIb,* in which a small duct connects

---

*Congenital esophageal atresia (EA) and trachea-esophageal fistula (TEF) may exist as separate entities, but most people have both, and therefore the classification systems group them together. Five types of congenital EA/TEF and two classification systems—Gross and Vogt classification systems—have been identified. Gross type C (Vogt type IIIb) EA/TEF, which consists of distal TEF with proximal EA, is the most common type (88.5%). Gross type A (Vogt type II) is isolated EA, and Gross type E (TEF without EA or H-type TEF) is less common (8% and 4%, respectively); the remainder consist of Gross types B (Vogt III a) (proximal TEF with distal EA) and D (Vogt IIIc) (proximal TEF and distal TEF) (*Chest.* 2004;126:915-925).

the trachea to the esophagus, frequently in a downward direction. The fistula is diagnosed most often in early childhood by accidental aspiration. Frequently, the fistula can be closed by endoscopic means such as electrocautery and/or sealing by glue. In rare instances, the fistula never causes problems and is found by chance in adulthood. Other types of fistulas are post-traumatic. These can result from difficult intubation or from interventional bronchoscopic procedures. Especially in post intubation trauma, the diagnosis is missed easily if the endotracheal tube cuff obstructs the lesion. Often, it is only the dislocation of the cuff or extubation that unmasks the defect, resulting in mediastinal emphysema and aspiration. Early diagnosis of this complication and its surgical repair by primary closure of the esophageal and tracheal leak are mandatory, in which case complications are infrequent. Delayed surgical intervention, however, may be accompanied by delayed postoperative healing due to infection. A third type of fistula is postsurgical, occurring most often after esophageal segmental resection. These usually occur at the site of anastomosis, especially in cases of complicated wound healing after preoperative chemo-radiotherapy. They are very difficult to surgically repair, even when bypass and transplant procedures, vascularized muscle flaps, or other techniques are used.

Many patients with fistulas require endoscopic palliation. This usually entails the insertion of various kinds of prostheses. If possible, we place tracheal stents without tracheostomy so that phonation is preserved. However, some patients do require tracheostomy and a Montgomery T-tube. In patients with malignancy, if no recurrence of tumor occurs, quality of life can be maintained with stents; we have many patients that we have been following now for longer than 10 years. The same is true for some patients after aggressive treatment for inoperable tracheal cancers such as adenoid-cystic carcinoma. In these patients, we used to propose extensive bronchoscopic resection using neodymium-doped yttrium aluminum garnet (Nd:YAG) laser followed by high-dose-rate (HDR) brachytherapy, but this was occasionally followed by fistula formation. Currently we simply restore enough airway lumen so that we can insert a stent, and we then perform brachytherapy from within the stent. Using this strategy, we no longer see fistula-type complications. Those malignant fistulas due to necrotic tumor growth are almost never treatable by open surgical resection, which is accompanied by an excessive complication rate and high mortality. From a frequency perspective, in our experience with 49 patients with aerodigestive fistulas treated between January 1997 and December 2002, 6 patients (12%) had prior surgery, 29 (59%) radiation, 4(8%) chemo-radiotherapy, and 10 (21%) no prior therapy.

Urgency of Treatment

In the case presented by the authors, the pathology was obvious. The malignant tracheo-broncho-esophageal fistula caused chronic aspiration with aspiration pneumonia and finally respiratory insufficiency. Already at the time of first diagnosis, the patient was suffering from dysphagia. Because no life-threatening symptoms occurred, sufficient time was available to perform a thorough clinical evaluation to ascertain local extent and exclude metastases. Unfortunately, the patient obviously had not agreed to this strategy. Besides general staging, including esophago-bronchoscopy, we would have applied endobronchial ultrasound (EBUS) and endoesophageal ultrasound (EUS) to determine the extent of the tumor, the involvement of lymph nodes, and, very important, the proximity of the fistula to large adjacent vessels. These procedures facilitate development of an interdisciplinary treatment plan, which in this case might have been a carefully calibrated regimen of combined chemo-radiotherapy to avoid a radiogenic aerodigestive fistula. In cases of significant dyspnea, a stent could have been placed additionally inside the left main bronchus. We strongly believe that in cases of life-threatening symptoms from high-grade tracheal obstruction, establishing a safe airway is mandatory before any other decisions are made, especially with regard to prognosis and quality of life.

Prognosis and Quality of Life

Especially in an emergency situation, which, according to our experience, is the case in 60% of patients at initial presentation, an individual assessment of prognosis and prospective quality of life can be impossible. Thus a decision must be made on the basis of experience. In our series of 49 patients suffering from aerodigestive fistulas, the median survival after intervention was 237 days (14 to 476 days). In only 6 patients, closure of the fistula was unsuccessful, decreasing mean survival to 39 days (2 to 62 days), and patients' quality of life was very poor. Of those 6 patients, 4 patients needed temporary intensive care after intervention and 2 died within 30 days after the intervention. Thus, overall prognosis is not so poor as to deter us from intervention. We believe that even a few weeks of a comparatively symptom-free life gives patients the chance to arrange their last will and take care of unsolved problems. It is only in the case of an obviously dismal situation, in which complications will lead to death within the next few days, that I refrain from any intervention, resorting instead to providing best supportive care (which includes sedation because constant severe aspiration is usually an intolerable situation). We can almost always assure the patient that he or she will not die from suffocation in full consciousness, and with patients we have cared for over many years, we frequently come to a mutual decision that regardless of procedures we might offer, life is no longer worthwhile, and we choose to stop all interventions. In my opinion, from examining the endoscopic image of the local extent of the fistula of the patient presented in the case scenario, noting destruction of the bifurcation as well as the left main bronchus, it is difficult to say whether we would have proceeded to place a stent. In some of these cases, I refrain from doing any procedure. Perhaps a more extensive explanation and discussion with the patient and his wife could have convinced him sooner that an early intervention could result in a better outcome with improved quality of life and longer survival.

Bronchoscopic Treatment Alternatives

With inoperable benign fistulas, the means for closure is de-epithelialization of the channel in cases of small fistulas, using a brush, argon plasma coagulation (APC), or laser before occlusion with fibrin glue. Sometimes decalcified spongiosa can also be implanted as a scaffold for fibroblasts. With larger fistulas, endoscopic suturing might become possible as new devices for natural orifices trans-endoscopic surgery (NOTES) are developed. With untreatable fistulas, especially those that form in malignant tissues, palliative occlusion by stent placement is the method of choice. Our strategy is as follows: If the fistula is combined with esophageal stenosis, we first try to reestablish the oral food passage in connection with closure of the fistula by placing an esophageal prosthesis. In contrast to the former cuffed rigid tubes, we nowadays prefer covered, self-expanding metallic stents. In our experience, stents made from stainless steel should be avoided because of their very high expanding pressures and tendency to perforate tissues. Stents made of Nitinol are preferred. Sometimes in the same session, we place an endoscopic percutaneous gastrostomy tube. Frequently, the fistula can thus be closed. This is confirmed during the procedure by instillation of contrast medium. In our experience, esophageal stents rarely cause airway compression requiring airway stent insertion. If necrosis of the esophagus is too extensive to establish safe fixation of an esophageal stent, we place one on the tracheobronchial side. In contrast with benign situations where removable silicone stents are warranted, in malignant tissues metallic stents can be used. Here too, the shape memory alloy Nitinol is ideal because it very closely resembles connective tissue in its physical behavior. For closure of fistulas, a covered stent is of course necessary. Self-expanding metallic bifurcation stents have recently become available, and in cases of malignant fistulas involving the bifurcation, I prefer to implant these instead of silicone Y prostheses because insertion is less traumatic and can be performed using the flexible bronchoscope. If the airway is narrowed by the esophageal stent, or if the fistula is not closed by the stent, an additional stent is placed inside the lumen of the organ that has not been stented. In our series, closure of the fistula was performed by placement of a tracheal stent in 28 (58%), an esophageal stent in 17 (33%), and double stenting in 4 (9%). Five patients needed an additional stent during follow-up.

Invasiveness and Risk

The main concern during stent placement is maintaining ventilation. Thus in the setting of a predominant obliteration of the airway, the stenosis must be treated first. We use a rigid bronchoscope with the patient under general anesthesia. After premedication with midazolam and remifentanil, general anesthesia is induced with propofol and relaxation by succinylcholine. I always prefer high-frequency jet ventilation at 100/min because airways are hardly moving and meticulous instrumentation is, in my opinion, facilitated. As the jet goes in centrally and a continuous backflow occurs along the walls, secretions are driven out rather than blown into the lung. Also, the risk of overinflating the stomach via the fistula is less than when controlled ventilation is used. I also find instrumentation via the open rigid bronchoscope much easier than through a closed system. Usually the procedure can be performed within 15 to 30 minutes. Carbon dioxide (CO_2) retention is of little concern, and oxygenation usually is not a problem. If patients need to be transferred to the intensive care unit, this usually occurs because of the prolonged action of muscle relaxants. Therefore in severely debilitated patients, we limit ourselves to using deep sedation with propofol without relaxation. Of course, all the necessary instruments for intervention in case of bleeding or emergency intubation must be at hand.

Cost-Effectiveness

Apart from the unbearable situation for the patient, the severe morbidity of recurrent pneumonia and respiratory insufficiency leads to repeated admissions with prolonged hospitalizations, all causing considerable costs. In contrast, after bronchoscopic intervention, most patients can be discharged quickly. In our case series, mean hospitalization lasted 3.1 days. Even given the cost of stents, which can amount to 2.500 to 3.000 Euros in Germany, particularly in cases of double stent insertion, bronchoscopic intervention is more cost-effective than palliative care and offers a comparatively better quality of life.

In closing, the procedures described in this case are reasonable and are supported by the literature and by my own experience. I would like to add that application of endobronchial ultrasound might have been useful for predicting the risk of fatal hemorrhage by detecting early erosion into the great vessels (such as the pulmonary artery and the aorta). In this case, implantation of a self-expanding covered stent might have been less traumatic but finally probably would not have prevented the fatal outcome. Recognition of the true extent of such a large, necrotic, tumor-related fistula might have led to a decision to not proceed with any intervention after all, or progression of the disease to the point that interventions were performed, according to my experience, could have been prevented. If patients receive all the information described as early as possible in the course of their disease, they may understand that prolonged life expectancy is feasible, in addition to a better quality of life, especially if general and endoscopic measures are taken before a catastrophic situation such as that described in this case occurs.

REFERENCES

1. Balazs A, Kupcsulik PK, Galambos Z. Esophagorespiratory fistulas of timorous origin: nonoperative management of 264 cases in a 20-year period. *Eur J Cardiothorac Surg.* 2008;34:1103-1107.
2. Choi MK, Park YH, Hong JY, et al. Clinical implications of esophagorespiratory fistulae in patients with esophageal squamous cell carcinoma (SCCA). *Med Oncol.* 2010;27:1234-1238.
3. Spigel DR, Hainsworth JD, Yardley DA, et al. Tracheoesophageal fistula formation in patients with lung cancer treated with chemoradiation and bevacizumab. *J Clin Oncol.* 2009;28:43-48.
4. Shen KR, Allen MS, Cassivi SD, et al. Surgical management of acquired nonmalignant tracheoesophageal and bronchoesophageal fistulae. *Ann Thorac Surg.* 2010;90:914-919.
5. Lee KE, Shin JH, Song HY, et al. Management of airway involvement of oesophageal cancer using covered retrievable Nitinol stents. *Clin Radiol.* 2009;64:133-141.
6. Kim KR, Shin JH, Song HY, et al. Palliative treatment of malignant esophagopulmonary fistulas with covered expandable metallic stents. *AJR Am J Roentgenol.* 2009;193:W278-W282.
7. Burt M, Diehl W, Martini N, et al. Malignant esophagorespiratory fistula: management options and survival. *Ann Thorac Surg.* 1991; 52:1222-1229.
8. Grebenik CR. Anaesthetic management of malignant tracheooesophageal fistula. *Br J Anaesth.* 1989;63:492-496.
9. Jaffe DH, Manor O, Eisenbach Z, et al. The protective effect of marriage on mortality in a dynamic society. *Ann Epidemiol.* 2007; 17:540-547.
10. Miller RC, Atherton PJ, Kabat BF, et al. Marital status and quality of life in patients with esophageal cancer or Barrett's esophagus: the Mayo Clinic Esophageal Adenocarcinoma and Barrett's Esophagus Registry study. *Dig Dis Sci.* 2010;55:2860-2868.
11. Chung SC, Stuart RC, Li AK. Surgical therapy for squamous-cell carcinoma of the oesophagus. *Lancet.* 1994;343:521-524.
12. Donnelly M, Anderson LA, Johnston BT, et al. Oesophageal cancer: caregiver mental health and strain. *Psycho-Oncology.* 2008;17: 1196-1201.
13. Reed MF, Mathisen DJ. Tracheoesophageal fistula. *Chest Surg Clin N Am.* 2003;13:271-289.
14. Fan ST, Lau WY, Yip WC, et al. Prediction of postoperative pulmonary complications in oesophagogastric cancer surgery. *Br J Surg.* 1987;74:408-410.
15. Nomori H, Horio H, Imazu Y, et al. Double stenting for esophageal and tracheobronchial stenoses. *Ann Thorac Surg.* 2000;70:1803-1807.
16. Mitsuoka M, Sakuragi T, Itoh T. Clinical benefits and complications of Dumon stent insertion for the treatment of severe central airway stenosis or airway fistula. *Gen Thorac Cardiovasc Surg.* 2007;55:275-280.
17. Hu Y, Zhao Y-F, Chen L-Q, et al. Comparative study of different treatments for malignant tracheoesophageal/bronchoesophageal fistulae. *Dis Esophagus.* 2009;22:526-531.
18. Rodriguez AN, Diaz-Jimenez JP. Malignant respiratory-digestive fistulas. *Curr Opin Pulm Med.* 2010;16:329-333.
19. Freitag L. Airway stents. In: Strausz J, Bolliger CT. *Interventional Pulmonology.* Lausanne, Switzerland: European Respiratory Society; 2010:190-217.
20. Meunier B, Stasik C, Raoul JL, et al. Gastric bypass for malignant esophagotracheal fistula: a series of 21 cases. *Eur J Cardiothorac Surg.* 1998;13:184-188.
21. Low DE, Kozarek RA. Comparison of conventional and wire mesh expandable prostheses and surgical bypass in patients with malignant esophagorespiratory fistulas. *Ann Thorac Surg.* 1998;65: 919-923.
22. Diaz-Jimenez P. New cufflink-shaped silicone prosthesis for the palliation of malignant tracheobronchial-esophageal fistula. *J Bronchol.* 2005;12:207-209.
23. Shin JH, Song HY, Ko GY, et al. Esophagorespiratory fistula: long-term results of palliative treatment with covered expandable metallic stents in 61 patients. *Radiology.* 2004;232:252-259.
24. Sharma P, Kozarek R; The Practice Parameters Committee of the American College of Gastroenterology. Role of esophageal stents in benign and malignant diseases. *Am J Gastroenterol.* 2010;105: 258-273.
25. Weigert N, Neuhaus H, Rosch T, et al. Treatment of esophagorespiratory fistulas with silicone-coated self-expanding metal stents. *Gastrointest Endosc.* 1995;41:490-496.
26. Kim YH, Shin JH, Song HY, et al. Treatment of tracheal strictures or fistulas using a barbed silicone-covered retrievable expandable Nitinol stent. *AJR Am J Roentgenol.* 2010;194:W232-W237.
27. Turkyilmaz A, Aydin Y, Eroglu A, et al. Palliative management of esophagorespiratory fistula in esophageal malignancy. *Surg Laparosc Endosc Percutan Tech.* 2009;19:364-367.
28. Ross WA, Alkassab F, Lynch PM, et al. Evolving role of self-expanding metal stents in the treatment of malignant dysphagia and fistulas. *Gastrointest Endosc.* 2007;65:70-76.
29. Colt HG, Meric B, Dumon JF. Double stents for carcinoma of the esophagus invading the tracheo-bronchial tree. *Gastrointest Endosc.* 1992;38:485-489.
30. Albes JM, Schafers HJ, Gebel M, et al. Tracheal stenting for malignant tracheoesophageal fistula. *Ann Thorac Surg.* 1994;57:1263-1266.
31. Freitag L, Tekolf E, Steveling H, et al. Management of malignant esophagotracheal fistulas with airway stenting and double stenting. *Chest.* 1996;110:1155-1160.
32. Nomori H, Horio H, Imazu Y, et al. Double stenting for esophageal and tracheobronchial stenoses. *Ann Thorac Surg.* 2000;70:1803-1807.
33. van den Bongard HJ, Boot H, Baas P, et al. The role of parallel stent insertion in patients with esophagorespiratory fistulas. *Gastrointest Endosc.* 2002;55:110-115.
34. Inada T, Umemoto M, Ohshima T, et al. Anesthesia for insertion of a Dumon stent in a patient with a large tracheo-esophageal fistula. *Can J Anaesth.* 1999;46:372-375.
35. Dutau H, Toutblanc B, Lamb C, et al. Use of the Dumon Y-stent in the management of malignant disease involving the carina: a retrospective review of 86 patients. *Chest.* 2004;126:951-958.
36. Alazemi S, Chatterji S, Ernst A, et al. Mediastinal migration of self-expanding bronchial stents in the management of malignant bronchoesophageal fistula. *Chest.* 2009;135:1353-1355.
37. Tomaselli F, Maier A, Sankin O, et al. Successful endoscopical sealing of malignant esophageotracheal fistulae by using a covered self-expandable stenting system. *Eur J Cardiothorac Surg.* 2001;20: 734-738.
38. Yamamoto R, Tada H, Kishi A, et al. Double stent for malignant combined esophago-airway lesions. *Jpn J Thorac Cardiovasc Surg.* 2002;50:1-5.
39. Kim JH, Shin JH, Song HY, et al. Esophagorespiratory fistula without stricture: palliative treatment with a barbed covered metallic stent in the central airway. *J Vasc Interv Radiol.* 2011;22:84-88.
40. Lagergren P, Fayers P, Conroy T, et al; European Organisation for Research Treatment of Cancer Gastrointestinal and Quality of Life Groups. Clinical and psychometric validation of a questionnaire module, the EORTC QLQ-OG25, to assess health-related quality of life in patients with cancer of the oesophagus, the oesophago-gastric junction and the stomach. *Eur J Cancer.* 2007;43:2066-2073.
41. Sharma S, Walsh D. Symptom management in esophageal cancer. *Chest Surg Clin N Am.* 1994;4:369-383.

Chapter 28

Rigid Bronchoscopic Intervention for Central Airway Obstruction and Concurrent Superior Vena Cava Syndrome Caused by Small Cell Carcinoma

This chapter emphasizes the following elements of the Four Box Approach: risk-benefit analyses and therapeutic alternatives; anesthesia and other perioperative care; and referrals to medical, surgical, or palliative/end-of-life subspecialty care.

CASE DESCRIPTION

An 85-year-old male with an extensive history of smoking (70 pack-years) developed shortness of breath, which worsened within the week before admission. He had excessive cough, which resulted in hemoptysis (estimated at a few teaspoons/day). Review of systems revealed weight loss (20 kg/6 mo), as well as facial and neck edema for several months. Vital signs showed blood pressure of 150/70 mm Hg, heart rate of 115/min, body temperature of 37.2° C, and respiratory rate of 22/min. On physical examination, the patient had prominent edema of the face, neck, and bilateral upper extremities, with neck vein distention and multiple engorged dilated vessels over the anterior aspect of the chest. Expiratory wheezing was heard on the left hemithorax, and no breath sounds were heard on the right. The rest of the physical examination was normal. Laboratory findings showed WBC count of 19,700 (neutrophils 81.3%, lymphocytes 2%), hemoglobin of 12.8 g/dL, and platelet count of 310,000/mm^3. Arterial blood gas analysis showed pH of 7.54, arterial carbon dioxide tension ($PaCO_2$) of 39 mm Hg, and partial pressure of oxygen in arterial blood (PaO_2) of 64 mm Hg (O_2 = 2 L/min on nasal prong). Electrolytes were within normal limits. Electrocardiography (ECG) showed sinus tachycardia with bifascicular block. Two-dimensional echocardiography showed a small secundum-type atrial septal defect, normal left ventricular function, and no evidence of right ventricular dysfunction. Chest radiograph revealed near complete opacification of the right hemithorax (Figure 28-1). Chest computed tomography showed a 7.3 × 5.7 cm large mediastinal and right hilar mass with near

complete occlusion of the superior vena cava (SVC); the mass had eroded into the right mainstem bronchus and lower trachea, causing near complete collapse of the right lung and a right pleural effusion (see Figure 28-1). Bronchoscopic biopsy and washings performed at an outside facility showed small cell carcinoma. The patient was placed on broad-spectrum antibiotics and was transferred to our hospital for consideration for bronchoscopic intervention to restore airway patency. On repeat bronchoscopic examination, the tumor involved the lower trachea above the main carina, completely occluding the entrance to the right main bronchus (see Figure 28-1). The patient was a retired clothing factory owner who lived with his wife. He had a very close family including several children who were actively involved in his care. His family wanted him to receive active and what was hoped would be effective treatment for this tumor. Emergency radiotherapy of first intention had not been recommended by a radiation oncologist because of concerns for worsening tracheal obstruction by radiation-induced edema and ongoing sepsis. Therefore urgent rigid bronchoscopy was scheduled to establish airway patency and to potentially avoid worsening sepsis and respiratory failure.

DISCUSSION POINTS

1. List two major complications during general anesthesia in patients with large mediastinal masses.
2. Comment on the safety of therapeutic rigid bronchoscopy in people 80 years of age and older.
3. Enumerate seven measures to reduce operative and anesthetic complications in patients with concurrent superior vena cava syndrome and central airway obstruction.
4. Describe three major complications during rigid bronchoscopy in patients with large carinal tumors completely occluding a mainstem bronchus.

CASE RESOLUTION

Initial Evaluations

Physical Examination, Complementary Tests, and Functional Status Assessment

This patient had a new diagnosis of small cell lung cancer (SCLC). The Veterans Affairs Lung Study Group (VALSG)* staging system has been used traditionally to

---

*Limited disease patients are characterized by (1) disease confined to one hemithorax, although local extensions may be present; (2) no extrathoracic metastases, except for possible ipsilateral, supraclavicular nodes if they can be included in the same portal as the primary tumor; and (3) primary tumor and regional nodes, which can be treated adequately and totally encompassed in every portal. Extensive disease patients are inoperable patients who cannot be classified as having limited disease.

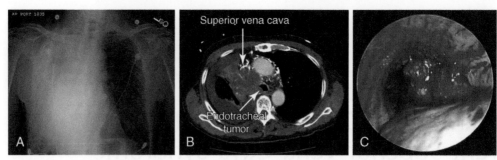

Figure 28-1 **A,** Chest radiograph shows near-complete opacification of the right hemithorax with slight ipsilateral shift of the trachea. **B,** Contrast-enhanced computed tomography shows near complete obstruction of the superior vena cava and lower endotracheal tumor completely closing the right main bronchus. **C,** Bronchoscopy confirmed these findings and revealed an actively bleeding, hypervascular "fleshy" tumor.

stage SCLC because of its simplicity. Based on this system, limited disease is seen in 30% to 40% at presentation, and extensive disease in 60% to 70% of patients. Accurate staging is clinically relevant because patients with limited-stage disease are treated with combined modality therapy, and those with extensive disease receive chemotherapy alone. Staging by the VALSG system is controversial in patients with locally advanced disease such as contralateral hilar or supraclavicular nodes, pericardial effusions, or malignant pleural effusions, as were seen in this case; for instance, this group is neither precisely defined (as limited or extended disease) nor uniformly managed by different investigators and is frequently excluded from protocols for limited-stage disease. In this regard, the consensus report from the International Association for the Study of Lung Cancer (IASLC) modified the VALSG classification based on the tumor-node-metastasis (TNM) staging system, and only patients with TxNxM1 were considered as having extended disease, so that IASLC criteria include more patients in the prognostically superior limited disease category than are assigned by the VALSG criteria.[1] The TNM staging system used for non–small cell lung cancer (NSCLC) has been increasingly advocated by the IASLC to stage SCLC because it describes the extent of disease more accurately than the VALSG system. In fact, the new IASLC M1a descriptors (pleural effusion, pericardial effusion, and contralateral/bilateral intrapulmonary metastasis) adequately prognosticate SCLC patients as having metastatic disease. In fact, the IASLC recommends the use of TNM for all cases of SCLC.[2]

Similar to our case, patients with advanced-stage lung cancer of any type may present with a variety of locoregional complications, including central airway obstruction (CAO), superior vena cava (SVC) syndrome, hemoptysis, and post obstructive pneumonia. Patients with CAO usually are not candidates for surgical resection for physiologic or oncologic reasons. Furthermore, chemotherapy and/or radiotherapy in the setting of post obstructive pneumonia may exacerbate the risk for sepsis. The prognosis is guarded, and in the presence of atelectasis, the ability of external beam radiation alone to restore airway patency was shown to be as low as 23%.[3] SVC obstruction by lymph node metastasis into the right paratracheal or precarinal station or by direct invasion

of lung cancer can cause SVC syndrome* in up to 10% of newly diagnosed cases of SCLC.[4] Tumor growth in most cases is gradual, allowing sufficient time for collateral circulation to develop, but many patients eventually present with headache, swelling of the face and neck, and even coma. However, SVC syndrome is no longer considered an emergency, and the use of intravascular stents is recommended only for relapsed or persistent SVC obstruction following chemotherapy or radiation therapy in SCLC.[5]

Comorbidities

SCLC is the most common malignancy associated with neurologic paraneoplastic syndromes produced by autoantibodies that cross-react with both SCLC cells and the central nervous system or the neuromuscular junction. These antibodies can cause the Lambert-Eaton myasthenic syndrome (LEMS)† in 3% of patients suffering from SCLC.[6] Our patient had no obvious neurologic symptoms suggesting LEMS or other paraneoplastic neurologic syndromes seen in SCLC such as limbic encephalitis,‡ paraneoplastic cerebellar degeneration, autonomic neuropathy, or subacute peripheral sensory neuropathy. SCLC cells can also produce a number of polypeptide hormones, including adrenocorticotropic hormone (ACTH) and antidiuretic hormone, resulting in the syndrome of inappropriate antidiuretic hormone and Cushing's syndrome, respectively. Our patient had no

---

*SVC syndrome is characterized by signs and symptoms of central venous obstruction (dyspnea, facial swelling, head fullness). Other symptoms include arm swelling, cough, chest pain, and dysphagia. Patients with cerebral edema may have headaches, confusion, or possibly coma.

†LEMS is an uncommon disorder of neuromuscular junction transmission with the primary clinical manifestation of progressive proximal muscle weakness, autonomic symptoms (dry mouth, blurred vision, constipation), and cranial nerve symptoms (dysarthria, dysphagia, and difficulty chewing). Antibodies directed against the voltage-gated calcium channel (VGCC), a large transmembrane protein with multiple subunits, play a central role in the pathophysiology of LEMS. These antibodies interfere with the normal calcium flux required for the release of acetylcholine.

‡This disorder is caused by SCLC in 40% to 50% of cases; it develops over days to months and is characterized by mood changes, hallucinations, and memory loss, and less commonly by hypothalamic symptoms such as hyperthermia, somnolence, and endocrine dysfunction.

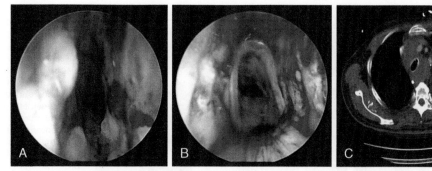

Figure 28-2   A, In a different patient, this severe tracheal obstruction is due to extrinsic compression from small cell lung cancer. **B,** Airway patency is improved after insertion of a straight studded silicone stent. **C,** Computed tomography after stent insertion shows a patent tracheal lumen that is circumferentially compressed by a large mediastinal tumor.

symptoms or laboratory markers suggesting these diagnoses, all of which could affect anesthesia and procedural planning.

Support System

Cancer treatment is emotionally and physically exhausting for patients, so it is important for them to have a good support system during this critical time of their lives. This patient had many family members who were eager to help. Strong family support and faith are noted to have a positive effect on response to cancer treatment.[7] If patients, friends, or family members have difficulty coping with the emotional aspects of the illness, experienced professionals in mental health services, social work services, and pastoral services, and local support groups can assist.[8]

Patient Preferences and Expectations

Although rigorous techniques are frequently used to evaluate survival and response, less rigor is often used when the impact of treatment on quality of life is assessed. Similar to our case, many patients with lung cancer are elderly with complex medical histories and multiple comorbidities. Given limited survival expectations, symptom palliation, quality of life, and convenience of therapy are especially important end points. This patient wished to be minimally involved in treatment decisions, deferring entirely to his family and the cancer care team. He expressed only his wish to not suffer from "chemo" like his brother had a few years previously. Other patients prefer that family members be excluded from treatment decisions and want to take charge themselves. Becoming actively involved in one's own cancer treatment may actually improve care and recovery after treatment. For instance, when patients are made fully aware of the potential side effects of treatment, they can promptly alert their cancer care team in case of problems.[8]

Procedural Strategies

Indications

The gold standard treatment for malignant CAO is surgical resection. Similar to this case, however, many patients are poor surgical candidates on the basis of their physiology or oncologic criteria (e.g., inoperable because of advanced tumor stage). Interventional bronchoscopic

procedures, when indicated in patients with inoperable NSCLC or SCLC, are expected to restore airway patency and improve lung function, symptoms, and functional status, thus allowing initiation of systemic therapy, which might improve survival.[9,10] Resectional techniques are used in cases of intraluminal disease. Airway stent insertion is performed in the setting of malignant CAO caused by severe extrinsic compression (Figure 28-2), or when more than 50% obstruction is present after debulking of the intraluminal component of the disease.[11]

Contraindications

No absolute contraindications to rigid bronchoscopy were noted. Because complete obstruction of the right upper lobe (RUL) bronchus occurred with no identifiable lumen and a potentially nonfunctioning distal lung parenchyma* (Figure 28-3), bronchoscopic attempts to restore RUL bronchial patency were contraindicated. SVC syndrome was a relative contraindication given concerns for hemodynamic instability.

Expected Results

This patient had complete obstruction of the right main bronchus and severe (70%) obstruction in the distal trachea. Palliating CAO was expected to improve dyspnea, lung function, and quality of life.[9,12,13] In patients with inoperable or recurrent NSCLC or SCLC occluding a central airway, studies showed no difference in overall survival between those who received both neodymium-doped yttrium aluminum garnet (Nd:YAG) laser treatment and radiation therapy (mean external dose, 53.1 Gy) as compared with historical controls treated with radiation therapy alone. In patients with restored airway lumen,[†] however, the time interval from treatment to

---

*No perfect method is available to assess this issue; radionuclide ventilation-perfusion studies can be performed, but reduced perfusion is expected in the lack of ventilation due to bronchial obstruction; in fact, studies show that ventilation and perfusion scores could improve after radiotherapy and/or laser therapy in inoperable patients with malignant bronchial obstruction.

†Complete restoration of airway patency (aka full recanalization) was assessed subjectively by bronchoscopy as restoration of the full shape of the obstructed bronchus and objectively by documenting normalization of peak expiratory flow (PEF); no recanalization was recorded when restoration of bronchial patency failed and distal lobar or segmental bronchi were not visible, and no improvement in PEF was observed.

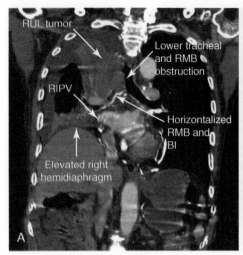
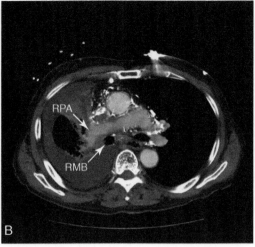

Figure 28-3 A, Anatomic relationships are altered because of the volume loss caused by complete right upper lobe obstruction and atelectasis. The right hemidiaphragm is elevated, and horizontalization of the right main bronchus and bronchus intermedius is evident. **B,** The right pulmonary artery is in close proximity and anterior and lateral to the right main bronchus. *BI,* Bronchus intermedius; *RMB,* right mainstem bronchus; *RIPV,* right inferior pulmonary vein; *RPA,* right pulmonary artery; *RUL,* right upper lobe.

death was prolonged by 4 months compared with those for whom a fully patent airway could not be restored.[14] Successful restoration of patency of a major airway occluded by intraluminal tumor using laser resection reduces the likelihood of respiratory failure as a cause of death and does not affect the likelihood of massive fatal hemorrhage, which was a major cause of death in these patients with or without laser treatment.[14] Therefore a major issue in these patients is whether they and their families should be warned of the possibility of major bleeding and informed of measures to take should this unfortunate event occur outside the hospital setting.*

Team Experience

Maintaining hemodynamic and respiratory stability during anesthesia requires constant communication between the bronchoscopist and the anesthesiologist. Procedures may be complicated by frequent periods of apnea, compromised airway seals, and the need for special ventilatory techniques such as spontaneous-assisted ventilation or high-frequency jet ventilation. Rigid bronchoscopic procedures involve repeated alternating periods of high and low stimulation requiring rapid titration of intravenous anesthetics to meet fluctuating demands.[15]

Coexisting SVC syndrome and CAO can cause life-threatening complications at any time during anesthesia in elderly patients with lung cancer undergoing rigid bronchoscopy. Working together as a team, anesthesiologists and bronchoscopists can anticipate problems and institute precautionary measures to ensure a safe and effective intervention. The procedural strategy, for example, should be shared with the anesthesiologist,

---

*Death by massive bleeding is traumatic for all involved. We ourselves have frequently witnessed this event in both hospital and home settings. Advance directives are essential to help guide the behaviors of family members and emergency health care personnel. Specific instructions may be required when patients and families elect to not proceed with resuscitative or life-prolonging measures. Children, if present at the scene, probably should be removed, and everything should be done to comfort the dying patient.

including expected duration of the procedure, whether hypoxemia or hypotension is expected, whether laser or electrocautery (which requires diminishing fraction of inspired oxygen [FiO_2] to below 40%) will be used, and whether intubation and mechanical ventilation will be required after the procedure.

Risk-Benefit Analysis

Because the goal of the procedure is palliation, treatment should have the least possible risk of side effects and discomfort. The risks of intervention warrant careful consideration when patients have significant comorbidities such as a large mediastinal mass, SVC syndrome, or very advanced age.[16,17] In our patient, the risks of further physiologic compromise, massive bleeding, and hemodynamic instability were considered to be outweighed by the potential benefit of restoring airway patency to improve functional status and offer systemic therapy. Therapeutic strategies should be elaborated on a case-by-case basis, and advantages and disadvantages of various alternatives discussed with the patient and family if desired, before or during the informed consent process.

Therapeutic Alternatives for Restoring Airway Patency

1. *Emergent external beam radiation therapy (EBRT)* could have been used for palliating the airway obstruction and the SVC syndrome.[18] Initiation of EBRT as primary treatment without attempts at restoration of airway patency in this patient in our opinion would have been of doubtful benefit. EBRT is only variably effective for cancer-induced CAO when the obstruction is severe enough to cause atelectasis, as occurred in our patient. In a study of 330 patients, EBRT palliated hemoptysis in 84% of patients and SVC syndrome in 86% of patients, but atelectasis in only 23%.[3] However, EBRT following effective laser treatment could potentially improve survival.[19] EBRT had not been recommended as the primary treatment in our patient because of concerns for worsening tracheal obstruction by radiation-induced edema and because of ongoing sepsis in the setting of post obstructive

pneumonia. It is noteworthy, from a systemic therapy perspective, that a meta-analysis showed no obvious benefit for combined chemotherapy and radiation therapy over chemotherapy alone in limited-stage SCLC patients older than 70 years. However, more recent trials have revealed a clear-cut benefit for physically "fit elderly"* patients to receive combined modality therapy versus chemotherapy alone, although outcome generally remains inferior to that of younger patients.[20]

2. *Chemotherapy for SCLC* involves cisplatin-etoposide regimens and in general is combined with chest radiotherapy for limited disease.[21] A systematic review of 29 trials involving 5530 patients found that platinum-based chemotherapy regimens did not offer a statistically significant survival benefit or overall tumor response compared with non–platinum-based regimens. However, platinum-based chemotherapy regimens did increase complete response rates[†] at the cost of more frequent adverse events, including nausea and vomiting, anemia, and thrombocytopenia.[22] CAO is present in as many as 20% to 30% of patients with lung cancer. These patients may develop post obstructive pneumonia.[23] Acute infection, as was seen in our patient, is a contraindication to administration of chemotherapy and is an exclusion criterion in most clinical trials.[24] We therefore decided to initially proceed with bronchoscopic restoration of airway patency with the patient under general anesthesia.

Cost-Effectiveness

Although no published literature is available regarding this issue, early bronchoscopic intervention in this patient with central airway obstruction was probably justified from an economic standpoint because prolonged hospitalization for post obstructive pneumonia might be prevented, and critical care hospitalization for impending respiratory failure might be avoided. From a clinical perspective, the literature supports bronchoscopic palliation of airway obstruction from small cell and non–small cell lung cancer before initiation of systemic or radiation therapy.

Informed Consent

This patient's family had good insight into his disease. Expectations were realistic. After they had been advised of all of the alternatives, the family elected to proceed with rigid bronchoscopy with the patient under general anesthesia. They were informed of potential failure to restore airway patency and were told about the risks

for bleeding, perforation, laryngeal edema, respiratory failure, temporary or prolonged mechanical ventilation, and death.

Techniques and Results

Anesthesia and Perioperative Care

In a patient with severe CAO, premedication with opiates or benzodiazepines in the preoperative period, along with concerns for airway obstruction, anxiety, pain, and periprocedural agitation, should be avoided, or these agents should be administered with caution because they can lead to tachypnea and high airflow velocity during breathing, which increases already turbulent flow in the narrowed airways, exacerbates the pressure drop along the stenosis, and worsens the work of breathing. If possible, patients should be transported to the operating room in a head-up sitting position to avoid worsening preexistent airway and vascular obstruction.[25] This simple maneuver can reduce the likelihood of precipitating airway obstruction.[26]

Careful preoperative assessment for neuromuscular weakness is important in patients with SCLC because approximately 8% of patients with LEMS develop respiratory failure requiring mechanical ventilation. This may develop spontaneously or may be induced by general anesthesia.[27] Patients are sensitive to neuromuscular blocking agents and volatile anesthetics, which may cause prolonged paralysis and residual muscle weakness.[15] Ideally, these agents should be avoided. Furthermore, the delivery of volatile anesthetics may be problematic when rigid bronchoscopy is performed using an open system with spontaneous-assisted ventilation because the quantity of anesthetic gas reaching the patient is uncertain, and the operating room personnel and operator are at risk for pollution from the escaped anesthetics.[15] Total intravenous anesthesia (TIVA) is a preferred technique for rigid bronchoscopy using an open system.*

Securing the airway by rigid bronchoscopic intubation in patients with a large mediastinal mass associated with SVC syndrome and CAO can be challenging. In patients with SVC syndrome, airway management can be complicated by upper airway edema, hemodynamic instability during general anesthesia, and procedure-related bleeding.[28] The same degree of edema that is seen externally in the face and neck can be present in the mouth, oropharynx, hypopharynx, and larynx.[29] Prompt and atraumatic insertion of the rigid bronchoscope prevents further worsening of preexisting upper airway edema related to severe SVC obstruction. By standing at the head of the patient's bed during induction, the bronchoscopist is ready and equipped to ensure airway control and, if necessary, to bypass the obstruction, especially in cases of tracheal lesions.[30]

---

*Patients older than 70 years of age with a good performance status (Karnofsky score >60).

[†]Tumor response for objective overall response and complete response were defined per World Health Organization (WHO) guidelines for tumor response evaluation. Objective response can be determined clinically, radiologically, or biochemically, or by surgico-pathologic restaging. Complete response represents the disappearance of all known disease, determined by two observations not less than 4 weeks apart. Partial response consists of a 50% or greater decrease in total tumor load of lesions that have been measured to determine the effect of therapy by two observations not less than 4 weeks apart. Overall tumor response refers to partial and complete response rates together.

---

*Open systems allow the use of jet ventilation to maintain effective gas exchange. Controlled ventilation with a closed system requires capping of the proximal end of the bronchoscope and any small side ports, as well as connecting the large side port to an anesthesia machine. Some method of preventing air leaking through the vocal cords must be provided (e.g., packing the pharynx with damp gauze). A totally closed system allows the use of inhalational anesthetics. Open systems allow the use of jet ventilation to maintain effective gas exchange.

Anesthesia in the supine position can lead to a decrease in the dimensions of the thoracic cage, a cephalad displacement of the dome of the diaphragm, and a reduction in thoracic volume. Although patients may be asymptomatic while awake, they may develop critical airway obstruction during anesthesia as the result of reduction in the dimensions of the chest wall. This limits the available space for the airways relative to the tumor and mediastinal structures. The decrease in tracheal distention pressure caused by the action of anesthetic agents on chest wall muscle tone also promotes central airway collapse,[26] and the supine position prompts an increase in central blood volume, which further increases tumor blood volume and size, worsening both the SVC syndrome and the CAO. Positional changes should certainly be initiated if inadequate ventilation is evident, because airway obstruction sometimes might be ameliorated by placing patients into a lateral decubitus or sitting position.

Although TIVA is used routinely in our institution, loss of airway control has been reported during induction using both intravenous and inhalation anesthesia for rigid bronchoscopy.[26,30,31] Muscle relaxants or a dose of propofol that produces apnea can be disastrous in a patient who cannot be ventilated because of CAO.[17] Anesthesia induction is the most dangerous period in terms of cardiovascular instability when drugs with a marked tendency for hemodynamic depression are used. Careful hemodynamic monitoring should be provided because patients with SVC syndrome are prone to decreased venous return, reduced cardiac output, and refractory hypotension. Acute worsening of symptoms has been reported as a result of overly generous fluid administration, prompting some authors to recommend diuresis in patients with clinically overt findings of SVC syndrome. It is assumed that diuresis will also decrease tumor volume,[25] but diuresis can decrease cardiac preload leading to hypotension, worsening a situation already complicated by compromised venous return.

Spontaneous-assisted ventilation* was shown to have a good cardiac safety profile in patients undergoing rigid bronchoscopy under general anesthesia.[31] Although a deeper level of anesthesia is required occasionally to avoid excessive cough and bucking secondary to bronchoscope-induced stimuli, light anesthesia allows spontaneous ventilation. This helps maintain hemodynamic stability and improve oxygenation. Again, we prefer to avoid using neuromuscular blocking agents because they eliminate airway muscular tone that helps maintain airway patency, which may result in prolonged weakness leading to postoperative respiratory failure.[30] Positive-pressure ventilation will increase the flow velocity and promote turbulent flow past the region of stenosis. Subsequently, the laminar flow pattern cannot be resumed, potentially resulting in ineffective ventilation of the distal airways and loss of effective gas exchange.[29]

Ideally, we like to see our patients waking up on the table, avoiding any need for postprocedural endotracheal intubation. During anesthesia maintenance, continuous positive-pressure ventilation and deep anesthesia are also avoided to preserve a normal transpulmonary pressure gradient and to maintain airway patency during spontaneous inspiration.[17] This may result in parts of the procedure being performed in a slightly moving or even an occasionally bucking patient. Although precautions are warranted to avoid airway trauma or excessive bronchoscope-related stimulation, short maneuvers are possible, and brief patient movements do not always warrant additional anesthetic to make the patient immobile.

Instrumentation

We chose a 12 mm Efer-Dumon rigid ventilating bronchoscope and an Nd:YAG laser for tumor coagulation and debulking. Various sizes of silicone and metal stents were readily available in case laser-assisted debulking failed to restore airway patency to less than 50% obstruction.

Anatomic Dangers and Other Risks

Because of complete RUL bronchial obstruction and volume loss, normal anatomic relationships in the mediastinum were altered; the right mainstem bronchus (RMB) was more horizontal, the right pulmonary artery was anterior to the proximal RMB, and the right inferior pulmonary vein was medial and posterior to the distal bronchus intermedius (BI) (see Figure 28-3). Therefore laser treatment had to be performed carefully in this area to avoid direct application onto the anterior or posteromedial walls. Because the tumor was hypervascular (see Figure 28-1), superficial absorption of laser energy was expected to be high. This would result in suboptimal deep coagulation and greater risk for bleeding during and after tumor debulking; this risk was probably further increased by the presence of collateral vessels and tumor congestion due to SVC syndrome. In addition, airway obstruction from blood and tumor debris could cause hypoxemia, which in this patient might have been poorly tolerated.

Results and Procedure-Related Complications

When general anesthesia was induced with intravenous propofol and remifentanil, the patient was difficult to ventilate with the bag mask, probably because of edema in the oropharynx and larynx. Therefore prompt intubation was performed using a 12 mm ventilating rigid bronchoscope. On bronchoscopic examination, the tumor involved the lower third of the trachea, starting 3 cm above the main carina. It completely occluded the entrance to the right main bronchus (see Figure 28-1). The carina was infiltrated, but the left bronchial tree was normal. Nd:YAG laser coagulation and tumor vaporization using a total of 7120 joules were followed by tumor debulking. Abundant thick secretions were suctioned from the previously obstructed right middle and lower lobe bronchi, and bleeding areas were treated using Nd:YAG laser photocoagulation. Flexible bronchoscopy at the end of the procedure confirmed patency of the right lower lobe and right middle lobe bronchi, but the right upper lobe remained completely occluded, and residual tumor was noted along the right lateral wall of the trachea (see video on ExpertConsult.com) (Video VI.28.1). At

---

*Spontaneous-assisted ventilation without the use of muscle relaxants requires an Ambu bag with a high-flow oxygen source, which is connected to the side port of the rigid bronchoscope.

Figure 28-4 A, The lower tracheal and mainstem bronchi immediately after intervention show improved airway patency. **B,** Improved atelectasis of the right lung immediately after therapeutic bronchoscopy while the patient was still intubated. **C,** Follow-up flexible bronchoscopy 4 weeks after therapeutic bronchoscopy reveals airway patency without recurrent tumor growth causing obstruction. **D,** After the second cycle of chemotherapy, 1 month after the intervention, near complete expansion of the previously atelectatic right lung was seen on a chest radiograph.

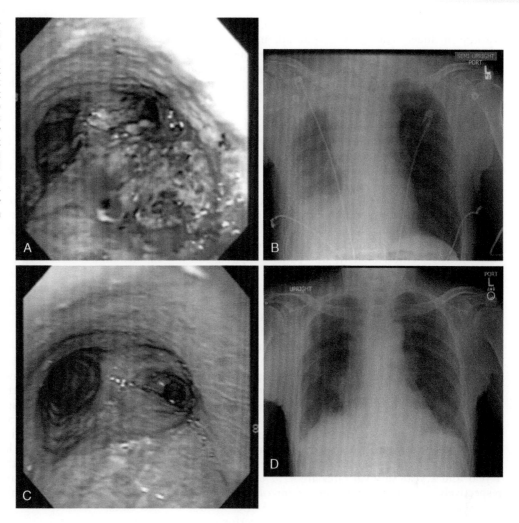

extubation, the presence of laryngeal edema prompted us to intubate the patient with a 7.5 mm endotracheal tube, given our concerns for postoperative respiratory failure. Corticosteroids and ventilatory support were provided overnight in the intensive care unit. We explained to the family that this temporary setback would most likely be corrected by the following morning. Indeed, the patient was fully awake with satisfactory weaning parameters and a good leak test, allowing extubation the next day. We did not extubate over a flexible bronchoscope, even though we had noted laryngeal edema at the time of rigid bronchoscopy. His chest radiograph showed improved aeration with re-expansion of a significant portion of the atelectatic right lung (Figure 28-4).

Long-Term Management

Outcome Assessment

Airway obstruction was partially relieved, and ventilation to the right lung was improved. Dyspnea subjectively improved such that the patient was transferred back to the referring facility within 48 hours to continue antibiotic treatment and immediately initiate systemic therapy.

Referral

Currently, the standard approach in limited-disease SCLC consists of four to six cycles of platinum-based polychemotherapy combined with radiotherapy of the tumor region and the mediastinum, followed by prophylactic cranial irradiation in case of complete remission. The most widely used chemotherapy regimen in limited-disease SCLC consists of cisplatin and etoposide.[32] Both radiation oncology and medical oncology services evaluated this patient, and a decision was made to initially proceed with chemotherapy. Even though it is recommended by American College of Chest Physicians (ACCP) lung cancer guidelines, the survival benefit of concurrent rather than sequential radiation delivery rests largely on findings of a single multicenter trial.[33] Emergent radiation therapy was not needed because airway patency had been restored. In fact, a meta-analysis showed no significant reductions in 2-year and 3-year mortality rates despite early thoracic radiotherapy.[33]

Follow-up Tests and Procedures

Systemic chemotherapy is advocated for both limited- and extensive-stage disease. Once a tissue diagnosis was made and airway patency was restored, the staging workup included chest, liver, and adrenal computed tomography, cranial magnetic resonance imaging (MRI), and a bone scan; in selected cases, unilateral or bilateral bone marrow aspirates and biopsies are also performed because bone marrow can be involved in 15% to 30% of patients at presentation.[34]

Our elderly patient had an improved but still poor performance status (Eastern Cooperative Oncology Group [ECOG] 2). He was offered combination chemotherapy with etoposide and carboplatin.[33] Follow-up bronchoscopy showed patent airways (see Figure 28-4), and chest radiograph showed marked improvement in right lung atelectasis 1 month later (see Figure 28-4). Symptoms, quality of life, and SVC syndrome–related clinical findings improved further after a second cycle of chemotherapy. Unfortunately, our patient expired suddenly from a suspected cardiovascular event while watching television in his home approximately 3 months after the rigid bronchoscopic intervention.

Median survival for SCLC patients without treatment is only 2 to 4 months from the time of diagnosis. For patients undergoing treatment, however, median ranges of survival for limited disease are 15 to 20 months, and for extensive-stage SCLC 8 to 13 months. Approximately 20% to 40% of patients with limited-stage disease and less than 5% of patients with extensive-stage disease survive 2 years.[35] The 5-year survival rates are 10% to 13%, and 1% to 2%, respectively.[36] For patients older than 75 years of age, median survival time for limited disease SCLC is reportedly 10.3 months. In these patients, 1 year and 2 year survival rates are 47.6% and 11.3%, respectively.[37] In addition to the extent of the disease, important adverse prognostic factors in SCLC include male sex (for unknown reasons), poor performance status, weight loss, and continuation of smoking, which may contribute to chemoresistance.[38]

Quality Improvement

Airway patency was restored, which allowed prompt initiation of chemotherapy. The patient's need for endotracheal intubation and overnight mechanical ventilatory support was considered a perioperative complication. We also discussed with our anesthesiologist our concerns regarding a transient inability to ventilate during induction. Remifentanil is an ultra-short-acting fentanyl derivative with a rapid onset time of 1 minute and a short duration of action (3 to 10 minutes). This drug is particularly useful for rigid bronchoscopic procedures because it allows active anesthetic management of fluctuating periods of high and low airway stimulation.[15] We wondered, however, whether safer alternatives to propofol were available for our elderly patient. Dexmedetomidine, for instance, is an α_2-agonist sedative-analgesic that inhibits endogenous norepinephrine release. Some anesthesiologists believe that this drug offers several physiologic benefits, including a reduced sympathetic response to a surgical stimulus, which can have cardioprotective effects in the elderly; other potential benefits of dexmedetomidine include a reduced rise in systemic and pulmonary vascular resistance and a potentially reduced occurrence of postoperative respiratory depression.[15] In

fact, case reports show that dexmedetomidine, almost without any additional anesthetic drug, maintained spontaneous ventilation in a patient with combined SVC syndrome and severe CAO.[39] Alternatively, ketamine, through its profound analgesic, sedative, and amnestic properties, could have been a valuable adjunct drug in our patient because ketamine does not suppress respiration, it reduces the narcotic requirement, and, through its sympathomimetic effects, it could have been useful if blood pressure had needed to be maintained in the presence of volume restriction.[15]

We realized that our patient's quality of life should have been objectively evaluated using a validated instrument. In one study, 269 patients undergoing combination chemotherapy and radiotherapy for SCLC of limited extent were asked to complete a Daily Diary Card that enabled an assessment of their quality of life during and after treatment. Results showed that although cytotoxic chemotherapy had an adverse effect on quality of life, the impairment affected only the first 2 or 3 days following each course of treatment. This information could have assisted us in counseling the patient about the likely effects of treatment.[40]

As an adjunct to general and cancer-specific diagnostic procedures, a comprehensive geriatric assessment (CGA) should be an integral part of cancer treatment in the elderly patient. CGA is based on standardized interviews and covers areas of physical and psychological dysfunction. The routine introduction of CGA in clinical research and daily practice might help clinicians identify those cancer patients for whom the greatest benefit from treatment is to be expected, and to formulate appropriate treatment and management strategies on an individualized basis.[32]

DISCUSSION POINTS

1. List two major complications during general anesthesia in patients with large mediastinal masses.
   - Loss of airway patency after induction due to severe compression of the trachea and mainstem bronchi
   - Hypotension caused by compression/obstruction of the superior vena cava and, potentially, compression of the pulmonary artery and heart[25]
2. Comment on the safety of therapeutic rigid bronchoscopy in people 80 years of age and older.
   - Octogenarians have multiple comorbidities and an advanced American Society of Anesthesiologists (ASA) class, which result in common cardiovascular and respiratory complications after rigid bronchoscopy. In this small case series, however, no increased perioperative mortality or postoperative respiratory failure required mechanical ventilation.[16]
   - To enhance safety, a thorough preoperative evaluation is warranted to address comorbidities. Bronchoscopists should do their best to shorten the duration of total anesthetic time. Patients may benefit from careful hemodynamic and respiratory monitoring during and after the intervention. Such monitoring might include end-tidal carbon dioxide (CO_2) measurements, arterial line placement, and bispectral index monitoring.

3. Enumerate seven measures to reduce operative and anesthetic complications in patients with concurrent superior vena cava syndrome and central airway obstruction.[29]
   - Schedule the operation after control of SVC syndrome has been attained (if possible).
   - Limit the amount of intravenous fluid administration and keep an intravenous access on lower extremities.
   - Maintain the patient in a sitting position preoperatively.
   - Use cautious anesthetic induction to avoid hemodynamic depression and loss of airway.
   - Maintain spontaneous-assisted ventilation and avoid muscle relaxants.
   - Beware of postoperative respiratory failure due to upper respiratory tract edema.
   - Provide careful monitoring for hemodynamic instability (e.g., arterial line).
4. Describe three major complications during rigid bronchoscopy in patients with large carinal tumors completely occluding a mainstem bronchus.
   - Perforation of the bronchial wall may result in broncho-mediastinal fistula.[41] Factors that might lead to this complication include the following:
     - Deviated axis of airway lumen by atelectasis and tumor (see Figure 28-3)
     - Misdirected laser beam (perpendicular to the airway wall)
     - Mechanical rupture by the rigid bronchoscope
   - Imprudent use of laser resection (high power) may lead to perforation of the airway wall and injury to the pulmonary artery, resulting in bronchovascular fistula and fatal hemorrhage.[42]
   - Hypoventilation or hypoxemia may be caused by contralateral airway obstruction from bleeding and tumor debris, or by an inability to ventilate through the rigid bronchoscope unless the rigid scope can be moved beyond the area of obstruction to remove secretions and ensure ventilation to the airways distal to the obstruction.

Expert Commentary

provided by D. John Doyle, MD, PhD

This case is far more complicated than most cases of malignant central airway obstruction in that the patient is quite elderly, has an occlusion of the superior vena cava (SVC) with venous engorgement and facial edema, and has a bifascicular cardiac conduction block, as well as an atrial septal defect (ASD). Such comorbid conditions suggest that the patient is at high risk for perioperative complications and even for succumbing during treatment. Two additional clinical constraints influence our management. First, definitive open surgical resection of the malignancy is not an appropriate option; second, avoiding the risks of general anesthesia is impractical. In particular, although the idea of initially treating the patient with radiotherapy is appealing, from clinical experience we know that the severe airway edema that such therapy produces can present

a significant danger to the patient in the absence of airway stent insertion.[43]

Without doubt, airway management is the greatest challenge in this case. Hence, the importance of the bronchoscopist and the anesthesiologist working together to plan and implement a management strategy cannot be overemphasized.[44] Airway edema resulting from SVC obstruction can render both intubation and ventilation difficult. One consideration, therefore, is whether general anesthesia should be preceded by awake intubation. A related issue is whether to immediately proceed to rigid bronchoscopy should it be decided to first induce general anesthesia. Yet another issue is whether bronchoscopy should be performed under general anesthesia with the patient breathing spontaneously, albeit with assistance. The bronchoscopy and anesthesia teams will find it necessary to discuss advantages and disadvantages of these various clinical options in light of the patient's condition, available equipment, and the preferences and training of the two clinical teams. In our experience, in cases such as this one, the bronchoscopy team often prefers to use a rigid bronchoscope with the assistance of muscle relaxants. In the United States, where sugammadex* still is not available, succinylcholine is often used as an initial relaxant. Its short duration of action adds a measure of safety should the patient become impossible to intubate or ventilate after its administration. Many Europeans would prefer to use rocuronium 0.6 mg/kg as a relaxant, followed by a "sugammadex rescue,"[45] should ventilation and intubation prove impossible after its administration.

Because of the presence of SVC syndrome, drugs administered via the upper body take longer to enter the central circulation. Consequently, placing an intravenous catheter in a lower body location such as the foot may be advantageous in severe cases of SVC obstruction. In this patient, the additional presence of an ASD makes the use of air trap devices† in the intravenous lines desirable.

Like the authors, we usually use total intravenous anesthesia (TIVA) in such cases because of worries regarding the reliability of delivering inhaled agents to the patient and because of concerns about polluting the operating room, especially with large fresh gas flows (e.g., >5 L/min) often required because of circuit

---

*Sugammadex (Bridion) is modified cyclodextrin used for reversal of rocuronium-induced neuromuscular blockade. It acts by encapsulating the rocuronium molecule, rendering it unable to bind to the acetylcholine receptor at the neuromuscular junction. The dosage varies between 2 and 16 mg/kg IV, depending on the degree of blockade to be reversed. The most common side effect is dysgeusia (metal or bitter taste); concerns about cardiac rhythm disturbances and hypersensitivity following sugammadex administration have caused the FDA to decline approval of the drug at this time.

†An air trap device captures air bubbles in intravenous lines to prevent them from entering the circulation. Unfortunately, protocol cannot be administered through them (at least in some models) because the traps will clog up. Although one solution might be to avoid the use of propofol (using ketamine, thiopental, or some other drug instead), most clinicians simply inject propofol via a stopcock distal to the filter to avoid this problem.

leaks and the use of airway suction. Preoperative anxiolytic medications are usually avoided, especially in frail patients with a compromised airway; however, an antisialagogue like glycopyrrolate can sometimes be helpful.

Our traditional TIVA recipe consists of propofol 500 mg (50 mL) to which 1 mg of remifentanil is added in a single 60 mL syringe. After induction with midazolam, fentanyl, propofol, and rocuronium, our usual starting dose of the propofol portion of this mixture is 100 mcg/kg/min, followed by titration to clinical effect. Note that a dose of 100 mcg/kg/min of propofol here produces a corresponding remifentanil dose of 0.2 mcg/kg/min. Although some clinicians prefer to use two separate infusion systems in such cases, with the possibility of controlling each infusion separately, we believe that our approach is simpler, has withstood the test of time, involves less chance for operator error, and requires less equipment and space.

In addition to standard monitors (e.g., electrocardiogram, pulse oximeter, capnograph, temperature, spirometry), two special monitors are worth considering. First, an arterial line, sometimes placed before the induction* of general anesthesia in patients with poor ventricular function or other severe cardiac problems, will allow early warning of hemodynamic difficulties. An arterial line will additionally facilitate the drawing of blood for blood gas studies† (useful in respiratory monitoring) and for hemoglobin levels (useful in the event of blood loss and blood transfusions). Second, in cases of TIVA, as in this case, we frequently employ electroencephalographic (EEG) monitoring of the depth of anesthesia, such as the use of bispectral index (BIS) monitoring (Aspect Medical Systems, Norwood, Mass), employing a target BIS score between 40 and 60.

In all cases such as this one, the possibility of massive blood loss during and after the procedure must be considered. Blood should be available on short notice, along with adequate venous access. A "type and screen" (for antibodies) will suffice in most cases. An interesting ethical issue concerns the degree to which blood should be administered in settings where the hemorrhage is so severe that all clinical efforts would be futile. A related issue concerns the "Do Not Resuscitate" status of such patients when the treatment offered is merely palliative.

Extubation in these cases can sometimes be challenging, and stridor and even frank respiratory failure sometimes follow. In awakening these patients, we sometimes transition from rigid bronchoscopy to an anesthesia face mask, but more frequently, we transition to a supraglottic airway such as a laryngeal mask airway or even an endotracheal tube before waking the patient, depending on the expected difficulty of

maintaining adequate spontaneous respiration. Most cases will benefit from routine administration of intravenous dexamethasone to reduce edema. Stridor is sometimes encountered after extubation; although this may require reintubation, we are often able to avoid this via the use of inhaled racemic epinephrine or the use of heliox, a mixture of helium (typically 70%) and oxygen.[46] Extubation over a tube exchanger can be helpful in cases where the need for reintubation is a concern and would be expected to be challenging.[47]

In summary, anesthesia-related considerations in this case include the patient's numerous comorbidities, the desirability of using total intravenous anesthesia, the possibility of significant blood loss, and the prospect of respiratory difficulties at the end of the procedure.

REFERENCES

1. Micke P, Faldum A, Metz T, et al. Staging small cell lung cancer: Veterans Administration Lung Study Group versus International Association for the Study of Lung Cancer—what limits limited disease? *Lung Cancer*. 2002;37:271-276.
2. Shepherd FA, Crowley J, Van Houtte P, et al. The International Association for the Study of Lung Cancer lung cancer staging project: proposals regarding the clinical staging of small cell lung cancer in the forthcoming (seventh) edition of the tumor, node, metastasis classification for lung cancer. *J Thorac Oncol*. 2007;2:1067-1077.
3. Slawson RG, Scott RM. Radiation therapy in bronchogenic carcinoma. *Radiology*. 1979;132:175-176.
4. Baker GL, Barnes HJ. Superior vena cava syndrome: etiology, diagnosis, and treatment. *Am J Crit Care*. 1992;1:54-64.
5. Gauden SJ. Superior vena cava syndrome induced by bronchogenic carcinoma: is this an oncological emergency? *Australas Radiol*. 1993;37:363-366.
6. Pelosof LC, Gerber DE. Paraneoplastic syndromes: an approach to diagnosis and treatment. *Mayo Clin Proc*. 2010;85:838-854.
7. Lissoni P, Messina G, Parolini D, et al. A spiritual approach in the treatment of cancer: relation between faith score and response to chemotherapy in advanced non-small cell lung cancer patients. *In Vivo*. 2008;22:577-581.
8. NCCN guidelines for patients; http://www.nccn.com/component/content/article/73-life-with-cancer-overview/854-things-to-consider-during-treatment.html. Accessed March 22, 2011.
9. Wood DE, Liu YH, Vallières E, et al. Airway stenting for malignant and benign tracheobronchial stenosis. *Ann Thorac Surg*. 2003;76:167-174.
10. Morris CD, Budde JM, Godette KD, et al. Palliative management of malignant airway obstruction. *Ann Thorac Surg*. 2002;74:1928-1933.
11. Bolliger CT. Multimodality treatment of advanced pulmonary malignancies. In Bolliger CT, Mathur PN, eds. *Interventional Bronchoscopy: Progress Respiratory Research*. Basel: Karger; 2000:187-196.
12. Mohsenifar Z, Jasper AC, Koerner SK. Physiologic assessment of lung function in patients undergoing laser photoresection of tracheobronchial tumors. *Chest*. 1988;93:65-69.
13. Vergnon JM, Costes F, Bayon MC, et al. Efficacy of tracheal and bronchial stent placement on respiratory functional tests. *Chest*. 1995;107:741-746.
14. Macha HN, Becker KO, Kemmer HP. Pattern of failure and survival in endobronchial laser resection: a matched pair study. *Chest*. 1994;105:1668-1672.
15. Puruggganan RV. Intravenous anesthesia for thoracic procedures. *Curr Opin Anaesthesiol*. 2008;21:1-7.
16. Davoudi M, Shakkottai S, Colt HG. Safety of therapeutic rigid bronchoscopy in people aged 80 and older: a retrospective cohort analysis. *J Am Geriatr Soc*. 2008;56:943-944.

---

*The arterial line can also be placed after induction; one should be prepared, however, for hemodynamic instability in patients with poor left ventricular function.

†The frequency of blood draws will depend on how the case proceeds and is very much a judgment issue.

17. Mackie AM, Watson CB. Anaesthesia and mediastinal masses: a case report and review of the literature. *Anaesthesia*. 1984;39:899-903.
18. Escalante CP. Causes and management of superior vena cava syndrome. *Oncology*. 1993;7:61-68; discussion 71-72, 75-77.
19. Eichenhorn MS, Kvale PA, Miks VM, et al. Initial combination therapy with YAG laser photoresection and irradiation for inoperable non-small cell carcinoma of the lung: a preliminary report. *Chest*. 1986;89:782-785.
20. Langer CJ. Elderly patients with lung cancer: biases and evidence. *Curr Treat Options Oncol*. 2002;3:85-102.
21. Paumier A, Le Péchoux C. Radiotherapy in small-cell lung cancer: where should it go? *Lung Cancer*. 2010;69:133-140.
22. Amarasena IU, Walters JA, Wood-Baker R, et al. Platinum versus non-platinum chemotherapy regimens for small cell lung cancer. *Cochrane Database Syst Rev*. 2008;(4):D006849.
23. Ernst A, Feller-Kopman D, Becker HD, et al. Central airway obstruction. *Am J Respir Crit Care Med*. 2004;169:1278-1297.
24. Thomas P, Robinet G, Gouva S, et al. Randomized multicentric phase II study of carboplatin/gemcitabine and cisplatin/vinorelbine in advanced non-small cell lung cancer GFPC 99-01 study. *Lung Cancer*. 2006;51:105-114.
25. Pullerits J, Holzman R. Anesthesia for patients with mediastinal masses. *Can J Anaesth*. 1989;36:681-690.
26. Conacher ID. Anaesthesia and tracheobronchial stenting for central airway obstruction in adults. *Br J Anaesth*. 2003;90:367-374.
27. O'Neill JH, Murray NM, Newsom-Davis J. The Lambert-Eaton myasthenic syndrome: a review of 50 cases. *Brain*. 1988;111:577.
28. Narang S, Harte BH, Body SC. Anesthesia for patients with a mediastinal mass. *Anesthesiol Clin North Am*. 2001;19:559-579.
29. Sibert KS, Biondi JW, Hirsch NP. Spontaneous respiration during thoracotomy in a patient with a mediastinal mass. *Anesth Analg*. 1987;66:904-907.
30. McMahon CC, Rainey L, Fulton B, et al. Central airway compression: anaesthetic and intensive care consequences. *Anaesthesia*. 1997;52:158-162.
31. Perrin G, Colt HG, Martin C, et al. Safety of interventional rigid bronchoscopy using intravenous anesthesia and spontaneous assisted ventilation: a prospective study. *Chest*. 1992;102:1526-1530.
32. Weinmann M, Jeremic B, Bamberg M, et al. Treatment of lung cancer in elderly part II: small cell lung cancer. *Lung Cancer*. 2003; 40:1-16.
33. Samson DJ, Seidenfeld J, Simon GR, et al; American College of Chest Physicians. Evidence for management of small cell lung cancer: ACCP evidence-based clinical practice guidelines (2nd edition). *Chest*. 2007;132:314S-323S.
34. Tritz DB, Doll DC, Ringenberg QS, et al. Bone marrow involvement in small cell lung cancer: clinical significance and correlation with routine laboratory variables. *Cancer*. 1989;63:763.
35. Osterlind K, Hansen HH, Hansen M, et al. Long-term disease-free survival in small-cell carcinoma of the lung: a study of clinical determinants. *J Clin Oncol*. 1986;4:1307.
36. Lassen U, Osterlind K, Hansen M, et al. Long-term survival in small-cell lung cancer: posttreatment characteristics in patients surviving 5 to 18+ years—an analysis of 1,714 consecutive patients. *J Clin Oncol*. 1995;13:1215.
37. Matsui K, Masuda N, Fukuoka M, et al. Phase II trial of carboplatin plus oral etoposide for elderly patients with small-cell lung cancer. *Br J Cancer*. 1998;77:1961-1965.
38. Martinez-Garciaz E, Irigoyen M, Gonzalez-Moreno O, et al. Repetitive nicotine exposure leads to a more malignant and metastasis-prone phenotype of SCLC: a molecular insight into the importance of quitting smoking during treatment. *Toxicol Sci*. 2010;116: 467-476.
39. Abdelmalak B, Marcanthony N, Abdelmalak J, et al. Dexmedetomidine for anesthetic management of anterior mediastinal mass. *J Anesth*. 2010;24:607-610.
40. Fayers PM, Bleehen NM, Girling DJ, et al. Assessment of quality of life in small-cell lung cancer using a Daily Diary Card developed by the Medical Research Council Lung Cancer Working Party. *Br J Cancer*. 1991;64:299-306.
41. Mohan A, Guleria R, Mohan C, et al. Laser bronchoscopy—current status. *J Assoc Physicians India*. 2004;52:915-920.
42. Vanderschueren RG, Westermann CJ. Complications of endobronchial neodymium-Yag (Nd:Yag) laser application. *Lung*. 1990;168: 1089-1094.
43. Casal RF. Update in airway stents. *Curr Opin Pulm Med*. 2010;16: 321-328.
44. Abernathy JH 3rd, Reeves ST. Airway catastrophes. *Curr Opin Anaesthesiol*. 2010;23:41-46.
45. Duvaldestin P, Plaud B. Sugammadex in anesthesia practice. *Expert Opin Pharmacother*. 2010;11:2759-2771.
46. Galway U, Doyle DJ, Gildea T. Anesthesia for endoscopic palliative management of a patient with a large anterior mediastinal mass. *J Clin Anesth*. 2009;21:150-151.
47. Cooper RM. The use of an endotracheal ventilation catheter in the management of difficult extubations. *Can J Anaesth*. 1996;43: 90-93.

Chapter 29

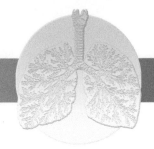

Bronchoscopic Treatment of a Large Right Mainstem Bronchial Stump Fistula

This chapter emphasizes the following elements of the Four Box Approach: risk-benefits analysis and therapeutic alternatives; techniques and instrumentation; and results and procedure-related complications.

CASE DESCRIPTION

The patient was a 79-year-old male referred for treatment of a large right pneumonectomy stump fistula. He had multiple comorbidities, including severe chronic obstructive lung disease (COPD), systemic hypertension, coronary artery disease, abdominal aortic aneurysm, and carotid artery stenosis, and a remote history of thyroid carcinoma. He had been diagnosed with squamous cell carcinoma 6 months earlier at another institution, where he had undergone right upper lobectomy and radical mediastinal lymph node dissection. Positive surgical margins prompted completion of pneumonectomy several days later. Postoperative hemorrhage required repeat thoracotomy within hours after the pneumonectomy had been performed. The postoperative course was complicated by prolonged mechanical ventilation for respiratory failure, pulmonary embolism, residual left femoral deep vein thrombosis warranting anticoagulation, and placement of an inferior vena cava filter. A tracheotomy was performed on postoperative day 7. Three weeks after surgery, the patient had developed increasing-right sided pleural effusion, copious secretions, and fever. Flexible bronchoscopy revealed a post pneumonectomy stump fistula. A 32-French chest tube was placed into the right hemithorax, and this revealed the presence of a large air leak. Sputum cultures were positive for *Pseudomonas aeruginosa,* and the patient was started odn intravenous imipenem and amikacin. He was considered inoperable and was referred to our institution for possible bronchoscopic treatment of his right post pneumonectomy stump fistula. Chest radiograph at admission showed an air-fluid level in the right hemithorax consistent with

---

*BPF can be classified into central and peripheral types. Central BPF involves segmental or larger airways and occurs most frequently after lung resection or trauma. This type of BPF is diagnosed by bronchoscopy and usually requires surgical repair. Peripheral BPF is a communication between the peripheral airway or lung parenchyma and the pleural space. Peripheral BPF has more diverse causes, including necrotizing pneumonia, trauma, lung surgery, bronchoscopic lung biopsy, and malignancy.

bronchopleural fistula (BPF). Bronchoscopy showed a large BPF due to dehiscence of the right mainstem bronchial stump (Figure 29-1).

DISCUSSION POINTS

1. List four risk factors associated with the development of bronchial stump fistula.
2. List three bronchoscopic treatment modalities for patients with large bronchial stump fistulas.
3. Describe and justify the use of three ventilator management strategies in patients with stump fistula and respiratory failure.

CASE RESOLUTION

Initial Evaluations

Physical Examination, Complementary Tests, and Functional Status Assessment

This patient had a central bronchopleural fistula (BPF).* Bronchial stump dehiscence (failure) represents BPF when disruption of a bronchial closure occurs after anatomic pulmonary resection. Early failure (within a few days to a few weeks following surgery) is usually the result of a technical problem such as a stapler misfiring, loose or broken sutures, or excessive tension with stump closure, causing poor apposition of tissues. Following pneumonectomy, bronchial stump dehiscence within the first few days to few weeks typically presents with a large air leak and coughing of copious quantities of secretions. Respiratory distress may occur secondary to spillage of pleural fluid through the bronchial stump into the contralateral lung or by loss of air into the empty pleural space, leading in some cases to a tension pneumothorax. Late stump failure (occurring later than 2 to 4 weeks after surgery but usually within 90 days of operation) is typically secondary to weak bronchial tissue and infection (bronchitis, empyema), which lead to loss of integrity of the bronchial stump.[1] Patients present with cough and expectoration of frothy, blood-tinged secretions. Fever is often present, and patients may have sweats and chills secondary to infection within the pleural space.

BPFs after pneumonectomy, as seen in this case, are not uncommon[2,3] and are associated with high mortality rates, usually resulting from empyema.[4] The estimated incidence of post pneumonectomy BPF ranges between 3% and 28%. Although the perioperative mortality of pneumonectomy overall is now less than 7%, this rises to 25% when complicated by empyema, and it may be

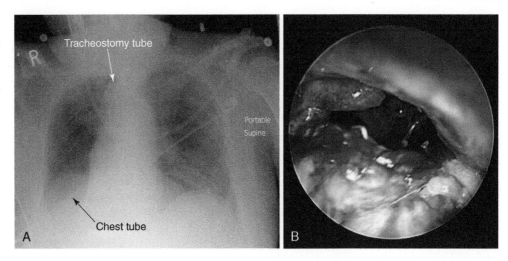

Figure 29-1 A, Chest radiograph obtained at the time of rigid bronchoscopy showing the right hydropneumothorax with fluid level present in the infrahilar region and the left lower lobe infiltrate. **B,** Rigid bronchoscopic view of complete right post pneumonectomy stump dehiscence.

as high as 50% when associated with fistula.*[3,5,6] In addition to empyema, the main complication of BPF is aspiration pneumonia caused by spillage of contaminated secretions into the contralateral healthy lung, potentially leading to adult respiratory distress syndrome (ARDS). The resulting impaired respiratory mechanics, contralateral lung contamination, and chronic pleural sepsis contribute to poor outcome.[7]

The bronchial stump after pneumonectomy or lobectomy could be fragile in cases of bronchial stump ischemia, extensive peribronchial dissection, inflammation at the suture line, or residual tumor at the bronchial stump margins. Several other risk factors also predispose to fistula formation and bronchial stump dehiscence, including preoperative chemotherapy or radiation therapy, right pneumonectomy, male gender, a large and long stump, postoperative mechanical ventilation, tracheostomy, and excessive dissection and tension at the bronchial suture line. Right-sided pneumonectomy, as performed in our case, is considered a major risk factor for stump disruption, in part because of the larger size and greater tendency of the right main bronchus to spring open, especially in the setting of positive-pressure ventilation, and because surgery-related alterations in the right bronchial microvasculature may lead to stump necrosis.[3] BPF after right pneumonectomy occurs with significantly increased frequency compared with left pneumonectomy (13.2% vs. 5.0%).[8] Pathophysiologically, this may be explained by at least two factors: First, the most common vascular supply to the right mainstem bronchus consists of a single bronchial artery, whereas the left mainstem bronchus is most commonly supplied by two bronchial arteries. Second, the left mainstem bronchus is protected beneath the aortic arch and surrounding vascularized mediastinal tissue. Another possible risk factor, present in our patient, is the use of sutures rather than staples for stump closure (Figure 29-1). In this regard, in a series of 713 pneumonectomies, Deschamps and colleagues observed an increased frequency of post pneumonectomy BPF following suture

closure versus stapled closure of the bronchus (incidence of 12.5% vs. 3.8%, respectively).[4]

As part of the initial evaluation, chest computed tomography (CT) may reveal a direct sign of BPF: A fistulous tract is noted between the bronchus or lung and the pleural space. Indirect signs include air bubbles beneath the bronchial stump and "suspected fistula" defined as a suspicious but not definite communication between the pleural space and the airway or lung parenchyma.[9] CT is useful not only for visualization and localization of BPF but also for identification of the cause, number, and size of the BPF and of underlying lung lesions (e.g., post lung resection, necrotizing pneumonia).[9]

Diagnosis on bronchoscopy is made by observing the direct signs of BPF. These are defined by the presence of a fistula opening at the bronchial stump or by the appearance of dye, previously injected into the airways during bronchoscopy, in the chest tube collection device. Air bubbling during the respiratory cycle (see video on ExpertConsult.com) (Video VI.29.1) and purulent secretions from the segmental airways are indirect signs of peripheral BPF. As part of an initial evaluation, even asymptomatic patients with clinically or radiographically suspected BPF should undergo flexible bronchoscopy for evaluation of the stump.* A fistula will often be visible, and a small amount of air bubbling may be observed with careful inspection of the stump (see video on Expert-Consult.com) (Video VI.29.1).† In our patient, bronchoscopy revealed a large BPF due to complete stump dehiscence (see Figure 29-1).

Comorbidities

Our patient had multiple cardiovascular and pulmonary comorbidities that increased the risk for myocardial infarction, stroke, and worsening respiratory failure

---

*The mortality rate ranges from 16% to 72%.

*Sometimes BPF can "hide" at the junction of the cartilage and the posterior membrane; a careful evaluation during both inspiration and expiration is necessary.

†If no fistula is demonstrable on bronchoscopy in a patient who is otherwise asymptomatic without leukocytosis, observation without pleural drainage may be warranted, but the presence of an occult fistula should remain highly suspected.

for procedures performed under general anesthesia. In fact, because of his poor functional status and comorbidities, he was not considered a candidate for repeat thoracotomy.

Support System

The patient had a very supportive wife. They had been married for 40 years and had three children and seven grandchildren. They were both independent in their activities of daily living.

Patient Preferences and Expectations

Because the patient's tumor was now completely resected, the wife expressed her wish to be aggressive and "do everything possible" to restore her husband's health. We did not consider her requests unrealistic. In today's health care environment, physicians' relationships with both patients and society have undergone important changes. For instance, patients are increasingly viewed as active "consumers" able to demand and are often encouraged to command and expect enhanced services, including extended hours and rapid access. In opposition to some examples in the managed care environment, where patients and health care providers might feel they are the victims of decreased access or have difficulty obtaining second opinions or referrals to specialists outside of their plans, the easy availability of health information coupled with a sense of entitlement is causing a power shift in the physician-patient relationship whereby patients might, on the basis of unrealistic expectations, impose their desire for costly tests and procedures in their attempt to do everything possible to reverse the effects of their illness, even if such tests or procedures are not believed to be medically indicated.[10]

Procedural Strategies

Indications

There was little doubt that without treatment of the BPF, this patient would have continued to deteriorate and eventually would have died from empyema and pneumonia in the contralateral lung. Given the reasonable reluctance to re-intervene surgically, a bronchoscopic attempt at closure of the fistula was warranted. Management strategies for BPF depend on a number of factors, including underlying cause, size, time of onset of the fistula post surgery, and health status of the patient. Surgery is the treatment of choice for this condition, but bronchoscopic techniques have been advocated as an option when surgery is not possible or has to be postponed.[7] Management of patients who have developed BPF and require mechanical ventilation is even more complex. Surgical repair is not a good option for these patients because postoperative mechanical ventilation is associated with a high failure rate owing to persistent barotrauma on the repaired stump.[7]

In general, nonsurgical, bronchoscopic strategies are categorized as follows: (1) occlusion with indwelling airway stents, (2) occlusion with glue or other materials, and (3) procedures that induce scar tissue formation at the fistula site. The goal of the stent, as chosen in this case, is to provide a tight seal in the airway to prevent spillage of infected pleural fluid into the contralateral lung. Because many types of stents with different biomechanical properties are available, selection of a stent requires consideration of the physical characteristics of the stent and potential associated short-term and long-term complications.[11] Several case reports of endobronchial stent insertion for isolated fistulas have been published, but case series of more than two patients are few.[12] Obviously, the effect of case selection is difficult to quantify from these publications. However, the feasibility of the technique in selected patients is encouraging. In one study, for instance, authors used specially designed covered metal stents (with a blind ending arm to fit the bronchial stump) in six patients. Patients underwent follow-up CT scan and bronchoscopy to confirm satisfactory stent placement. The mortality rate (mean follow-up, 316 days) was 0% with 67% of patients having the fistula closed; this led to resolution of the empyema.[12]

In our case, a large stent was needed to seal the large stump fistula as tightly as possible to prevent aspiration pneumonia to the left lung and to allow satisfactory single-lung ventilation in case mechanical ventilation needed to be continued. We therefore decided to use a Y silicone stent (with occlusion of one of the bronchial limbs) in an attempt to close the large bronchial stump fistula in this critically ill patient, who was not a surgical candidate. This approach can also be used as a permanent solution for patients with poor life expectancy to improve quality of life, or as a temporary bridge until a patient's clinical condition improves sufficiently to allow repeat thoracotomy.

Contraindications

No absolute contraindications to rigid bronchoscopy were noted, but general anesthesia was obviously risky in this patient with sepsis from empyema, pulmonary embolism, and multiple cardiovascular problems. In this regard, the physical status classification system of the American Society of Anesthesiologists (ASA) is a relatively simple system that has proved effective in stratifying overall preoperative risks of morbidity and mortality for patients undergoing anesthesia and surgery.[13] Complications are much more likely to occur in patients with preexisting disease states. For example, an ASA class 1 patient has no underlying conditions or limitations, but a class 5 patient is not expected to survive the next 24 hours without the proposed intervention. Risks inherent to a specific procedure are not incorporated into the ASA class. The relative risk of serious perioperative complications is 4.4 for ASA patient status 4, as was assigned to ours (i.e., a severe incapacitating disease process that is a constant threat to life), illustrating that increasing serious comorbidities reflected in the ASA classification increase perioperative morbidity.[14] Our patient was considered nonoperable because of his poor clinical status and high operative risk. Surgical contraindication was determined by consensus at our multidisciplinary meeting, which included critical care physicians, the interventional pulmonologist, and the consulting thoracic surgeon. The choice of using stent insertion, rather than repeat surgical repair, was thus based on the patient's unstable respiratory status, poor general health status, and inflamed appearance of BPF margins (see Figure 29-1).

Expected Results

Most published experience related to airway fistulas describes occlusion of tracheal or bronchoesophageal fistulas,[15,16] as well as case reports, small case series, and a few review articles pertaining to postsurgical bronchial stump fistulas.[17-21] In addition to their described use in patients with an inoperable or unresectable tumor involving the mainstem bronchi and lower trachea, Y stents have been used successfully in patients with tracheabroncho-esophageal fistulas, resulting in improved dyspnea and quality of life and a reduced rate of recurrent infection.[22] A Y stent has been reported to successfully cover a BPF in a patient who underwent right upper lobectomy for lung cancer.[23] However, the Y stent has patent distal bronchial limbs and thus cannot completely occlude a major post pneumonectomy stump dehiscence. For this purpose, modified versions of the Y stent have involved occlusion of one of the bronchial limbs to occlude or cover the airway defect in patients who are not surgical candidates. In one report, the authors shortened the right limb of a studded Dumon Y stent (Novatech, Cedex, France) and closed the right distal bronchial limb with silicone material cut out from the stent itself.[17] This resulted in successful occlusion of a 2 mm bronchial stump fistula. Another modified version of the Y stent is obtained by requesting the manufacturer to customize the stent at the time of manufacture by shortening the right bronchial limb and sealing its distal aspect. Such a stent was used successfully in a patient with a major right bronchial stump fistula and respiratory failure.[21] The fact that such a customized stent must be ordered and manufactured, however, may limit wider applicability and may delay scheduling of the therapeutic intervention.

Team Experience

Rigid bronchoscopy is performed at this institution on a weekly basis by a team of experienced physicians and nurses. Patients with BPF who require bronchoscopic treatment are encountered several times a year.

Therapeutic Alternatives for Sealing Off the Fistula

In general, treatment options for this problem depend on the initial type of surgery performed (pneumonectomy, lobectomy, sleeve or wedge resection), fistula size, the patient's physiologic status, and the overall condition of the remaining lung.

Surgical treatment options include bronchial stump revision with omental or muscular flap coverage. Surgeons usually advocate immediate thoracoplasty and open window thoracostomy when a major bronchial stump dehiscence is suspected, to prevent empyema and aspiration pneumonia on the contralateral side.[24,25] At the time of our evaluation, the patient was not considered to be a surgical candidate.

Minimally invasive techniques such as thoracoscopic and bronchoscopic procedures using different glues, coils, and sealants have been performed to attempt closure of BPFs in patients who are deemed to be poor candidates for repeat thoracotomy. Successful bronchoscopic closure of fistulas has been described with the use of ethanol, polyethylene glycol–based gel, fibrin, acrylic glue, cellulose, and gel foam, and placement of angiographic occlusion metallic coils, polidocanol, decalcified spongy calf bone, or unidirectional endobronchial valves or spigots.[7] Scar-forming techniques have been reported, in which thermal energy was provided by neodymium-doped yttrium aluminum garnet (Nd:YAG) laser or electrocautery (Figure 29-2). In the absence of tumor or infection, the laser beam or electrocautery probe is directed toward the mucosa surrounding the fistula to induce tissue edema, protein denaturation, and inflammation, eventually facilitating closure of the fistula by fibrosis.[26] Scar tissue and BPF closure can also be achieved by submucosal injection of the vein sclerosant polidocanol.[27] According to published studies, resolution of BPF using these bronchoscopic techniques ranges from 33% to 58%. These techniques involve repeated bronchoscopic interventions in most patients.[26,28,29] Furthermore, they are usually

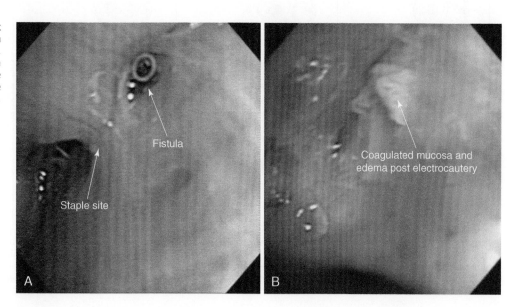

Figure 29-2 A, A 3 mm right upper lobe bronchopleural fistula (BPF) in a different patient. **B,** Closed BPF after treatment with electrocautery; in this case, the leak ceased during the procedure but reopened several weeks later, necessitating repeat intervention.

Fistula

Staple site

Coagulated mucosa and edema post electrocautery

A

B

reserved for patients with small fistulas measuring less than 5 mm and for those with fistulas that occur in more distal bronchial regions. The absence of evidence supporting the use of one technique versus another justifies a multidisciplinary approach in which interventional bronchoscopists and thoracic surgeons choose a specific product or technique based on their experience and product availability.

For closing large stump fistulas, in addition to our approach, other bronchoscopic treatments have been proposed:

1. *Gluing techniques:* Fibrin glue occlusion with spongy calf bone was used in a large series of 45 post resection fistulas (40 post pneumonectomy) up to 8 mm in diameter.[30] Only 20% of cases were cured using this technique, with resolution of both fistula and empyema. Most patients had an adverse outcome, with 20% dying as inpatients, 35.6% necessitating surgery, and 15.6% left with a chronic empyema. Another series in which synthetic glue was used in 12 post pneumonectomy fistulas had a better fistula resolution rate (66.7%) and survival of 83%, but it was disappointing that only 10% of empyemas resolved.[31] In another series, cyanoacrylate glue was used in three patients, with no mortality, but resolution of BPF and empyema was achieved in only one patient (33%).[32]

2. *Amplatzer double-disk occluders:* These represent a group of devices designed originally for transcatheter closure of cardiac septal defects or patent ductus arteriosus. These devices are made of Nitinol mesh with a central connector between the disks. The presence of two disks, one on either side of the lesion (Figure 29-3), leads to greater coverage and increases the likelihood of closure, as opposed to the use of glue, which is applied to the internal aspect alone. In the bronchial tree, the device

induces local granulation tissue formation that potentiates its occluding properties without compromising airway patency.[33] Endobronchial closure using an Amplatzer device was shown to be a safe and effective method of treating postoperative BPF in nonsurgical candidates. In one series, the authors inserted Amplatzer devices during flexible bronchoscopy under moderate sedation in 10 patients with 11 BPFs. In 9 patients, symptoms related to the BPF disappeared. Results were maintained over a median follow-up period of 9 months.[33]

3. *Expandable metallic stent insertion:* This technique has been used successfully for sealing BPFs. A large and long, straight, fully or partially covered expandable metal stent can be inserted, so that the covered portion of the main body of the stent occludes the bronchial stump fistula, while the distal aspect of the stent extends distally into the contralateral healthy bronchus and the proximal portion of the stent extends proximally into the trachea[18] (see Figure 29-3). In one case series, results from seven nonoperable patients who presented with large post pneumonectomy BPF (6 to 12 mm) are reported. The authors used a dedicated customized covered conical self-expandable metallic stent.[11] Cessation of the air leak and clinical improvement were achieved in all patients after stent placement. Stent-related complications (two migrations with recurrence of the leak and one stent rupture) were managed using bronchoscopic techniques in two patients and surgery in one. Mortality related to overwhelming sepsis was 57%, but definitive surgery was ultimately possible in three patients (43%).[11]

4. *Partially covered Nitinol stent with a closed distal aspect:* This device has been specifically designed and used for the treatment of bronchial stump fistula[12] (see Figure 29-3).

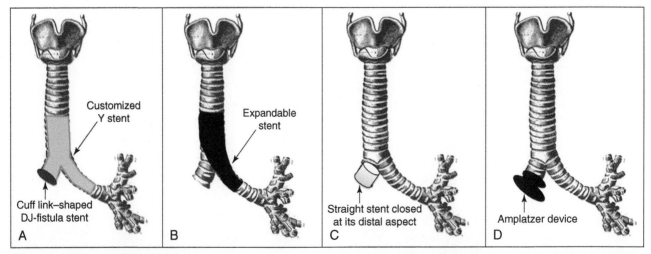

Figure 29-3 Diagram showing positioning of various stents in the airway for sealing off large stump fistulas. **A,** The cufflink-shaped DJ fistula stent is attached to the distal extremity of the right bronchial limb of the customized Y stent. **B,** Customized covered conical self-expandable metallic stent with the distal aspect of the stent extending down into the contralateral healthy bronchus and the proximal portion of the stent extending up into the trachea. **C,** Partially or fully covered metallic or silicone stent with a closed distal aspect. **D,** The Amplatzer device consists of two disks, one on either side of the fistula.

Cost-Effectiveness

Options available to treat BPF include medical therapies, bronchoscopic techniques, and surgical procedures. No controlled studies have compared different sealants or described surgical versus bronchoscopic treatment. Apparently, when surgery is feasible, it is performed, and attempts at bronchoscopic management are not necessary. Lack of published consensus among experts suggests that no single treatment modality is optimal. Given the limited published experience describing bronchoscopic management of large BPFs, it is unclear which bronchoscopic method or device is most effective.

In one review of the literature, the question addressed was whether bronchoscopic approaches to the closure of BPFs were effective compared with conventional re-thoracotomy; only six case series including more than two post pneumonectomy BPF patients were identified, resulting in an overview of 85 patients with post pneumonectomy BPFs who underwent bronchoscopic repair. Success was noted in 30% of cases with use of a wide range of bronchoscopic techniques.* Mortality was 40%. Many patients required multiple bronchoscopic procedures and additional drainage procedures of their empyemas. As of this writing, it seems that bronchoscopic treatments are offered most often to patients who are too unwell to undergo re-thoracotomy.[28]

Informed Consent

Informed consent was obtained from the patient's wife. She was informed about the risk of death from hemodynamic instability due to general anesthesia in the setting of empyema-induced sepsis; the risks of cardiac ischemia and stroke given the patient's previous cardiovascular history; and the risk that we might fail in our attempts to close the fistula.

Techniques and Results

Anesthesia and Perioperative Care

As part of their supportive management, patients with BPF and empyema require chest tubes to drain the air accumulating in the pleural space and the empyema cavity; this leads to a continuous leak of air from the airway to the external environment, resulting in loss of airway pressure, decreased tidal volume, and potentially progressive alveolar collapse.† In some BPF patients requiring mechanical ventilation, leaks can exceed 500 mL per breath.[34] For patients receiving volume-controlled ventilation, the volume of the leak is estimated as the difference between exhaled and set minute volume, assuming an intact circuit.‡ The length of the chest tube and its radius are important determinants of flow as governed by the *Fanning equation*, which describes turbulent flow of moist gases through a tube:

$$V = \Pi^2 r^5 P/fl$$

where V = flow, P = pressure, f = friction factor, l = length of the tube, and r = radius of the tube. The smallest internal diameter of a tube that would allow a maximal flow of 15 L/min at −10 cm H_2O suction is 6 mm.[35] Increasing negative airway pressure to compensate for lost volume while the patient is on mechanical ventilation only worsens the magnitude of the fistula. Also, negative pressures applied to a chest tube to assist drainage of the pleural space may increase flow through the fistula by increasing transpulmonary pressures and inducing auto-triggering of the ventilator. If not considered, auto-triggering may lead to inappropriate use of sedatives and paralytic agents to suppress hyperventilation. This can be avoided by decreasing sensitivity and minimizing airway pressure.[36] Alternatively, separation of the lungs by means of independent lung ventilation allows appropriate ventilation and minimizes air passing through the BPF.[37]

Instrumentation

The Y stent we used had a large, 16 mm wide tracheal limb and two 13 mm wide bronchial limbs. The stent was cut, then was sculpted in such a way that the tracheal limb was 3 cm long, the right bronchial limb only 1 cm long, and the left bronchial limb 3 cm long. The right bronchial limb was cut so that its distal aspect barely entered the right pneumonectomy stump lumen. We added a cufflink-shaped silicone prosthesis known as a tracheo-esophageal DJ fistula stent, which was developed specifically to palliate small tracheo-esophageal fistulas.[38] This stent was sutured onto the distal right bronchial limb of a studded Y-shaped stent to occlude the large right pneumonectomy stump fistula (Figure 29-4). The cufflink-shaped prosthesis is made of three portions: a 20 mm mushroom-shaped top, a 4 mm central limb, and a 10 mm elliptical distal aspect. The mushroom-shaped limb was pushed into the distal portion of the right bronchial limb of the Y stent, after which four 0 silk sutures were placed to tie the mushroom-shaped aspect to the Y stent, securing the cufflink-shaped prosthesis to the distal

---

*Bronchoscopic techniques included cyanoacrylate or fibrin glue application, YAG laser therapy, injection of the vein sclerosant polidocanol, and tracheobronchial stenting.

†Three compartment drainage systems are used for BPFs; these systems can handle flows from 10 to 42 L/min at a suction pressure of −20 cm H_2O. Increasing the suction pressure to −40 cm H_2O does not improve maximal flow.

‡Air leaks may vary from less than a liter to in excess of 16 L/min.

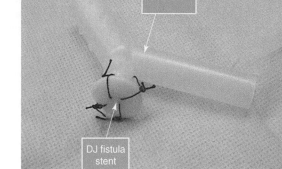

Figure 29-4 The cufflink-shaped DJ fistula stent sutured to the right bronchial arm of a silicone Y stent.

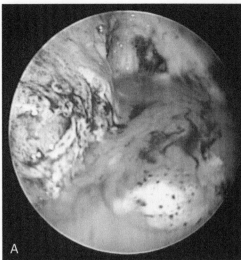
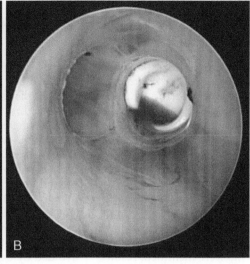

Figure 29-5 A, The right thoracic cavity with purulent fluid is seen through the right bronchial stump. **B,** Postoperatively, the combined stent is inside the airway and is completely covering the fistula.

aspect of the right bronchial limb of the Y stent (see Figure 29-4). This combined studded Y-shaped and DJ fistula silicone stent was then inserted using a rigid bronchoscope and large forceps.

Anatomic Dangers and Other Risks

Our patient had already contaminated his left lung. This was noted on the admission chest radiograph (see Figure 29-1). Once contamination of the contralateral (residual) lung occurs in a septic patient, acute respiratory failure can occur from ARDS and worsening lung compliance. In our case, during rigid bronchoscopic intervention, care was taken to prevent further spillage of pus from the empyema cavity into the left bronchial tree. One initial maneuver in the management of patients with BPF is urgent positioning in the reverse Trendelenburg position (head up). Another is to place the patient in a slightly lateral decubitus position, pneumonectomy side down, to prevent spillage of pleural fluid from the post pneumonectomy space into the airway of the remaining lung.

Results and Procedure-Related Complications

Bronchoscopy revealed a large pneumonectomy stump dehiscence. The flexible bronchoscope and a 12 mm EFER ventilating rigid bronchoscope (Bryan Corp., Woburn, Mass) could be moved easily through the fistulous tract into the right hemithorax, where a large volume of purulent fluid was noted (see video on ExpertConsult.com) (Video VI.29.2) (Figure 29-5). The fluid was removed by aspiration. The stump itself was severely inflamed, explaining its dehiscence. Necrotic debris was removed using forceps. The stump opening was at least 10 mm in diameter (see video on ExpertConsult.com) (Video VI.29.3). The rigid bronchoscope, which had been inserted through the patient's tracheostomy, was removed, and with rigid forceps, the stent was folded and inserted through the open tracheostomy and was positioned by feel onto the carina, such that the left bronchial limb could be guided down into the left main bronchus, and the right bronchial limb could be guided into the open

right pneumonectomy stump. The patient's tracheostomy allowed us to insert a stent that was large enough to completely occlude the large stump dehiscence.* The rigid bronchoscope was once more inserted into the airways, and the right bronchial limb–cufflink-shaped stent was gently pushed into position within the stump with the use of rigid forceps, completely occluding the fistulous tract (see video on ExpertConsult.com) (Video VI.29.4). Fibrin sealant was administered to prevent micro leaks around the stent itself. The patient then was extubated, and a No. 8 Shiley tracheotomy tube was inserted. The distal aspect of the tube was positioned such that its distal aspect was 2 cm above the proximal aspect of the indwelling Y stent. The patient was connected to the ventilator and was moved to the medical intensive care unit.

Long-Term Management

Outcome Assessment

Closure of the stump fistula was performed safely and without procedure-related complications. Immediately postoperatively, the patient's large air leak ceased. Broad-spectrum antibiotics were continued,[†] and the patient was transferred back to the referring hospital in stable condition, where he was successfully weaned from mechanical ventilation. Referring physicians were asked to perform occasional flexible bronchoscopy for secretion management.

Follow-up Tests and Procedures

Follow-up bronchoscopies revealed minimal secretions and a clean stent. One week after our bronchoscopic intervention, the patient's air leak had resolved

---

*Otherwise, with Rusch forceps, the stent can be grasped and promptly inserted under direct laryngoscopy using the push technique of Y-stent deployment.
    †Pleural fluid microbiology results had revealed *Pseudomonas aeruginosa*, which was treated with piperacillin/tazobactam and levofloxacin.

completely, and the empyema cavity had been drained, allowing removal of the large-bore chest tube. The patient was rapidly weaned from mechanical ventilation, a Passy Muir speaking valve was placed on the tracheostomy tube, and the patient was subsequently discharged home 27 days after his rigid bronchoscopy. Three months later, the tracheostomy tube was removed.

We were concerned that the silk sutures used to secure the DJ stent to the Y stent might not endure over the long term. Follow-up bronchoscopy performed 10 months later at an outside institution, however, showed these sutures to be intact. One year after the stent placement, after extensive nutritional and functional rehabilitation, this patient underwent uneventful thoracotomy with removal of the stent and definitive surgical closure of the fistula.

Quality Improvement

In this case, closure of the fistula was performed without complications in a patient at high risk for general anesthesia. This facilitated removal from mechanical ventilation and improved functional status. We considered that care was appropriate because the inserted stent had acted as a bridge, allowing significant improvement in the patient's clinical status, so that he could eventually undergo definitive surgery successfully.

DISCUSSION POINTS

1. List four risk factors associated with development of bronchial stump fistula.

   Predisposition to bronchial stump dehiscence can occur as the result of preoperative (related to patient-specific characteristics), intraoperative, and postoperative risk factors.[1] These include the following:
   - Comorbidities (diabetes, malnutrition)
   - Medications (steroids, antimetabolites)
   - Prior treatments (radiation)
   - Positive-pressure mechanical ventilation*
2. List three bronchoscopic treatment modalities for patients with large bronchial stump fistulas.
   - Silicone stents
   - Self-expandable metallic stents
   - Amplatzer devices
3. Describe and justify the use of three ventilator management strategies in patients with stump fistula and respiratory failure.

   In general, ventilatory management strategies for BPF include fistula exclusion from ventilation using a double-lumen endotracheal tube or advancing a conventional tube into the contralateral airway with the cuff distal to the fistula. If this is not possible, ensuring that the air leak is well drained from the pleural space with one or multiple chest tubes is required. Unless impractical, ventilator settings should be adjusted to minimize positive airway pressure.

- *Conventional ventilation:* This setting can be attempted in volume or pressure control modes, but spontaneous ventilation should be maintained whenever feasible because the primary goals in these circumstances are to keep airway pressure below the critical opening pressure of the fistula and to optimize pleural suction pressures and prevent further lung injury. To reduce flow across a BPF, minimal levels of positive end-expiratory pressure (PEEP), a short inspiratory time, low tidal volumes, and a low respiratory rate are useful.[36] No controlled studies have compared various modes of conventional mechanical ventilation in the setting of a BPF. Regardless of the mode, peak airway pressures should be maintained below 30 cm H_2O because higher pressures are associated with increased air leak.[39]
- *Independent lung ventilation (ILV):* In the setting of a BPF, this modality facilitates optimal ventilation of the contralateral, less diseased or normal lung while maintaining lower airway pressures on the affected side to reduce the air leak. ILV necessitates functional lung separation. Various techniques such as deliberate endobronchial intubation with or without bronchoscopic assistance, endobronchial blockade (e.g., bronchial blockers), and double-lumen endotracheal tubes (DLTs) enable ventilation and, depending on the types of tubes used, suctioning of each lung separately.* ILV is technically demanding and increases resource utilization in terms of equipment, monitoring, and skilled nursing care.[39]
- *High-frequency ventilation (HFV):* This setting has been shown to provide adequate gas exchange at lower airway pressures.
  - In *high-frequency jet ventilation (HFJV),* gas under high pressure is delivered through a small-bore cannula inserted into the endotracheal tube. Tidal volume is determined by jet pressure and inspiratory time. Tidal volumes of 2 to 5 mL/kg are delivered at frequencies of 100 to 200 breaths/min. In the largest reported series of patients with BPF occurring as a sequela of ARDS, HFJV was no better than conventional ventilation, and no significant changes in air leaks were observed.[40]
  - *High-frequency oscillatory ventilation (HFOV)* allows constant use of higher mean airway pressures, minimizing dead space and inducing reductions in peak airway pressures. HFOV creates pressure oscillations in the airways, thus generating small tidal volumes while maintaining relatively constant mean airway pressure. One study reported an improvement in oxygenation, lower mean airway pressure, and diminished air leak in patients with BPFs.[41]

---

*Positive-pressure ventilation is the most important risk factor for BPF. Early return to spontaneous respiration without positive-pressure mechanical assistance should be a priority after surgery to avoid inherent barotraumas and risk to the bronchial stump closure.

*They may be placed using direct laryngoscopy or fiberoptic bronchoscopy or through a tracheostomy. It should be emphasized that insertion of a DLT can be challenging, especially in hypoxic patients with or without difficult airways.

Expert Commentary

provided by Hiroaki Osada, MD, PhD

This has been an interesting case with an excellent outcome. Discharge home in 27 days after the bronchoscopic intervention, during which a novel, cufflink-shaped DJ fistula stent was used in conjunction with a Y stent, was indeed an excellent way to repair this right post pneumonectomy BPF in a patient with five substantial comorbidities. The conclusion made at the multidisciplinary conference to choose an attempt at bronchoscopic intervention and not to proceed to re-thoracotomy for fistula closure, therefore, seems reasonable. Allow me, however, to think about some possible alternatives because there is no single best way of treating this type of complex problem.

An aggressive open surgical intervention can serve as an optimal method of management for patients with post pneumonectomy empyema secondary to an associated bronchopleural fistula.[42] One of these surgical interventions consists of the addition of a muscle flap to cover the fistula. For this procedure, the right thoracic cavity must first be sterilized as much as possible. In my opinion, using a chest tube alone is not enough. Not only is pleural lavage via the chest tube needed, but also or instead, an open window thoracostomy[43,44] placed in the posterior aspect of the chest wall should be considered and might be more effective. To do this under general anesthesia, a double-lumen endotracheal tube should be inserted into the left main bronchus with the proximal cuff inflated in the lower trachea to establish unilateral ventilation.

Surgeons look to the chest radiograph with great interest when evaluating the stability of the mediastinum* (tendency to shift away from the midline after pneumonectomy) and whenever BPF is encountered in the early postoperative period, regardless of whether it is associated with empyema. This patient had an already stabilized mediastinum more than 3 weeks after his initial surgery. This means that his right hemithorax could be opened to atmospheric pressure.†

After central venous hyperalimentation for several days with the patient under anesthesia with intercostal nerve block, a window may be created in a short time. Open drainage and changing sponges for several days could bring the thoracic empyema under control. Then a muscle flap using the latissimus dorsi or the pectoralis major could be placed over the fistula, with or without limited thoracoplasty. With thoracoplasty

avoided, Clagett's procedure* may be considered after the pleural cavity becomes healthy and granulated.[44] An omental flap can also be used and is often ideal, but it is probably not indicated in this case because the patient has an aortic aneurysm.

It is certainly risky to perform such an invasive procedure, but it seems that eventually, the patient tolerated such surgery at the end of his entire treatment course. Therefore I wonder whether this patient could have tolerated this alternative way of treatment earlier in the course of his disease.

Although outside the scope of this discussion, I wonder why this patient had not undergone a bronchoplastic procedure to save the middle and lower lobes when the upper lobe stump had turned out to be pathologically positive. From a surgical perspective, I also wonder whether the right main bronchial stump had been reinforced with some vital tissue. A pedicled flap[45] of the latissimus dorsi muscle, a pericardium[46] for example, or at least a good intercostal muscle flap is usually available. Such preventive methods are very important, although they are not done routinely.

REFERENCES

1. Liberman M, Cassivi SD. Bronchial stump dehiscence: update on prevention and management. *Semin Thorac Cardiovasc Surg.* 2007;9:366-373.
2. Wright CD, Wain JC, Mathisen DJ, et al. Postpneumonectomy bronchopleural fistula after sutured bronchial closure: incidence, risk factors, and management. *J Thorac Cardiovasc Surg.* 1996;112:1367-1371.
3. Sirbu H, Busch T, Aleksic I, et al. Bronchopleural fistula in the surgery of non-small cell lung cancer: incidence, risk factors, and management. *Ann Thorac Cardiovasc Surg.* 2001;7:330-336.
4. Deschamps C, Bernard A, Nichols 3rd FC, et al. Empyema and bronchopleural fistula after pneumonectomy: factors affecting incidence. *Ann Thorac Surg.* 2001;72:243-247.
5. Wong PS, Goldstraw P. Post-pneumonectomy empyema. *Eur J Cardiothorac Surg.* 1994;8:345-350.
6. Sonobe M, Nakagawa M, Ichinose M, et al. Analysis of risk factors in bronchopleural fistula after pulmonary resection for primary lung cancer. *Eur J Cardiothorac Surg.* 2000;18:519-523.
7. Lois M, Noppen M. Bronchopleural fistulas: an overview of the problem with a special focus on endoscopic management. *Chest.* 2005;128:3955-3965.
8. Darling GE, Abdurahman A, Yi Q-L, et al. Risk of right pneumonectomy: role of bronchopleural fistula. *Ann Thorac Surg.* 2005;79:433-437.
9. Seo H, Kim TJ, Jin KN, et al. Multi-detector row computed tomographic evaluation of bronchopleural fistula: correlation with clinical, bronchoscopic, and surgical findings. *J Comput Assist Tomogr.* 2010;34:13-18.
10. Edwards N, Kornacki MJ, Silversin J. Unhappy doctors: what are the causes and what can be done? *Br Med J.* 2002;324:835-838.
11. Dutau H, Breen DP, Gomez C, et al. The integrated place of tracheobronchial stents in the multidisciplinary management of large post-pneumonectomy fistulas: our experience using a novel customised conical self-expandable metallic stent. *Eur J Cardiothorac Surg.* 2011;39:185-189.

---

*After lung removal, the mediastinum is not supported on one side and may shift. The residual pleural space should fill after surgery through a combination of mediastinal shift, diaphragm elevation, coagulation of serous drainage, and development of fibrotic tissue. If mediastinal shift is excessive, than decreased cardiac output may occur and may require mediastinal stabilization.

†Most surgeons attempt to prevent acute shift of the mediastinum by avoiding chest tubes after pneumonectomy. If they are used, tubes are clamped or are left to the water seal drainage only.

---

*It is a two-stage surgical procedure for treatment of empyema; the first stage involves creating an open window thoracostomy by resecting parts of ribs to create an opening into the thorax to allow drainage and antiseptic irrigation of the space. During the second stage, when the pleural space is clean and sterile, the space is filled with antibiotic solution and is closed surgically.

12. Han X, Wu G, Li Y, et al. A novel approach: treatment of bronchial stump fistula with a plugged, bullet-shaped, angled stent. *Ann Thorac Surg.* 2006;81:1867-1871.

13. Cohen MM, Duncan PG, Tate RB. Does anesthesia contribute to operative mortality? *JAMA.* 1988;260:2859.

14. Wolters U, Wolf T, Stutzer H, et al. ASA classification and perioperative variables as predictors of postoperative outcome. *Br J Anaesth.* 1996;77:217-222.

15. Colt HG, Meric B, Dumon JF. Double stents for carcinoma of the esophagus invading the tracheo-bronchial tree. *Gastrointest Endosc.* 1992;38:485-489.

16. Freitag L, Tekolf E, Steveling H, et al. Management of malignant esophagotracheal fistulas with airway stenting and double stenting. *Chest.* 1996;110:1155-1160.

17. Ferraroli GM, Testori A, Cioffi U, et al. Healing of a bronchopleural fistula using a modified Dumon stent: a case report. *J Cardiovasc Surg.* 2006;1:16.

18. Garcia Franco CE, Aldeyturriaga JF, Gavira JZ. Ultraflex expandable metallic stent for the treatment of a bronchopleural fistula after pneumonectomy. *Ann Thorac Surg.* 2005;79:386.

19. Tayama K, Eriguchi N, Futamata Y, et al. Modified Dumon stent for the treatment of a bronchopleural fistula after pneumonectomy. *Ann Thorac Surg.* 2003;75:290-292.

20. Madden BP, Sheth A, Ho TB, et al. A novel approach to the management of persistent postpneumonectomy bronchopleural fistula. *Ann Thorac Surg.* 2005;79:2128-2130.

21. Tuskada H, Osada H. The use of a modified Dumon stent for postoperative bronchopleural fistula. *Ann Thorac Surg.* 2005;80:1928-1930.

22. Shiraishi T, Kawahara K, Shirakusa T, et al. Stenting for airway obstruction in the carinal region. *Ann Thorac Surg.* 1998;66:1925-1929.

23. Watanabe S, Shimokawa S, Yotsumoto G, et al. The use of a Dumon stent for the treatment of bronchopleural fistula. *Ann Thorac Surg.* 2001;72:276-278.

24. Hankins JR, Miller JE, Attar S, et al. Bronchopleural fistula: thirteen-year experience with 77 cases. *J Thorac Cardiovasc Surg.* 1978;76:755-762.

25. Baldwin JC, Mark JB. Treatment of bronchopleural fistula after pneumonectomy. *J Thorac Cardiovasc Surg.* 1985;90:813-817.

26. Kiriyama M, Fujii Y, Yamakawa Y, et al. Endobronchial neodymium:yttrium-aluminum garnet laser for non-invasive closure of small proximal bronchopleural fistula after lung resection. *Ann Thorac Surg.* 2002;73:945-949.

27. Varoli F, Roviaro G, Grignani F, et al. Endoscopic treatment of bronchopleural fistulas. *Ann Thorac Surg.* 1998;65:807-809.

28. West D, Togo A, Kirk AJ. Are bronchoscopic approaches to postpneumonectomy bronchopleural fistula an effective alternative to repeat thoracotomy? *Interact Cardiovasc Thorac Surg.* 2007;6:547-550.

29. Wang KP, Schaeffer L, Heitmiller R, et al. Nd:YAG laser closure of a bronchopleural fistula. *Monaldi Arch Chest Dis.* 1993;48:301-303.

30. Hollaus PH, Lax F, Janakiev D, et al. Endoscopic treatment of postoperative bronchopleural fistula: experience with 45 cases. *Ann Thorac Surg.* 1998;66:923-927.

31. Scappaticci E, Ardissone F, Ruffini E, et al. Postoperative bronchopleural fistula: endoscopic closure in 12 patients. *Ann Thorac Surg.* 2000;69:1629-1630.

32. Sabanathan S, Richardson J. Management of postpneumonectomy bronchopleural fistulae: a review. *J Cardiovasc Surg.* 1994;35:449-457.

33. Fruchter O, Kramer MR, Dagan T, et al. Endobronchial closure of bronchopleural fistulae using Amplatzer devices: our experience and literature review. *Chest.* 2011;139:682-687.

34. Pierson DJ, Horton CA, Bates PW. Persistent bronchopleural air leak during mechanical ventilation: a review of 39 cases. *Chest.* 1986;90:321-323.

35. Powner DJ, Cline D, Rodman GH. Effect of chest tube suction on gas through a BPF. *Crit Care Med.* 1985;13:99-101.

36. Shekar K, Foot C, Fraser J, et al. Bronchopleural fistula: an update for intensivists. *J Crit Care.* 2010;25:47-55.

37. Konstantinov IE, Saxena P. Independent lung ventilation in the postoperative management of large bronchopleural fistula. *J Thorac Cardiovasc Surg.* 2010;139:e21-e22.

38. Diaz-Jimenez P. New cufflink-shaped silicone prosthesis for the palliation of malignant tracheobronchial-esophageal fistula. *J Bronchol.* 2005;12:207-209.

39. Dennis JW, Eigen H, Ballantine TV, et al. The relationship between peak inspiratory pressure and positive end expiratory pressure on the volume of air lost through bronchopleural fistula. *J Pediatr Surg.* 1980;15:971-976.

40. Bishop MJ, Benson MS, Sato P, et al. Comparison of high frequency jet ventilation with conventional mechanical ventilation for bronchopleural fistula. *Anesth Analg.* 1987;66:833-838.

41. Ha DV, Johnson D. High frequency oscillatory ventilation in the management of a high output bronchopleural fistula: a case report. *Can J Anaesth.* 2004;51:78-83.

42. Wain JC. Management of late postpneumonectomy empyema and bronchopleural fistula. *Chest Surg Clin N Am.* 1996;6:529-541.

43. Regnard JF, Alifano M, Puyo P, et al. Open window thoracostomy followed by intrathoracic flap transposition in the treatment of empyema complicating pulmonary resection. *J Thorac Cardiovasc Surg.* 2000;120:270-275.

44. Massera F, Robustellini M, Pona CD, et al. Predictors of successful closure of open window thoracostomy for postpneumonectomy empyema. *Ann Thorac Surg.* 2006;82:288-292.

45. Abolhoda A, Bui TD, Milliken JC, et al. Pedicled latissimus dorsi muscle flap: routine use in high-risk thoracic surgery. *Tex Heart Inst J.* 2009;36:298-302.

46. Taghavi S, Marta GM, Lang G, et al. Bronchial stump coverage with a pedicled pericardial flap: an effective method for prevention of postpneumonectomy bronchopleural fistula. *Ann Thorac Surg.* 2005;79:284-288.

Chapter 30

Hemoptysis Caused by Distal Left Main Bronchial Tumor in a Patient with Primary Lung Adenocarcinoma

This chapter emphasizes the following elements of the Four Box Approach: techniques and instrumentation; results and procedure-related complications; risk-benefit analyses and therapeutic alternatives; and referrals to medical, surgical, or palliative/end-of-life subspecialty care.

CASE DESCRIPTION

A 62-year-old female who had been diagnosed 6 weeks earlier with stage IV primary adenocarcinoma with rib and brain metastasis came to the emergency department with respiratory distress and hemoptysis. Hemoptysis was described as 4 to 6 tablespoons of bright red blood within 24 hours. She had a history of GERD and COPD requiring 2 L of home oxygen. She had smoked 1 pack per day for 20 years but quit 10 years earlier. At the time of her presentation, she had just completed a cycle of bevacizumab therapy and 10 days of brain radiotherapy. On physical examination, she was awake, alert, and oriented, without neurologic deficits; air entry in the left hemithorax was diminished. Her ECOG (Zubrod score)* before the hemoptysis was 1.[1] Her heart rate was 110, blood pressure 160/90, and respiratory rate 28/min. She required 5 L of oxygen by nasal cannula to maintain oxygen saturation of 92%. Chest radiograph showed left-sided tracheal deviation and atelectasis of the left lower lobe and lingula. Aeration in the upper lung field zone was maintained (Figure 30-1, A). The patient consented to bronchoscopy

with electrocautery; a large blood clot was noted completely occluding the distal left main bronchus (Figure 30-1, B). After clot removal, patency to the left upper lobe was restored, but active bleeding was noted coming from the tumor that was completely occluding the left lower lobe bronchus (Figure 30-1, C). The tumor was cauterized using an electrocautery probe (Figures 30-1, D and E). During the following hours, this controlled her hemoptysis. Follow-up chest radiograph post procedure shows improved aeration to the left upper lobe and persistent atelectasis in the left lower lobe (Figure 30-1, F).

DISCUSSION POINTS

1. List two alternative bronchoscopic procedures that can be applied to control this patient's hemoptysis.
2. List three contraindications to electrocautery performed through the flexible bronchoscope.
3. Describe and justify a diagnostic approach to a patient with lung cancer involving the mediastinum who presents with recurrent hemoptysis after bronchial artery embolization.

CASE RESOLUTION

Initial Evaluations

Physical Examination, Complementary Tests, and Functional Status Assessment

This patient with underlying chronic obstructive pulmonary disease (COPD) and stage IV lung adenocarcinoma presented with respiratory distress likely exacerbated by the left main bronchial obstruction caused by tumor-related bleeding. Several definitions have been put forth for what "major" airway bleeding (hemoptysis) represents, as well as for quantifying the degree and amount of bleeding, but the actual practical and clinical implications of such definitions based on amounts of expectorated blood are unknown. According to one classification schema, bleeding is considered nonmassive for less than 600 mL/24 hr, massive for more than 600 mL/24 hr, exsanguinating for more than 1000 mL/24 hr or for a rate greater than 150 mL/hr, and catastrophic when it causes an immediate threat to life. Based on this system, our patient had a nonmassive hemoptysis (4 to 6 tablespoons is the equivalent of 60 to 90 mL). This is similar to what is considered a significant bronchoscopy-related bleeding in other classification schemas, defined in studies

---

*The Eastern Cooperative Oncology Group (ECOG) score, also called the World Health Organization (WHO) or Zubrod score, runs from 0 to 5, with 0 denoting perfect health and 5 death. 0: asymptomatic (fully active; able to carry on all predisease activities without restriction); 1: symptomatic but completely ambulatory (restricted in physically strenuous activity but ambulatory and able to carry out work of a light or sedentary nature); 2: symptomatic, <50% in bed during the day (ambulatory and capable of all self-care but unable to carry out any work activities; up and about more than 50% of waking hours); 3: symptomatic, >50% in bed, but not bedbound (capable of only limited self-care, confined to bed or chair 50% or more of waking hours); 4: bedbound (completely disabled; cannot carry on any self-care; totally confined to bed or chair); 5: death.

Figure 30-1 A, Chest radiograph pre-bronchoscopy shows left-sided tracheal deviation and atelectasis of the left lower lobe and lingula but maintained aeration in the upper lung field zone. **B**, A large blood clot occludes the distal left main bronchus. **C**. After clot removal, evidence shows active bleeding from the tumor completely occluding the left lower lobe bronchus. **D**, Electrocautery probe in contact with the oozing tumor. **E**, Charring is noted on the surface of the tumor closing the lower lobe bronchus, but no active bleeding is seen. **F**, Chest radiograph post procedure shows improved aeration to the left upper lobe but expected persistent atelectasis in the left lower lobe.

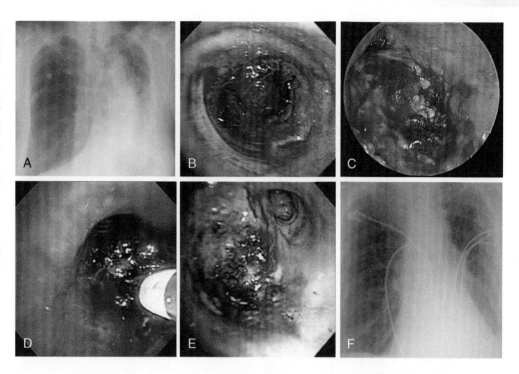

as more than 50 mL.*[2] It appears that when it comes to hemoptysis, no uniform cutoff value is agreed upon in the literature to define "massive" (Table 30-1).[3-10]

Lack of consensus regarding this cutoff volume, the known to be unreliable estimation of expectorated volume (e.g., half a cup, a few teaspoons, two tablespoons), and the indiscriminate use of descriptive criteria independent of common nomenclature, as well as other major determinants of morbidity and mortality such as rate of bleeding, the patient's ability to maintain patent airways, and the extent and severity of cardiopulmonary comorbidities, have led investigators to propose more clinically relevant definitions for what constitutes a major airway bleed.[11] These definitions rely on clinical consequences of hemoptysis such as airway obstruction and hemodynamic instability (Table 30-2).[12-15] Based on this classification, our patient had massive hemoptysis, in that she required hospitalization for respiratory distress and hypoxemia. It is estimated that it takes approximately 400 mL of blood in the alveolar space to decrease gas exchange significantly, but less is probably required in someone with previously compromised lung function.[16] In fact, the cause of death in patients with hemoptysis is usually asphyxiation rather than exsanguination.[17] Regardless of how it is defined, massive hemoptysis assessed subjectively or objectively is a major distressing clinical problem for both the patient and the treating physician. In one survey, 86% of responding chest physicians had treated

Table 30-1   Definitions for "Massive" Hemoptysis Based on the Amount or Rate of Expectorated Blood

Defining Terms	Amount or Rate of Expectorated blood	Reference
Massive hemoptysis	≥200 mL/24 hr	3
Major hemoptysis	≥200 mL/24 hr	4, 5
Severe hemoptysis	≥150 mL/12 hr	6
Severe hemoptysis	>400 mL/24 hr	7
Exsanguinating hemoptysis	≥1000 mL or ≥150 mL/hr	8
Life-threatening hemoptysis	≥600 mL/24 hr	9
Life-threatening hemoptysis	>200 mL/hr in a patient with normal or nearly normal lung function, or >50 mL/hr in a patient with chronic respiratory failure or >2 episodes of moderate hemoptysis (>30 mL) occurring within 24 hours in spite of administration of intravenous vasopressin	10

Table 30-2   Definitions for "Massive" Hemoptysis Based on Clinical Impact

Defining Term	Clinical Consequence	Reference
Massive hemoptysis	Transfusion requirement	12
Massive hemoptysis	Hospitalization	13
Massive hemoptysis	Endotracheal intubation	14
Exsanguinating hemoptysis	Aspiration and airway obstruction	8
Life-threatening hemoptysis	Hypoxemia (PaO_2 <60 mm Hg)	15

PaO_2, Partial pressure of oxygen in arterial blood.

*Using this definition, bronchoscopy-induced hemoptysis is seen in approximately 0.7% of all flexible bronchoscopies, with a higher prevalence of 1.6% to 4.4% for transbronchial lung biopsy. Most agree that routine prebronchoscopy coagulation testing is unjustified, but certain societies such as the British Thoracic Society recommend preoperative verification in patients with known risk factors even if no biopsy is planned.

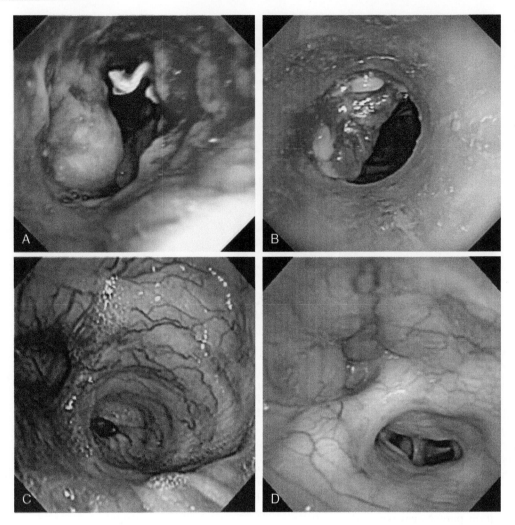

Figure 30-2 A, Bleeding from tumor growth through the uncovered part of an Ultraflex stent. **B,** Bleeding granulation tissue distal to a straight studded silicone stent. **C,** Neovascularization and erythema in a patient with adenocarcinoma. **D,** Mucosal infiltration and neovascularization in a patient with non-Hodgkin's lymphoma.

patients with massive hemoptysis during the previous year, and 28% had seen patients die from hemoptysis.[18]

In addition to intrinsic lung disease, increased risks for hemoptysis include a variety of coagulopathic disturbances—congenital, acquired (i.e., uremia), or medication-related (e.g., clopidogrel, bevacizumab). The cause of hemoptysis also tends to be population and region specific. For instance, in Africa and China,* tuberculosis remains a common cause of massive hemoptysis, but this is uncommon in the United States[19]; in the United States, in fact, the most common causes for hemoptysis are chronic bronchitis, bronchiectasis, and bronchogenic carcinoma, as seen in this patient. These are followed by tuberculosis, fungal infection (e.g., aspergilloma), bacterial pneumonia and abscess, and pulmonary infarction.†

The bronchoscopist might encounter hemoptysis caused by granulation tissue overgrowth and erosion of tracheobronchial mucosa from indwelling metal, hybrid, and silicone airway stents (Figure 30-2). Relevant to this patient's clinical presentation is that hemoptysis occurs in 20% of lung cancer patients at some point during their disease course, with massive episodes developing as the terminal event in 3%.[20] Reported mortality rates for massive hemoptysis range from 9% to 38% and depend on rate of bleeding* and cause; the highest mortality rate (38%) was reported in a case series that included a high proportion of patients with advanced carcinoma.†[21] In patients with cancer and non–tumor-related hemoptysis (e.g., infection, bronchiectasis), median survival (33 months) was better in comparison with patients who had

---

*Present in 55% of Chinese patients and in 85% of South Africans with massive hemoptysis.

†Less common causes of hemoptysis include mitral stenosis, Goodpasture's syndrome, endobronchial foreign bodies, broncholithiasis, airway stents, bronchial adenoma, pulmonary arteriovenous (AV) malformations, Behçet's disease, Wegener's granulomatosis, drugs (cocaine, anticoagulants, penicillamine), cystic fibrosis, lymphangioleiomyomatosis, laceration of the pulmonary artery by a balloon-tipped catheter, and lung parasites.

---

*One older study reported a 71% mortality rate in patients who lost more than 600 mL of blood in 4 hours, a mortality rate of 22% in patients losing more than 600 mL within 4 to 16 hours, and of 5% in those with 600 mL of hemoptysis within 16 to 48 hours.[17]

†Higher mortality has been associated with aspiration of blood in the contralateral lung, massive bleeding requiring single-lung ventilation, and bronchogenic carcinoma.

tumor-related bleeding (2.7 months) following endovascular management.[22] These data justify the need to identify the exact cause of hemoptysis in patients in whom cancer has been diagnosed.

Therefore during the initial evaluation of a patient with hemoptysis, a careful bronchoscopic inspection may reveal findings that suggest increased risk for bleeding or findings that could explain the hemoptysis, such as hypervascularization, aberrant vessels, and submucosal arterioles (see Figure 30-2). Pathogenically, the airway inflammation/infiltration associated with carcinoma can cause hypervascularity of bronchial arteries and stimulation of collateral circulation development. Further inflammation or severe coughing causes erosion of these abnormal vascular networks and can result in hemoptysis. Furthermore, in the setting of cancer, angiogenic growth factors may be produced. These promote neovascularization and recruitment of collateral circulation from systemic blood vessels. In this regard, our patient did receive bevacizumab, which was reported to cause hemoptysis (potentially fatal) in 2.3% of patients.*[23] Bronchoarterial fistula is of particular concern in patients with tumors invading mediastinal structures. In general, however, a pulmonary arterial origin is responsible for approximately 5% of cases of hemoptysis.[24] Large mediastinal vessel rupture secondary to blood vessel wall invasion is very rare but may lead to fatal massive hemoptysis, especially in patients treated with brachytherapy or external beam radiation therapy.[25] Multidetector chest computed tomography (MDCT)[†] with intravenous contrast[‡] is very accurate for predicting involvement of nonbronchial systemic arteries in patients with massive bleeding.[§] Tumor invasion of the pulmonary artery should not be misread as pulmonary embolism because anticoagulation in this setting could be catastrophic. MDCT is also useful for planning arterial embolization by providing information about bronchial and nonbronchial systemic arteries.[24] Although some authors suggest that computed tomography (CT) can replace bronchoscopy as a first-line diagnostic approach in patients with large (<300 mL/24 hr) or massive hemoptysis (>300 mL/24 hr) because of its higher diagnostic yield,[7] others find it complementary to bronchoscopy for bleeding site identification.[26] MDCT is of considerable diagnostic value for diagnosing

underlying disease, and used alone can localize the site of bleeding in 63% to 100% of patients. Combining bronchoscopy and CT increases this yield even further.[21] Bronchoscopy is particularly useful in unstable patients with active bleeding who might require endobronchial treatment. Bronchoscopy identifies the site of bleeding 73% to 93% of the time in cases of massive hemoptysis,* but localization rates are significantly lower in cases of mild or moderate hemoptysis.[19]

Comorbidities

In a patient with underlying COPD, the physiologic consequences of hemoptysis can be significant, even when it is not massive. Blood filling of anatomic dead space (≈150 mL) occurs quickly, and any further blood spilling into an already abnormal parenchyma leads to tachypnea, hypoxemia, tachycardia, bradycardia, hypotension, respiratory failure, arrhythmia, and even cardiac arrest. Airway obstruction from bleeding is obviously very poorly tolerated in patients with significant comorbidities such as severe COPD or history of pneumonectomy and in the critically ill.

Support System

Our patient was divorced; she had two children who were very supportive. They were quite distraught about their mother's respiratory distress and bleeding and were wondering whether the chemotherapy was helpful for her disease. They had begun inquiries about supportive care measures. They were told that our interpretation of the published evidence was that chemotherapy improves overall survival in patients with advanced non–small cell lung carcinoma (NSCLC) and that those who are fit enough, as their mother had been before this episode (Eastern Cooperative Oncology Group [ECOG] 1), should receive chemotherapy if it is offered. A meta-analysis (2714 patients from 16 randomized controlled studies) of chemotherapy and supportive care versus supportive care alone for NSCLC showed a significant benefit for chemotherapy equivalent to a relative increase in survival of 23%, and an absolute increase in survival of 9% at 12 months. Overall, survival was increased from 20% to 29%, with an absolute increase in median survival of 1.5 months (extending survival from 4.5 months to 6 months).[27]

Patient Preferences and Expectations

During our conversation, our patient stated that she would undergo any treatments as long as they continued to offer her a good quality of life. She agreed to bronchoscopy with electrocautery to cease the bleeding if possible, but not to intubation and mechanical ventilation, even if respiratory failure was triggered by the bronchoscopy itself. When we asked her why, she said that deep down inside, she believed that intubation

---

*It is possible that by antagonizing vascular endothelial growth factor (VEGF), bevacizumab might decrease the renewal capacity of the endothelial cell, which in turn causes endothelial dysfunction in the supporting layers of blood vessels. Consequently, anti-VEGF therapy might present a tendency for bleeding; in lung cancer, this is seen most often with squamous cell carcinoma, for which it is considered contraindicated.

†CT might be superior to chest radiography and comparable with bronchoscopy for detecting the site of bleeding in massive hemoptysis, with correct localization in 70% to 88.5% of cases.[19]

‡MDCT may also detect vascular lesions such as aneurysms, arteriovenous malformations, bronchiectases, and lung cavities as alternative explanations.

§Signs of pulmonary artery bleeding consisted of the following: (1) pulmonary artery (PA) pseudoaneurysm, or (2) aneurysm, or (3) the presence of a pulmonary artery in the inner wall of a cavitary lesion. MDCT findings of associated bronchial arterial hypertrophy predicted the need for simultaneous bronchial artery and PA embolization.

---

*Although the likelihood of visualizing the site of bleeding was significantly better with early versus delayed fiberoptic bronchoscopy (FOB), the timing of the procedure did not alter therapeutic decisions or clinical outcome in nonmassive hemoptysis.

was too invasive and was probably "futile." Sitting at her bedside, surrounded by her family and several physicians-in-training, we asked her what she meant by that. She quoted *Star Trek* in saying, "resistance is futile,"* and she told us that eventually, death must be accepted. She did not think intubation would prevent her from dying in the very near future, and if anything would probably cause both her and her loved ones to suffer. She insisted that she did not want her daughters to have memories of her on a breathing machine.

According to principles of autonomy and self-determination, patients or their surrogates have the right to refuse procedures regardless of the opinions of their health care providers, so long as they are considered capable of making such decisions, even if the treatment is considered to be life-sustaining. However, the opposite, that is, their right to demand a treatment—especially one that is regarded as "futile" by heath care providers—is much more controversial.[28] In this regard, the Texas Advance Directives Act of 1999 provided an extrajudicial conduit for a health care facility to discontinue life-sustaining procedures against patient (or surrogate) wishes.[†]

Although futility has been described in both qualitative and quantitative terms, today almost all experts would agree that futility cannot be viewed solely as having a single definition but must be considered in context, based on the knowledge, biases, values, and experiences of the individuals involved, and taking into account perceived and accepted goals of care that have been identified for a particular individual. Several succinct definitions have been offered, however, to help clarify the futility issue. One proposed definition for a futile action refers to an action that cannot achieve its goals, no matter how often it is repeated.[29] In this sense, however, futility does not refer to something that is impossible to do (as of this writing, systemic chemotherapy is not curative for stage IV lung cancer).

We believe that our patient's refusal of intubation, regardless of the cause or indication, was likely a reflection of hopelessness and not necessarily a demonstration of her understanding of futility concepts, although her reference to resistance and acceptance can be quite pertinent. Hopelessness is subjective, but futility refers to the objective quality of an action.[29] Futility refers to "the expectation of success that is predictably or empirically so unlikely that its exact probability is often incalculable."[29] We respected our patient's choice, but we took the liberty of explaining to both her and her family that intubation in the setting of hemoptysis causing respiratory distress is not a futile intervention[‡] because it could allow us to secure her airway, prevent further damage from ipsilateral or contralateral aspiration, stabilize her respiratory status, and potentially treat her hemoptysis using additional bronchoscopic techniques, or by providing time to perform emergent bronchial artery embolization. We emphasized that these procedures not only would stabilize her condition but could, and in our experience often did, allow extubation and discharge to home.

Procedural Strategies

Indications

The primary goal of treating an airway bleed is to establish and maintain an open airway to avoid severe hypoxemia and asphyxiation. This is achieved by performing bronchoscopic suction, using large-bore suctioning (e.g., Yankauer suction catheter) of the oral pharynx, and placing the patient in a lateral safety position with the bleeding side down.* This allows face-to-face contact with the patient if the bronchoscopy team is working from the front or side of the patient (Figure 30-3). The lateral position makes it easier for blood and secretions to flow out from the larynx, then into and out of the corner of the mouth. It is easier to suction the mouth and hypopharynx, and the epiglottis does not collapse onto the glottic opening, as it does in the supine position. It also helps avoid excessive collapse of the larynx and prevents upper airway obstruction by the tongue or an edematous upper airway, especially in patients with obstructive sleep apnea (OSA) or in those who have been administered moderate sedation or anxiolytics (these drugs might be beneficial in patients who are fighting for breath, coughing, or becoming increasingly anxious, frightened, and combative because of ongoing hemoptysis).

The second goal of bronchoscopic intervention is to stop the bleeding. This can be attempted by tamponade of the bleeding bronchus using continuous bronchoscopic suction, but in severe, difficult to control cases, unilateral intubation or double-lumen intubation may be necessary.[†] If intubation is considered, the largest endotracheal tube possible should be inserted. If double-lumen intubation is considered, often times, a flexible bronchoscope with a satisfactorily sized suction channel cannot be inserted, making bronchoscopic aspiration of blood and secretions difficult. Obviously, intubation of the bleeding airway requires practice and additional expertise.

Bleeding can be slowed by using balloons or the rigid bronchoscope (when used) or cotton pledgets for tamponading the airway, or by instilling vasoconstriction

---

*Used as the tagline for *Star Trek: First Contact* (1996), the eighth feature film in the *Star Trek* science fiction series by Paramount films, and the first to showcase the talents of the actors from *Star Trek: The Next Generation* television series.
†Texas Advance Directives Act, 1999. Texas Health and Safety Code §166.046. The process is initiated when a physician believes that he is being asked to provide what in the physician's judgment is futile care.
‡Schneiderman et al. had defined as futile "in the last 100 cases a medical treatment has been useless."[29]

*In the setting of active bleeding, the patient or the table is tilted 45 degrees toward the bleeding side.
†Use of a double-lumen tube permits adequate suctioning of blood, but its placement requires experienced personnel, and tube insertion can be difficult, especially in the actively bleeding patient. It may be wiser to first insert a large endotracheal tube, if necessary, selectively intubating the patient's good lung while turning the patient onto the lateral decubitus position (bleeding site downward) or using a bronchial blocker.

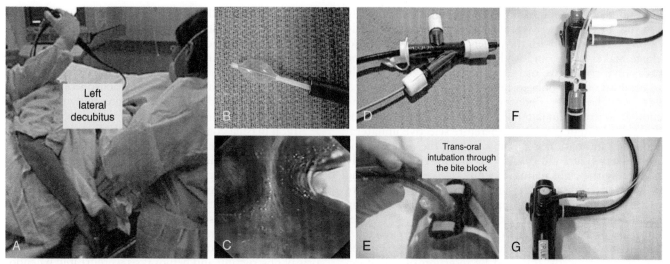

Figure 30-3 **A,** The safety (lateral decubitus) position in a patient with massive hemoptysis after left lung transbronchial biopsy. **B,** Fogarty catheter through the flexible bronchoscope. **C,** Fogarty catheter inflated and wedged in a lobar bronchus. **D,** Endotracheal tube (ETT) adapter for placing the Arndt bronchial blocker. **E,** Bronchoscopic intubation using an 8 mm ETT though the patient's mouth after an oral bite block is secured. **F,** Oxygen supplementation using oxygen tubing connected through a three-way stopcock to the working channel of the bronchoscope. **G,** Oxygen supplementation using oxygen tubing connected to the suction port of the bronchoscope.

agents such as epinephrine (1: 20,000)[*][30] and cold saline solution.[†][31] Lavage with normal saline at 4° C in 50 mL aliquots (average volume, 500 mL; range, 300 to 750 mL) stopped the bleeding in 23 patients with massive hemoptysis (>600 mL/24 hr).[†][31] Endobronchial instillation of tranexamic acid (500 to 1000 mg) was reported to immediately (within seconds) control airway bleeding (estimated at 600 to 750 mL), which did not respond to initial conservative therapy (cold saline, epinephrine).[32] To further enhance clot formation, the lateral decubitus position is probably useful through its gravity effect. Topical hemostatic tamponade using oxidized regenerated cellulose mesh, a sterile kitted fabric, has also been tried successfully in 56 of 57 (98%) patients with "life-threatening" hemoptysis.[§][15] If a tamponade balloon or a

---

[*]Local instillation of topical vasoconstrictive agents in the bleeding airway can be effective in mild to moderate hemoptysis following bronchial brushing and biopsy procedures. This approach is not useful for massive bleeding, however, because the drug is diluted and washed away. Significant cardiovascular effects can occur in the form of acute hypertension and tachyarrhythmias.[33] Intravenous vasopressin (0.2 to 0.4 units/min) causes bronchial arterial vasoconstriction, which presents danger if the patient has coronary artery disease and hypertension. In a trial comparing intravenous and endobronchial administration of terlipressin during bronchoscopy-induced bleeding, a similar hemostatic effect was observed for the two routes; however, drug plasma levels were 251-fold higher and diastolic pressure was significantly increased following intravenous administration.

[†]Saline lavage: Immediate administration of large aliquots of iced saline using a wedged or a partially wedged bronchoscope and continuous or intermittent suction and gravity-dependent clot formation stops bleeding in most cases.

[‡]One patient experienced transient sinus bradycardia during the procedure.

[§]The oxidized regenerated cellulose mesh was grasped with a biopsy forceps that had already been inserted into a flexible fiberoptic bronchoscope. It was then pulled back into the bronchoscope and was introduced into the bleeding airway, ranging from lobar to subsegmental bronchi.

Fogarty catheter (these can be used in segmental airways but usually are too small to occlude a lobar bronchus), a pulmonary artery balloon catheter (these Swan-Ganz catheters also are usually too small), or an endobronchial blocker (see Figure 30-3) is inserted into a bleeding segmental, lobar, or mainstem bronchus, its position should be verified by flexible bronchoscopy and chest radiograph because these items have a tendency to easily migrate out of the target airway. These devices can remain in place for several days if necessary. As has been mentioned, when these devices are considered, the bronchoscopist and assistants should first verify that the balloon diameter will be sufficient to completely occlude the target segmental, lobar, or mainstem bronchial airway, and that the balloon catheter fits through the working channel of the bronchoscope. The Cook (Arndt) bronchial blocker, for instance, does not fit through the working channel of a flexible bronchoscope, but if necessary, it can be placed using a dedicated adapter (see Figure 30-3) by inserting the catheter alongside (Video VI.30.1) or through (Video VI.30.2) a large endotracheal tube (see videos on ExpertConsult.com). In our experience, after a clot forms, it is wise to not immediately remove it, especially if bleeding has stopped. Inspection bronchoscopy, with or without clot removal, can be performed at a later time.

The third goal in managing hemoptysis is to prevent and treat respiratory, cardiac, and hemodynamic complications resulting from severe hypoxemia and hypercarbia. During flexible bronchoscopy, overuse of anxiolytics and narcotics should be avoided, if possible, when patients have significant hemoptysis, because these drugs will suppress cough, reduce minute ventilation, and thus worsen gas exchange. In addition, reduced consciousness and cough suppression may contribute to aspiration of upper airway secretions and aspiration pneumonia. Sedation or anxiolysis might warrant intubation even after bleeding is controlled. If intubation is warranted, a large single-lumen endotracheal tube usually can be inserted over the bronchoscope,* preferably through the mouth with the patient wearing a bite block. Haste makes waste, and we have seen on more than one occasion a combative or fearful patient spit out a poorly secured bite block only to bite down on the fragile flexible bronchoscope. Endotracheal tubes are not long enough to extend unilaterally into a mainstem bronchus if placed through the nares. Therefore selective unilateral bronchial intubation is possible only if the oral route is used[†] (see Figure 30-3). We do not advise selectively intubating the right main bronchus in a case of bleeding originating from the left lung, because this procedure usually occludes the right upper lobe bronchus, allowing ventilation to the right middle lobe and lower lobes only, and potentially further compromising gas exchange. Instead, we suggest that tracheal intubation be performed for left-sided bleeds, followed by insertion of a balloon catheter through or adjacent to the endotracheal tube, with subsequent introduction into the left main bronchus under bronchoscopic visualization.

Contraindications

We decided to attempt to control this patient's hemoptysis by using electrocautery. Electrocautery and argon plasma coagulation are contraindicated in a bleeding patient with a pacemaker/implanted autodefibrillator (unless they are deactivated temporarily) with high oxygen requirements (because of the risk for airway fire) or active massive hemoptysis for which electrocautery would be impractical (the treated field needs to be relatively dry for electrocautery to be efficacious). At the time of bronchoscopy, our patient had moderate mucosal hemorrhage, which we considered appropriate for electrocautery treatment.

Expected Results

Most mild to moderate mucosal bleeding can be controlled by using electrocautery via flexible or rigid bronchoscopy when lesions are visible. Several studies have showed an immediate response in controlling hemoptysis in 70% to 100% of patients.[34,35] The main disadvantage of using electrocautery for managing hemoptysis is loss of effectiveness due to diffusion of the current across a large surface area and wet tissues. The procedure may be more time-consuming than with laser because it is a contact mode therapy with more superficial tissue coagulation (2 to 3 mm for electrocautery vs. 5 to 10 mm penetration depth for neodymium-doped yttrium aluminum garnet [Nd:YAG] laser). Thus more debridement and probe cleaning are required. With any electrosurgery, there is a need for smoke evacuation. This requires intermittent suctioning, which may decrease tidal volumes and worsen hypoxemia in an already frail patient undergoing flexible bronchoscopy. Airway perforation, endobronchial fires and bronchoscope damage, bronchomalacia and stenosis, and pacemaker and automated implantable

cardioverter/defibrillator (AICD) dysfunction are rarely reported complications of electrosurgery.[36,37] During the electrocautery application, the bronchoscopist should be aware that cough induced when the probe touches the tumor can promote additional bleeding, and that blood can easily spread throughout the tracheobronchial tree, obscuring the bleeding site and potentially leading to severe hypoxemia and asphyxiation.

Argon plasma coagulation (APC) as a noncontact electrocautery mode could be chosen instead of contact probe electrocautery because it provides easy access to lesions located laterally or around anatomic corners (Figure 30-4).[38] In addition, APC allows homogeneous tissue desiccation (see video on ExpertConsult.com) (Video VI.30.3) because it seeks areas with higher water content and less electrical impedance. In a retrospective study, 31 patients with hemoptysis and 25 patients with both airway obstruction and hemoptysis were treated by endobronchial APC therapy. Bleeding was quantified as severe (>200 mL/24 hr) in 6 patients, moderate (50 to 200 mL/24 hr) in 23 patients, and mild (<50 mL/24 hr) but persistent for more than a week in 27 patients. Airway hemorrhage stopped immediately after the procedure in all patients with an endoluminal tumor responsible for the bleeding.[38]

Team Experience

A bronchoscopy team well experienced in their response to emergency situations should be available. We advise that teams practice procedures using inanimate models or high-fidelity simulation. Communication skills can be practiced, and bronchoscopists and their assistants should be familiar with various instruments and techniques. A hemoptysis protocol can be developed and placed into the policy and procedure manual of an interventional bronchoscopy unit. PowerPoint presentations can be designed for in-services and to ensure that all assistants are familiar with techniques and instruments. Crisis management is best performed when practitioners are familiar with and have practiced management procedures.* Overall, bronchoscopy in a moderately or massively bleeding patient should not be taken lightly. Patients probably should be hospitalized in the intensive care unit (sometimes, a small amount of hemoptysis is a sentinel event, eventually followed by a massive bleed), and the threshold for intubation with a large endotracheal tube should be low if it is believed that the airway needs to be protected.[†]

---

*Many teaching tools, checklists, PowerPoint presentations, and descriptions of techniques and instruments are available on the Bronchoscopy International website at www.Bronchoscopy.org, and in various manuals of the Bronchoscopy Education Project, officially endorsed by numerous national and international bronchology and interventional pulmonology societies, including the American, European, and World Associations for Bronchology and Interventional Pulmonology (AABIP, EABIP, and WABIP) and the South American Association for Respiratory Endoscopy (ASER).

[†]The debate regarding intubation is ongoing. Some believe that intubation protects the airway; others believe that cough is the better protector, and that the large caliber of a normal trachea is superior to the limited diameter of an endotracheal tube when it comes to clearing blood from the bleeding airway.

---

*A bite block should always be inserted to prevent patients from biting down on the bronchoscope (regardless of level of sedation).

[†]Nasal intubation will secure the airway by having the tip of the tube in the trachea.

Figure 30-4 Tracheal squamous cell carcinoma causing hemoptysis *(upper left)* is treated using a side port argon plasma coagulation (APC) probe *(upper right)*. Hemoptysis caused by an obstructing mucosal tumor in the left main bronchus *(lower left)*. After tumor debulking, a straight silicone stent was placed, which maintained airway patency and provided tamponade of the bleeding infiltrated bronchial mucosa *(lower right)*.

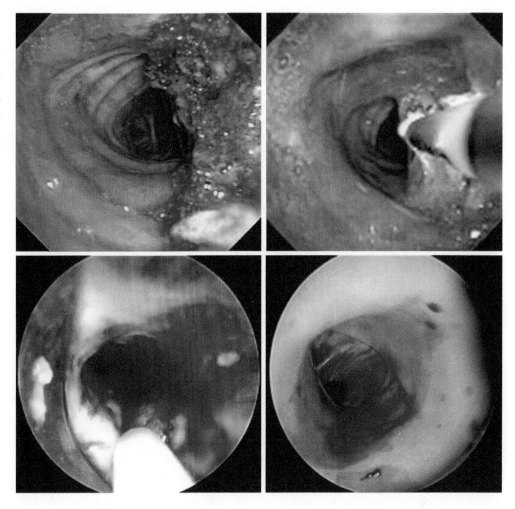

Therapeutic Alternatives

• *Rigid bronchoscopy:* This treatment is indicated for patients with massive hemoptysis resulting in respiratory compromise when the bleeding site is known or is highly suspected to be manageable by bronchoscopic interventions (based on imaging studies or flexible bronchoscopy). For instance, in this patient with known lung cancer and a chest radiograph showing left lower lobe (LLL) atelectasis, LLL obstruction was suspected and rigid bronchoscopy would have been a reasonable treatment alternative. The rigid bronchoscope allows good visualization of the airways, suctioning of blood clots and secretions through its large working channel and large suction catheters, the potential for effective tamponade of accessible bleeding sites using the rigid tube itself or various accessory instruments (see video on ExpertConsult.com) (Video VI.30.4), and isolation of the nonaffected lung by selectively intubating that particular mainstem bronchus. Furthermore, we believe that Nd:YAG laser applications and bronchial blocking techniques using a variety of devices are more readily performed through the wider lumen of a rigid bronchoscope.

• *Laser photocoagulation:* Nd:YAG laser coagulation can be an effective treatment option for hemoptysis when the source of bleeding is bronchoscopically visible. It allows photocoagulation of the bleeding abnormal mucosa, causing vasoconstriction of vessels feeding the bleeding site. The 1034 nm wavelength is, however, highly absorbed by dark pigments and therefore is absorbed by blood. This makes laser application ineffective and may cause superficial charring. Charred tissue easily adheres to laser fibers, creating a fire hazard (see video on ExpertConsult.com) (Video VI.30.5). Furthermore, current videotechnology saturates in red, making visibility problematic in the face of a large bleed. When a laser is used, a dry field is necessary. Often, two large suction catheters can be introduced through the rigid tube and placed onto and around the bleeding site. One catheter can be placed directly onto the bleeding vessel itself if visible. As blood rushes into the catheter, laser energy is applied around the bleeding site, blanching tissues and halting the bleed by vasoconstriction. Subsequently, laser energy can be applied directly onto the bleeding site, taking care to avoid overpenetration. Laser also provides an opportunity to vaporize underlying lesions or to assist with debulking after coagulation is optimized. Residual tumor and granulation bleed frequently. Often, the best treatment consists of removal of these tissues, followed by coagulation treatment of underlying mucosa.

Hemoptysis is seldom the sole indication for laser treatment because most patients with lung malignancy present with concomitant airway obstruction. Published results of laser photocoagulation for malignancy-induced hemoptysis are variable, but in a larger series of 24 patients, immediate control of hemoptysis was achieved in 67% of cases.[39]

- *Cryotherapy:* This technique has proved effective in managing mild hemoptysis in patients with endoluminal tumors and as a temporizing measure in patients with brisk bleeding. Blood clots can also be removed. Cryotherapy can be used to treat tumors because freezing causes vasoconstriction and microthrombi in venules and capillaries, and this results in tumor necrosis,[40] but probably has no role in patients with near total obstruction because the effects are delayed.[20]
- *Brachytherapy:* Although effective as a palliative treatment for mild, tumor-related hemoptysis in advanced lung cancer, this is not a treatment option for massive bleeding.[19]
- *Airway stent insertion:* Reports have described placing covered self-expanding airway stents (i.e., Polyflex, Ultraflex) to control bleeding and allow initiation of palliative radiotherapy.[41] We have occasionally used airway stents for tamponade of a bleeding site in patients with massive hemoptysis (especially if stent insertion was additionally indicated to maintain airway patency) (see Figure 30-4).
- *Surgical resection:* This approach requires clear identification of the bleeding site and a patient able to tolerate thoracotomy,* which was not the case in our patient with stage IV NSCLC and COPD. When performed, surgery has high morbidity and mortality ranging between 20% and 30% but up to 40% in the emergency setting. Because of this, surgical resection for massive hemoptysis has been mostly replaced by less invasive measures such as bronchoscopic treatments and bronchial artery embolization (BAE).† Surgery-related morbidity and mortality during an episode of acute hemorrhage are mostly related to operative bleeding, asphyxia, bronchopleural fistula, and respiratory failure.[42] In one survey from the American College of Chest Physicians, most respondents preferred bronchial artery embolization over conservative or surgical management for controlling hemoptysis.[43]

- *Bronchial artery embolization (BAE):* Immediate control of hemoptysis with BAE has been reported in 57% to 100% of patients,*[19] although bleeding recurrence after BAE has been described in 10% to 29% of patients at 1 month follow-up. The most extensive experience with BAE comes from studies of patients with hemoptysis caused by bronchiectasis, aspergilloma, and pulmonary arteriovenous malformation.[19] Hemoptysis related to bronchogenic carcinoma has a higher recurrence rate than that from other causes.[44-46] Success rates for malignancy- and aspergillosis-related hemoptysis are lower (58% to 67%) than those for other causes of hemoptysis such as cystic fibrosis (95%). One study of 19 patients with lung cancer and hemoptysis showed that BAE was technically and clinically successful in 100% and 79%, respectively, but had a recurrence rate of 33%.[47] Persistent or recurrent hemoptysis following BAE warrants consideration for bleeding of pulmonary artery origin.[48] If this is confirmed, PA embolization can be performed. Early recurrence after BAE is usually the result of incomplete embolization; late recurrence probably is caused by recanalization of previously embolized vessels, revascularization, or disease progression.[49] Bronchial arteries supply the bronchi and vasa vasorum of the aorta and pulmonary vessels, but also contribute to the esophagus, diaphragmatic and mediastinal visceral pleura, and spinal cord.† Inadvertent occlusion of these branches is responsible for BAE complications. The most common side effects are chest pain and dysphagia, reported in 24% to 91% and 1% to 18%, respectively. Inadvertent embolization of spinal arteries is a rare but significant complication of BAE and may be seen when spinal arteries branch off from the bronchial arteries being embolized.‡[19]

Cost-Effectiveness

No direct cost-effectiveness analyses have been performed for BAE and bronchoscopy for managing massive hemoptysis. Other published evidence suggests that identification of the bleeding source and isolation of the lobe or lung involved are matters of priority; rigid bronchoscopy is warranted because it is efficient at safeguarding airway patency, ensuring ventilation, and allowing good clearance of blood and debris from the airways.[31] A rigid bronchoscopy procedure for airway clearance before surgery may contribute to improving surgical outcome,

---

*Surgical resection is not an option for patients with poor functional status, moderate to severe lung function impairment, bilateral pulmonary disease, or other comorbidities.

†Surgery also remains the strategy of choice when management is needed for massive hemoptysis caused by diffuse and complex arteriovenous malformations, iatrogenic pulmonary artery rupture, chest trauma, and mycetoma not responding to other therapeutic strategies; when other therapeutic interventions are not readily available; or when all efforts to control bleeding medically (e.g., strict bed rest, no chest percussion or spirometric testing, aggressive cough suppression, bronchoscopic intervention, BAE) are unsuccessful.

---

*Actual visualization of a bleeding blush during arteriography is rare, but localization is inferential from visualization of the abnormal vascularity of reactive bronchial arterial networks. Vessels greater than 2 mm in diameter are considered abnormal and usually are embolized using Gelfoam, steel coils, polyvinyl alcohol, and isobutyl-2-cyanoacrylate or gelatin cross-linked particles called *tris-acryl microspheres*.

†Anatomic variations of the numbers and sites of origin of the bronchial arteries have been described in healthy individuals. About 20% of bronchial arteries have an aberrant origin from other systemic nonbronchial arteries. In 5% of patients, a spinal artery originates from a bronchial artery.

‡The incidence of this complication has significantly decreased since the "super-selective" technique, which enables distal cannulation of the target vessel, beyond the origin of spinal branches, became widely used.

probably because hemodynamics are stabilized, and airway hygiene is performed because bronchoscopy helps identify the bleeding site before surgery. In another study, a multidisciplinary approach favored BAE as first-line therapy, with surgery undertaken only when BAE failed.* The decision to prefer one specific modality over another is believed to be affected by the underlying cause of the hemoptysis and by the expertise of the thoracic surgery, interventional radiology, and bronchoscopy services at the center providing care.[9] In our opinion, care can be individualized, but our protocol pertaining to patients with hemoptysis includes making sure that each of these subspecialty services is informed of the patient's admission, and that all review patient data and images and participate in the multidisciplinary decision-making process.

Informed Consent

Our patient and her family had a clear understanding of the indications, contraindications, and alternatives for flexible bronchoscopic intervention. They agreed to proceed with the flexible bronchoscopy, and potentially to proceed with rigid bronchoscopy and BAE. The patient refused to consider an open surgical intervention.

Techniques and Results

Anesthesia and Perioperative Care

Before bronchoscopy is performed, cardiac monitoring and supplemental oxygen (the fraction of inspired oxygen [FiO_2] will need to be reduced to less than 0.4 during the actual electrocautery application) are necessary. The bronchoscopist should ensure that space in the procedure room is sufficient for staff members to move around should an emergency arise, and that medication and hemodynamic resuscitation equipment are readily available; in particular, airway resuscitation equipment should include a variety of endotracheal tubes, large-bore/Yankauer suction catheters, oral airways, and bite blocks. Because hypoxemia may occur, supplemental oxygen can be provided not only via face mask but also through the bronchoscope. The team should be well versed in the use of all necessary accessories, which ideally should be prepared before the procedure is begun (see Figure 30-3). Performing bronchoscopy in the patient with or at risk for massive hemoptysis provides the perfect case example for a strategy and planning, techniques, and results and response to complications study of team dynamics and procedure-related skills.

Instrumentation

We used a large-channel bronchoscope (2.8 mm) to accommodate the passage of electrocautery probes and to facilitate suctioning of blood and bloody secretions. An oral airway, a bite block, large-bore suction tubing, and an Arndt endobronchial blocker were readily available.

Anatomic Dangers and Other Risks

Inserting a flexible bronchoscope into the airway through the transnasal route causes a 17% rise in the functional residual capacity of the lungs, potentially altering gas exchange.[50] In a patient with COPD, this may lead to further air trapping and hypoventilation. Therefore, operators should watch for initial signs of hypercarbia. These include agitation, tachycardia, and hypertension, all of which develop before severe acidosis occurs. Once severe respiratory acidosis has been established, the patient's mental status is altered; bradycardia and hypotension can quickly lead to cardiorespiratory arrest. In our patient, who by the time of the procedure had become extremely fearful and anxious despite the bedside attentions of our nurses, a total of 5 mg of midazolam and 50 mcg of fentanyl was administered intravenously, in addition to 300 mg of 1% topical lidocaine onto the vocal cords and lower airways.

Results and Procedure-Related Complications

With the patient receiving oxygen via face mask, the flexible bronchoscope was advanced through the right nostril. The nasopharynx and the larynx were normal. The vocal cords were normal and symmetric. After local laryngeal anesthesia was obtained, the scope was advanced into the patient's subglottis, then to the level of the main carina. No tracheal abnormalities were noted, except for bloody secretions, which were easily aspirated. The main carina looked sharp. Two milliliters of lidocaine was instilled into the right and left mainstem bronchi, respectively, followed by inspection of the right bronchial tree. This was performed first to ascertain normal or abnormal airways, before our attention was turned to the left bronchial tree, where we suspected airway obstruction; no mucosal abnormalities were evident on the right, but bloody secretions were present, which were suctioned without difficulty. On the left, hemorrhagic secretions were observed in the mainstem bronchus, and distally, complete obstruction by a large blood clot was noted (see Figure 30-1). Before the clot was removed bronchoscopically, the patient was placed in the left decubitus position. When the patient is turned onto this "safety position" (bleeding side down), the contralateral airway is better protected from spillage of blood into the normal lung. With the use of saline washes, the clot was gently removed. Once this had been done, it was noted that the left upper lobe was completely patent, but the lower lobe was completely closed by infiltrating tumor involving the secondary left carina. Active hemorrhage was evident at the surface of the tumor. Five milliliters of epinephrine (1:20,000) was instilled locally, the FiO_2 was reduced to an estimated value of less than 0.4 (3 L via face mask), and electrocautery with a contact probe was initiated at 30 W power using 1 to 3 second bursts (see video on ExpertConsult.com) (Video VI.30.6). After bleeding had been controlled (see Figure 30-1), the airways were re-inspected. No evidence suggested spillage of bloody secretions into the right bronchial tree. The scope was removed and the procedure was terminated. Our patient had no evidence of hemodynamic instability or worsened

---

*Old tuberculosis and bronchiectasis were the main underlying diseases in that series, with only 4 of 49 patients given a diagnosis of lung cancer.

oxygen desaturation during the procedure. She was transferred to the intensive care unit (ICU) for monitoring.

Long-Term Management

Outcome Assessment

The chest radiograph post procedure showed improved aeration in the upper lung zone (see Figure 30-1). We thought that in addition to her airway tumor, the bleeding might have been exacerbated by her bevacizumab treatment. We contacted the patient's oncologist, who arranged for a follow-up clinic visit to discuss options for further chemotherapy.

Follow-up Tests and Procedures

The coagulation effect from electrocautery is superficial (maximum, 2 to 3 mm). We feared that once the charred layer at the surface of the tumor was expectorated, her hemoptysis might recur. We scheduled her for a BAE after consulting with our interventional radiology department. Several hours after her bronchosocopy, she underwent selective left parabronchial artery embolization. A single left bronchial artery was identified, and a selective angiogram revealed abnormal vascularity (Figure 30-5) and a blush in the hilar region of the left lung, corresponding to the hilar mass seen on CT and to the bleeding area

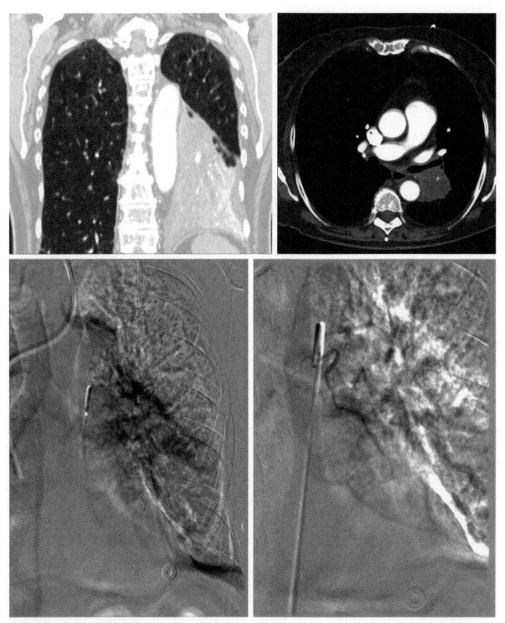

Figure 30-5 Coronal chest computed tomography (lung window view) showed upper lobe–predominant emphysema and complete left lower lobe atelectasis *(upper left)*. The contrast-enhanced axial mediastinal view showed complete closure of the left lower lobe bronchus by the infrahilar lung mass *(upper right)*. Selective angiograms of the left bronchial artery before *(lower left)* and after *(lower right)* embolization; note the hypervascular area and the blush in the left lung before embolization, which resolved after the intervention.

seen on bronchoscopy. Selective embolization was performed by slow injection of a mixture of microparticles (embosphere 300 to 500 microns) with water-soluble contrast. Intermittent fluoroscopy was performed during the injection to assess progression of the embolization until satisfactory flow stasis and obliteration of the abnormal vascularity and blush were achieved. Post embolization angiograms showed satisfactory obliteration of the abnormal vascularity (see Figure 30-5). The procedure was terminated, the catheter and the right femoral sheath were removed, and an arteriotomy closure device was placed on the right groin for hemostasis. No immediate complications were reported.

By the next day, the patient's hemoptysis had completely resolved. Three days post embolization, a flexible bronchoscopy was performed, which revealed hyperemic infiltrated mucosa but no active bleeding. She was discharged home with a plan to undergo follow-up with her pulmonologist and oncologist, and to undergo flexible bronchoscopy on an as needed basis only. Six weeks later, however, she presented again with hemoptysis. She was

again transferred to our institution, and we assured her that although immediate control of hemoptysis can be achieved in 73% to 99% of patients treated with BAE, recurrent hemoptysis on long-term follow-up is not uncommon, occurring in 10% to 55.3%. We did not tell her that higher mortality rates have been reported in patients who experienced recurrent bleeding following BAE for massive hemoptysis. In those studies, the following risk factors were identified for recurrence of hemoptysis: (1) residual mild bleeding beyond the first week after BAE; (2) blood transfusion before the procedure; and (3) diagnosis of aspergilloma as the underlying cause.[51] Our patient had none of these, but on repeat flexible bronchoscopy, she showed rapid progression of her endobronchial disease with now near complete occlusion of the left main bronchus by tumor and blood clot. Indeed, late recurrence post BAE can result from recanalization of previously embolized vessels, revascularization, or disease progression.[49] We proceeded with rigid bronchoscopy, tumor debulking, and Y stent placement at the left secondary carina (Figure 30-6) because we had

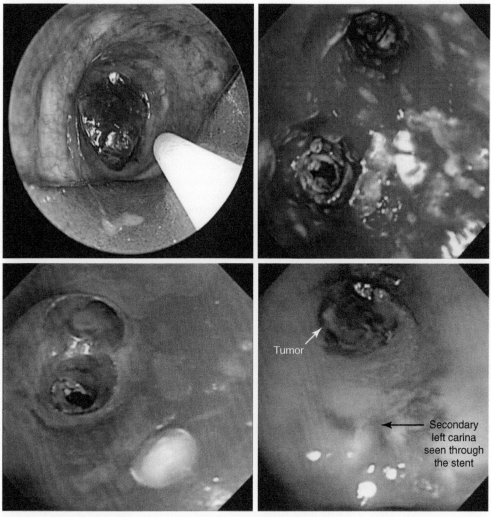

Figure 30-6 Rigid bronchoscopic view at the time of recurrent hemoptysis showed complete closure of the distal left main bronchus by a large exophytic tumor *(upper left)*. Once this has been removed, the upper and lower lobe bronchi were visualized, but the mucosa was circumferentially infiltrated by tumor *(upper right)*. A Y stent (12 × 10 × 10) was trimmed and sculpted to fit into the upper and lower lobe bronchi *(lower left)*. Flexible bronchoscopy 2 weeks later showed tumor growth distal to the left upper lobe limb of the Y stent *(lower right)*.

noted some airway patency to the lower lobe after the distal left main bronchus (LMB) tumor was debulked. During the next 2 months, our patient underwent two additional flexible bronchoscopies to remove tumor overgrowth distal to the limbs of the Y stent (see Figure 30-6), but she had no additional episodes of hemoptysis. We last saw her in our emergency department as she was being admitted for excessive weakness, malnutrition, post obstructive pneumonia, and impending respiratory failure. The patient and her family wanted supportive care and had declined invasive procedures, intubation, noninvasive mechanical ventilation, and ICU admission. She thanked us for having prolonged her life and was admitted to our palliative and end-of-life care service. She passed away quietly several hours later on comfort care measures.

Referrals

We believe that consultation with interventional radiology was effective and had been in this patient's best interest because her hemoptysis was controlled for several months after combined bronchoscopic and BAE procedures. Thoracic surgery consultation was not deemed necessary in this patient because of her advanced lung cancer and severe COPD, which precluded surgical intervention. Furthermore, she was unwilling to consider any form of open surgical intervention.

Quality Improvement

We discussed whether a second embolization would have benefited this patient when her hemoptysis recurred. Evidence suggests that BAE can be safely performed in such circumstances.[49] However, mucosal bleeding was controlled by electrocautery during repeat flexible bronchoscopy. The cause of her death was progressive cancer-related cachexia and tumor progression with obstruction of the segmental airways distal to the stent; death was not due to hemoptysis. One could propose that the application of delayed effect bronchoscopic interventions such as photodynamic therapy (PDT) or brachytherapy might have maintained distal airway patency. Indeed, PDT was considered during our encounters with the patient, but the need to avoid sun exposure for 6 weeks was against this patient's goals of care. Brachytherapy was not offered to this patient because of our concerns for causing massive hemoptysis in a territory (left upper lobe [LUL]) at high risk for bronchoarterial fistula formation.[25]

DISCUSSION POINTS

1. List two alternative bronchoscopic procedures that can be applied to control this patient's hemoptysis.
   - Argon plasma coagulation[38]
   - Nd:YAG laser[39]
2. List three contraindications to electrocautery performed through the flexible bronchoscope.
   - High oxygen requirements (because of the risk for airway fire)
   - Active massive hemoptysis (requires first lung isolation and better airway control)
   - Pacer-dependent cardiac arrhythmia (because pacer deactivation could lead to dangerous arrhythmias,

and application of electrocautery without temporary pacer deactivation could lead to pacer dysfunction and permanent damage)
3. Describe and justify a diagnostic approach to a patient with lung cancer involving the mediastinum who presents with recurrent hemoptysis *after* bronchial artery embolization.
   - The lungs have a dual arterial supply: the pulmonary and bronchial systems. The pulmonary arteries account for 99% of the arterial supply and are responsible for gas exchange; bronchial arteries constitute the remaining 1% and supply nutrient branches to the bronchi, vasa vasorum to the pulmonary arteries and veins, and smaller bronchopulmonary branches to the lung parenchyma.[49]
   - The systemic arterial system is the primary source of bleeding in hemoptysis, but bleeding may result from a pulmonary arterial source in approximately 5% of cases. Pulmonary angiography has therefore been proposed in patients with early recurrent hemoptysis *after* systemic arterial embolization. Results from one study of 306 patients showed that the pulmonary artery was the source of bleeding in 93% of patients in whom immediate control of hemoptysis was not achieved. Underlying diagnoses included lung abscess, tuberculosis, and lung cancer.[52]

Expert Commentary

provided by Laura Findeiss, MD, FSIR

This case involves moderate hemoptysis secondary to metastatic bronchogenic carcinoma in a 62-year-old female. Important features of the case include patient expectations and prognosis relative to the underlying condition, volume of bleeding and projected risk from the acute event, and the risk-benefit ratio of available treatment modalities. In this patient, bronchoscopy was chosen as the initial diagnostic and therapeutic modality, with embolization used as an adjunctive treatment following bronchoscopic electrocautery of the visualized hemorrhage.

No algorithm for approaching the patient with hemoptysis has been universally accepted. Early referral for surgery, the historical mainstay of therapy, has fallen out of favor. Published recommendations range from prompt use of bronchoscopy for diagnosis, localization, and pulmonary toilet to no bronchoscopy, with CT recommended as the primary diagnostic modality before BAE. A trend toward multidisciplinary approaches has been noted,[9] and most contemporary management strategies incorporate BAE as a strategy for temporizing or definitively treating hemoptysis. New bronchoscopically mediated technologies for achieving hemostasis are promising, but as of this writing, no directly comparative literature exists to guide selection of treatment modality.

Guidelines for performance of bronchial artery embolization are not well defined, and bleeding thresholds vary in the literature. A threshold volume of 300 mL/24 hr is often referenced in the interventional radiology literature. However, some studies have used much lower thresholds, and Mal et al. have used "hemoptysis that poses a threat to life" as the trigger for proceeding to embolization in their practice.[10] In general, threshold criteria for performance of interventions should be based on a risk-benefit analysis, whereby a benefit is projected, and the risk of the intervention does not exceed the risk of no intervention.

In a large study of outcomes of hemoptysis, Hirschberg et al. described mortality rates for different volumes of hemoptysis.[21] This group defined "trivial" hemoptysis as drops of blood or bloody sputum, moderate as less than 500 mL/24 hr or 1 to 2 cups, and massive as greater than 500 mL/24 hr or more than 2 cups. Most patients with malignancy presented with trivial or moderate hemoptysis. A small number of therapeutic bronchoscopies and surgeries, but no BAE, were performed. In-hospital mortality rates of 2.5% and 6% were reported in the trivial and moderate groups, respectively. A higher total mortality of 21% in the malignancy group was not specifically attributable to bleeding.

Complications from BAE range from femoral artery access complications, as seen with any transarterial procedure, dissection of aorta or bronchial arteries, bronchial infarction, and nontarget embolization. The most feared complication of BAE continues to be inadvertent embolization of the arteries to the spinal cord. The anterior spinal artery may arise from common trunks with the bronchial arteries, or may have well-developed anastomotic connections with the bronchial arteries. Although the risk is considered to be very low (<1% to 2.7%), the complication of paraplegia is devastating and warrants careful consideration of alternatives, as well as thorough discussion with the patient of risks and benefits of the embolization procedure. In all patients, it is imperative to perform careful angiography with close inspection for spinal arteries, especially when interrogating a right intercostobronchial trunk, from which the anterior spinal artery may commonly arise. If any opacification of the spinal artery is observed, many authors recommend against embolization. Super-selective technique using a microcatheter positioned well distal to the origin of the bronchial artery is recommended for improved efficacy and decreased complication rates[53] (Figure 30-7). Physicians considering referral of patients for BAE should be made aware of the degree of expertise within their institutions, and of overall complication rates. This information is essential if one is to carefully weigh advantages and disadvantages of the various therapeutic modalities being considered before treating the patient with hemoptysis.

The reported volume of hemoptysis of 4 to 6 tablespoons over a 24 hour period in the patient described in this scenario was below the threshold traditionally considered appropriate for performance of BAE. However, a trend toward more liberal use of BAE has been observed for lower volumes of hemoptysis as a palliative measure, with some evidence of improved survival in patients with malignancy who undergo

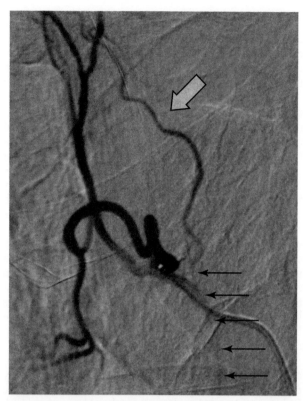

Figure 30-7 Oblique digital subtraction angiogram of right intercostobronchial trunk during embolization; careful scrutiny of late phase images is critical in evaluating for collateral filling of small arteries that may represent the anterior spinal artery. A collateral vessel filling from the distal territory of the intercostobronchial distribution *(large open arrow)* provides collateral supply to a small straight artery in the midline *(multiple small arrows)* that is suspicious for the anterior spinal artery.

BAE. In 2000, Witt et al. evaluated a series of 30 patients with malignancy-related pulmonary hemorrhage who underwent BAE and found improved survival of 139 days in this group compared with 62 days in a historical cohort managed conservatively for hemoptysis.[54] Such findings encourage use of BAE in this group not only as a palliative measure, but as a therapeutic maneuver that may prolong survival. Little is known about tumor response to embolization beyond cessation of bleeding. However, transarterial embolization has become the standard treatment for hepatic malignancy, and some published research describes the use of pulmonary chemoembolization with evidence of improved control of disease.[55]

Some authors have described worse prognosis following BAE in patients with malignancy compared with cohorts with other causes of hemoptysis. However, there is a relative paucity of literature specific to the response of tumor-related bleeding to interventional techniques. A large portion of the data on the response of tumor bleeding to embolization is based on subgroup analyses in small retrospective studies. However, results with three series of patients with malignancy undergoing BAE have been published,[22,47,54] and early results of embolization are similar to those of historical cohorts of patients with inflammatory and infectious causes of hemoptysis. In the series by Wang et al., cumulative hemoptysis control in patients with tumor-related bleeding was not statistically different from that seen with benign causes of hemoptysis $(P = .77)$.[22]

In a patient who is stable and oxygenating adequately, CT is excellent as a primary noninvasive diagnostic modality and may be used for localization of tumor and identification of feeding arteries in preparation for transcatheter embolization. In my opinion, a potential disadvantage of bronchoscopy in the stable patient is disruption of the thrombus, leading to exacerbation of bleeding that may be difficult to control with electrocautery or other techniques. This phenomenon is seen frequently in GI endoscopy whereby stable patients may become unstable after bleeding is "stirred up" by the diagnostic procedure. Under these circumstances, a potentially urgent elective embolization becomes an emergent procedure in a patient with immediate threat to life. As the authors describe, electrocautery becomes less feasible when tissues are very wet, as from massive bleeding, or when there is a high ongoing oxygen requirement, raising the risk for endobronchial fire.

This patient had control of her bleeding with bronchoscopy and electrocautery, and her bronchial artery embolization was performed in an urgent, elective fashion with good technical results. Her return with hemoptysis 6 weeks after the initial treatment is not unusual because reported recurrence of hemoptysis after bronchial artery embolization of all causes ranges from 14% to 42%. Her recurrent hemoptysis was again treated bronchoscopically. One might wonder, based on the data from Witt et al. reporting prolonged survival in patients with malignancy who underwent embolization, whether she may have benefitted from repeat embolization for her clearly aggressive tumor.

REFERENCES

1. Oken MM, Creech RH, Tormey DC, et al. Toxicity and response criteria of the Eastern Cooperative Oncology Group. *Am J Clin Oncol.* 1982;5:649-655.
2. Mitchell D. Transbronchial lung biopsy with the fiberoptic bronchoscope. *Br J Dis Chest.* 1981;75:258-262.
3. Knott-Craig CJ, Oostuizen G, Rossouw G, et al. Management and prognosis of massive hemoptysis: recent experience with 120 patients. *J Thorac Cardiovasc Surg.* 1993;105:394-397.
4. Corey R, Hla KM. Major and massive hemoptysis: reassessment of conservative management. *Am J Med Sci.* 1987;294:301-309.
5. Brinson GM, Noone PG, Mauro MA, et al. Bronchial artery embolization for the treatment of hemoptysis in patients with cystic fibrosis. *Am J Respir Crit Care Med.* 1998;157:1951-1958.
6. de Gracia J, de la Rosa D, Catallan E, et al. Use of endoscopic fibrinogen-thrombin in the treatment of severe hemoptysis. *Respir Med.* 2003;97:790-795.
7. Khalil A, Soussan M, Mangiapan G, et al. Utility of high-resolution chest CT scan in the emergency management of hemoptysis in the intensive care unit: severity, localization and aetiology. *Br J Radiol.* 2007;80:21-25.
8. Garzon AA, Cerruti MM, Golding ME. Exsanguinating hemoptysis. *J Thorac Cardiovasc Surg.* 1982;84:829-833.
9. Shigemura N, Wan IY, Yu SCH. Multidisciplinary management of life-threatening massive hemoptysis: a 10-year experience. *Ann Thorac Surg.* 2009;87:849-853.
10. Mal H, Rullon I, Mellot F, et al. Immediate and long-term results of bronchial artery embolization for life-threatening hemoptysis. *Chest.* 1999;115:996-1001.
11. Ibrahim WH. Massive hemoptysis: the definition should be revised. *Eur Respir J.* 2008;32:1131-1132.
12. Flume PA, Yankaskas JR, Ebeling M, et al. Massive hemoptysis in cystic fibrosis. *Chest.* 2005;128:729-738.
13. Holsclaw DS, Grand RJ, Shwachman H. Massive hemoptysis in cystic fibrosis. *J Pediatr.* 1970;76:829-838.
14. Ong TH, Eng P. Massive hemoptysis requiring intensive care. *Intensive Care Med.* 2003;29:317-320.
15. Valipour A, Kreuzer A, Koller H, et al. Bronchoscopy-guided topical hemostatic tamponade therapy for the management of life-threatening hemoptysis. *Chest.* 2005;127:2113-2118.
16. Jean-Baptiste E. Clinical assessment and management of massive hemoptysis. *Crit Care Med.* 2000;28:1642-1647.
17. Crocco JA, Rooney JJ, Fankushen DS, et al. Massive hemoptysis. *Arch Intern Med.* 1968;121:495-498.
18. Haponik EF, Fein A, Chin R. Managing life-threatening hemoptysis: has anything really changed? *Chest.* 2000;118:1431-1435.
19. Sakr L, Dutau H. Massive hemoptysis: an update on the role of bronchoscopy in diagnosis and management. *Respiration.* 2010;80: 38-58.
20. Kvale PA, Selecky PA, Prakash UB; American College of Chest Physicians. Palliative care in lung cancer: ACCP evidence-based clinical practice guidelines (2nd edition). *Chest.* 2007;132(suppl): 368S-403S.
21. Hirshberg B, Biran I, Glazer M, et al. Hemoptysis: etiology, evaluation, and outcome in a tertiary referral hospital. *Chest.* 1997;112: 440-444.
22. Wang GR, Ensor JE, Gupta S, et al. Bronchial artery embolization for the management of hemoptysis in oncology patients: utility and prognostic factors. *J Vasc Interv Radiol.* 2009;20:722-729.
23. Cho YJ, Murgu SD, Colt HG. Bronchoscopy for bevacizumab-related hemoptysis. *Lung Cancer.* 2007;56:465-474.
24. Khalil A, Parrot A, Nedelcu C, et al. Severe hemoptysis of pulmonary arterial origin: signs and role of multidetector row CT. *Chest.* 2008;133:212-219.
25. Tendulkar RD, Fleming PA, Reddy CA, et al. High-dose-rate endobronchial brachytherapy for recurrent airway obstruction from hyperplastic granulation tissue. *Int J Radiat Oncol Biol Phys.* 2008;70:701-706.
26. Revel MP, Fournier LS, Hennebicque AS, et al. Can CT replace bronchoscopy in the detection of the site and cause of bleeding in patients with large or massive hemoptysis? *AJR Am J Roentgenol.* 2002;179:1217-1224.
27. Non-Small Cell Lung Cancer Collaborative Group. Chemotherapy and supportive care versus supportive care alone for advanced non-small cell lung cancer. *Cochrane Database Syst Rev.* 2010;12:(5): CD007309.
28. Mayo TWJ. Futility: my life. In: Colt HG, Quadrelli S, Friedman L, eds. *The Picture of Health: Medical Ethics and the Movies.* New York: Oxford University Press; 2011.
29. Schneiderman LJ, Jecker NS, Jonsen AR. Medical futility: its meaning and ethical implications. *Ann Intern Med.* 1990;112: 949-954.
30. Zavala DC. Pulmonary hemorrhage in fiberoptic transbronchial biopsy. *Chest.* 1976;70:584-588.
31. Conlan AA, Hurwitz SS. Management of massive haemoptysis with the rigid bronchoscope and cold saline lavage. *Thorax.* 1980;35: 901-904.
32. Wong LT, Lillquist YP, Culham G, et al. Treatment of recurrent hemoptysis in a child with cystic fibrosis by repeated bronchial artery embolizations and long-term tranexamic acid. *Pediatr Pulmonol.* 1996;22:275-279.
33. Mazkereth R, Paret G, Ezra D, et al. Epinephrine blood concentrations after peripheral bronchial versus endotracheal administration of epinephrine in dogs. *Crit Care Med.* 1992;20:1582-1587.
34. Homasson JP. Endobronchial electrocautery. *Semin Respir Crit Care.* 1997;18:535-543.
35. Sutedja G, van Kralingen K, Schramel FM, et al. Fiberoptic bronchoscopic electrosurgery under local anaesthesia for rapid palliation in patients with central airway malignancies: a preliminary report. *Thorax.* 1994;49:1243-1246.
36. Hooper RG, Jackson FN. Endobronchial electrocautery. *Chest.* 1988;94:595-598.

37. Coulter TD, Mehta AC. The heat is on: impact of endobronchial electrosurgery on the need for Nd-YAG laser photoresection. *Chest.* 2000;118:516-521.

38. Morice RC, Ece T, Ece F, et al. Endobronchial argon plasma coagulation for treatment of hemoptysis and neoplastic airway obstruction. *Chest.* 2001;119:781-787.

39. Hetzel MR, Smith SGT. Endoscopic palliation of tracheobronchial malignancies. *Thorax.* 1991;46:325-333.

40. Mathur PN, Wolf KM, Busk MF, et al. Fiberoptic bronchoscopic cryotherapy in the management of tracheobronchial obstruction. *Chest.* 1996;110:718-723.

41. Brandes JC, Schmidt E, Yung R. Occlusive endobronchial stent placement as a novel management approach to massive hemoptysis from lung cancer. *J Thorac Oncol.* 2008;3:1071-1072.

42. Garzon AA, Cerruti M, Gourin A, et al. Pulmonary resection for massive hemoptysis. *Surgery.* 1970;67:633-638.

43. Haponik EF, Chin R. Hemoptysis: clinicians' perspectives. *Chest.* 1990;97:469-475.

44. Fartoukh M, Khalil A, Louis L, et al. An integrated approach to diagnosis and management of severe haemoptysis in patients admitted to the intensive care unit: a case series from a referral centre. *Respir Res.* 2007;8:11-20.

45. Swanson KL, Johnson M, Prakash UBS, et al. Bronchial artery embolization, experience with 54 patients. *Chest.* 2002;121:789-795.

46. Hayakawa K, Tanaka F, Torizuka T. Bronchial artery embolization for hemoptysis: immediate and long-term results. *Cardiovasc Intervent Radiol.* 1992;15:154-159.

47. Park HS, Kim YI, Kim HY, et al. Bronchial artery and systemic artery embolization in the management of primary lung cancer patients with hemoptysis. *Cardiovasc Intervent Radiol.* 2007;30:638-643.

48. Remy J, Lemaitre L, Lafitte JJ, et al. Massive hemoptysis of pulmonary arterial origin: diagnosis and treatment. *AJR Am J Roentgenol.* 1984;143:963-969.

49. Chun JY, Morgan R, Belli AM. Radiological management of hemoptysis: a comprehensive review of diagnostic imaging and bronchial arterial embolization. *Cardiovasc Intervent Radiol.* 2010;33:240-250.

50. Matsushima Y, Jones RL, King EG, et al. Alterations in pulmonary mechanics and gas exchange during routine fiberoptic bronchoscopy. *Chest.* 1984;86:184-188.

51. Van den Heuvel MM, Els Z, Koegelenberg CF. Risk factors for recurrence of haemoptysis following bronchial artery embolization for life-threatening haemoptysis. *Int J Tuberc Lung Dis.* 2007;11:909-914.

52. Rabkin JE, Astafjev VI, Gothman LN, et al. Transcatheter embolization in the management of pulmonary hemorrhage. *Radiology.* 1987;163:361-365.

53. Tanaka N, Yamakado K, Murashima S, et al. Superselective bronchial artery embolization for hemoptysis with a coaxial microcatheter system. *J Vasc Interv Radiol.* 1997;8:65-70.

54. Witt CH, Schmidt B, Geisler A, et al. Value of bronchial artery embolisation with platinum coils in tumorous pulmonary bleeding. *Eur J Cancer.* 2000;36:1949-1954.

55. Vogl TJ, Wetter A, Lindemayr S, et al. Treatment of unresectable lung metastases with transpulmonary chemoembolization: preliminary experience. *Radiology.* 2005;234:917-922.

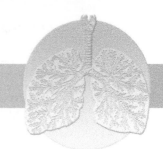

Section 7

Case-Based Self-Assessment Questions

CLINICAL SCENARIO

A 55-year-old white male with a 20–pack-year history of smoking presented with syncope, a 2 month history of increasing exertional dyspnea, and a cough that had been refractory to bronchodilators and antibiotics. He was married and lived with his wife. The patient's father and one brother had died of lung cancer. The emergency department physician believed that the patient was disabled, required special care and assistance, and warranted immediate hospitalization. The physical examination, however, was normal except for stridor heard over the trachea during forced expiration. The workup for syncope included an electrocardiogram, two-dimensional echocardiogram, bilateral carotid duplex ultrasonography, and computed tomography (CT) of the head, all of which were normal. A pulmonary consultant ordered a CT scan of the chest, which revealed a 1.5 cm right upper lung (RUL) nodule and a 4 cm right paratracheal mass invading the trachea (Figure 1).

Question 1: If this patient is proven to have primary lung malignancy, which of the following is the most accurate predictor of survival?

A. Stridor

B. Exertional dyspnea

C. Syncope

D. Performance status

Answer: D

Estimated survival is an important factor for decision making in all disease processes. If this patient has primary lung cancer, he would be clinically staged IIIB because of tracheal involvement (T4 tumor). In such cases of advanced cancer, prognostic considerations are especially important because treatment goals nearing the end of life may change from efforts to prolong life at all costs, to those of palliating symptoms, preserving quality of life, and maintaining dignity. Estimating survival based on objective data is warranted because physicians' subjective assessments of predicted survival are often incorrect, with the direction of error being usually optimistic.*[1] Patients, in most circumstances, want their doctors to be realistic when it comes to prognosis. Although exact numbers may not be requested by patients or their families, having knowledge of relatively accurate prognostic indicators helps physicians conduct meaningful and honest discussions.

A clinical symptom such as stridor, although a sign of severe laryngeal or tracheal obstruction,[2] does not delineate a benign or malignant disease process. In general, stridor and other symptoms of upper or central airway obstruction (CAO), including exertional dyspnea, wheezing, or even syncope, are nonspecific.[3] In fact, results from analysis of 100 variables from several studies showed that only dyspnea, dysphagia, weight loss, xerostomia, anorexia, and cognitive impairment were strongly and independently associated with cancer patient survival. These signs and symptoms were outranked, however, by assessment of performance status,[1] which deservedly has become a "sixth vital sign" in clinical oncology.† Because performance status is the strongest prognostic indicator of survival in patients with cancer, it is frequently used as an entry criterion and adjustment factor in clinical trials of anticancer treatment.[1] One commonly used measure of performance is the Karnofsky Performance Status score (range, 0 to 100 in 10 point increments, where 0 is death and 100 is perfect health), a general measure of functional impairment in which the lower the score, the worse is survival for most serious illnesses.[1]

This patient was assigned a Karnofsky score of only 40. In the setting of lung cancer, known central airway obstruction, and Karnofsky scores below 50, a combination of interventional bronchoscopy and external beam radiation therapy (EBRT) to relieve the airway obstruction has been shown to be the therapeutic option of choice, often resulting in rapid restoration of airway patency, improved symptoms, improved performance status, and increased survival.[4]

The case continues

Several hours after admission, the patient lost consciousness while standing to go to the restroom. He was promptly intubated with a 7.5 mm endotracheal tube (ETT) and was placed on mechanical ventilation assist control–volume control mode (ACVC): tidal volume was 500 mL, respiratory rate 14/min, fraction of inspired oxygen (FiO₂) 1.0 and flow 80 L/min, and positive end-expiratory pressure (PEEP) 5 cm H₂O. On these settings, the peak airway pressure was 60 cm H₂O and plateau pressure was 20 cm H₂O. Flexible bronchoscopy was planned to determine the pattern of tracheal obstruction, to identify associated mucosal changes, and to potentially support the indication for a therapeutic airway procedure. The only flexible bronchoscope available had an outside diameter of 6 mm.

---

*Physicians tend to believe that their patients will live longer than they actually do.

†The other five vital signs are heart rate, blood pressure, temperature, respiratory rate, and pain level.

Figure 1 A, Normal tracheal lumen proximal to the tumor. **B,** Right paratracheal mass compressing and invading the lower trachea below the aortic arch. **C,** The normal tracheal lumen is seen at the level of the main carina distal to the tumor. **D,** Right upper lobe spiculated pulmonary nodule.

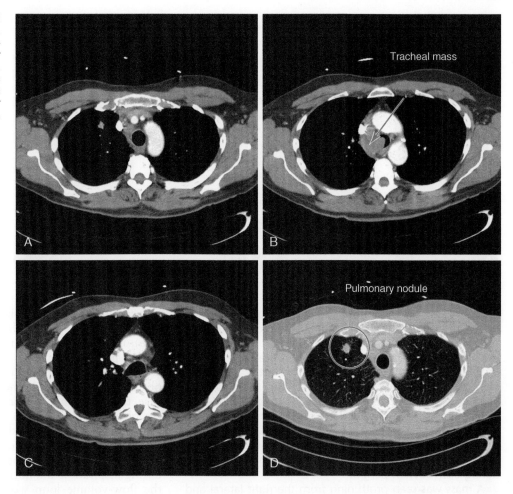

Question 2: The next appropriate step is to:

A. Postpone the procedure until bronchodilator treatments result in decreased peak airway pressure

B. Change the endotracheal tube to a larger diameter (e.g., 8 or 8.5 mm), which will accommodate the 6 mm outer diameter flexible bronchoscope

C. Cancel the procedure because peak airway pressures are too high

D. Perform inspection bronchoscopy quickly at the bedside

Answer: D

In the absence of evidence that the endotracheal tube is kinked, or that the patient's high peak airway pressures are due to mucus plugging or bronchospasm, it is likely that the obstructing tracheal mass itself is responsible for elevated peak airway and normal plateau pressures. Bronchodilators, therefore, would not be expected to improve respiratory status. Bronchoscopy should be rapidly performed, given that ventilation may be difficult because of a less than 2 mm difference between the size of the outer diameter of the bronchoscope and the internal lumen of the endotracheal tube.

Ideally, a No. 8 or larger ETT is preferred for bronchoscopy because it allows proper ventilation during the procedure and potentially prevents a further increase in peak airway pressure or development of auto-PEEP.

These tubes provide at least a 2 mm difference between the scope and the ETT diameter, preventing critical alterations in ventilatory parameters.[5] Changing the ETT, however, by extubation and repeat laryngoscopy or by use of a tube exchanger is hazardous in a patient with critical tracheal obstruction. Reintubation may be difficult, and should the airway be lost, ventilation cannot be ensured. A safer approach may be to perform inspection flexible bronchoscopy through the existing ETT while monitoring peak airway pressures, tidal volumes, heart rate, and oxygenation. In case of tachycardia, a rise in blood pressure, or oxygen desaturation during the procedure, the bronchoscope can be immediately withdrawn until stable vital signs return.

The case continues

Flexible bronchoscopy was performed after a bite block was inserted into the mouth and was secured around the existing ETT. A swivel adapter with a fitted rubber cap was attached, allowing bronchoscopy with minimal loss of tidal volume. The FiO_2 was increased to 1.0, starting 5 minutes before the procedure, and continued until after the procedure, then was titrated down to prebronchoscopy levels. PEEP was removed during bronchoscopy to avoid raising peak airway pressures by as much as 25 mm Hg.[6] If discontinuation of PEEP had not been feasible, it would have been reduced by 50%. Volume control ventilatory mode was preferred so that the increasing airway resistance secondary to the bronchoscopy would not result in reduced tidal volume. If pressure-controlled ventilation had been

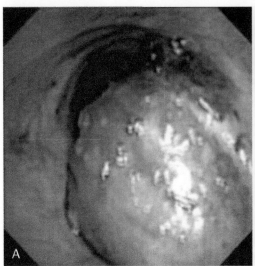
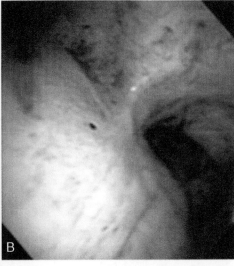

Figure 2 A, Flexible broncho-scopic view of the mass showing 70% obstruction of the airway lumen. **B,** Bronchoscopic view distal to the tumor shows patent airways and normal main carina.

used, the peak pressure setting would have been increased to compensate for the loss of tidal volume consequent to the increased resistance. Moderate sedation was achieved with 2 mg intravenous midazolam. Had the patient been unable to cooperate or otherwise tolerate the procedure comfortably, supplemental doses may have been needed in 1- to 2-minute increments and according to moderate sedation guidelines used in our institution. To remove airway secretions, bronchoscopic suction was applied using short, 3 second or less bursts, because as much as 200 to 300 cm^3 of the patient's tidal volume can be removed during each suction period.[6]

A mass was seen protruding from the right lateral and posterior walls of the lower trachea. The tracheal lumen was narrowed by more than 70%. A severe mixed extrinsic compression and endoluminal obstruction pattern was noted. The remaining airways were normal except for an enlarged carina (Figure 2). The procedure lasted only 1 minute, during which the peak airway pressure increased to 80 cm H$_2$O but without hypoxemia or hemodynamic instability.

Question 3: Had this patient undergone physiologic testing during his initial workup, which of the following patterns would have been expected on the flow-volume loop?

    A. Flattening of the inspiratory curve

    B. Flattening of the expiratory curve

    C. Flattening of the inspiratory and expiratory curves

    D. Airway collapse pattern

Answer: C

In cases of extrathoracic tracheomalacia, laryngomalacia, or vocal cord processes, the flow-volume loop pattern may be that of flattening of the inspiratory curve (Figure 3, *A*). This is due to the fact that intraluminal pressure during inspiration (PL) is lower than extraluminal pressure (Pm = atmospheric pressure) for the extrathoracic airway. Therefore, any obstruction in this airway segment will be made worse during inspiration and will cause limitation of the inspiratory flow. During expiration,

however, to have an expiratory flow, the intraluminal pressure (PL) is higher than the atmospheric pressure (Pm), the extrathoracic airway will dilate, and the flow will be normal.

The opposite is true in cases of variable intrathoracic obstruction such as intrathoracic tracheomalacia. In this case, the obstruction is worsened during expiration when the pleural pressures (Ppl) exceed the intraluminal pressure (PL) (Figure 3, *B*), and there will be flattening of the expiratory curve of the flow-volume loop.

Our patient had a tracheal mass limiting airflow both during inspiration and during exhalation. The pattern on the flow-volume loop would likely have been that of blunting of both inspiratory and expiratory curves (Figure 3, *C*), the so-called square pattern. This pattern may be seen before spirometry yields abnormal results but may not be appreciated until the airway diameter is already narrowed to about 8 to 10 mm and is often masked in severe COPD.

The airway collapse pattern (Figure 3, *D*) is usually seen in severe COPD and may suggest excessive dynamic airway collapse. This flow-volume loop pattern suggests compression of the mainstem bronchi and trachea. The sudden drop in flow velocity occurs early during expiration when intrathoracic pressure is still increasing, as documented by esophageal pressure measurements. Because there is no reduction of force expelling air from the lungs, the sudden fall in velocity can be explained only by a sudden increase in resistance to airflow, which occurs because of collapse of the central airways. The small, relatively constant flow (i.e., plateau) that occurs after the sudden drop in velocity is consistent with air being forced through a narrow airway.

The case continues

This patient was married and had good social support. He had previously expressed his desire for diagnosis and was ready to consider all available treatment options, including mechanical ventilation, surgery, and other treatment modalities. He very likely had lung cancer and thus required tissue diagnosis. Alternatives presented to the patient's wife included rigid bronchoscopy, flexible bronchoscopy with biopsy, and percutaneous needle aspiration of the pulmonary nodule.

Figure 3 **A,** Dynamic (i.e., variable) extrathoracic obstruction with flow limitation and flattening of the inspiratory limb of the loop. **B,** Dynamic (i.e., variable) intrathoracic obstruction with flow limitation and flattening of the expiratory limb of the loop. **C,** Fixed upper/central airway obstruction with flow limitation and flattening of both inspiratory and expiratory limbs of the flow-volume loop. **D,** In the "airway collapse" pattern, maximal flow is reached quickly after expiration of a small volume of air. Following maximal flow, a large fall in flow occurs, although only a small volume is exhaled. In a subsequent phase, the flow rate falls very little during the remainder of expiration. This phase is responsible for the long plateau. *PL,* Intraluminal pressure; *Pm,* atmospheric pressure; *Ppl,* pleural pressure.

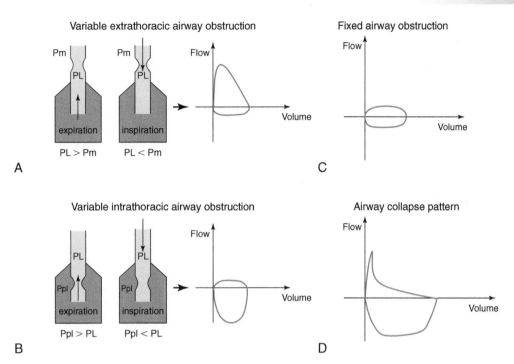

Variable extrathoracic airway obstruction

Pm   Pm   Flow

PL   PL

expiration   inspiration   Volume

PL > Pm   PL < Pm

A

Variable intrathoracic airway obstruction

PL   PL   Flow

Ppl   Ppl

expiration   inspiration   Volume

Ppl > PL   Ppl < PL

B

Fixed airway obstruction

Flow

Volume

C

Airway collapse pattern

Flow

Volume

D

Question 4: Which of the following reasons for recommending rigid bronchoscopy should be given during the informed consent process?

A. Rigid bronchoscopy and restoration of airway patency might allow subsequent systemic therapy in a more stable and spontaneously breathing patient.

B. Rigid bronchoscopy and restoration of airway patency will improve exercise capacity and dyspnea.

C. Rigid bronchoscopy and restoration of airway patency might allow removal from mechanical ventilatory support and discharge from the intensive care unit.

D. All of the above

Answer: D

Patients with respiratory failure and malignant CAO treated by bronchoscopic intervention, who subsequently underwent definitive systemic therapy, were shown to have improved dyspnea and longer survival (median, 38.2 months; range, 1.7 to 57.0 months) compared with those who did not undergo bronchoscopic intervention (median, 6.2 months; range, 0.1 to 33.7 months; P < .001).[7] Restoring airway patency also improves exercise capacity and dyspnea.[7] In this study, a significant improvement in symptoms was noted in 94% of patients undergoing airway stent insertion, although ultimately 40% of patients required multiple bronchoscopic procedures. This raises concerns about the cost per quality of life-years gained in patients with advanced disease.[8] The expense of palliative interventional procedures such as bronchoscopic laser resection and stent insertion, however, is probably small compared with the costs of repeated external beam radiation therapy or prolonged hospitalization in the intensive care unit. Rapid tissue diagnosis, restoration of airway patency, subsequent extubation and removal from mechanical ventilation, and discharge from

the intensive care unit to a ward or even outpatient setting because of this single procedure likely result in considerable savings that positively impact health care costs and resource utilization.

Evidence that removal from mechanical ventilation in critically ill patients with airway obstruction and respiratory failure is possible because of interventional bronchoscopic procedures is limited but reproducible. Lo et al. successfully extubated 7 of 7 patients who were on mechanical ventilation for respiratory failure from malignant obstruction.[9] Colt and Harrell successfully removed ventilatory support in 10 of 19 patients (52.6%) with malignant and benign obstruction,[10] suggesting that when procedures were unsuccessful, immediate referral to hospice and comfort care was justified. Schaffer and Allen inserted metal stents in 6 patients with malignant CAO and in 2 with benign CAO, successfully extubating 6 of them 2 to 11 days later.[11] Furthermore, successful removal from mechanical ventilation has been associated with prolonged survival when systemic treatment is also administered (98 vs. 8.5 days).[12]

The case continues

During our dialogue with the patient's wife, it was believed that the risks of further airway compromise and clinical deterioration were outweighed by the benefit of restoring airway patency with an ability to immediately diagnose the abnormality, wean the patient from mechanical ventilation, and offer systemic therapy. Although we planned to make the diagnosis on frozen section of the tumor removed from the airway, we could have also chosen to perform endobronchial needle aspiration (EBNA), brushing, or endobronchial forceps biopsy. In our experience, EBNA has a lower risk of bleeding than brushing or biopsy, and it provides immediate diagnosis when on-site cytologic examination is available. On-site cytology is not yet the standard of practice in many institutions; however, it may increase procedure-related costs, and, contrary to endobronchial biopsy, tissue architecture is not seen.[13]

Question 5: Had rigid bronchoscopic resection not been offered, which procedure would you have chosen to make a diagnosis in this patient?

A. CT-guided percutaneous needle aspiration of the right upper lobe nodule

B. Endobronchial ultrasound (EBUS) radial probe-guided transbronchial biopsy of the nodule

C. Electromagnetic navigation (EMN) for guiding transbronchial biopsy of the nodule

D. Surgical consultation for video-assisted thoracic surgery (VATS) or thoracotomy

E. Flexible bronchoscopy with EBNA at the bedside in the intensive care unit (ICU)

Answer: E

Rather than approaching the tracheal mass, some might address the pulmonary nodule for diagnosis. CT-guided percutaneous needle aspiration of the right upper lobe nodule has a high diagnostic rate (91%) but would not provide information on staging, and it carries an increased risk for pneumothorax, especially in patients on positive-pressure ventilation (5% to 60%).[14] Endobronchial ultrasound (EBUS) radial probe-guided transbronchial biopsy has a diagnostic yield of 70%[15] but requires special training for image acquisition and interpretation and is not universally available. Electromagnetic navigation (EMN) in addition to EBUS radial probe biopsy increases the yield to 88%. Pneumothorax occurs in about 5%[16] of patients, but this rate might be higher (14%) in mechanically ventilated patients.[17]

Video-assisted thoracic surgery (VATS) or thoracotomy has excellent diagnostic yields for solitary pulmonary nodules, especially when curative surgery is subsequently warranted. This patient's mediastinal adenopathy and tracheal involvement made him ineligible for curative surgery. Furthermore, these surgical procedures require general anesthesia with placement of a double-lumen tube to allow independent lung ventilation, which would not have been feasible until tracheal patency was restored.

In patients with visible endobronchial lesions, endobronchial needle aspiration (EBNA) with on-site cytology examination has a diagnostic yield of 96% when combined with biopsy, washings, and brushing, compared with about 76% using any of these procedures alone.[13] Therefore EBNA at the bedside in the ICU is a reasonable alternative, particularly if diagnosis is desired before consideration for rigid or flexible bronchoscopic resection.[18]

The case continues

Rigid bronchoscopy with Nd:YAG laser standby was immediately scheduled to restore airway patency and provide diagnosis.

Question 6: If rigid bronchoscopy had not been available, what therapeutic alternative would you have chosen to restore airway patency in this patient?

A. Brachytherapy

B. Photodynamic therapy (PDT)

C. Cryotherapy

D. Electrocautery or argon plasma coagulation (APC)

E. Covered metal stent insertion

Answer: E

Systemic therapies such as EBRT and systemic chemotherapy might be appropriate treatment strategies once a tissue diagnosis has been obtained. In case of non–small cell lung carcinoma (NSCLC), this tumor would be a clinical stage IIIB with an estimated median survival of 10 months and a 5 year survival of 7%.[19] Current evidence shows that for individuals with unresectable disease, good performance score, and minimal weight loss, treatment with combined chemoradiotherapy results in better survival than radiotherapy alone. Concurrent chemoradiotherapy seems to be associated with improved survival compared with sequential chemoradiotherapy.[20] Restoration of airway patency should improve performance score and accelerate appropriate initiation of systemic therapy. Therefore even in the absence of rigid bronchoscopy, restoration of airway patency is warranted.

Brachytherapy is an endobronchial therapy with proven efficacy in patients with endoluminal tumor and a substantial extrabronchial component. A Cochrane meta-analysis concluded, however, that for palliation of NSCLC symptoms, endobronchial brachytherapy (EBB) alone was less effective than EBRT. For patients previously treated by EBRT who are symptomatic from recurrent endobronchial central obstruction, EBB may be considered.[21] Tissue effects are delayed and necrotic debris after radiation can worsen airway obstruction.

Photodynamic therapy (PDT) has resulted in successful weaning from mechanical ventilation of a small number of patients with malignant CAO and respiratory failure.[22] The therapeutic effect of PDT is delayed, however, for at least 48 hours, and this might actually worsen airway obstruction during the initial post-treatment period because of sloughing of airway mucosa and retained tumor debris. PDT usually is not indicated in patients with critical tracheal narrowing but appears to be most effective when there is more than 50% narrowing from lobar or segmental bronchial mucosal disease.[23]

Cryotherapy results in thrombosis and necrosis of tumor tissues and would address only the exophytic, endoluminal component of the obstructing airway lesion. Cryotherapy has been shown to be most effective when performed in combination with EBRT.[24] Similar to PDT and EBB, the effect is delayed and initially might worsen airway obstruction.

Electrocautery and argon plasma coagulation (APC) remove the exophytic component and allow superficial cauterization (3 to 6 mm), which may not suffice to stop large airway bleeding in cases of obstructing tracheal tumor. As gas is forced into the airway wall, it can collect in a blood vessel, causing embolism or perforation. Argon gas is heavy, inert, and 17 times less soluble in the body than carbon dioxide. Thus, it may also pass into the systemic circulation.[25] Although the tracheal wall is fairly dense, erosion from tumor presents a risk to major vessels. Systemic, life-threatening gas embolism occurring as a complication of bronchoscopic application of APC has been reported[26] and might be of particular risk in view of the highly vascular pattern of this patient's particular tracheal lesion.

Fully or partially covered metal stent insertion is a plausible alternative in cases of malignant CAO. This can be performed through the ETT in the ICU.[27] It is also a suitable alternative in patients with significant comorbidities precluding general anesthesia. These stents are more costly than silicone stents and can be difficult to remove. Because the bulk of the obstruction resulted from malignant extrinsic compression, the need for excessive debulking was unlikely,[28] and stent insertion alone could probably restore airway patency. These stents can be placed with or without fluoroscopic guidance.[27,29]

The case continues

The patient's family had good insight into his disease. Expectations were realistic, and we had learned from the patient's wife that they had cared for his dying father and brother, both of whom had lung cancer. After they had been advised of all of the alternatives, the family elected to proceed with rigid bronchoscopy under general anesthesia. They were informed of the possibility of failure to restore airway patency and were told about the risks for bleeding, perforation, worsening respiratory distress, temporary or prolonged mechanical ventilation, and death.

Question 7: Which type of anesthesia method would you suggest for this patient's rigid bronchoscopy?

   A. Spontaneous-assisted ventilation with total intravenous anesthesia

   B. Spontaneous-assisted ventilation with inhalational anesthetics

   C. Conventional positive-pressure ventilation

   D. Jet ventilation

Answer: A

Concern for loss of airway during induction exists because of critical tracheal narrowing.[30] Induction should be cautious and preferably should be conducted without neuromuscular blockers; use of these might result in complete loss of muscular tone of the posterior membrane, possibly worsening an already critically narrowed airway.[31] Spontaneous-assisted ventilation with intravenous anesthetics has been shown to have a good cardiac safety profile in patients undergoing rigid bronchoscopy under general anesthesia. Spontaneous-assisted ventilation is provided through an open circuit during the rigid bronchoscopic procedure.[32] This usually is done without the use of muscle relaxants and requires an Ambu bag with a high-flow oxygen source connected to the side port of the rigid bronchoscope. In case of an air leak resulting in an inability to ventilate and oxygenate satisfactorily, the mouth and nose can be packed with gauze and Vaseline nasal packing.

The delivery of volatile anesthetics may be problematic when rigid bronchoscopy is performed using an open system with spontaneous-assisted ventilation because the quantity of anesthetic gas reaching the patient is uncertain, and operating room personnel and the operator are at risk for pollution from escaped anesthetics.[33]

Positive-pressure ventilation will increase flow velocity and turbulent flow past the region of stenosis. Subsequently, a laminar flow pattern cannot be resumed, potentially resulting in ineffective ventilation of the distal airways and loss of effective gas exchange.[34]

Jet ventilation can be considered for severe tracheal obstruction.[35] High-frequency jet ventilation (HFJV) or intermittent low-frequency jet ventilation can be delivered through a rigid or flexible bronchoscope. HFJV through catheters with internal diameters as small as 2.0 mm placed beyond the tracheal obstruction allows safe levels of oxygenation, provided an adequate expiratory passage is present.[36] Jet ventilation poses a risk for barotrauma and pneumothorax and therefore was not our method of choice for this patient.

The case continues

Rigid bronchoscopy with spontaneous ventilation was performed. The patient was extubated and under direct visualization was intubated with a 12 mm Efer-Dumon rigid nonventilating bronchoscope (Bryan Corp., Woburn, Mass). Neodymium-doped yttrium aluminum garnet (Nd:YAG) laser was available on standby in case of bleeding or for tumor coagulation. Various types and sizes of silicone stents were also readily available (Figure 4).

Potential dangers during bronchoscopic resection of a lesion in this location involve the superior vena cava and azygos vein located adjacent to the anterior and lateral wall of the lower trachea. The aorta is anterior (Figure 5).

Moderate bleeding occurred when the tumor was probed with the suction catheter (Figure 6). This stopped after instillation of 60 mL of saline. The tumor was debulked using the beveled edge of the rigid bronchoscope. Laser was not necessary. A 14 × 50 mm straight studded silicone stent was inserted into the lower trachea so that the distal aspect of the stent was located 1 cm above the main carina (see Figure 6). Preliminary tissue diagnosis was non–small cell carcinoma.

The case lasted 40 minutes. No additional intravenous anesthesia was given 10 minutes before rigid extubation, after which the patient was breathing well spontaneously. Reintubation with an endotracheal tube was not necessary. The patient was transferred to the ICU for 24 hours, during which no postoperative complications were noted. He was discharged home 48 hours after the rigid bronchoscopic intervention. Final diagnosis was squamous cell carcinoma. He returned to work and was fully ambulatory when seen in our clinic 1 week later.

Question 8: What is the most appropriate next step?

   A. Compete staging, including whole body PET/CT and brain MRI

   B. Consult palliative care medicine

   C. Make arrangements for hospice care

   D. Refer the patient to thoracic surgery for resection

Answer: A

Complete staging should be performed to better assess prognosis and treatment strategy. This includes a whole body positron emission tomography (PET)/computed tomography (CT) scan and brain magnetic resonance

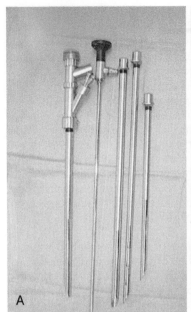

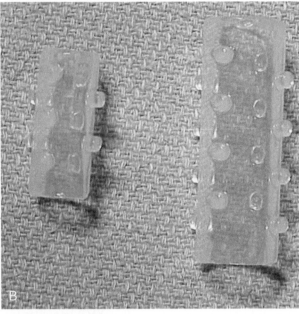

Figure 4 A, Efer-Dumon rigid bronchoscopes of different sizes with a rigid telescope *(second instrument from the left).* **B,** Two straight studded silicone stents (12 × 20 mm and 14 × 40 mm, respectively).

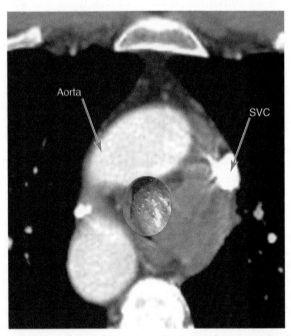

Figure 5 Fused bronchoscopic and computed tomography (CT) image at the level of the tumor, showing the adjacent superior vena cava (SVC) and aorta.

imaging (MRI), which in this patient showed no extra-thoracic disease. Because this patient had stage IIIB NSCLC (T4 tumor due to tracheal involvement), he was not a surgical candidate. Optimal treatment for stage IIIB NSCLC depends on several variables, including extent of disease, age, comorbidities, performance scores, and weight loss.[20] This patient's Karnofsky performance status score post procedure had increased to 90; therefore referral for palliative or hospice care was considered premature. Concurrent chemoradiotherapy, which prolongs survival and is at the present time considered to be the standard of care for inoperable locally

advanced NSCLC,[37] is usually restricted to healthy cancer patients who maintain a good performance status. Because this patient's status had significantly improved,[38] concurrent chemoradiotherapy was offered following discussion in our multidisciplinary chest conference (with representatives from cardiothoracic surgery, oncology, critical care medicine, interventional pulmonology, and radiation oncology).

The case continues

While on systemic therapy (1 month after the procedure), the patient developed acute shortness of breath and an inability to raise secretions.

Question 9: The most appropriate next step is to:

    A. Perform flexible bronchoscopy

    B. Obtain a three-dimensional computed tomography

    C. Perform pulmonary function tests

    D. Consult palliative care medicine

Answer: A

Acute onset of shortness of breath and difficulty raising secretions are likely due to a stent-related complication, rather than to progression of disease or pulmonary embolism. Stent migration should be expected after radiation therapy, especially in cases of tumor shrinkage, causing loss of intimate contact between the stent and the airway wall. In one report, indwelling airway stents could be removed in 50% of patients with malignant CAO at a median of 31.7 days after successful systemic therapy.[39] The risk of stent migration has an estimated incidence of 1% to 5%.[28] Other stent-related complications include kinking, obstruction by tumor or granulation tissue overgrowth, bacterial colonization, and impaired mucociliary clearance causing retained secretions and stent obstruction. Repeat flexible bronchoscopies are reportedly necessary to remove secretions in up to 40% of patients with indwelling stents.[8] Additional rigid bronchoscopic

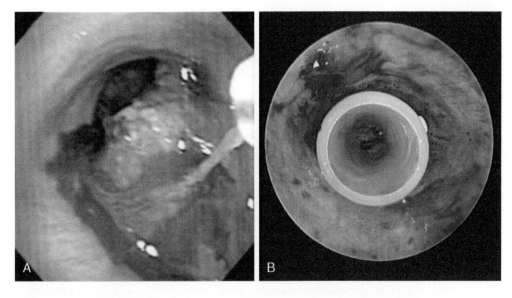

Figure 6 A, Hemorrhagic secretions after probing with a suction catheter. **B,** A 14×50 mm straight studded silicone stent in the lower trachea restored airway patency.

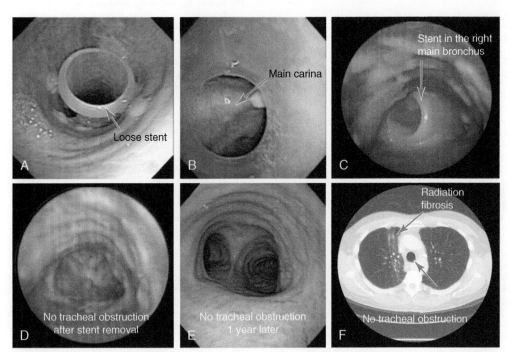

Figure 7 A, Stent dislodged from the lower trachea 1 month after insertion, signaling successful concurrent chemoradiotherapy. **B,** The stent had migrated 1 cm distally and was sitting on the main carina, partially occluding the entrance to the right and left mainstem bronchi. **C,** Rigid bronchoscopic view of the stent migrated farther down into the right mainstem bronchus and causing near complete occlusion of the left mainstem bronchus. **D,** Rigid bronchoscopic view after stent removal shows patent airway and no evidence of obstruction. **E,** Flexible bronchoscopic view 1 year after the initial procedure and after completion of systemic therapy shows maintained airway patency and no evidence of tumor. **F,** Computed tomography 1 year after the procedure shows a patent trachea, no mediastinal tumor, and mild radiation fibrosis within the field of prior external beam radiation.

procedures are seldom required in patients with malignant CAO, in part because of their limited survival.[10,28]

In this patient's case, pulmonary function testing might reveal reduced expiratory flows, but findings are nonspecific and would not preclude a diagnostic bronchoscopy. Computed tomography might identify stent migration, tumor shrinkage, or obstruction by mucus, but would not be therapeutic. Consulting palliative care medicine could be premature because a reversible stent-related complication is most likely.

In fact, outpatient flexible bronchoscopy showed that the stent had migrated distally to the main carina (Figure 7). Rigid bronchoscopy with stent revision was promptly scheduled for the same morning. The patient had begun to cough violently. By the time of rigid bronchoscopy, the stent had partially migrated into the right main bronchus, crossing over the carina and nearly occluding the entrance of the left main bronchus. The stent was removed with rigid forceps. The airway was patent, and no evidence of recurrent endoluminal disease was found (see Figure 7). One year later, the patient continued to do well, had not required stent reinsertion or repeat bronchoscopic interventions, and had no respiratory complaints. Chest CT showed only chronic radiation pneumonitis changes with fibrosis (see Figure 7).

REFERENCES

1. Lamont EB, Christakis NA. Survival estimates in advanced cancer. www.UpToDate.com. Accessed March 16, 2010.
2. Hollingsworth HM. Wheezing and stridor. *Clin Chest Med.* 1987; 8:231-240.
3. Fries MR, Galindo RL, Flint PW, et al. Giant fibrovascular polyp of the esophagus: a lesion causing upper airway obstruction and syncope. *Arch Pathol Lab Med.* 2003;127:485-487.
4. Canak V, Zarić B, Milovancev A, et al. Combination of interventional pulmonology techniques (Nd:YAG laser resection and brachytherapy) with external beam radiotherapy in the treatment of lung cancer patients with Karnofsky Index < or = 50. *J BUON.* 2006;11:447-456.
5. Lawson RW, Peters JI, Shelledy DC. Effects of fiberoptic bronchoscopy during mechanical ventilation in a lung model. *Chest.* 2000; 118:824-831.
6. Tai DY. Bronchoscopy in the intensive care unit (ICU). *Ann Acad Med Singapore.* 1998;27:552-559.
7. Jeon K, Kim H, Yu CM, et al. Rigid bronchoscopic intervention in patients with respiratory failure caused by malignant central airway obstruction. *J Thorac Oncol.* 2006;1:319-323.
8. Wood DE, Liu YH, Vallières E, et al. Airway stenting for malignant and benign tracheobronchial stenosis. *Ann Thorac Surg.* 2003;76:167-174.
9. Lo CP, Hsu AA, Eng P. Endobronchial stenting in patients requiring mechanical ventilation for major airway obstruction. *Ann Acad Med Singapore.* 2000;29:66-70.
10. Colt HC, Harrell J. Therapeutic rigid bronchoscopy allows level of care changes in patients with acute respiratory failure from central airways obstruction. *Chest.* 1997;112:202-206.
11. Shaffer JP, Allen JN. The use of expandable metal stents to facilitate extubation in patients with large airway obstruction. *Chest.* 1998; 114:1378-1382.
12. Stanopoulos IT, Beamis Jr JF, Martinez FJ, et al. Laser bronchoscopy in respiratory failure from malignant airway obstruction. *Crit Care Med.* 1993;21:386-391.
13. Mazzone P, Jain P, Arroliga AC, et al. Bronchoscopy and needle biopsy techniques for diagnosis and staging of lung cancer. *Clin Chest Med.* 2002;23:137-158.
14. Toloza EM, Harpole L, Detterbeck F, et al. Invasive staging of non-small cell lung cancer: a review of the current evidence. *Chest.* 2003;123:157S-166S.
15. Herth FJ, Eberhardt R, Becker HD, et al. Endobronchial ultrasound-guided transbronchial lung biopsy in fluoroscopically invisible solitary pulmonary nodules: a prospective trial. *Chest.* 2006;129: 147-150.
16. Eberhardt R, Anantham D, Ernst A, et al. Multimodality bronchoscopic diagnosis of peripheral lung lesions: a randomized controlled trial. *Am J Respir Crit Care Med.* 2007;176:36-41.
17. O'Brien JD, Ettinger NA, Shevlin D, et al. Safety and yield of transbronchial biopsy in mechanically ventilated patients. *Crit Care Med.* 1997;25:440-446.
18. Colt H, Prakash U, Offord K. Bronchoscopy in North America: survey by the American Association for Bronchology, 1999. *J Bronchol.* 2000;7:8-25.
19. Goldstraw P, Crowley J, Chanksy K, et al. The IASLC Lung Cancer Staging Project: proposals for the revision of the TNM stage groupings in the forthcoming (seventh) edition of the TNM classification of malignant tumours. *J Thorac Oncol.* 2007;2: 704-706.
20. Jett JR, Schild SE, Keith RL, et al; American College of Chest Physicians. Treatment of non-small cell lung cancer, stage IIIB: ACCP evidence-based clinical practice guidelines (2nd edition). *Chest.* 2007;132:266S-276S.
21. Cardona AF, Reveiz L, Ospina EG, et al. Palliative endobronchial brachytherapy for non-small cell lung cancer. *Cochrane Database Syst Rev.* 2008;(2):CD004284.
22. Shah SK, Ost D. Photodynamic therapy: a case series demonstrating its role in patients receiving mechanical ventilation. *Chest.* 2000; 118:1419-1423.
23. Edell ES, Cortese DA. Photodynamic therapy: its use in the management of bronchogenic carcinoma. *Clin Chest Med.* 1995;16: 455-463.
24. Vergnon JM, Schmitt T, Alamartine E, et al. Initial combined cryotherapy and irradiation for unresectable non-small cell lung cancer: preliminary results. *Chest.* 1992;102:1436-1440.
25. Kono M, Yahagi N, Kitahara M, et al. Cardiac arrest associated with use of an argon beam coagulator during laparoscopic cholecystectomy. *Br J Anaesth.* 2001;87:644-646.
26. Reddy C, Majid A, Michaud G, et al. Gas embolism following bronchoscopic argon plasma coagulation: a case series. *Chest.* 2008;134:1066-1069.
27. Chung FT, Lin SM, Chen HC, et al. Factors leading to tracheobronchial self-expandable metallic stent fracture. *J Thorac Cardiovasc Surg.* 2008;136:1328-1335.
28. Lemaire A, Burfeind WR, Toloza E, et al. Outcomes of tracheobronchial stents in patients with malignant airway disease. *Ann Thorac Surg.* 2005;80:434-438.
29. Saad CP, Murthy S, Krizmanich G, et al. Self-expandable metallic airway stents and flexible bronchoscopy: long-term outcomes analysis. *Chest.* 2003;124:1993-1999.
30. McMahon CC, Rainey L, Fulton B, et al. Central airway compression: anaesthetic and intensive care consequences. *Anaesthesia.* 1997;52:158-162.
31. Pullerits J, Holzman R. Anaesthesia for patients with mediastinal masses. *Can J Anaesth.* 1989;36:681-688.
32. Perrin G, Colt HG, Martin C, et al. Safety of interventional rigid bronchoscopy using intravenous anesthesia and spontaneous assisted ventilation: a prospective study. *Chest.* 1992;102:1526-1530.
33. Purugganan RV. Intravenous anesthesia for thoracic procedures. *Curr Opin Anaesthesiol.* 2008;21:1-7.
34. Sibert KS, Biondi JW, Hirsch NP. Spontaneous respiration during thoracotomy in a patient with a mediastinal mass. *Anesth Analg.* 1987;66:904-907.
35. Baraka AS, Siddik SS, Taha SK, et al. Low frequency jet ventilation for stent insertion in a patient with tracheal stenosis. *Can J Anaesth.* 2001;48:701-704.
36. Brodsky JB. Bronchoscopic procedures for central airway obstruction. *J Cardiothorac Vasc Anesth.* 2003;17:638-646.
37. Trodella L, D'Angelillo RM, Ramella S, et al. Multimodality treatment in locally advanced non-small cell lung cancer. *Ann Oncol.* 2006;17:ii32-ii33.
38. Spira A, Ettinger DS. Multidisciplinary management of lung cancer. *N Engl J Med.* 2004;350:379-392.
39. Witt C, Dinges S, Schmidt B, et al. Temporary tracheobronchial stenting in malignant stenoses. *Eur J Cancer.* 1997;33:204-208.

Index

Page numbers followed by "f" indicate figures, "t" indicate tables, and "b" indicate boxes.